Lung Cancer

Lung Cancer

EDITED BY

Jack A. Roth, MD, F.A.C.S.

Professor and Bud Johnson Clinical Distinguished Chair
Department of Thoracic and Cardiovascular Surgery
Professor of Molecular and Cellular Oncology
Director, W.M. Keck Center for Innovative Cancer Therapies
Chief, Section of Thoracic Molecular Oncology
The University of Texas M.D. Anderson Cancer Center
Houston, Texas, USA

James D. Cox, MD

Professor and Head
Division of Radiation Oncology
The University of Texas M. D. Anderson Cancer Center
Houston, Texas, USA

Waun Ki Hong, MD, D.M.Sc. (Hon.)

American Cancer Society Professor
Samsung Distinguished University Chair in Cancer Medicine
Professor and Head, Division of Cancer Medicine
Professor, Department of Thoracic/Head and Neck Medical Oncology
The University of Texas M.D. Anderson Cancer Center
Houston, Texas, USA

THIRD EDITION

Blackwell
Publishing

Blackwell Publishing, Inc., 350 Main Street, Malden, Massachusetts 02148-5020, USA
Blackwell Publishing Ltd, 9600 Garsington Road, Oxford OX4 2DQ, UK
Blackwell Publishing Asia Pty Ltd, 550 Swanston Street, Carlton, Victoria 3053, Australia

First published 1998
Third edition 2008

1   2008

Library of Congress Cataloging-in-Publication Data

Lung cancer / edited by Jack A. Roth, James D. Cox, Waun Ki Hong. – 3rd ed.
     p.   ;   cm.
   Includes bibliographical references and index.
   ISBN 978-1-4051-5112-2 (alk. paper)
   1. Lungs–Cancer.   I. Roth, Jack A.   II. Cox, James D. (James Daniel), 1938–
   III. Hong, Waun Ki.
   [DNLM: 1. Lung Neoplasms–therapy.   2. Lung Neoplasms–diagnosis.   3. Lung Neoplasms–genetics.
   WF 658 L9604 2008]
RC280.L8L765 2008
616.99′424–dc22

ISBN: 978-1-4051-5112-2

A catalogue record for this title is available from the British Library

Set in 9.5/12pt Meridien by Aptara Inc., New Delhi, India
Printed and bound in Singapore by Fabulous Printers Pte Ltd

For further information on Blackwell Publishing, visit our website:
http://www.blackwellpublishing.com

Contents

Contributors

Miguel Alvelo-Rivera, MD
Assistant Professor of Surgery,
Division of Thoracic Surgery
University of Pittsburgh Medical Center,
Pittsburgh, PA, USA

Vladimir Badmaev, MD
Vice President, Scientific and Medical Affairs
Sabinsa Pharmaceutical, Inc.,
New Jersey, NJ, USA

Joan E. Bailey-Wilson, PhD
Senior Investigator and Co-Branch Chief,
National Human Genome Research Institute,
National Institutes of Health,
Baltimore, MD, USA

Benjamin Besse, MD
Assistant Professor,
Department of Medicine,
Institut Gustave Roussy,
Villejuif, France

Nishin Bhadkamkar
Resident, House Staff Doctor
Emory University School of Medicine
Atlanta, GA, USA

David P. Carbone, MD, PhD
Professor of Medicine and Cancer Biology,
Vanderbilt-Ingram Cancer Center,
Nashville, TN, USA

Joe Y. Chang, MD, PhD
Assistant Professor,
Director of Translation Research in
   Thoracic Radiation Oncology,
Department of Radiation Oncology,
The University of Texas M. D. Anderson Cancer Center,
Houston, TX, USA

Thierry Le Chevalier, MD
Department of Medicine,
Institut Gustave Roussy,
Villejuif, France

James D. Cox, MD
Professor and Head, Division of Radiation Oncology
The University of Texas,
M.D. Anderson Cancer Center,
Houston, TX, USA

Philippe G. Dartevelle, MD
Professor of Thoracic and Cardiovascular Surgery
   at Paris Sud University
Head of the Department of Thoracic
   and Vascular Surgery and Heart Lung Tansplantation
Hôpital Marie Lannelongue Le Plessis
   Robinson France

Burton Dickey, MD
Professor and Chair,
Department of Pulmonary Medicine
The University of Texas
M. D. Anderson Cancer Center
Houston, TX, USA

Steven M. Dubinett, MD
Professor and Chief
Division of Pulmonary and Critical Care Medicine,
Department of Medicine,
Director, UCLA Lung Cancer Research Program,
Jonsson Comprehensive Cancer Center,
David Geffen School of Medicine at UCLA,
Los Angeles, CA, USA

Kentya H. Ford, PhD
Postdoctoral Fellow,
Department of Behavioral Sicence,
The University of Texas,
M. D. Anderson Cancer Center,
Houston, TX, USA

Frank Fosella, MD
Medical Director, Thoracic Oncology
   Multidisciplinary Care Center;
Professor, Department of Thoracic/Head
   and Neck Medical Oncology
The University of Texas,
M.D. Anderson Cancer Center
Houston, TX , USA

Wilbur A. Franklin, MD
Professor, Department of Pathology,
University of Colorado Health Sciences Center,
Aurora, CO, USA

Adi F. Gazdar, MD
Professor of Pathology and Deputy Director,
Hamon Center for Therapeutic Oncology Research,
The University of Texas Southwestern Medical Center,
Dallas, TX, USA

Ji-Youn Han, MD, PhD
Chief Scientist, Lung Cancer Branch,
National Cancer Center
Goyang, Gyeonggi, Korea

Emer O. Hanrahan, MB, BCh, MRCPI
Medical Oncology Fellow,
Department of Thoracic/Head and
    Neck Medical Oncology,
The University of Texas M.D. Anderson
    Cancer Center,
Houston, TX, USA

John Heymach, MD, PhD
Assistant Professor,
Department of Thoracic/Head and Neck Medical Oncology
    and Cancer Biology
The University of Texas,
M.D. Anderson Cancer Center
Houston, TX , USA

Karen Suchanek Hudmon, Dr PH, MS, BS Pharm
Associate Professor,
Department of Pharmacy Practice,
Purdue University School of Pharmacy &
    Pharmaceutical Sciences,
West, Lafavette,
IN, USA

Minh Huynh, MD
Staff Oncologist
Kaiser Permanente Walnut Creek Medical Center,
Walnut Creek, CA

Jacob M. Kaufman, MD, PhD
Candidate, Predoctoral Trainee
Vanderbilt University School of Medicine
Vanderbilt University Cancer Center,
Nashville, TN, USA

Brian D. Kavanagh, MD, MPH
Professor and Vice Chairman,
Department of Radiation Oncology,
University of Colorado Comprehensive Cancer Center,
Aurora, CO, USA

Michael Kent, MD
Surgical Resident, Department of
    Thoracic Surgery,
Beth Israel Deaconess Medical Center,
Boston, MA, USA

Fadlo R. Khuri, MD
Professor of Hematology and Oncology,
Winship Cancer Institute,
Emory University,
Atlanta, GA, USA

Ritsuko Komaki, MD
Professor, Department of Radiation
    Oncology,
Gloria Lupton Tennison Distinguished
    Professorship for Lung Cancer Resarch
The University of Texas,
M. D. Anderson Cancer Center,
Houston, TX, USA

Jonathan Kurie, MD
Professor, Department of Thoracic/Head
    and Neck Medical Oncology
The University of Texas,
M.D. Anderson Cancer Center
Houston, TX, USA

Stephen Lam, MD, FRCPC
Professor of Medicine,
University of British Columbia;
and Chair, Lung Tumor Group,
British Columbia Cancer Agency,
Vancouver, British Columbia, Canada

Primo N. Lara Jr, MD
Professor of Medicine,
University of California Davis
Cancer Center, Sacramento, CA, USA

Dae Ho Lee, MD
Assistant Professor,
Division of Oncology,
Department of Internal Medicine,
College of Medicine,
University of Ulsan and Asan Medical
    Center,
Seoul, Korea

Jay M. Lee, MD
Surgical Director, Thoracic Oncology Program
Assistant Professor of Surgery
Division of Cardiothoracic Surgery
David Geffen School of Medicine at UCLA
Los Angeles, CA, USA

Jin Soo Lee, MD
Director,
Research Institute,
National Cancer Center,
Goyang, Gyeonggi, Korea

Zhongxing Liao, MD
Associate Professor,
The University of Texas M.D.
Anderson Cancer Center,
Houston, TX, USA

Jie Lin, PhD
Instructor, Department of Epidemiology,
The University of Texas M.D. Anderson Cancer Center,
Houston, TX, USA

James D. Luketich, MD
Sampson Endowed Professor of Surgery;
    and Chief, Heart,
Lung and Esophageal Surgery Institute,
University of Pittsburgh
Medical Center,
Pittsburgh, PA, USA

Thomas J. Lynch
Chief of Hematology–Oncology,
Massachusetts General Hospital,
Boston, MA, USA

Annette McWilliams, MD, FRCPC
Clinical Assistant Professor,
Department of Medicine,
University of British Columbia;
    and Respiratory Physician,
Department of Cancer Imaging,
BC Cancer Research Centre,
Vancouver, BC, Canada

John D. Minna, MD
Professor of Internal Medicine and Pharmacology;
    and Director, Hamon Center for Therapeutic
    Oncology Research,
The University of Texas Southwestern Medical Center,
Dallas, TX, USA

Seyed Javad Moghaddam, MD
Instructor, Department of Pulmonary Medicine
The University of Texas,
M.D. Anderson Cancer Center,
Houston, TX, USA

James L. Mulshine, MD
Professor, Internal Medicine and Associate Provost
    for Research,
Rush University Medical Center,
Chicago, IL, USA

Sacha Mussot, MD
Thoracic and Vascular Surgeon and Staff Member
Department of Thoracic and Vascular Surgery
    and Heart Lung Transplantation
Hôpital Marie Lannelongue – Le Plessis Robinson – France

Monique B. Nilsson, PhD
Research Scientist,
Department of Cancer Biology,
The University of Texas M.D. Anderson Cancer Center,
Houston, TX, USA

Katherine M.W. Pisters, MD
Professor of Medicine,
Department of Thoracic/Head & Neck Medical
    Oncology,
Division of Cancer Medicine,
The University of Texas M.D. Anderson Cancer
    Center,
Houston, TX, USA

Alexander V. Prokhorov, MD, PhD
Professor, Department of Behavioral Science,
The University of Texas M.D. Anderson Cancer
    Center,
Houston, TX, USA

Carolyn E. Reed, MD
Professor of Surgery and Chief,
Section of General Thoracic Surgery,
Medical University of South Carolina,
Charleston, SC, USA

Kenneth E. Rosenzweig, MD
Associate Attending,
Department of Radiation Oncology,
Memorial Sloan–Kettering Cancer Center,
New York, NY, USA

Jack Roth, MD
Professor and Bud Johnson Clinical Distinguished Chair
Department of Thoracic and Cardiovascular Surgery
Professor of Molecular and Cellular Oncology
Director, W.M. Keck Center for Innovative Cancer
    Therapies
Chief, Section of Thoracic Molecular Oncology
The University of Texas,
M.D. Anderson Cancer Center
Houston, TX, USA

Mitsuo Sato, MD, PhD
Postdoctoral Researcher,
Hamon Center for Therapeutic Oncology Research
    and the Simmons Cancer Center,
The University of Texas Southwestern Medical Center,
Dallas, TX, USA

Lecia Sequist, MD, MPH
Instructor in Medicine,
Harvard Medical School,
MGH Cancer Center,
Boston, MA, USA

David S. Shames, PhD
Postdoctoral Fellow
Hamon Center for Therapeutic Oncology Research
The University of Texas Southwestern Medical Center,
Dallas, TX, USA

Amir Sharafkhaneh, MD
Assistant Professor of Medicine at Baylor College
   of Medicine and Staff,
Physician at the Michael E. DeBakey VA Medical Center,
Houston, TX, USA

Sherven Sharma, PhD
Associate Professor,
Division of Pulmonary and Critical
   Care Medicine,
Department of Medicine,
UCLA Lung Cancer Research Program,
David Geffen School of Medicine at UCLA,
West Los Angeles VA,
Los Angeles, CA, USA

Alfred R. Smith, PhD
Professor, The University of Texas
M.D. Anderson Proton Therapy Center,
Houston, TX, USA

Margaret R. Spitz, MD, MPH
Professor and Chair,
Department of Epidemiology,
The University of Texas
M.D. Anderson Cancer Center,
Houston, TX, USA

Sonal Sura, MD
Radiation Oncology Resident,
New York City, NY, USA

Robert D. Timmerman, MD
Professor and Vice Chairman,
Effie Marie Cain Distinguished Chair
   in Cancer Therapy Research,
Department of Radiation Oncology,
University of Texas
Southwestern Medical Center,
Dallas, TX, USA

Anne S. Tsao, MD
Assistant Professor,
Department of Thoracic/Head and
   Neck Medical Oncology,
The University of Texas
M.D. Anderson Cancer Center,
Houston, TX, USA

Suryakanta Velamuri, MD
Assistant Professor of Medicine,
Balor College of Medicine;
   and Staff Physician,
Michael E. Debakey VA Medical Center,
Houston, TX, USA

Ignacio I. Wistuba, MD
Associate Professor of Pathology
and Thoracic/Head & Neck Medical
   Oncology,
The University of Texas
M.D. Anderson Cancer Center,
Houston, TX, USA

Xifeng Wu, MD, PhD
Professor, Department of Epidemiology,
The University of Texas
M.D. Anderson Cancer Center,
Houston, TX, USA

Bedrettin Yildizeli, MD
Associated Professor of Thoracic Surgery,
Department of Thoracic Surgery,
Marmara University Hospital,
Istanbul, Turkey

Preface

When the first edition of *Lung Cancer* was published 14 years ago, the editors were optimistic that progress in reducing the mortality from this disease would result from insights in the biology of cancer and new treatment strategies. Rapid progress in the biology, prevention, diagnosis, and treatment of lung cancer convinced us that a third edition was warranted. This book is not intended as a comprehensive textbook, but as a concise summary of advances in lung cancer clinical research and treatment for the clinician.

Over 20 years of research on the biology of lung cancer has culminated in the clinical application of targeted therapies. These agents disable specific oncogenic pathways in the lung cancer cell and can mediate tumor regression with fewer adverse events. Several chapters are devoted to summarizing the most recent work in this field. Much research is attempting to identify biomarkers to predict a high risk for developing lung cancer. This will be important for implementing screening and prevention strategies. New techniques have emerged for lung cancer staging that improve accuracy. A variety of surgical and radiation therapy techniques have been developed which will make local tumor control more effective and less invasive. Combined modality therapy and new chemotherapeutic agents are yielding higher response rates and improved survival when used in the adjuvant setting. The final section of the book describes novel approaches that may emerge as important preventative, diagnostic, and therapeutic modalities in the near future.

The editors emphasize that these advances are possible because of the work of those dedicated to translational research and rigorously conducted clinical trials. We are optimistic that progress will continue at a rapid pace and that deaths from lung cancer will continue to decrease.

Jack A. Roth
James D. Cox
Waun Ki Hong

CHAPTER 1
Smoking Cessation

Alexander V. Prokhorov, Kentya H. Ford, and Karen Suchanek Hudmon

Overview

Tobacco use is a public health issue of enormous importance, and smoking is the primary risk factor for the development of lung cancer. Considerable knowledge has been gained with respect to biobehavioral factors leading to smoking initiation and development of nicotine dependence. Smoking cessation provides extensive health benefits for everyone. State-of-the-art treatment for smoking cessation includes behavioral counseling in conjunction with one or more FDA-approved pharmaceutical aids for cessation. The US Public Health Service *Clinical Practice Guideline for Treating Tobacco Use and Dependence* advocates a five-step approach to smoking cessation (Ask about tobacco use, Advise patients to quit, Assess readiness to quit, Assist with quitting, and Arrange follow-up). Health care providers are encouraged to provide at least brief interventions at each encounter with a patient who uses tobacco.

Introduction

More than two decades ago, the former US Surgeon General C. Everett Koop stated that cigarette smoking is the "chief, single, avoidable cause of death in our society and the most important public health issue of our time" [1]. This statement remains true today. In the United States, cigarette smoking is the primary known cause of preventable deaths [2],

resulting in nearly 440,000 deaths each year [3]. The economic implications are enormous: more than $75 billion in medical expenses and over $81 billion in loss of productivity as a result of premature death are attributed to smoking each year [4–8]. While the public often associates tobacco use with elevated cancer risk, the negative health consequences are much broader. The 2004 Surgeon General's Report on the health consequences of smoking [9] provides compelling evidence of the adverse impact of smoking and concluded that smoking harms nearly every organ in the body (Table 1.1). In 2000, 8.6 million persons in the United States were living with an estimated 12.7 million smoking-attributable medical conditions [10]. There is convincing evidence that stopping smoking is associated with immediate as well as long-term health benefits, including reduced cumulative risk for cancer. This is true even in older individuals, and in patients who have been diagnosed with cancer [11].

Smoking and lung cancer

In the United States, approximately 85% of all lung cancers are in people who smoke or who have smoked [3]. Lung cancer is fatal for most patients. The estimated number of deaths of lung cancer will exceed 1.3 million annually early in the third millennium [12]. Lung cancer is the leading cause of cancer-related deaths among Americans of both genders, with 174,470 estimated newly diagnosed cases and 162,460 deaths [13,14]. The number of deaths due to lung cancer exceeds the

Lung Cancer, 3rd edition. Edited by Jack A. Roth, James D. Cox, and Waun Ki Hong. © 2008 Blackwell Publishing, ISBN: 978-1-4051-5112-2.

Table 1.1 Health consequences of smoking.

Cancer	Acute myeloid leukemia Bladder Cervical Esophageal Gastric Kidney Laryngeal Lung Oral cavity and pharyngeal Pancreatic
Cardiovascular diseases	Abdominal aortic aneurysm Coronary heart disease (angina pectoris, ischemic heart disease, myocardial infarction, sudden death) Cerebrovascular disease (transient ischemic attacks, stroke) Peripheral arterial disease
Pulmonary diseases	Acute respiratory illnesses Pneumonia Chronic respiratory illnesses Chronic obstructive pulmonary disease Respiratory symptoms (cough, phlegm, wheezing, dyspnea) Poor asthma control Reduced lung function in infants exposed (in utero) to maternal smoking
Reproductive effects	Reduced fertility in women Pregnancy and pregnancy outcomes Premature rupture of membranes Placenta previa Placental abruption Preterm delivery Low infant birth weight Infant mortality (sudden infant death syndrome)
Other effects	Cataract Osteoporosis (reduced bone density in postmenopausal women, increased risk of hip fracture) Periodontitis Peptic ulcer disease (in patients who are infected with *Helicobacter pylori*) Surgical outcomes Poor wound healing Respiratory complications

Source: Reference [9].

annual number of deaths from breast, colon, and prostate cancer combined [15]. Recent advances in technology have enabled earlier diagnoses, and advances in surgery, radiation therapy, imaging, and chemotherapy have produced improved responses rates. However, despite these efforts, overall survival has not been appreciably affected in 30 years, and only 12–15% of patients with lung cancer are being cured with current treatment approaches [16]. The prognosis of lung cancer depends largely on early detection and immediate, premetastasis stage treatment [17]. Prevention of lung cancer is the most desirable and cost-efficient approach to eradicating this deadly condition. Numerous epidemiologic studies consistently define smoking as the major risk factor for lung cancer (e.g. [18–20]). The causal role of cigarette smoking in lung cancer mortality has been irrefutably established in longitudinal studies, one of which lasted as long as 50 years [21]. Tobacco smoke, which is inhaled either directly or as second-hand smoke, contains an estimated 4000 chemical compounds, including over 60 substances that are known to cause cancer [22]. Tobacco irritants and carcinogens damage the cells in the lungs, and over time the damaged cells may become cancerous. Cigarette smokers have lower levels of lung function than nonsmokers [9,23], and quitting smoking greatly reduces cumulative risk for developing lung cancer [24].

The association of smoking with the development of lung cancer is the most thoroughly documented causal relationship in biomedical history [25]. The link was first observed in the early 1950s through the research of Sir Richard Doll, whose pioneering research has, perhaps more so than any other epidemiologist of his time, altered the landscape of disease prevention and consequently saved millions of lives worldwide. In two landmark US Surgeon Generals' reports published within a 20-year interval (in 1964 [26] and in 2004 [9]), literature syntheses further documented the strong link between smoking and cancer. Compared to never smokers, smokers have a 20-fold risk of developing lung cancer, and more than 87% of lung cancers are attributable to smoking [27]. The risk for developing lung cancer increases with younger age at initiation of smoking, greater number of cigarettes smoked, and greater number of years smoked [11]. Women smoking the same amount as men experience twice the risk of developing lung cancer [28,29].

Second-hand smoke and lung cancer

While active smoking has been shown to be the main preventable cause of lung cancer, second-hand smoke contains the same carcinogens that are inhaled by smokers [30]. Consequently, there has been a concern since release of the 1986 US Surgeon General's report [31] concluding that second-hand smoke causes cancer among nonsmokers and smokers. Although estimates vary by exposure location (e.g., workplace, car, home), the 2000 National Household Interview Survey estimates that a quarter of the US population is exposed to second-hand smoke [32]. Second-hand smoke is the third leading cause of preventable deaths in the United States [33], and it has been estimated that exposure to second-hand smoke kills more than 3000 adult nonsmokers from lung cancer [34]. According to Glantz and colleagues, for every eight smokers who die from a smoking-attributable illness, one additional nonsmoker dies because of second-hand smoke exposure [35].

Since 1986, numerous additional studies have been conducted and summarized in the 2006 US Surgeon General's report on *"The Health Consequences of Involuntary Exposure of Tobacco Smoke."* The report's conclusions based on this additional evidence are consistent with the previous reports: exposure to second-hand smoke increases risk of lung cancer. More than 50 epidemiologic studies of nonsmokers' cigarette smoke exposure at the household and/or in the workplace showed an increased risk of lung cancer associated with second-hand smoke exposure [34]. This means that 20 years after second-hand smoke was first established as a cause of lung cancer in lifetime nonsmokers, the evidence supporting smoking cessation and reduction of second-hand smoke exposure continues to mount. Eliminating second-hand smoke exposure at home, in the workplaces, and other public places appears to be essential for reducing the risk of lung cancer development among nonsmokers.

Smoking among lung cancer patients

Tobacco use among patients with cancer is a serious health problem with significant implications for morbidity and mortality [36–39]. Evidence indicates that continued smoking after a diagnosis with cancer has substantial adverse effects on treatment effectiveness [40], overall survival [41], risk of second primary malignancy [42], and increases the rate and severity of treatment-related complications such as pulmonary and circulatory problems, infections, impaired would healing, mucositis, and Xerostomia [43,44].

Despite the strong evidence for the role of smoking in the development of cancer, many cancer patients continue to smoke. Specifically, about one third of cancer patients who smoked prior to their diagnoses continue to smoke [45] and among patients received surgical treatment of stage I nonsmall cell lung cancer [46] found only 40% who were abstinent 2 years after surgery. Davison and Duffy [47] reported that 48% of former smokers had resumed regular smoking after surgical treatment of lung cancer. Therefore, among patients with smoking-related malignancies, the likelihood of a positive smoking history at and after diagnosis is high.

Patients who are diagnosed with lung cancer may face tremendous challenges and motivation to quit after a cancer diagnosis can be influenced by a range of psychological variables. Schnoll and colleagues [48] reported that continued smoking among patients with head and neck and lung cancer is associated with lesser readiness to quit, having relatives who smoke at home, greater time between diagnoses and assessment, greater nicotine dependence, lower self-efficacy, lower risk perception, fewer perceived pros and greater cons to quitting, more fatalistic beliefs, and higher emotional distress. Lung cancer patients should be advised to quit smoking, but once they are diagnosed, some might feel that there is nothing to be gained from quitting [49]. Smoking cessation should be a matter of special concern throughout cancer diagnosis, treatment, and the survival continuum, and the diagnosis of cancer should be used as a "teachable moment" to encourage smoking cessation among patients, family members, and significant others [37]. The

Table 1.2 Percentage of current cigarette smokers[a] aged ≥18 years, by selected characteristics—National Health Interview Survey, United States, 2005.

Characteristic	Category	Men (n = 13,762)	Women (n = 17,666)	Total (n = 31,428)
Race/ethnicity[b]	White, non-Hispanic	24.0	20.0	21.9
	Black, non-Hispanic	26.7	17.3	21.5
	Hispanic	21.1	11.1	16.2
	American Indian/Alaska Native	37.5	26.8	32.0
	Asian[c]	20.6	6.1	13.3
Education[d]	0–12 years (no diploma)	29.5	21.9	25.5
	GED[e] (diploma)	47.5	38.8	43.2
	High school graduate	28.8	20.7	24.6
	Associate degree	26.1	17.1	20.9
	Some college (no degree)	26.2	19.5	22.5
	Undergraduate degree	11.9	9.6	10.7
	Graduate degree	6.9	7.4	7.1
Age group (yrs)	18–24	28.0	20.7	24.4
	25–44	26.8	21.4	24.1
	45–64	25.2	18.8	21.9
	≥65	8.9	8.3	8.6
Poverty level[f]	At or above	23.7	17.6	20.6
	Below	34.3	26.9	29.9
	Unknown	21.2	16.1	18.4
Total		23.9	18.1	20.9

[a]Persons who reported having smoked at least 100 cigarettes during their lifetime and at the time of the interview reported smoking every day or some days; excludes 296 respondents whose smoking status was unknown.
[b]Excludes 314 respondents of unknown or multiple racial/ethnic categories or whose racial/ethnic category was unknown.
[c]Excludes Native Hawaiians or other Pacific Islanders.
[d]Persons aged ≥25 years, excluding 339 persons with unknown level of education.
[e]General Educational Development.
[f]Calculated on the basis of US Census Bureau 2004 poverty thresholds.
Source: Reference [7].

medical, psychosocial, and general health benefits of smoking cessation for cancer patients provide a clear rationale for intervention.

Forms of tobacco

Smoked tobacco

Cigarettes have been the most widely used form of tobacco in the United States for several decades [51], yet in recent years, cigarette smoking has been declining steadily among most population subgroups. In 2005, just over half of ever smokers reported being former smokers [3]. However, a considerable proportion of the population continues to smoke. In 2005, an estimated 45.1 million adult Americans (20.9%) were current smokers; of these, 80.8% reported to smoking every day, and 19.2% reported smoking some days [7]. The prevalence of smoking varies considerably across populations (Table 1.2), with a greater proportion of men (23.9%) than women (18.1%) reporting current smoking. Persons of Asian or Hispanic origin exhibit the lowest prevalence of smoking (13.3 and 16.2%, respectively), and American Indian/Alaska natives exhibit the highest prevalence (32.0%). Also, the prevalence of smoking among adults varies widely across the United States, ranging from 11.5% in Utah to

28.7% in Kentucky [51]. Twenty-three percent of high school students report current smoking, and among boys, 13.6% report current use of smokeless tobacco, and 19.2% currently smoke cigars [52]. These figures are of particular concern, because nearly 90% of smokers begin smoking before the age of 18 years [53].

Other common forms of burned tobacco in the United States include cigars, pipe tobacco, and bidis. Cigars represent a roll of tobacco wrapped in leaf tobacco or in any substance containing tobacco [54]. Cigars' popularity has somewhat increased over the past decade [55]. The latter phenomenon is likely to be explained by a certain proportion of smokers switching cigarettes for cigars and by adolescents' experimentation with cigars [56]. In 1998, approximately 5% of adults had smoked at least one cigar in the past month [57]. The nicotine content of cigars sold in the United States ranged from 5.9 to 335.2 mg per cigar [58] while cigarettes have a narrow range of total nicotine content, between 7.2 and 13.4 mg per cigarette [59]. Therefore, one large cigar, which could contain as much tobacco as an entire pack of cigarettes is able to deliver enough nicotine to establish and maintain physical dependence [59].

Pipe smoking has been declining steadily over the past 50 years [60]. It is a form of tobacco use seen among less than 1% of Americans [60]. Bidi smoking is a more recent phenomenon in the United States. Bidis are hand-rolled brown cigarettes imported mostly from Southeast Asian countries. Bidis are wrapped in a *tendu* or *temburni* leaf [61]. Visually, they somewhat resemble marijuana joints, which might make them attractive to certain groups of the populations. Bidis are available in multiple flavors (e.g., chocolate, vanilla, cinnamon, strawberry, cherry, mango, etc.), which might make them particularly attractive to younger smokers. A survey of nearly 64,000 people in 15 states in the United States revealed that young people (18–24 years of age) reported higher rates of ever (16.5%) and current (1.4%) use of bidis then among older adults (ages 25 plus years). With respect to sociodemographic characteristics, the use of bidis is most common among males, African Americans, and concomitant cigarette smokers [62]. Although featuring

less tobacco than standard cigarettes, bidis expose their smokers to considerable amounts of hazardous compounds. A smoking machine-based investigation found that bidis deliver three times the amount of carbon monoxide and nicotine and almost five times the amount of tar found in conventional cigarettes [63].

Smokeless tobacco

Smokeless tobacco products, also commonly called "spit tobacco," are placed in the mouth to allow absorption of nicotine through the buccal mucosa. Spit tobacco includes chewing tobacco and snuff. Chewing tobacco, which is typically available in loose leaf, plug, and twist formulations, is chewed or parked in the cheek or lower lip. Snuff, commonly available as loose particles or sachets (resembling tea bags), has a much finer consistency and is generally held in the mouth and not chewed. Most snuff products in the United States are classified as moist snuff. The users park a "pinch" (small amount) of snuff between the cheek and gum (also known as dipping) for 30 minutes or longer. Dry snuff is typically sniffed or inhaled through the nostrils; it is used less commonly [64].

In 2004, an estimated 3.0% of Americans 12 years of age and older had used spit tobacco in the past month. Men used it at higher rates (5.8%) than women (0.3%) [60]. The prevalence of spit tobacco is the highest among 18- to 25-year-olds and is substantially higher among American Indians, Alaska natives, residents of the southern states, and rural residents [61,66]. The consumption of chewing tobacco has been declining since the mid-1980s; conversely, in 2005, snuff consumption increased by approximately 2% over the previous year [66], possibly because tobacco users are consuming snuff instead of cigarettes in locations and situations where smoking is banned.

Factors explaining tobacco use

Smoking initiation

In the United States, smoking initiation typically occurs during adolescence. About 90% of adult smokers have tried their first cigarette by 18 years of age and 70% of daily smokers have become regular smokers by that age [67,68]. Because most adolescents who smoke at least monthly continue to smoke into adulthood, youth-oriented tobacco preventions and cessation strategies are warranted [67,68]. Since the mid-1990s, by 2004, the past-month prevalence had decreased by 56% in 8th graders, 47% in 10th graders, and 32% in 12th graders [69]. In recent years, however, this downward trend has decelerated [69]. The downward trend is unlikely to be sustained without steady and systematic efforts by health care providers in preventing initiation of tobacco use and assisting young smokers in quitting.

A wide range of sociodemographic, behavioral, personal, and environmental factors have been examined as potential predictors of tobacco experimentation and initiation of regular tobacco use among adolescents. For example, it has been suggested that the prevalence of adolescent smoking is related inversely to parental socioeconomic status and adolescent academic performance [68]. Other identified predictors of adolescent smoking include social influence and normative beliefs, negative affect, outcome expectations associated with smoking, resistance skills (self-efficacy), engaging in other risk-taking behaviors, exposure to smoking in movies, and having friends who smoke [70–75].

Although numerous studies have been successful in identifying predictors of smoking initiation, few studies have identified successful methods for promoting cessation among youth, despite the finding that in 2005, more than half of high school cigarette smokers have tried to quit smoking in the past year and failed [52]. These results confirm the highly addictive nature of tobacco emphasizing the need for more effective methods for facilitating cessation among the young.

Nicotine addiction

Nicotine has come to be regarded as a highly addictive substance. Judging by the current diagnostic criteria, tobacco dependence appears to be quite prevalent among cigarette smokers; more than 90% of smokers meet the DSM-IV (Diagnostic and Statistical Manual of Mental Disorders) criteria for nicotine dependence [76]. Research has shown that nicotine acts on the brain to produce a number of effects [77,78] and immediately after exposure, nicotine induces a wide range of central nervous system, cardiovascular, and metabolic effects. Nicotine stimulates the release of neurotransmitters, inducing pharmacologic effects, such as pleasure and reward (dopamine), arousal (acetylcholine, norepinephrine), cognitive enhancement (acetylcholine), appetite suppression (norepinephrine), learning and memory enhancement (glutamate), mood modulation and appetite suppression (serotonin), and reduction of anxiety and tension (β-endorphin and GABA) [78]. Upon entering the brain, a bolus of nicotine activates the dopamine reward pathway, a network of nervous tissue in the brain that elicits feelings of pleasure and stimulates the release of dopamine.

Although withdrawal symptoms are not the only consequence of abstinence, most cigarette smokers do experience craving and withdrawal on cessation [79], and, therefore, relapse is common [80]. The calming effect of nicotine reported by many users is usually associated with a decline in withdrawal effects rather than direct effects on nicotine [53]. This rapid dose-response, along with the short half-life of nicotine ($t^1/_2 = 2$ h), underlies tobacco users' frequent, repeated administration, thereby perpetuating tobacco use and dependence. Tobacco users become proficient in titrating their nicotine levels throughout the day to avoid withdrawal symptoms, to maintain pleasure and arousal, and to modulate mood. Withdrawal symptoms include depression, insomnia, irritability/frustration/anger, anxiety, difficulty concentrating, restlessness, increased appetite/weight gain, and decreased heart rate [81,82].

The assumption that heavy daily use (i.e., 15–30 cigarettes per day), is necessary for dependence to develop is derived from observations of "chippers," adult smokers who have not developed dependence despite smoking up to five cigarettes per day for many years [83,84]. Chippers do not tend to differ from other smokers in their absorption and metabolism of nicotine, causing some investigators to suggest that this level of consumption may be too low to cause nicotine dependence. However, these atypical smokers are usually eliminated from most studies, which are routinely limited to smokers of at least 10 cigarettes per day [83].

Signs of dependence on nicotine have been reported among adolescent smokers, with approximately one fifth of them exhibiting adult-like dependence [85]. Although, lengthy and regular tobacco use has been considered necessary for nicotine dependence to develop [68], recent reports have raised concerns that nicotine dependence symptoms can develop soon after initiation, and that these symptoms might lead to smoking intensification [79,86]. Adolescent smokers, who use tobacco regularly, tend to exhibit high craving for cigarettes and substantial levels of withdrawal symptoms [87].

Genetics of tobacco use and dependence

As early as 1958, Fisher hypothesized that the link between smoking and lung cancer could be explained at least in part by shared genes that predispose individuals to begin smoking as young adults and to develop lung cancer later in adulthood [88]. More recently, tobacco researchers have begun to explore whether genetic factors do in fact contribute toward tobacco use and dependence.

Tobacco use and dependence are hypothesized to result from an interplay of many factors (including pharmacologic, environmental and physiologic) [77]. Some of these factors are shared within families, either environmentally or genetically. Studies of families consistently demonstrate that, compared to family members of nonsmokers, family members of smokers are more likely to be smokers also. However, in addition to shared genetic predispositions, it is important to consider environmental factors that promote tobacco use—siblings within the same family share many of the same environmental influences as well as the same genes. To differentiate the genetic from the environmental influences, epidemiologists use adoption, twin, twins reared apart, and linkage study designs [89].

Key to the adoption studies is the assumption that if a genetic link for tobacco use exists, then tobacco use behaviors (e.g., smoking status, number of years smoked, number of cigarettes smoked per day) will be more similar for persons who are related genetically (i.e., biologically) than for persons who are not related genetically. Hence, one would expect to observe greater similarities between children and their biological parents and siblings than would be observed between children and their adoptive parents or adopted siblings. Indeed, research has demonstrated stronger associations (i.e., higher correlation coefficients) between biologically-related individuals, compared to nonbiologically-related individuals, for the reported number of cigarettes consumed [90]. In recent years, it has become more difficult to conduct adoption studies, because of the reduced number of intranational children available for adoption [91]. Additionally, delayed adoption (i.e., time elapsed between birth and entry into the new family) is common with international adoptions and might lead to an overestimation of genetic effects if early environmental influences are attributed to genetic influences [92].

In twin studies, identical (monozygotic) twins and fraternal (dizygotic) twins are compared. Identical twins share the same genes; fraternal twins, like ordinary siblings, share approximately 50% of their genes. If a genetic link exists for the phenomenon under study, then one would expect to see a greater concordance in identical twins than in fraternal twins. Thus, in the case of tobacco use, one would expect to see a greater proportion of identical twins with the same tobacco use behavior than would be seen with fraternal twins. Statistically, twin studies aim to estimate the percentage of the variance in the behavior that is due to (1) genes (referred to as the "heritability"), (2) shared (within the family) environmental experiences, and (3) nonshared (external from the family) environmental experiences [91]. A number of twin studies of tobacco use have been conducted in recent years. These studies have largely supported a genetic role [91,93]; higher concordance of tobacco use behavior is evident in identical twins than in fraternal twins. The estimated average heritability for smoking is 0.53 (range, 0.28–0.84) [93,94]; approximately half of the variance in smoking appears to be attributable to genetic factors.

Recent advances in the mapping of the human genome have enabled researchers to search for genes associated with specific disorders, including tobacco use. Using a statistical technique called linkage analysis, it is possible to identify genes that predict a trait or disorder. This process is not based on prior knowledge of a gene's function, but rather it is determined by examining whether the trait or disorder is coinherited with markers found in specified chromosomal regions. Typically, these types of investigations involve collection of large family pedigrees, which are studied to determine inheritance of the trait or disorder. This method works well when a single gene is responsible for the outcome; however, it becomes more difficult when multiple genes have an impact, such as with tobacco use. In linkage studies of smoking, it is common for investigators to identify families, ideally with two or more biologically-related relatives that have the trait or disorder under study (referred to as affected individuals, in this case, smokers) and other unaffected relatives. For example, data from affected sibling pairs with parents is a common design in linkage analysis. A tissue sample (typically blood) is taken from each individual, and the sample undergoes genotyping to obtain information about the study participant's unique genetic code. If a gene in a specific region of a chromosome is associated with smoking, and if a genetic marker is linked (i.e., in proximity), then the affected pairs (such as affected sibling pairs) will have increased odds for sharing the same paternal/maternal gene [91].

As genetic research moves forward, new clues provide insight into which genes might be promising "candidates" as contributors to tobacco use and dependence. Currently, there are two general lines of research related to candidate genes for smoking. One examines genes that affect nicotine pharmacodynamics (the way that nicotine affects the body) and the other examines genes that affect nicotine pharmacokinetics (the way that the body affects nicotine). A long list of candidate genes are being examined—some of the most extensively explored involve (a) the dopamine reward pathway (e.g., those related to dopamine synthesis, receptor activation, reuptake, and metabolism) and (b) nicotine metabolism via the cytochrome P450 liver enzymes (specifically, CYP2A6 and CYP2D6).

In summary, each of these types of study designs supports the hypothesis that genetics influence the risk for a wide range of tobacco-related phenotypes, such as ever smoking, age at smoking onset, level of smoking, ability to quit, and the metabolic pathways of nicotine (e.g., see [45,89,95–99]). But given that there are many predictors of tobacco use and dependence, of which genetic predisposition is just one piece of a complex puzzle, it is unlikely that society will move toward widespread genotyping for early identification of individuals who are at risk for tobacco use. Perhaps a more likely use of genetics as related to tobacco use is its potential for improving our treatment for dependence [91]. If genetic research leads to new knowledge regarding the mechanisms underlying the development and maintenance of dependence, it is possible that new, more effective medications might be created. Furthermore, through pharmacogenomics research we might gain improved knowledge as to which patients, based on their genetic profiles, would be best treated with which medications. Researchers are beginning to examine how DNA variants affect health outcome with pharmacologic treatments, with a goal of determining which genetic profiles respond most favorably to specific pharmaceutical aids for cessation (e.g. [98,100–103]).

Benefits of quitting

The reports of the US Surgeon General on the health consequences of smoking, released in 1990 and 2004, summarize abundant and significant health benefits associated with giving up tobacco [9,104]. Benefits noticed shortly after quitting (e.g., within 2 weeks to 3 months), include improvements in pulmonary function and circulation. Within 1–9 months of quitting, the ciliary function of the lung epithelium is restored. Initially, patients might experience increased coughing as the lungs clear excess mucus and tobacco smoke particulates. In several months, smoking cessation results in measurable improvements of lung function. Over time, patients experience decreased coughing, sinus congestion, fatigue, shortness of breath, and risk for pulmonary infection and 1 year postcessation, the excess risk for coronary heart disease is reduced to half that of continuing smokers. After 5–15 years, the risk for stroke is reduced to a rate similar to that of people who are lifetime nonsmokers, and 10 years after quitting, an individual's chance of dying of lung cancer is approximately half that of continuing smokers. Additionally, the risk of developing mouth, larynx, pharynx, esophagus, bladder, kidney, or pancreatic cancer is decreased. Finally, 15 years after quitting, a risk for coronary heart disease is reduced to a rate similar of that of people who have never smoked. Smoking cessation can also lead to a significant reduction in the cumulative risk for death from lung cancer, for males and females.

Smokers who are able to quit by age 35 can be expected to live an additional 6–9 years compared to those who continue to smoke [105]. Ossip-Klein *et al.* [106] recently named tobacco use a "geriatric health issue." Indeed, a considerable proportion of tobacco users continue to smoke well into their 70s and 80s, despite the widespread knowledge of the tobacco health hazards. Elderly smokers frequently claim that the "damage is done," and it is "too late to quit;" however, a considerable body of evidence refutes these statements. Even individuals who postpone quitting until age 65 can incur up to four additional years of life, compared with those who continued to smoke [24,106]. Therefore, elderly smokers should not be ignored as a potential target for cessation efforts. Health care providers ought to remember that it is never too late to advise their elderly patients to quit and to incur health benefits.

A growing body of evidence indicates that continued smoking after a diagnosis of cancer has substantial adverse effects. For example, these studies indicate that smoking reduces the overall effectiveness of treatment, while causing complications with healing as well as exacerbating treatment side effects, increases risk of developing second primary malignancy, and decreases overall survival rates [36–38,107–109]. On the other hand, the medical, health, and psychosocial benefits of smoking cessation among cancer patients are promising. Gritz *et al.* [37] indicated that stopping smoking prior to diagnosis and treatment can have a positive influence on survival rates. Although many smoking cessation interventions are aimed at primary prevention of cancer, these results indicate that there can be substantial medical benefits for individuals who quit smoking after they are diagnosed with cancer.

Smoking cessation interventions

Effective and timely administration of smoking cessation interventions can significantly reduce the risk of smoking-related disease [110]. Recognizing the complexity of tobacco use is a necessary first step in developing effective interventions and trials for cessation and prevention. The biobehavioral model of nicotine addiction and tobacco-related cancers presents the complex interplay of social, psychological, and biological factors that influence tobacco use and addiction (Figure 1.1). These factors in turn mediate dependence, cessation, and relapse in most individuals, and treatment has been developed to address many of the factors noted in the model [38].

The health care provider's role and responsibility

Health care providers are uniquely positioned to assist patients with quitting, having both access to quitting aids and commanding a level of respect that renders them particularly influential in advising patients on health-related issues. To date, physicians have received the greatest attention in the scientific community as providers of tobacco cessation treatment. Although less attention has been paid to other health care providers such as pharmacists and nurses, they too are in a unique position to serve the public and situated to initiate behavior change among patients or complement the efforts of other providers [64,111].

Fiore and associates conducted a meta-analysis of 29 investigations in which they estimated that compared with smokers who do not receive an intervention from a clinician, patients who receive a tobacco cessation intervention from a physician clinician or a nonphysician clinician are 2.2 and 1.7 times as likely to quit smoking at 5 or more months postcessation, respectively [112]. Although brief advice from a clinician has been shown to

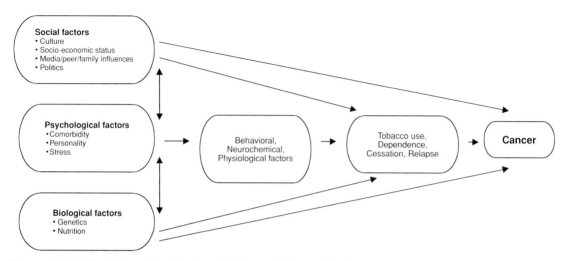

Figure 1.1 Biobehavioral model of nicotine addiction and tobacco-related cancers. (Adapted from [38].)

lead to increased likelihood of quitting, more intensive counseling leads to more dramatic increases in quit rates [112]. Because the use of pharmacotherapy agents approximately doubles the odds of quitting [7,112], smoking cessation interventions should consider combining pharmacotherapy with behavioral counseling.

To assist clinicians and other health care providers in providing cessation treatment, the US Public Health Service has produced a *Clinical Practice Guideline for the Treatment of Tobacco Use and Dependence* [112]. The *Guideline* is based on a systematic review and analysis of scientific literature which yields a series of recommendations and strategies to assist health care providers in delivering smoking cessation treatment. The *Guideline* emphasizes the importance of systematic identification of tobacco users by health care workers and offering at least brief treatment interventions to every patient who uses tobacco. Among the most effective approaches for quitting are behavioral counseling and pharmacotherapy, used alone or, preferably, in combination [112].

Behavioral counseling

Behavioral interventions play an integral role in smoking cessation treatment, either alone or in conjunction with pharmacotherapy. These interventions, which include a variety of methods ranging from self-help materials to individual cognitive–behavioral therapy, enable individuals to more effectively recognize high-risk smoking situations, develop alternative coping strategies, manage stress, improve problem-solving skills, and increase social support [113]. The *Clinical Practice Guideline* outlines a five-step framework that clinicians can apply when assisting patients with quitting. Health care providers should: (a) systematically identify all tobacco users, (b) strongly advise all tobacco users to quit, (c) assess readiness to make a quit attempt, (d) assist patients in quitting, and (e) arrange follow-up contact. The steps have been described as the 5 A's: Ask, Advise, Assess, Assist, and Arrange follow-up (Table 1.3). Due to the possibility of relapse, health care providers should also provide patients with brief relapse prevention treatment. Relapse prevention reinforces the patient's decision to quit, reviews the benefits of quitting, and assists the patient in resolving any problems arising from quitting [112]. The outlined strategy has been termed the 5 R's (Table 1.3): Relevance, Risks, Rewards, Roadblocks, and Repetition. In the absence of time or expertise for providing more comprehensive counseling, clinicians are advised to (at a minimum), ask about tobacco use, advise tobacco users to quit, and refer these patients to other resources for quitting, such as a toll-free tobacco cessation quitline (1-800-QUIT NOW, in the US).

Table 1.3 The 5 A's and 5 R's for smoking cessation interventions.

5 A's	Ask about tobacco use	Identify and document tobacco use status for every patient at every visit
	Advise to quit	Urge every tobacco user to quit in a clear, strong, and personalized manner
	Assess readiness to make a quit attempt	Assess whether or not the tobacco user is ready to make a quit attempt in the next 30 days
	Assist in quit attempt	Use counseling and/or pharmacotherapy with the patient willing to make a quit attempt to help him or her quit
	Arrange follow-up	Schedule follow-up contact, preferably within the first week after the quit date
5 R's	Relevance	Encourage the patient to indicate why quitting is personally relevant, being specific as possible
	Risk	Ask the patient to identify the negative consequences of tobacco use, including acute risks (e.g., short breath), long-term risks (e.g., cancer, and environmental risks, e.g., cancer among family)
	Rewards	Request that the patient identify potential benefits of stopping tobacco use (e.g., improved health)
	Roadblocks	Ask the patient to identify barriers or impediments to quitting and note the elements of treatment that could address such barriers (e.g., withdrawal symptoms, fear of failure, lack of support)
	Repetition	Repeat the motivational intervention every time an unmotivated patient visits the clinic setting

Adapted from [112].

Pharmaceutical aids for smoking cessation

According to the *Clinical Practice Guideline* [112], all patients attempting to quit should be encouraged to use one or more effective pharmacotherapy agents for cessation except in the presence of special circumstances. These recommendations are supported by the results of more than 100 controlled trials demonstrating that patients receiving pharmacotherapy are approximately twice as likely to remain abstinent long-term (greater than 5 mo) when compared to patients receiving placebo (Figure 1.2). Although one would argue that pharmacotherapy is costly and might not be a necessary component of a treatment plan for each patient, it is the most effective known method for maximizing the odds of success for any given quit attempt, particularly when combined with behavioral counseling [112].

Currently, seven marketed agents have an FDA-approved indication for smoking cessation in the US: five nicotine replacement therapy (NRT) formulations (nicotine gum, nicotine lozenge, transdermal nicotine patches, nicotine nasal spray, and nicotine oral inhaler), sustained-release bupropion, and varenicline tartrate. These are described in brief below, and summaries of the prescribing information for each medication are provided in Table 1.4.

Nicotine replacement therapy

In clinical trials, patients who use NRT products are 1.77 times as likely to quit smoking than are those who receive placebo [7]. The main mechanism of action of NRT products is thought to be a stimulation of nicotine receptors in the ventral tegmental area of the brain, which results in dopamine release in the nucleus accumbens. The use of NRT is to reduce the physical withdrawal symptoms and to alleviate the physiologic symptoms of withdrawal, so the smoker can focus on the behavioral and psychological aspects of quitting before fully abstaining nicotine. Key advantages of NRT are that patients are not exposed to the carcinogens and other toxic compounds found in tobacco and tobacco smoke, and NRT provides slower onset of action than nicotine delivered via cigarettes, thereby eliminating the near-immediate reinforcing effects of nicotine obtained through smoking (Figure 1.3). NRT products

Table 1.4 FDA-approved medications for smoking cessation.

	Nicotine replacement therapy (NRT) formulations[1]						Bupropion SR	Varenicline
	Gum	Lozenge	Transdermal preparations[1]		Nasal spray	Oral inhaler		
			Nicoderm CQ[2]	Generic Patch				
Product	Nicorette[2], Generic OTC 2 mg, 4 mg: original, FreshMint[2], Fruit Chill[2], mint, orange[2]	Commit[2], Generic OTC 2 mg, 4 mg; mint	Nicoderm CQ[2] OTC 24-hour release 7 mg, 14 mg, 21 mg	Generic Patch OTC/Rx (formerly Habitrol) 24-hour release 7 mg, 14 mg, 21 mg	Nicotrol NS[3] Rx Metered spray 0.5 mg nicotine in 50 μL aqueous nicotine solution	Nicotrol inhaler[3] Rx 10 mg cartridge delivers 4 mg inhaled nicotine vapor	Zyban[2], Generic Rx 150 mg sustained-release tablet	Chantix[3] Rx 0.5 mg, 1 mg tablet
Dosing	≥25 cigarettes/day: 4 mg <25 cigarettes/day: 2 mg Week 1–6: 1 piece q 1–2 hours Week 7–9: 1 piece q 2–4 hours Week 10–12: 1 piece q 4–8 hours • Maximum, 24 pieces/day • Chew each piece slowly • Park between cheek and gum when peppery or tingling sensation appears (~15–30 chews) • Resume chewing when taste or tingle fades • Repeat chew/park steps until most of the nicotine is gone (taste or tingle does not return; generally 30 min) • Park in different areas of mouth • No food or beverages 15 min before or during use • Duration: up to 12 weeks	1st cigarette ≤30 minutes after waking: 4 mg 1st cigarette >30 minutes after waking: 2 mg Week 1–6: 1 lozenge q 1–2 hours Week 7–9: 1 lozenge q 2–4 hours Week 10–12: 1 lozenge q 4–8 hours • Maximum, 20 lozenges/day • Allow to dissolve slowly (20–30 min) • Nicotine release may cause a warm, tingling sensation • Do not chew or swallow • Occasionally rotate to different areas of the mouth • No food or beverages 15 minutes before or during use • Duration: up to 12 weeks	>10 cigarettes/day: 21 mg/day × 6 weeks 14 mg/day × 2 weeks 7 mg/day × 2 weeks ≤10 cigarettes/day: 14 mg/day × 6 weeks 7 mg/day × 2 weeks • May wear patch for 16 hours if patient experiences sleep disturbances (remove at bedtime) • Duration: 8–10 weeks	>10 cigarettes/day: 21 mg/day × 4 weeks 14 mg/day × 2 weeks 7 mg/day × 2 weeks ≤10 cigarettes/day: 14 mg/day × 6 weeks 7 mg/day × 2 weeks • May wear patch for 16 hours, if patient experiences sleep disturbances (remove at bedtime) • Duration: 8 weeks	1–2 doses/hour (8–40 doses/day) One dose = 2 sprays (one in **each** nostril); each spray delivers 0.5 mg of nicotine to the nasal mucosa • Maximum – 5 doses/hour – 40 doses/day • For best results, initially use at least 8 doses/day • Patients should not sniff, swallow, or inhale through the nose as the spray is being administered • Duration: 3–6 mo	6–16 cartridges/day; individualized dosing • Initially, use at least 6 cartridges/day • Best effects with continuous puffing for 20 minutes • Nicotine in cartridge is depleted after 20 minutes of active puffing • Patient should inhale into back of throat or puff in short breaths • Do not inhale into the lungs (like a cigarette) but "puff" as if lighting a pipe • Open cartridge retains potency for 24 hours • Duration: up to 6 months	150 mg po q AM × 3 days, then increase to 150 mg po bid • Do not exceed 300 mg/day • Treatment should be initiated while patient is still smoking • Set quit date 1–2 weeks **after** initiation of therapy • Allow at least 8 hours between doses • Avoid bedtime dosing to minimize insomnia • Dose tapering is not necessary • Can be used safely with NRT • Duration: 7–12 weeks, with maintenance up to 6 months in selected patients	Days 1–3: 0.5 mg po q AM Days 4–7: 0.5 mg po bid Weeks 2–12: 1 mg po bid • Patients should begin therapy 1 week prior to quit date • Take dose after eating with a full glass of water • Dose tapering is not necessary • Nausea and insomnia are side effects that are usually temporary • Duration: 12 weeks; an additional 12 week course may be used in selected patients
Adverse effects	• Mouth/jaw soreness • Hiccups • Dyspepsia • Hypersalivation • Effects associated with incorrect chewing technique: – Lightheadedness – Nausea/vomiting – Throat and mouth irritation	• Nausea • Hiccups • Cough • Heartburn • Headache • Flatulence • Insomnia	• Local skin reactions (erythema, pruritus, burning) • Headache • Sleep disturbances (insomnia) or abnormal/vivid dreams (associated with nocturnal nicotine absorption)		• Nasal and/or throat irritation (hot, peppery, or burning sensation) • Rhinitis • Tearing • Sneezing • Cough • Headache	• Mouth and/or throat irritation • Unpleasant taste • Cough • Rhinitis • Dyspepsia • Hiccups • Headache	• Insomnia • Dry mouth • Nervousness/difficulty concentrating • Rash • Constipation • Seizures (risk is 1/1000 [0.1%])	• Nausea • Sleep disturbances (insomnia, abnormal dreams) • Constipation • Flatulence • Vomiting

Nicotine replacement therapy (NRT) formulations

	Gum	Lozenge	Transdermal preparations		Nasal spray	Oral inhaler	Bupropion SR	Varenicline
			Nicoderm CQ	Generic Patch				
Advantages	• Gum use might satisfy oral cravings • Gum use may delay weight gain • Patients can titrate therapy to manage withdrawal symptoms	• Lozenge use might satisfy oral cravings • Patients can titrate therapy to manage withdrawal symptoms	• Provides consistent nicotine levels over 24 hours • Easy to use and conceal • Once-a-day dosing associated with fewer compliance problems		• Patients can titrate therapy to manage withdrawal symptoms	• Patients can titrate therapy to manage withdrawal symptoms • Mimics hand-to-mouth ritual of smoking	• Easy to use; oral formulation might be associated with fewer compliance problems • Can be used with NRT • Might be beneficial in patients with depression	• Easy to use; oral formulation might be associated with fewer compliance problems • Offers a new mechanism of action for patients who have failed other agents
Disadvantages	• Gum chewing may not be socially acceptable • Gum is difficult to use with dentures • Patients must use proper chewing technique to minimize adverse effects	• Gastrointestinal side effects (nausea, hiccups, heartburn) might be bothersome	• Patients cannot titrate the dose • Allergic reactions to adhesive might occur • Patients with dermatologic conditions should not use the patch		• Nasal/throat irritation may be bothersome • Dependence can result • Patients must wait 5 minutes before driving or operating heavy machinery • Patients with chronic nasal disorders or severe reactive airway disease should not use the spray	• Initial throat or mouth irritation can be bothersome • Cartridges should not be stored in very warm conditions or used in very cold conditions • Patients with underlying bronchospastic disease must use the inhaler with caution	• Seizure risk is increased • Several contraindications and precautions preclude use (see Precautions, above)	• May induce nausea in up to one third of patients • Post-marketing surveillance data not yet available
Cost/day[4]	2 mg: $3.28–$6.57 (9 pieces) 4 mg: $4.31–$6.57 (9 pieces)	2 mg: $3.66–$5.26 (9 pieces) 4 mg: $3.66–$5.26 (9 pieces)	$2.24–$3.89 (1 patch)	$1.90–$2.94 (1 patch)	$3.67 (8 doses)	$5.29 (6 cartridges)	$3.62–$6.04 (2 tablets)	$4.00–$4.22 (2 tablets)

From: Rx for Change: [8] Copyright © 1999–2007, with permission.

[1]Transdermal patch formulations previously marketed, but no longer available: Nicotrol 5 mg, 10 mg, 15 mg delivered over 16 hours (Pfizer) and generic patch (formerly Prostep) 11 mg and 22 mg delivered over 24 hours.

[2]Marketed by GlaxoSmithKline.

[3]Marketed by Pfizer.

[4]Average wholesale price from 2006 Drug Topics Redbook. Montvale, NJ: Medical Economics Company, Inc., June 2007.

Abbreviations : Hx, history; MAO, monoamine oxidase; NRT, nicotine replacement therapy; OTC, (over-the-counter) non-prescription product; Rx, prescription product.

For complete prescribing information, please refer to the manufacturers' package inserts.

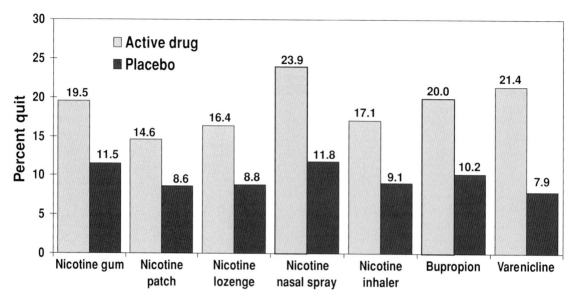

Figure 1.2 Long-term (≥6 mo) quit rates for FDA-approved medications for smoking cessation. (Data adapted from [4–7].) (*From Rx for Change*: [114] Copyright © 1999–2007, with permission.)

should be used with caution in patients who have underlying serious arrhythmias, serious or worsening angina pectoris, or a recent (within 2 weeks) myocardial infarction [112]. Animal data suggest that nicotine is harmful to the developing fetus, and as such prescription formulations of nicotine are classified by the Food and Drug Administration as pregnancy category D agents. Yet despite these concerns, most experts perceive the risks of NRT to be small relative to the risks of continued smoking. Use of NRT may be appropriate in patients with underlying cardiovascular disease or in women who

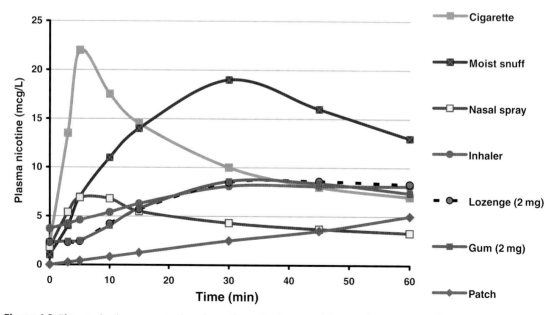

Figure 1.3 Plasma nicotine concentrations for various nicotine-containing products. (*From Rx for Change*: [114];) Copyright © 1999–2007, with permission.)

are pregnant if these patients are under medical supervision [112]. Patients with temporomandibular joint disease should not use the nicotine gum, and patients smoking fewer than 10 cigarettes daily should initiate NRT with caution and generally at reduced dosages [112]. The safety and efficacy of NRT have not been established in adolescents, and currently none of the NRT products are indicated for use in this population [112,115].

Sustained-release bupropion (Zyban)

Initially marketed as an atypical antidepressant, sustained-release bupropion is hypothesized to promote smoking cessation by inhibiting the reuptake of dopamine and norepinephrine in the central nervous system [116] and acting as a nicotinic acetylcholine receptor antagonist [117]. These neurochemical effects are believed to modulate the dopamine reward pathway and reduce the cravings for nicotine and symptoms of withdrawal [112].

Because seizures are a dose-related toxicity associated with bupropion, this medication is contraindicated in patients with underlying seizure disorders and in patients receiving concurrent therapy with other forms of bupropion (Wellbutrin, Wellbutrin SR, and Wellbutrin XL). Bupropion also is contraindicated in patients with anorexia or bulimia nervosa and in patients who are undergoing abrupt discontinuation of alcohol or sedatives (including benzodiazepines) due to the increased risk for seizures. The concurrent administration of bupropion and a monoamine oxidase (MAO) inhibitor is contraindicated and at least 14 days should elapse between discontinuation of an MAO inhibitor and initiation of treatment with bupropion [118]. Although seizures were not reported in the smoking cessation clinical trials, the incidence of seizures with the sustained-release formulation (Wellbutrin) used in the treatment of depression was 0.1% among patients without a previous history of seizures [119]. For this reason, bupropion should be used with extreme caution in patients with a history of seizure, cranial trauma, patients receiving medications known to lower the seizure threshold, and patients with underlying severe hepatic cirrhosis. Bupropion is classified as a pregnancy category C drug, meaning that either (a) animal studies have demonstrated that the drug exerts ani-

mal teratogenic or embryocidal effects, but there are no controlled studies in women, or (b) no studies are available in either animals or women. Correspondingly, the manufacturer recommends that this agent be used during pregnancy only if clearly necessary [118].

Varenicline tartrate (Chantix)

The efficacy of varenicline, a partial agonist selective for the a4b2 nicotinic acetylcholine receptor [120,121], is believed to be the result of sustained, low-level agonist activity at the receptor site combined with competitive inhibition of nicotine binding. The partial agonist activity induces modest receptor stimulation, which leads to increased dopamine levels, thereby attenuating the symptoms of nicotine withdrawal. In addition, by competitively blocking the binding of nicotine to nicotinic acetylcholine receptors in the central nervous system, varenicline inhibits the surges of dopamine release that occur following the inhalation of tobacco smoke. The latter effect might be effective in preventing relapse by reducing the reinforcing and rewarding effects of smoking [120]. The FDA classifies varenicline as a pregnancy category C drug, and the manufacturer recommends that this medication be used during pregnancy only if the potential benefit justifies the potential risk to the fetus [121].

Summary

Tobacco use remains prevalent among the population and represents a matter of special public health concern. It is the primary risk factor for the development of lung cancer. It has been shown to cause malignancies in other locations, as well as numerous other diseases. The body of knowledge of various aspects of smoking behavior has largely increased over the past two decades. Studies of factors predisposing to smoking initiation among youth may provide important clues for the development of feasible and effective smoking prevention activities. The knowledge of biobehavioral factors leading to development of nicotine dependence may assist in providing more effective treatments to patients who use tobacco products. The five A's approach (Ask about tobacco use, Advise patients to quit, Assess readiness to quit, Assist with quitting, and Arrange follow-up) is described in the US Public Health Service

Clinical Practice Guideline for Treating Tobacco Use and Dependence. Health care providers are encouraged to implement at least brief interventions at each encounter with a patient who uses tobacco.

References

1 USDHHS. *Cancer.A Report of the Surgeon General.* Rockville, MD: Office of Smoking and Health, 1982.

2 Mokdad AH, Marks JS, Stroup DF, Gerberding JL. Actual causes of death in the United States, 2000 [Special Communication]. *JAMA* 2004; **291(10)**:1238–45.

3 Centers for Disease Control and Prevention. Tobacco use among adults—United States, 2005. *MMWR* 2006; **55**:1145–1148.

4 Gonzales D, Rennard SI, Nides M *et al.* Varenicline, an a4β2 nicotinic acetylcholine receptor partial agonist, vs sustained-release bupropion and placebo for smoking cessation: a randomized controlled trial. *JAMA* 2006; **296**:47–55.

5 Hughes JR, Stead LF, Lancaster T. Antidepressants for smoking cessation; Art. No. CD000031. DOI: 10.1002/14651858.CD000031.pub3, 2004.

6 Jorenby DE, Hays JT, Rigotti NA *et al.* for Varenicline Phase 3 Study Group. Efficacy of varenicline, an a4β2 nicotinic acetylcholine receptor partial agonist, vs placebo or sustained-release bupropion for smoking cessation: a randomized controlled trial. *JAMA* 2006; **296**:56–63.

7 Silagy C, Lancaster T, Stead L, Mant D, Fowler G. Nicotine replacement therapy for smoking cessation. *Cochrane Database Syst Rev* 2004; **3**:CD000146.

8 CDC. Annual smoking-attributable mortality, years of potential life lost, and economic costs—United States, 1995–1999. *MMWR* 2002; **51**:300–3.

9 USDHHS. *The Health Consequences of Smoking: A Report of the Surgeon General.* Bethesda, MD: US Department of Health and Human Services, Centers for Disease Control and Prevention, National Center for Chronic disease Prevention and Health Promotion, 2004.

10 Center for Disease Control. Cigarette smoking attributable mortality—United States. *MMWR* 2003; **52(35)**:842–4.

11 Gotay C. Behavior and cancer prevention. *J Clin Oncol* 2005; **23**:301–10.

12 Peto R, Lopez AD, Thurn M, Heath C, Doll R. Mortality from smoking worldwide. *BMJ* 1996; **52**:12–21.

13 Yoder L. Lung cancer epidemiology. *Medsurg Nurs* 2006; **15(3)**:171–5.

14 Jemel A, Siegel R, Ward E *et al.* Cancer statistics 2006. *Cancer J Clin* 2006; **56(2)**:106–30.

15 Spiro SG, Silvestri GA. One hundred years of lung cancer. *Am J Respir Crit Care Med* 2005; **172**:523–39.

16 Knop C. *Lung Cancer.* Boston, MA: Hones and Barlett, 2005.

17 Pastorino U. Early detection of lung cancer. *Thematic Rev Ser* 2006; **73**:5–13.

18 Thun M, Day-Lally C, Myers D *et al.* Trends in Tobacco Smoking and Mortality from Cigarette Use in Cancer Prevention Studies I (1959 through 1965) and II (1982 through 1988). Washington, DC: National Cancer Institute, 1997.

19 Thun MJ, Lally CA, Flannery JT, Calle EE, Flanders WD, Heath CW, Jr. Cigarette smoking and changes in the histopathology of lung cancer. *J Natl Cancer Inst* 1997; **89**:1580–6.

20 Wynder E, Muscat JE. The changing epidemiology of smoking and lung cancer. *Environ Health Perspect* 1995; **103(Suppl 8)**:143–8.

21 Stampfer M. New insights from British doctors study. *Br Med J* 2004; **328(7455)**:1507.

22 National Cancer Institute. *Cigarette Smoking and Cancer.* Questions and Answers, 2004 [cited October 12, 2006]. Available from http://www.cancer.gov/cancertopics/factsheet/Tobacco/cancer.

23 Kamholz SL. Pulmonary and cardiovascular consequences of smoking. *Med Clin North Am* 2004; **88**:1415–30.

24 Peto R, Darby S, Deo H *et al.* Smoking, smoking cessation, and lung cancer in the UK since 1950: combination of national statistics with two case–control studies. *BMJ* 2000; **321(7257)**:329.

25 Albert A, Samet J. Epidemiology of lung cancer. *Chest* 2003; **123(Suppl 1)**:21S–49S.

26 US Public Health Service. *Surgeon General's Advisory Committee on Smoking and Health.* Washington, DC: US Public Health Service, 1964.

27 American Cancer Society. *Cancer Facts and Figures.* Atlanta, GA: American Cancer Society, 2004.

28 Mackay J, Amos A. Women and tobacco. *Respirology* 2003; **8**:123–30.

29 Siegfriend J. Woman and lung cancer: does estrogen play a role? *Lancet Oncol* 2001; **2(8)**:606–13.

30 US Environmental Protection Agency. *Respiratory Health Effects of Passive Smoking: Lung Cancer and Other Disorders.* Washington, DC: US EPA, 1992. Report No.: Publication EPA/600/6-90/006F.

31 USDHHS. *The Health Consequences of Using Smokeless Tobacco. A Report of the Advisory Committee to the Surgeon General.* NIH Publication No 86-2874 1986 [cited May 8, 2006]. Available from http://profiles.nlm.nih.gov/NN/B/B/F/C/_/nnbbfc.pdf.

32 Center for Disease Control. State-specific prevalence of cigarette smoking among adults, and policies and attitudes about second-hand smoke—United States, 2000. *MMWR* 2001; **50(49)**:1101–6.

33 Evans WN, Crankshaw E, Nimsch C *et al.* Media and secondhand smoke exposure: results from a national survey. *Am J Health Behav* 2006; **30(1)**:62–71.

34 USDHHS. *The Health Consequences of Involuntary Exposure to Tobacco Smoke: A Report of the Surgeon General.* Atlanta, GA: USDHHS, 2006.

35 Glantz S, Parmley W. Passive smoking and heart disease: epidemiology, physiology and biochemistry. *Circulation* 1991; **83(1)**:1–12.

36 Cox L, Patten C, Ebbert J *et al.* Tobacco use outcomes among patients with lung cancer treated for nicotine dependence. *J Clin Oncol* 2002; **20**:3461–9.

37 Gritz E, Fingeret M, Vidrine D, Lazev A, Mehta N, Reece G. Successes and failures of the teachable moment. *Cancer* 2005; **106**:17–27.

38 Gritz E, Vidrine D, Lazev A. *Smoking Cessation in Cancer Patients: Never too Late to Quit.* New York, NY: Springer Publishing, 2003.

39 Schnoll R, Rothman R, Wielt D *et al.* A randomized pilot study of cognitive–behavioral therapy versus basic health education for smoking cessation among cancer patients. *Ann Behav Med* 2004; **30(1)**:1–11.

40 Vander Ark W, DiNardo LJ, Oliver D. Factors affecting smoking cessation in patients with head and neck cancer. *Laryngoscope* 1997; **107**:888–92.

41 DeBoer M, Van den Borne B, Pruyne J *et al.* Psychosocial and physical correlates of survival and recurrence in patients with head and neck carcinoma: results of a 6-year longitudinal study. *Cancer* 1998; **83**:2567–629.

42 Tucker M, Murray N, Shaw E *et al.* Second primary cancers related to smoking and treatment of small-cell lung cancer. *J Natl Cancer Inst* 1997; **89**:1782–8.

43 Benowitz NL. Pharmacologic aspects of cigarette smoking and nicotine addiction. *N Engl J Med* 1988; **319**:1318–30.

44 Moller A, Villebro N, Pedersen T, Tonnesen H. Effects of preoperative smoking intervention on post-operative complications: a randomized clinical trial. *Lancet* 2002; **359**:1114–7.

45 Spitz MR, Fueger JJ, Chamberlain R, Goepfert H, Newell G. Cigarette smoking patterns in patients after treatment of upper aerodigestive tract cancers. *J Cancer Educ* 1990; **5**:109–13.

46 Gritz ER, Nisenbaum R, Elashoff RE, Holmes EC. Smoking behavior following diagnosis in patients with stage I non-small cell lung cancer. *Cancer Causes Control* 1991; **2**:105–12.

47 Davison A, Duffy M. Smoking habits of long-term survivors of surgery for lung cancer. *Thorax* 1982; **37**:331–3.

48 Schnoll R, Malstrom M, James C *et al.* Correlates of tobacco use among smokers and recent quitters diagnosed with cancer. *Patient Educ Couns* 2002; **46**:137–45.

49 Dresler C, Bailey M, Roper C, Patterson G, Cooper J. Smoking cessation and lung cancer resection. *Chest* 1996; **110**:1199–202.

50 Thun MJ, Henley SJ, Calle EE. Tobacco use and cancer: an epidemiologic perspective for geneticists. *Oncogene* 2002; **21**:7307–25.

51 Center for Disease Control and Prevention (CDC). State-specific prevalence of cigarette smoking among adults and secondhand smoke rules and policies in homes and workplaces—United States, 2005. *MMWR* 2006; **55**:1148–51.

52 Center for Disease Control. Youth risk behavior surveillance, United States, 2005. *MMWR* 2006; **55**:SS–55.

53 USDHHS. *Tobacco Addiction.* Atlanta, GA: USDHHS, 2006. (Printed 1998, reprinted 2001, Revised 2006)

54 Baker F, Ainsworth S, Dye JT *et al.* Health risks associated with cigar smoking. *JAMA* 2000; **284**:735–40.

55 US Department of Agriculture. *Tobacco Outlook.* Report TBS-258, 2005 [cited April 22, 2005]. Available from http://www.ers.usda.gov/publications/soview.aspf=speciality/tbs-bb/.

56 National Cancer Institute. *Cigars. Health Effects and Trends.* Bethesda, MD: National Cancer Institute, 1998. Report No.: NIH Publication No. 98–4302.

57 CDC. State-specific prevalence of current cigarette and cigar smoking among adults—United States, 1998. *MMWR Morb Mortal Wkly Rep* 1999; **48(45)**:1034–9.

58 Henningfield JE, Fant R, Radzius A *et al.* Nicotine concentration, smoke pH and whole tobacco aqueous pH of some cigar brands and types popular in the US. *Nicotine Tob Res* 1999; **1(2)**:163–8.

59 Kozlowski LT, Mehta N, Sweeney C *et al.* Filter ventilation and nicotine content of tobacco in cigarettes from Canada, The United Kingdom, and the United States. *Tob Control* 1998; **7(4)**:369.

60 U.S. Department of Health and Human Services, Substance Abuse and Mental Health Services Administration. *Results from the 2004 National Survey on Drug Use and Health: National Findings* (Office of Applied Studies, NHSDA Seris H-28, DHHS Publication No. SMA 05–4062), 2005.

61 Center for Disease Control. Bidi use among urban youth—Massachusetts, March–April 1999. *MMWR* 1999; **48(36)**:796–9.

62 Delnevo C, Pevzner E, Hrywna M *et al.* Bidi cigarette use among young adults in 15 states. *Prev Med* 2004; **39(1)**:207–11.

63 Rickert WS. *Determination of Yields of "Tar", Nicotine and Carbon Monoxide from Bidi Cigarettes: Final Report.* Ontario, Canada: Lab Stat International, Inc., 1999.

64 Hudmon K, Kilfoy B, Prokhorov A. The epidemiology of tobacco use and dependence. *Crit Care Nurs Clin N Am* 2006; **18**:1–11.

65 Ebbert J, Carr A, Dale L. Smokeless tobacco: an emerging addiction. *Med Clin N Am* 2004; **88(6)**:1593–605.

66 US Department of Agriculture. *Tobacco Outlook.* Report TBS-260. Available from http://usda.mannlib.cornell.edu/usda/ers/TBS//2000s/2006/TBS-04-28-2006.pdf.

67 Gilpin E, Choi W, Berry C *et al.* How many adolescents start smoking each day in the US? *J Adolesc Health* 1999; **24(4)**:248–55.

68 USDHHS. *Preventing Tobacco Use Among Young People: A Report of the Surgeon General.* Atlanta, GA: United States Department of Health and Human Service, Public Health Service, Centers for Disease Control and Prevention, National Center for Chronic Disease Prevention and Health Promotion, Office on Smoking and Health, 1994.

69 Johnston L, O'Malley PM, Bachman J, Schulenberg J. *Monitoring the Future National Results on Adolescent Drug Use: Overview of Key Findings, 2005.* Bethesda, MD: National Institute on Drug Abuse, 2006.

70 Biglan A, Duncan TE, Ary DV, Smolkowski K. Peer and parental influences on adolescent tobacco use. *J Behav Med* Aug 1995; **18(4)**:315–30.

71 Gritz ER, Prokhorov AV, Hudmon KS *et al.* Predictors of susceptibility to smoking and ever smoking: a longitudinal study in a triethnic sample of adolescents. *Nicotine Tob Res* Aug 2003; **5(4)**:493–506.

72 Hansen WB. Pilot test results comparing the All Stars program with seventh grade D.A.R.E.: program integrity and mediating variable analysis. *Subst Use Misuse* Aug 1996; **31(10)**:1359–77.

73 MacKinnon DP. Analysis of mediating variables in prevention and intervention research. *NIDA Res Monogr* 1994; **139**:127–53.

74 Sargent J. Smoking in movies: impact on adolescent smoking. *Adolesc Med Clin* 2005; **16(2)**:345–70.

75 Wahlgren DR, Hovell MF, Slymen DJ, Conway TL, Hofstetter CR, Jones JA. Predictors of tobacco use initiation in adolescents: a two-year prospective study and theoretical discussion. *Tob Control* 1997; **6(2)**:95–103.

76 APA. *Diagnostic and Statistical Manual of Mental Disorders*, 4th edn. Washington, DC: American Psychiatric Association, 2000.

77 Benowtiz N. Cigarette smoking and nicotine addiction. *Med Clin N Am* 1992; **76**:415–37.

78 Benowtiz N. The biology of nicotine dependence: from the 188 Surgeon General's Report to the present and into the future. *Nicotine Tob Res* 1999; **1(Suppl 2)**:S159–63.

79 DiFranza J, Rigotti N, McNeill A *et al.* Initial symptoms of nicotine dependence in adolescents. *Tob Control* 2000; **9**:313–9.

80 Brown R, Lejuez C, Kahler C, Strong D, Zwolensky M. Distress tolerance and early smoking lapse. *Clin Psychol Rev* 2005; **25(6)**:713–33.

81 APA. *Diagnostic and Statistical Manual of Mental Disorders*, 4th edn. Washington, DC: American Psychiatric Association, 1994.

82 DiFranza JR, Wellman RJ. A sensitization-homeostasis model of nicotine craving, withdrawal, and tolerance: integrating the clinical and basis science literature. *Nicotine Tob Res* 2005; **7(1)**:9–26.

83 Shiffman S. Tobacco chippers—individual differences in tobacco dependence. *Psychopharmacology* 1989; **97**:539–47.

84 Shiffman S, Fischer LB, Zettler-Segal M, Benowitz NL. Nicotine exposure among nondependent smokers. *Arch Gen Psychiatry* 1990; **47**:333–6.

85 Prokhorov A, Pallonen U, Fava J, Ding L, Niaura R. Measuring nicotine dependence among high-risk adolescent smokers. *J Addict Behav* 1996; **21**:117–27.

86 DiFranza J, Wellman R. Preventing cancer by controlling youth tobacco use. *Semin Oncol Nurs* 2003; **19**:261–7.

87 Prokhorov A, Hudmon KS, Cinciripini P, Marani S. "Withdrawal symptoms" in adolescents: a comparison of former smokers and never-smokers. *Nicotine Tob Res* 2005; **7(6)**:909–13.

88 Fisher RA. Cigarettes, cancer and statistics. *Centennial Rev* 1958; **2**:151–66.

89 Sullivan PF, Kendler KS. The genetic epidemiology of smoking. *Nicotine Tob Res* 1999; **1**:S51–S7.

90 Eysenck HJ. *The Causes and Effects of Smoking.* Beverly Hills, CA: Sage, 1980.

91 Hall W, Madden P, Lynskey M. The genetics of tobacco use: methods, findings and policy implications. *Tob Control* 2002; **11**:119–24.

92 Rutter M, Pickles A, Murray R *et al.* Testing hypotheses on specific environmental causal effects on behavior. *Psychol Bull* 2001; **127**:291–324.

93 Hughes JR. Genetics of smoking: a brief review. *Behav Ther* 1986; **17**:335–45.

94 Carmelli D, Swan GE, Robinette D, Fabsitz R. Genetic influences on smoking—a study of male twins. *N Engl J Med* 1992; **327**:829–33.

95 Heath A, Kirk K, Meyer J, Martin N. Genetic and social determinants of initiation and age at onset of smoking in Australian twins. *Behav Genet* 1999; **29**:395–407.

96 Koudsi N, Tyndale R. Genetic influences on smoking. *Drug Monit* 2005; **27(6)**:704–9.

97 Lerman C, Tyndale R, Patterson F *et al.* Nicotine metabolite ratio predicts efficacy of transdermal nicotine for smoking cessation. *Clin Pharmacol Ther* 2006; **79**:600–8.

98 Swan GE, Hops H, Wilhelmsen KC *et al.* A genome-wide screen for nicotine dependence susceptibility loci. *Am J Med Genet B Neuropsychiatr Genet* June 5, 2006; **141(4)**:354–60.

99 Xian H, Scherrer J, Madden P *et al.* The heritability of failed smoking cessation and nicotine withdrawal in twins who smoked and attempted to quit. *Nicotine Tob Res* 2003; **5**:245–54.

100 Berrettini WH, Lerman CE. Pharmacotherapy and pharmacogenetics of nicotine dependence. *Am J Psychiatry* 2005; **152**:1441–51.

101 Lerman C, Jepson C, Wileyto EP *et al.* Role of functional genetic variation in the dopamine D2 receptor (DRD2) in response to bupropion and nicotine replacement therapy for tobacco dependence: results of two randomized clinical trials. *Neuropsychopharmacology* [online] 2006; **31(1)**:231–42.

102 Lerman C, Shields PG, Wileyto EP *et al.* Pharmacogenetic investigation of smoking cessation treatment. *Pharmacogenetics* 2002; **12(8)**:627–34.

103 Munafo MR, Lerman C, Niaura R, Shields AE, Swan GE. Smoking cessation treatment: pharmacogenetic assessment. *Curr Opin Mol Ther* 2005; **7**:202–8.

104 USDHHS. *The Health Benefits of Smoking Cessation: A Report of the Surgeon General.* Atlanta, GA: United States Department of Health and Human Services, Public Health Service, Centers for Disease Control, Center for Chronic Disease Prevention and Health Promotion, 1990. Office on Smoking and Health, United States Government Printing Office, CDC Publication No.: 90–8416.

105 Taylor DH, Jr, Hasselblad V, Henley J, Thus MJ, Sloan FA. Benefits of smoking cessation for longevity. *Am J Public Health* 2002; **92(6)**:990–6.

106 Ossip-Klein D, Pearson T, McIntosh S *et al.* Smoking is a geriatric disease. *Nicotine Tob Res* 1999; **1(4)**:299–300.

107 Pinto B, Trunzo J. Health behaviors during and after cancer diagnosis. *Cancer* 2005; **104(Suppl 11)**:2614–23.

108 Schnoll R, Rothman R, Wielt D *et al.* A randomized pilot study of cognitive–behavioral therapy versus basic health education for smoking cessation among cancer patients. *Ann Behav Med* 2005; **30(1)**:1–11.

109 Walker MC, Larsen R, Zona D, Govindan R, Fisher E. Smoking urges and relapse among lung cancer patients: findings from a preliminary retrospective study. *Prev Med* 2004; **39**:449–57.

110 Prokhorov AV, Hudmon KS, Gritz ER. Promoting smoking cessation among cancer patients: a behavioral model. *Oncology (Huntingt)* Dec 1997; **11(12)**:1807–13; discussion 13–4.

111 Corelli R, Hudmon K. Pharmacologic interventions for smoking cessation. *Crit Care Nurs Clin N Am* 2006; **18**:39–51.

112 Fiore MC, Bailey WC, Cohen SJ *et al. Treating Tobacco Use and Dependence: Clinical Practice Guideline.* Rockville, MD: US Department of Health and Human Services, 2000.

113 West R, McNeill A, Raw M. Smoking cessation guidelines for health professionals: an update. *Thorax* 2000; **55**:987–99.

114 *Rx for Change: Clinician-Assisted Tobacco Cessation.* San Francisco, CA: University of California San Francisco, University of Southern California, and Western University of Health Sciences, 1999–2007.

115 Prokhorov AV, Hudmon KS, Stancic N. Adolescent smoking: epidemiology and approaches for achieving cessation. *Paediatr Drugs* 2003; **5(1)**:1–10.

116 Ascher JA, Cole JO, Colin J *et al.* Bupropion: a review of its mechanism of antidepressant activity. *J Clin Psychiatry* 1995; **56**:395–401.

117 Slemmer JE, Martin BR, Damaj MI. Bupropion is a nicotinic antagonist. *J Pharmacol Exp Ther* 2000; **295**:321–7.

118 GlaxoSmithKline Inc. *Zyban Package Insert.* Research Triangle Park, NC: GlaxoSmithKline Inc., 2006.

119 Dunner DL, Zisook S, Billow AA, Batey SR, Johnston JA, Ascher JA. A prospective safety surveillance study for bupropion sustained-release in the treatment of depression. *J Clin Psychiatry* 1998; **59**:366–73.

120 Foulds J. The neurobiological basis for partial agonist treatment of nicotine dependence: varenicline. *Int J Clin Pract* 2006; **60**:571–6.

121 Pfizer Inc. *Chantix Package Insert.* New York, NY: Pfizer Inc., 2006.

CHAPTER 2

Lung Cancer Susceptibility Genes

Joan E. Bailey-Wilson

Introduction

After heart disease, cancer is the most common cause of death and lung cancer is the most common cause of cancer death in the United States [1]. From 1950 to 1988, lung cancer experienced the largest increase in mortality rate of all the cancers and lung cancer caused an estimated 146,000 deaths in the United States in 1992 [2]. Lung cancer became the leading cause of cancer death in men in the early 1950s and in women in 1987.

Cancer of the lung has frequently been cited as an example of a malignancy that is solely determined by the environment [3,4] and the risks associated with cigarette smoking [3–7] and certain occupations, such as mining [8], asbestos exposure, shipbuilding, and petroleum refining [9–14], are well established. Most lung cancers are attributable to cigarette smoking (e.g. [15]). Dietary studies have found reduction in risk associated with high compared to low consumption of carotene-containing fruits and vegetables (for reviews see [16–19]). At least one recent, very large meta-analysis [20] has found significant protective effects of increased levels of dietary β-cryptoxanthin although recent trials of beta-carotene and vitamin A supplements have not shown any significant reduction in lung cancer risk; instead they showed an increased risk of lung cancer death in the treated group [21–24]. Environmental tobacco smoke (ETS, passive smoking) has also been shown to be associated with increased risk

of lung cancer (for review see [3,4,25–27]) with a recent prospective European study estimating that between 16 and 24% of lung cancers in nonsmokers and long-term ex-smokers were attributable to ETS [28]. A recent meta-analysis of 22 studies showed that exposure to workplace ETS increased risk of lung cancer in workers by 24% and that this risk was highly correlated with duration of exposure [29]. These environmental risk factors cannot be reviewed in detail here. There is little doubt that the majority of lung cancer cases are attributable to (i.e., would not occur in the absence of) cigarette smoking and other behavioral and environmental risk factors [2,7,25,30]. However, some investigators have long hypothesized that individuals differ in their susceptibility to these environmental insults (e.g. [31–34]). It is well known that mutations and loss of heterozygosity at genetic loci such as oncogenes and tumor suppressor genes are involved in lung carcinogenesis (see [35,36] for reviews) but most of these changes are thought to be accumulated at the somatic cell level. However, evidence has been mounting that certain allelic variants at some genetic loci may affect susceptibility to lung cancer, although these effects may be small. Furthermore, mounting epidemiologic evidence has suggested lung cancer may show familial aggregation after adjusting for cigarette smoking and other risk factors, and that differential susceptibility to lung cancer may be inherited in a Mendelian fashion. There is evidence that both lung cancer and smoking-associated cancer in general have an inherited genetic component, but the existence of such a genetic component has not been definitely proven. This chapter will detail the evidence

Lung Cancer, 3rd edition. Edited by Jack A. Roth, James D. Cox, and Waun Ki Hong. © 2008 Blackwell Publishing, ISBN: 978-1-4051-5112-2.

suggesting the existence of inherited major susceptibility loci for lung cancer risk, and will relate these risks to the well-known risks due to environmental risk factors, particularly personal cigarette smoking.

Inhalation of tobacco smoke

The association between cigarette smoking and lung cancer is strong and well established (e.g. [3,5,6,37–42]). The incidence of lung cancer is correlated with the cumulative amount and duration of cigarettes smoked in a dose–response relationship [7,38,43] and smoking cessation results in decreased risk of the disease, with the amount of decrease being related to time elapsed since the individual stopped smoking [7,44]. Lung cancer rates and smoking rates are also highly correlated in different geographic regions [45]. In 1991, Shopland *et al.* [46] showed that the relative risk of lung cancer for male smokers versus nonsmokers is 22.36 and that for female smokers versus female nonsmokers is 11.94. They also estimated that 90% of lung cancers in men and 78% in women were directly attributable to tobacco smoking. Kondo *et al.* [47] showed a significant ($p < 0.001$) dose–response relationship between number of cigarettes smoked and the frequency of p53 mutations in tumors of lung cancer patients, suggesting that somatic p53 mutations may be caused in some way by exposure to a carcinogen/mutagen in tobacco smoke or its metabolites. A review by Anberg and Samet [30] discusses this evidence of the role of cigarette smoking in lung cancer causation in more detail. None of the evidence given below for genetic susceptibility loci should be construed as suggesting that cigarette smoking is not the main cause of lung cancer.

Biologic risk factors

In general, all studies suggesting genetic susceptibility have also shown strong risk due to cigarette smoking and often have shown an interaction of high-risk genotype and smoking on lung cancer risk. When trying to determine whether a complex disease or trait such as lung cancer has a genetic susceptibility, one asks three major questions:

1 Does the disease (lung cancer) cluster in families? If some risk for lung cancer is inherited, then one would expect to see clustering of that trait in some families above what would be expected by chance.

2 If the aggregation of lung cancer does occur in some families, can the observation be explained by shared environmental/cultural risk factors? In this disease, one needs to assess whether the familial clustering of lung cancer is solely due to clustering of smoking behaviors or other environmental exposures within families.

3 If the excess clustering in families is not explained by measured environmental risk factors, is the pattern of disease consistent with Mendelian transmission of a major gene (i.e., of transmission through some families of a moderately high penetrance risk allele) and can this gene(s) be localized and identified in the human genome.

Evidence for familial aggregation of lung cancer

Tokuhata and Lilienfeld [48,49] provided epidemiologic evidence for familial aggregation of lung cancer over 40 years ago. After accounting for personal smoking, their results suggested the possible interaction of genes, shared environment, and common life-style factors in the etiology of lung cancer. In their study of 270 lung cancer patients and 270 age-, sex-, race-, and location-matched controls and their relatives, they found a relative risk of 2–2.5 for mortality due to lung cancer in cigarette-smoking relatives of cases as compared to smoking relatives of controls. Nonsmoking relatives of lung cancer cases were also at higher risk when compared to nonsmoking relatives of controls. Smoking was a more important risk factor for males but family history was the more important risk factor for females. They also noted a synergistic interaction between familial and smoking factors on the risk of lung cancer in relatives, with smoking relatives of lung cancer patients having much higher risk of lung cancer than either nonsmoking relatives of patients or smoking relatives of controls. They observed a substantial increase in mortality due to noncancerous respiratory diseases in relatives of patients as compared to relatives of controls, suggesting that the case relatives have a common susceptibility to respiratory diseases. However, they found no significant differences between the spouses of the lung cancer cases and controls for lung cancer mortality, mortality from noncancerous respiratory diseases, or smoking habits.

The major weakness of this study was that smoking status alone was used, as no measures of amount or duration of smoking in the relatives were available. Therefore, some of the familial aggregation could be due to familial correlation in smoking levels or age at starting smoking. However, nonsmoking relatives of cases were at higher risk than nonsmoking relatives of controls.

Since this time, many other studies have shown evidence of familial aggregation of lung cancer. In 1975, Fraumeni *et al.* [50] reported an increased risk of lung cancer mortality in siblings of lung cancer probands. In 1982, Goffman *et al.* [51] reported families with excess lung cancer of diverse histologic types. Lynch *et al.* [52] reported evidence for increased risk of cancer at all anatomic sites for relatives of lung cancer patients but no significant increased risk for lung cancer alone in these relatives. Leonard *et al.* [53] reported that survivors of familial retinoblastoma may also be at increased risk for small cell lung cancer.

In southern Louisiana, our retrospective case–control studies reported an increased familial risk for lung cancer [54] and nonlung cancers [55] among relatives of lung cancer probands after allowing for the effects of age, sex, occupation, and smoking. In these two studies, familial aggregation analyses were performed on a set of 337 lung cancer probands (cases), their spouse controls, and the parents, siblings, half-siblings, and offspring of both the probands and the controls. The probands were male and female Caucasians who died from lung cancer during the period 1976–1979 in a 10-parish (county) area of southern Louisiana, a region noted for its high lung cancer mortality rates. There were about 3.5 male probands to every female lung cancer proband in the dataset. A strong excess risk for lung cancer was detected among first-degree relatives of probands compared to relatives of spouse controls, after adjusting for age, sex, smoking status,

total duration of smoking, cigarette pack-years, and a cumulative index of occupational/industrial exposures. Parents of probands had a fourfold risk of having developed lung cancer as opposed to parents of spouses, after adjusting for the effects of age, sex, smoking, and occupational exposures. Females over 40 years old who were relatives of probands were at nine times higher risk than similar female relatives of spouses, even among nonsmokers who had not reported excessive exposure to hazardous occupations. Among female heavy smokers who were relatives of probands, the risk was increased four- to sixfold. Overall, male relatives of probands had a greater risk of lung cancer than their female counterparts. After controlling for the confounding effects of the measured environmental risk factors, relationship to a proband remained a significant determinant of lung cancer, with a 2.4 odds in favor of relatives of probands.

These same families were reanalyzed [55] to determine if nonlung cancers exhibited similar familial aggregation. When analyzing the number of cancers at any site that occurred in a family, proband families were found to be 1.67 times more likely than spouse families to have one family member (other than the proband) with cancer, and 2.16 times more likely to have two family members with cancer. For three cancers and four or more cancers, the relative risk increased to 3.66 and 5.04, respectively. Each risk estimate was significant at the 0.01 level. The most striking differences in cancer prevalence between proband and control families were noted for cancer of the nasal cavity/sinus, mid-ear, and larynx (odds ratio, OR = 4.6); trachea, bronchus and lung (OR = 3.0); skin (OR = 2.8); and uterus, placenta, ovary, and other female organs (OR = 2.1). After controlling for age, sex, cigarette smoking, and occupational/industrial exposures, relatives of lung cancer probands maintained an increased risk of nonlung cancer ($p < 0.05$) when compared to relatives of spouse controls.

A family case–control study, drawn from a population-based registry in Saskatchewan, Canada, was reported by McDuffie [56]. A total of 359 cases and 234 age- and gender-matched community controls were included in the study. Most families reported at least one member with a history of neoplastic disease exclusive of the proband (62% of patients' families and 57% of control families). However, the families of the lung cancer cases were more likely (30%) to have two or more family members affected with any cancer than the families of the controls. The case families were also significantly more likely to have two or more relatives with lung cancer than were the control families. In addition, a higher percentage of all primary tumors were lung tumors (16.5%) in patients' relatives as compared to controls' relatives (10%). The progression of increased risks for observing 1, 2, 3, and 4+ affected relatives in case families versus control families was slightly smaller than in the Sellers *et al.* study [55] but showed the same type of progression.

Family history data from an incident case–control study in Texas were analyzed for evidence of familial aggregation by Shaw *et al.* [57]. A total of 943 histologically confirmed lung cancer cases and 955 age-, gender-, vital-status-, and ethnicity-matched controls were interviewed regarding smoking, alcohol use, cancer in first-degree relatives, medical history, and demographic characteristics. After adjusting for personal smoking status, passive smoking exposure (ever/never), and gender, participants with at least one first-degree relative with lung cancer had a lung cancer risk of 1.8 compared to those with no relatives with lung cancer. Lung cancer risk increased as the number of relatives with cancer increased and was highest when only relatives with lung cancer were considered (odds ratios of 1.7 and 2.8 for one and two or more relatives with lung cancer, respectively). Lung cancer was diagnosed at a significantly younger age among cases who had first-degree relatives with lung cancer than among those who had no relatives with lung cancer. However, no such age difference was seen between cases who had first-degree relatives with any cancer versus those who had no relatives with cancer. This study also examined histologic subtypes of lung cancer cases and found that for each histologic type, there were significant risks associated with having any relatives with lung cancer, with odds ratios of 2.1 for adenocarcinoma, 1.9 for squamous cell carcinoma, and 1.7 for small cell lung cancer. Finally, in this study, only current and former smokers had an increased

lung cancer risk associated with lung cancer in relatives.

Cannon-Albright *et al.* [58] examined the degree of relatedness of all pairs of lung cancer patients in the Utah Population Database. By comparing this to the degree of relatedness in sets of matched controls, they showed that lung cancer exhibited excess familiality, and three of four histological tumor types still showed excess familiality when considered separately. In the same population, but using different methodology, Goldgar *et al.* [59] studied lung cancer probands and controls who had died in Utah and their first-degree relatives. They found that 2.55 times more lung cancers occurred in first-degree relatives of lung cancer probands than expected based on rates in control relatives. When they stratified by gender, they observed higher relative risks for female relatives of female probands (FRR = 4.02) versus male relatives of male probands (FRR = 2.5). No adjustment was made in these analyses for personal smoking or other environmental risk factors, so these results may simply reflect the familiality of smoking behaviors. However, this is a largely nonsmoking population and Utah has the lowest smoking rates of any state in the United States.

The number of lung cancers observed in some twin studies have been too small to draw conclusions regarding familiality of lung cancer [60] although possible aggregation of bronchoalveolar carcinoma has been suggested in twin and family studies [61,62]. However, this effect may be due to aggregation of cigarette smoking as risk of this cancer is linked to tobacco consumption [63]. In 1995, a study using a large twin registry, the National Academy of Sciences—National Research Council Twin Registry, Braun *et al.* [64] reported that the observed concordance rates of monozygotic (MZ) twins for death from lung cancer compared to that of dizygotic (DZ) twins was 1.1 (95% confidence interval, 0.6–1.9) although this did not adjust for smoking behaviors in the twins. These results suggest that, as expected, on a population level, smoking behavior is probably a much stronger risk factor than inherited genetic susceptibility.

Studies of familial risk of lung cancer in nonsmokers [65–67] have also shown increased risk of lung cancer associated with a family history of lung cancer. The study by Schwartz *et al.* [65] found increased risk of lung cancer among relatives of younger, nonsmoking lung cancer cases as compared with relatives of younger controls after adjusting for smoking, occupational and medical histories of each family member, suggesting increased susceptibility to lung cancer among relatives of early-onset nonsmoking lung cancer patients. Wu *et al.* [66] found an increased risk of lung cancer in persons with a history of lung or aerodigestive tract cancer in first-degree relatives after adjustment for ETS exposure, which was significant for affected mothers and sisters. Mayne *et al.* [67], in a population-based study of nonsmokers (45% never smokers and 55% former smokers who had quit at least 10 years prior to diagnosis or interview; 437 lung cancer cases and 437 matched population controls) in New York State, found that after adjusting for age and smoking status (yes, no) in the relatives, a positive history in first-degree relatives of any cancer or lung cancer or aerodigestive tract cancer or breast cancer were each associated with significantly increased risk of lung cancer.

In 2000, Bromen *et al.* [68], in a population-based case–control study in Germany, showed that lung cancer in parents or siblings was significantly associated with an increased risk of lung cancer and that this risk was much stronger in younger participants. In 2003, Etzel *et al.* [69] evaluated whether first-degree relatives of lung cancer cases were at increased risk for lung cancer and for other smoking-related cancers (bladder, head and neck, kidney, and pancreas). They studied 806 hospital-based lung cancer patients and 663 controls matched on age, sex, ethnicity, and smoking history, all from the Houston, Texas, area. After adjustment for smoking history of patients and their relatives, there was significant evidence for familial aggregation of lung cancer and of smoking-related cancers. However, they did not find increased aggregation in the families of young onset (less than or equal to age 55) lung cancer cases or in families of never-smokers.

Two studies in China [70,71] found, after adjusting for age, sex, birth order, residence, family size, chronic obstructive pulmonary disease (COPD), smoking and cumulative index of smoky coal exposure or occupational/industrial exposure index,

that first-degree relatives of lung cancer patients were at significantly increased risk for lung cancer compared to the same relatives of controls. They also observed that families of the lung cancer patients were significantly more likely to have three or more affected relatives than were control families.

A series of studies using the Swedish Family-Cancer Database [72–75], which totals over 10.2 million individuals, found that a high proportion of lung cancers diagnosed before the age of 50 appear to be heritable, and that lung cancer patients with a family history of lung cancer were at a significantly increased risk of subsequent primary lung cancers.

In the United Kingdom, a case–control study of lung cancer prevalence in first-degree relatives of 1482 female lung cancer cases and 1079 female controls [76] was performed, adjusting for age and tobacco exposure (pack-years) in the cases and controls. They found that lung cancer in any first-degree relative was associated with a significant increase in lung cancer risk, and that the increase in risk was stronger in relatives of cases with onset less than 60 years or cases with three or more affected relatives. However, this study was not able to adjust for personal smoking in the relatives since these data were not available.

A study of white and black relatives of early-onset lung cancer cases and of 773 frequency-matched controls in Detroit, Michigan [77], showed that smokers with a family history of early-onset lung cancer had a higher risk of lung cancer with increasing age than smokers without a family history, and that relatives of black cases were at higher risk than relatives of white cases, after adjusting for age, sex, pack-years of cigarette smoking, pneumonia, and COPD.

A recent study [78] utilizing the Icelandic Cancer Registry calculated risk ratios of lung cancer in first-, second-, and third-degree relatives of 2756 lung cancer patients diagnosed between 1955 and 2002. Relative risks were significantly elevated for all three classes of relatives, and this increased risk was stronger in relatives of early-onset lung cancer patients (age at onset less than or equal to 60 years). The effect did not appear to be solely due to the effects of smoking in all relative types, except for cousins and spouses.

A review in 2005 by Matakidou *et al.* [79] of 28 case–control, 17 cohort and 7 twin studies of the relationship between family history and risk of lung cancer and a meta-analysis of risk estimates, concluded that the case–control and cohort studies consistently show an increased risk of lung cancer given a family history of lung cancer, and that risk appears to be increased given a history of early-onset lung cancer or of multiple affected relatives. However, the results of the twin studies and the observed increased risk of disease in spouses highlighted the importance of environmental risk factors, such as smoking, in this disease.

Segregation analyses of lung- and smoking-associated cancers

Given the evidence for familial aggregation of lung and other smoking-associated cancers, after accounting for personal tobacco use and occupational/industrial risk factors, segregation analyses have been performed to determine whether patterns of transmission consistent with at least one major, high-penetrance genetic locus may be involved in lung cancer risk.

Sellers *et al.* [80] performed genetic segregation analyses on the lung cancer proband families of Ooi *et al.* [54] described above. The trait was expressed as a dichotomy, affected or unaffected with lung cancer. The analyses used the general transmission probability model [81], which allows for variable age of onset of the lung cancer [82–84]. The likelihood of the models was calculated using a correction factor appropriate for single ascertainment [85,86], i.e., conditioning the likelihood of each pedigree on the probands being affected by their ages at examination or death.

Age of onset of lung cancer was assumed to follow a logistic distribution that depended on pack-years of cigarette consumption and its square, an age coefficient and a baseline parameter. Results indicated compatibility of the data with Mendelian codominant inheritance of a rare major autosomal gene that produces earlier age of onset of the cancer. Segregation at this putative locus could account for 69 and 47% of the cumulative incidence of lung cancer in individuals up to ages 50 and 60, respectively. The gene was predicted to be involved in only

22% of all lung cancers in persons up to age 70, a reflection of an increasing proportion of noncarriers succumbing to the effects of long-term exposure to tobacco [80,87].

Additional segregation analysis of these families was performed to determine whether evidence exists for a major gene that increases susceptibility to a group of smoking-associated cancers rather than just lung cancer alone. The trait was defined as unaffected or affected with cancer at any of the following sites: lung, lip, oral cavity, esophagus, nasopharynx, trachea, bronchus, larynx, cervix, bladder, kidney, colon/rectum, and pancreas. The results were compatible with segregation of a major gene that influences age-of-onset of cancer. The hypotheses of Mendelian dominant, codominant, and recessive inheritance could not be rejected but, according to Akaike's Information Criterion [88], Mendelian codominant inheritance provided the best fit to the data [89]. Additional analyses suggest that better fit of Mendelian inheritance of an allele that acts with smoking to influence the risk of cancer is obtained if a somewhat different cluster of smoking-associated cancers is considered "affected": lung, oral cavity, esophagus, nasopharynx, larynx, pancreas, bladder, kidney, and uterine cervix [90].

Segregation analyses of these data ([91] and our unpublished results) using Class A regressive models showed significant evidence for a polygenic/multifactorial component in addition to the major gene component described above. Inclusion of this polygenic/multifactorial component significantly improved the fit of the model to the data without changing the basic conclusions of the previous analyses, i.e., that evidence exists for a major locus with a codominant susceptibility allele that acts in conjunction with smoking, and that all models excluding such a major gene effect were rejected. Gauderman *et al.* [92] reanalyzed these same data using a Gibbs sampler method to examine gene by environment interactions and found evidence for a major dominant susceptibility locus that acts in conjunction with cigarette smoking to increase risk; this model was very similar to the previous results since the codominant Mendelian models predicted very small numbers of homozygous susceptibility allele carriers.

Yang and her coworkers performed complex segregation analysis on the families of nonsmoking lung cancer probands in metropolitan Detroit [93]. Evidence was found for Mendelian codominant inheritance with modifying effects of smoking and chronic bronchitis in families of nonsmoking cases diagnosed at ages 40–59. The estimated risk allele frequency was 0.004. While homozygous individuals with the risk allele are rare in the study population, penetrance was very high for early-onset lung cancer (85% in males and 74% in females by age 60). The probability of developing lung cancer by age 60 in individuals heterozygous for the rare allele was low in the absence of smoking and chronic bronchitis (7% in males and 4% in females) but in the presence of these risk factors it increased to 85% in males and 74% in females, which was the same level predicted for homozygotes. The attributable risk associated with the high-risk allele declines with age, when the role of tobacco smoking and chronic bronchitis become more important.

Wu *et al.* [94] performed complex segregation analysis of families of 125 female, nonsmoking lung cancer probands in Taiwan. These lung cancer probands were diagnosed with lung cancer between 1992 and 2002 at two hospitals in Taiwan. Complete data on patients, spouses and first-degree relatives were collected for 108 families. Data collected on the patients and their relatives included demographic, life-style, and medical history variables. Complex segregation analysis using logistic models for age at onset, including pack-years of cigarette smoking in the model was performed on 58 of these families. An ascertainment correction was made using the phenotype of the probands, but this may have been inadequate since the 58 families were a subset of the 108 families where there was at least one additional affected relative in the family. The Mendelian codominant model that included risk due to personal smoking fit the data best, significantly better than the sporadic or purely environmental models. This model was not rejected against the general model in an early-onset (less than 60 years) subset of the families but was rejected in the later-onset families and the total dataset.

Taken together, the Taiwan, Detroit, and Louisiana studies share remarkably similar results and demonstrate statistical evidence for at least one major gene that acts in conjunction with personal smoking and possibly chronic bronchitis to increase risk of lung cancer.

Weaknesses of familial aggregation and segregation analyses

While most of these studies included measures of personal smoking on the cases (or probands) and controls in the models, some of the aggregation studies did not include measures of amount of cigarette smoking in the relatives and only one included measures of passive smoking. The segregation analyses did not include passive smoking or occupational risk factors in the models, and only one of these three studies collected data on history of chronic bronchitis. Furthermore, segregation analyses are not sufficient to prove the existence of a major locus because only a subset of all possible models can be tested. These segregation analyses did not, for example, model the large number of possible oligogenic cases where two or three major loci act in conjunction with smoking to affect risk of lung cancer.

Oncogenes and tumor suppressor genes

In addition to epidemiological evidence, experimental evidence of the role of genes in lung cancer causation has been accumulating. First, it seems probable that genetic changes are responsible for the pathogenesis of most, if not all, human malignancies [95]. In particular, lung carcinogenesis is the result of a series of genetic mutations that accumulate progressively in the bronchial epithelium, first generating histologically identifiable premalignant lesions and finally resulting in an invasive carcinoma. The premalignant genetic changes may occur many years before the appearance of invasive carcinoma.

Cytogenetic and molecular studies have shown that mutations in protooncogenes and tumor suppressor genes (TSGs) are critical in the multistep development and progression of lung tumors. Allele loss analyses have implicated the presence of other tumor suppressor genes involved in lung tumorigenesis. These studies revealed frequent occurrences of chromosomal deletions including regions of 3p,

5q, 8p, 9p, 9q, 11p, 11q, and 17q. These studies are outside the scope of this chapter (see e.g. [96–98] for reviews).

Linkage analysis of lung cancer

Linkage analysis is a statistical analysis of pedigree data that looks for evidence of cosegregation through the generations in human pedigrees of alleles at a genetic "susceptibility" locus and some known genetic "marker" locus (usually a DNA polymorphism). Linkage analysis is a very powerful method for detecting genetic loci that are highly penetrant (after adjusting for environmental risk factors). However, power decreases as the susceptibility allele becomes more common and less penetrant. Since cigarette smoking is an extremely strong risk factor for lung cancer (e.g., 4), it is important that one looks for a major gene after controlling for at least personal smoking, as this will increase the power to detect linkage.

Bailey-Wilson *et al.* [99] published the first evidence of linkage of a putative lung cancer susceptibility locus to a region of chromosome 6q. Data were collected at eight recruitment sites of the Genetic Epidemiology of Lung Cancer Consortium (GELCC): the University of Cincinnati, University of Colorado, Johns Hopkins School of Public Health, Karmanos Cancer Institute, Saccomanno Research Institute, Louisiana State University Health Sciences Center, Mayo Clinic, and Medical College of Ohio. Of the 26,108 lung cancer cases screened at GELCC sites for this study, 13.7% had at least one first-degree relative with lung cancer. Following the initial family history screening process, we collected additional information from the 3541 families with at least one first-degree relative with lung cancer. We interviewed probands and/or their family representatives to collect data regarding additional persons affected with any cancers in the extended family, vital status of affected individuals, availability of archival tissue, and willingness of family members to participate in the study. Further pedigree development and biospecimen collection (blood, buccal cells, or fixed tissue) were performed on 771 families with three or more first-degree relatives affected

with lung cancer. Cancers were verified by medical records, pathology reports, cancer registry records, or death certificates for 69% of individuals affected with either lung or throat cancer (LT), and by reports of multiple family members for the other 31% of family members affected with LT. Of these families, only 52 had enough biospecimens available to make them informative for linkage analyses. DNA isolated from blood was genotyped at the Center for Inherited Disease Research (CIDR, a National Institutes of Health-supported core research facility), and DNA from buccal cells and archival tissue and sputum were genotyped at the University of Cincinnati, for a panel of 392 microsatellite (short tandem repeat polymorphism, STRP) marker loci. The data were checked for errors and then analyzed using parametric and nonparametric linkage methods. Marker allele frequencies were calculated separately and linkage analyses were performed separately for the white American and African American families, with the results combined in overall tests of linkage.

Our primary analytical approach assumed a model with 10% penetrance in carriers and 1% penetrance in the noncarriers. This analytical approach weights information only from the affected subjects. For this analysis we used FASTLINK for two-point analysis and SIMWALK2 for multipoint analysis. We chose this linkage model as our primary analytical approach because of uncertainty about the strength of relationship between smoking behavior and lung cancer risk in the high-risk families we are studying, and because the complex "gene + environment" models from the published segregation analyses were not currently available in any multipoint linkage analysis program. In addition, since about 90% of the affected family members in our studies smoked, weighting only the affected individuals in our simple dominant, low penetrance model has the effect of jointly allowing for smoking status, while ignoring information from unaffected subjects. We allowed for genetic heterogeneity (different families having different genetic causation) in the analysis. Secondary analyses used more complex models that included age and pack-years of cigarette smoking to modify the penetrances. Our standard for this analysis was LODLINK, which uses the genetic regressive model, obtained from segregation analyses by

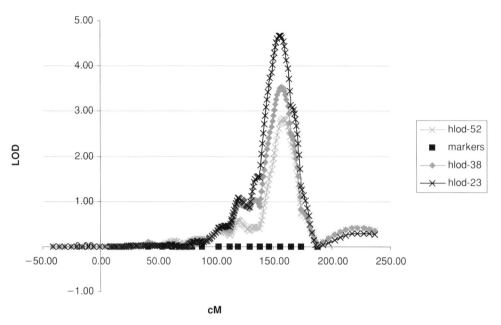

Figure 2.1 Plot of chromosome 6 parametric multipoint HLOD scores (lung cancer affected only analysis) from SIMWALK2 in all 52 families, in the 38 families with 4 or more affected individuals, and in the 23 multigenerational families with 5 or more affected individuals.

Sellers *et al.* [80] and Bailey-Wilson *et al.* [91]. The current implementation of LODLINK only permitted two-point analysis when a covariate is included and it is well known that two-point linkage is less powerful in general than multipoint linkage analysis. Nonparametric analyses were also performed as secondary analyses with variance components models using SOLAR (binary trait option) and mixed effects Cox regression models, in which time to onset of disease is modeled as a quantitative trait.

Multipoint parametric linkage under the simple dominant low-penetrance affected-only model (Figure 2.1) yielded a maximum heterogeneity LOD score (HLOD) of 2.79 at 155 cM (marker D6S2436) on chromosome 6q23–25 in the 52 families, with 67% of families estimated to be linked. Multipoint analysis of a subset of 38 families with four affected relatives gave an HLOD of 3.47 at this same location, with 78% of families estimated to be linked, whereas for the 23 highest risk families (five or more affected in two or more generations), the multipoint HLOD score was 4.26, with 94% of these families

estimated to be linked to this region. Our nonparametric analyses and the two-point parametric analyses that used the Sellers *et al.* model [80,91] all provided additional support for linkage to this region.

Additional families are now being collected by the GELCC to attempt to confirm this linkage result in an independent sample and to narrow the critical region that may contain a susceptibility gene. In addition, several other regions showed suggestive evidence of linkage and these are being pursued.

Association of common alleles of small effect (polymorphisms) with lung cancer risk

Results of hundreds of studies using association analysis to evaluate the effects of various polymorphisms, in metabolic genes, growth factors, growth factor receptors, markers of DNA damage and repair and genomic instability, and in oncogenes and tumor suppressor loci have been published. Many of these studies have yielded inconsistent results. The effects of risk alleles at these loci are expected to be individually small, and they may interact with smoking and/or other loci to increase lung cancer risk. These association studies are beyond the scope of this chapter. Two recent reviews [100,101] can help the reader obtain an overview of these studies.

Discussion

All these lines of evidence suggest that there may be one or several genes causing inherited increased risk to lung cancer in the general population. While association studies have given evidence that alleles at various genetic loci may influence lung cancer risk, there has frequently been disagreement between studies. The first linkage study of lung cancer has given significant evidence of linkage to a region on chromosome 6q. If a susceptibility locus is identified in this region, it will be of major public health importance as it will allow identification of individuals at especially high risk who can then be targeted for intensive efforts at environmental risk reduction. In addition, identification of such a gene will lead to better understanding of the mechanism of carcinogenesis in general, perhaps eventually leading to better methods of prevention and treatment.

Confirmation of a genetic predisposition for lung cancer can be obtained by finding evidence for linkage of the putative susceptibility gene(s) to genetic marker loci in a specific chromosomal region(s). One potential problem in the search for such a linkage is heterogeneity. There are different types of heterogeneity of this disease and of its etiological factors: (1) there is heterogeneity at the level of histological types of lung cancer, (2) there is heterogeneity at the level of exposure to a variety of environmental risk factors, and (3) there could be heterogeneity at the level of inherited susceptibility loci, i.e., there could be one locus involved in susceptibility for one family and a different locus involved in susceptibility for another family. All of these types of heterogeneity could possibly confound the identification of a susceptibility locus (or loci) for lung cancer. The suggestive evidence in the published linkage study [99] for susceptibility loci

at several other regions of the genome supports the possibility of locus heterogeneity in lung cancer.

If, through linkage and positional cloning techniques, a genetic locus or loci that contributes to inheritable risk for lung cancer can be identified, or one of the candidate loci suggested to modify risk by association studies can be confirmed as a susceptibility locus, then the effects of the alleles at this locus and its interaction with cigarette smoking and the other well-known environmental risk factors for lung cancer can be elucidated with much more accuracy than presently possible and our understanding of lung carcinogenesis in general may be increased.

Acknowledgments

This work was supported by the intramural program of the National Human Genome Research Institute, NIH.

References

1 Ries LAG, Harkins D, Krapcho M *et al.* (eds). *SEER Cancer Statistics Review, 1975–2003*. Bethesda, MD: National Cancer Institute. http://seer.cancer.gov/csr/1975_2003/, based on November 2005 SEER data submission, posted to the SEER web site, 2006.
2 Beckett WS. Epidemiology and etiology of lung cancer. *Clin Chest Med* 1993; **14**:1–15.
3 Doll R, Peto R. *The Causes of Cancer: Quantitative Estimates of Avoidable Risks of Cancer in the United States Today*. New York: Oxford University Press, 1981.
4 Doll R, Peto R. *The Causes of Cancer*. Oxford: Oxford University Press, 1981.
5 Burch PR. Smoking and lung cancer. Tests of a causal hypothesis. *J Chron Dis* 1980; **33**:221–38.
6 Carbone D. Smoking and cancer. *Am J Med* 1992; **93(1A)**:13S–17S.
7 Doll R, Peto R, Wheatley K, Gray R, Sutherland I. Mortality in relation to smoking: 40 years' observations on male British doctors. *BMJ* 1994; **309**:901–11.
8 Seaton A. Occupational pulmonary neoplasms. In: *Occupational Lung Disease*. Philadelphia: Saunders, 1975.
9 Seaton A. Occupational pulmonary neoplasms. In: Morgan WKC, Seaton A (eds). *Occupational Lung Diseases*, 2nd edn. Philadelphia: Saunders, 1984:657–75.

10 Blot WJ, Fraumeni JF. Geographic patterns of lung cancer: industrial correlations. *Am J Epidemiol* 1976; **103**:539–50.

11 Blot WJ, Harrington JM, Toledo A *et al.* Lung cancer after employment in shipyards during World War II. *N Engl J Med* 1979; **229**:620–4.

12 Gottlieb MS, Steadman R. Lung cancer in Shipbuilding and related industries in Louisiana. *South Med J* 1979; **72**:1099–101.

13 Whitesell PL, Drage CW. Occupational lung cancer. *Mayo Clin Proc* 1993; **68**:183–8.

14 Cullen MR, Barnett MJ, Balmes JR *et al.* Predictors of lung cancer among asbestos-exposed men in the {beta}-carotene and retinol efficacy trial. *Am J Epidemiol* 2005; **161(3)**:260–70.

15 Mattson ME, Pollack ES, Cullen JW. What are the odds that smoking will kill you? *Am J Public Health* 1987; **77**:425–31.

16 Fontham ETH. Protective dietary factors and lung cancer. *Int J Epidemiol* 1990; **19**:S32–42.

17 Donaldson MS. Nutrition and cancer: a review of the evidence for an anti-cancer diet. *Nutr J* Oct 20, 2004; **3**:19.

18 Gonzalez CA. Nutrition and cancer: the current epidemiological evidence. *Br J Nutr* 2006; **96(Suppl 1)**: S42–5.

19 Divisi D, Di Tommaso S, Salvemini S, Garramone M, Crisci R. Diet and cancer. *Acta Biomed* Aug 2006; **77(2)**:118–23.

20 Mannisto S, Smith-Warner SA, Spiegelman D *et al.* Dietary carotenoids and risk of lung cancer in a pooled analysis of seven cohort studies. *Cancer Epidemiol Biomarkers Prev* 2004; **13**:40–8.

21 Omenn GS, Goodman G, Thornquist M *et al.* The beta-carotene and retinol efficacy trial (CARET) for chemoprevention of lung cancer in high risk populations: smokers and asbestos-exposed workers. *Cancer Res* 1994; **54**:2038s–43s.

22 Marwick C. Trials reveal no benefit, possible harm of beta carotene and vitamin A for lung cancer prevention [News]. *JAMA* 1996; **275**:422.

23 Smigel K. Beta carotene fails to prevent cancer in two major studies; CARET intervention stopped [News]. *J Natl Cancer Inst* 1996; **88**:145.

24 Goodman GE, Thornquist MD, Balmes J *et al.* The Beta-Carotene and Retinol Efficacy Trial: incidence of lung cancer and cardiovascular disease mortality during 6-year follow-up after stopping beta-carotene and retinol supplements. *J Natl Cancer Inst* 2004; **96(23)**:1743–50.

25 Davila DG, Williams DE. The etiology of lung cancer. *Mayo Clin Proc* 1993; **68**:170–82.

26 Fontham ETH, Correa P, Chen VW. Passive smoking and lung cancer. *J La State Med Soc* 1993; **145**:133–6.

27 Subramanian J, Govindan R. Lung cancer in never smokers: a review. *J Clin Oncol* 2007; **25(5)**:561–70.

28 Vineis P, Hoek G, Krzyzanowski M *et al.* Lung cancers attributable to environmental tobacco smoke and air pollution in non-smokers in different European countries: a prospective study. *Environ Health* 2007; **6**:7.

29 Stayner L, Bena J, Sasco AJ *et al.* Lung cancer risk and workplace exposure to environmental tobacco smoke. *Am J Public Health* 2007; **97(3)**:545–51.

30 Anberg A, Samet J. Epidemiology of lung cancer. In: Kane M, Kelly K, Miller Y, Bunn P (eds). *The Biology of Lung Cancer. Volume 122 of the Lung Biology in Health and Disease Series*. New York: Marcel Dekker, 1998.

31 Parnell RW. Smoking and cancer [Letter]. *Lancet* 1951; **1**:963.

32 Heath CW: Differences between smokers and non-smokers. *Arch Intern Med* 1958; **101**:377–88.

33 Friberg L. Smoking habits of monozygotic and dizygotic twins. *Br Med J* 1959; **1**:1090–2.

34 Motulsky AG. Drug reactions, enzymes, and biochemical genetics. *JAMA* 1957; **165**:835–7.

35 Niklinski J, Niklinska W, Chyczewski L, Becker HD, Pluygers E. Molecular genetic abnormalities in premalignant lung lesions: biological and clinical implications. *Eur J Cancer Prev* 2001; **10(3)**:213–26.

36 Panani AD, Roussos C. Cytogenetic and molecular aspects of lung cancer. *Cancer Lett* 2006; **239(1)**:1–9.

37 Hammond EC. Smoking in relation to the death rates of one million men and women. *Natl Cancer Inst Monogr* 1966; **19**:127–204.

38 Doll R, Peto R. Cigarette smoking and bronchial carcinoma: dose and time relationships among regular smokers and lifelong non-smokers. *J Epidemiol Community Health* 1978; **32**:303–13.

39 Garfinkel L. Selection, follow-up, and analysis in the American Cancer Society prospective studies. *Natl Cancer Inst Monogr* 1985; **67**:49–52.

40 Department of Health and Human Services, Public Health Service. *Health Consequences of Smoking, Cancer: A Report of the Surgeon General*. Washington, DC: US Government Printing Office, 1972.

41 Department of Health and Human Services, Public Health Service. *Reducing the Health Consequences of Smoking: 25 Years of Progress; A Report of the Surgeon General*. Washington, DC: US Government Printing Office, 1989 (Publication No. CDC 89-8411).

42 International Agency for Research on Cancer. Tobacco smoking. *IARC Monogr Eval Carcinog Risks Hum* 1986; **38**:15–395.

43 Damber LA, Larsson L-G. Smoking and lung cancer with special regard to type of smoking and type of cancer: a case–control study in north Sweden. *Br J Cancer* 1986; **53**:673–81.

44 Centers for Disease Control, Office on Smoking and Health. *Health Benefits of Smoking Cessation: A Report of the Surgeon General, 1990.* Washington, DC: US Government Printing Office, 1990 (Publication No. 90-8416).

45 Silverberg E. Cancer statstics, 1980. *CA Cancer J Clin* 1980; **30**:23–38.

46 Shopland DR, Eyre HJ, Pechacek TF. Smoking-attributable cancer mortality in 1991: is lung cancer now the leading cause of death among smokers in the United States? *J Natl Cancer Inst* 1991; **83**:1142–8.

47 Kondo K, Tsuzuki H, Sasa M, Sumitomo M, Uyama T, Monden Y. A dose–response relationship between the frequency of p53 mutations and tobacco consumption in lung cancer patients. *J Surg Oncol* 1996; **61**:20–6.

48 Tokuhata GK, Lilienfeld AM. Familial aggregation of lung cancer in humans. *J Natl Cancer Inst* 1963; **30**:289–312.

49 Tokuhata GK, Lilienfeld AM. Familial aggregation of lung cancer among hospital patients. *Public Health Rep* 1963; **78**:277–83.

50 Fraumeni JF, Wertelecki W, Blattner WA *et al.* Varied manifestations of a familial lymphoproliferative disorder. *Am J Med* 1975; **59**:145–51.

51 Goffman TE, Hassinger DD, Mulvihill JJ. Familial respiratory tract cancer, opportunities for research and prevention. *JAMA* 1982; **247**:1020–3.

52 Lynch HT, Kimberling WJ, Markvicka SE *et al.* Genetics and smoking-associated cancers. A study of 485 families. *Cancer* 1986; **57**:1640–6.

53 Leonard RCF, Mackay T, Brown A, Gregory A, Crompton GK, Smyth JF. Small-cell lung cancer after retinoblastoma. *Lancet* 1988; **II**:1503.

54 Ooi WL, Elston RC, Chen VW, Bailey-Wilson JE, Rothschild H. Increased familial risk for lung cancer. *J Natl Cancer Inst* 1986; **76**:217–22.

55 Sellers TA, Ooi WL, Elston RC *et al.* Increased familial risk for non-lung cancer among relatives of lung cancer patients. *Am J Epidemiol* 1987; **126**:237–46.

56 McDuffie HH. Clustering of cancer in families with primary lung cancer. *J Clin Epidemiol* 1991; **44**:69–76.

57 Shaw GL, Falk RT, Pickle LW, Mason TJ, Buffler PA. Lung cancer risk associated with cancer in relatives. *J Clin Epidemiol* 1991; **44**:429–37.

58 Cannon-Albright LA, Thomas A, Goldgar DE *et al.* Familiality of cancer in Utah. *Cancer Res* 1994; **54**:2378–85.

59 Goldgar DE, Easton DF, Cannon-Albright LA, Skolnick MH. Systematic population-based assessment of cancer risk in first-degree relatives of cancer probands. *J Natl Cancer Inst* 1994; **86(21)**:1600–8.

60 Hrubec A, Neel JV. Contribution of familial factors to the occurrence of cancer before old age in twin veterans. *Am J Hum Genet* 1982; **34**:658–71.

61 Joishy SK, Cooper RA, Rowley PT. Alveolar cell carcinoma in identical twins: similarity in time of onset, histochemistry, and site of metastasis. *Ann Intern Med* 1977; **87**:447–50.

62 Paul SM, Bacharach B, Goepp C. A genetic influence on alveolar cell carcinoma. *J Surg Oncol* 1987; **36**:249–52.

63 Falk RT, Pickle LW, Fontham ETH *et al.* Epidemiology of bronchioloalveolar carcinoma. *Cancer Epidemiol Biomarkers Prev* 1992; **1**:339–44.

64 Braun MM, Caporaso NE, Page WF, Hoover RN. A cohort study of twins and cancer. *Cancer Epidemiol Biomarkers Prev* 1995; **4**:469–73.

65 Schwartz AG, Yang P, Swanson GM. Familial risk of lung cancer among nonsmokers and their relatives. *Am J Epidemiol* 1996; **114**:554–62.

66 Wu AH, Fontham ET, Reynolds P *et al.* Family history of cancer and risk of lung cancer among lifetime nonsmoking women in the United States. *Am J Epidemiol* 1996; **143**:535–42.

67 Mayne ST, Buenconsejo J, Janerich DT. Familial cancer history and lung cancer risk in United States nonsmoking men and women. *Cancer Epidemiol Biomarkers Prev* 1999; **8(12)**:1065–9.

68 Bromen K, Pohlabeln H, Jahn I, Ahrens W, Jockel KH. Aggregation of lung cancer in families: results from a population-based case–control study in Germany. *Am J Epidemiol* 2000; **152(6)**:497–505.

69 Etzel CJ, Amos CI, Spitz MR. Risk for smoking-related cancer among relatives of lung cancer patients. *Cancer Res* 2003; **63(23)**:8531–5.

70 Jin Y, Xu Y, Xu M, Xue S. Increased risk of cancer among relatives of patients with lung cancer in China. *BMC Cancer* 2005; **5**:146.

71 Jin YT, Xu YC, Yang RD, Huang CF, Xu CW, He XZ. Familial aggregation of lung cancer in a high incidence area in China. *Br J Cancer* 2005; **92(7)**:1321–5.

72 Li X, Hemminki K. Familial and second lung cancers: a nation-wide epidemiologic study from Sweden. *Lung Cancer* 2003; **39(3)**:255–63.

73 Li X, Hemminki K. Inherited predisposition to early onset lung cancer according to histological type. *Int J Cancer* 2004; **112(3)**:451–7.

74 Li X, Hemminki K. Familial multiple primary lung cancers: a population-based analysis from Sweden. *Lung Cancer* 2005; **47(3)**:301–7.

75 Hemminki K, Li X. Familial risk for lung cancer by histology and age of onset: evidence for recessive inheritance. *Exp Lung Res* 2005; **31(2)**:205–15.

76 Matakidou A, Eisen T, Bridle H, O'Brien M, Mutch R, Houlston RS. Case–control study of familial lung cancer risks in UK women. *Int J Cancer* 2005; **116(3)**:445–50.

77 Cote ML, Kardia SL, Wenzlaff AS, Ruckdeschel JC, Schwartz AG. Risk of lung cancer among white and black relatives of individuals with early-onset lung cancer. *JAMA* 2005; **293(24)**:3036–42.

78 Jonsson S, Thorsteinsdottir U, Gudbjartsson DF *et al.* Familial risk of lung carcinoma in the Icelandic population. *JAMA* 2004; **292(24)**:2977–83. [Erratum in: *JAMA* 2005; **293(2)**:163.]

79 Matakidou A, Eisen T, Houlston RS. Systematic review of the relationship between family history and lung cancer risk. *Br J Cancer* 2005; **93(7)**:825–33.

80 Sellers TA, Bailey-Wilson JE, Elston RC, Wilson AF, Ooi WL, Rothschild H. Evidence for mendelian inheritance in the pathogenesis of lung cancer. *J Natl Cancer Inst* 1990; **82**:1272–9.

81 Elston RC, Stewart J. A general model for the genetic analysis of pedigree data. *Hum Hered* 1971; **21**:523–42.

82 Elston RC, Yelverton KC. General models for segregation analysis. *Am J Hum Genet* 1975; **27**:31–45.

83 Bonney GE. Regressive logistic models for familial disease and other binary traits. *Biometrics* 1986; **42**:611–25.

84 Elston RC, George VT. Age of onset, age at examination, and other covariates in the analysis of family data. *Genet Epidemiol* 1989; **6**:217–20.

85 Cannings C, Thompson EA. Ascertainment in the sequential sampling of pedigrees. *Clin Genet* 1977; **12**:208–12.

86 Elston RC, Sobel E. Sampling considerations in the gathering and analysis of pedigree data. *Am J Hum Genet* 1979; **31**:62–9.

87 Sellers TA, Bailey-Wilson JE, Elston RC, Rothschild H. Evidence for Mendelian factors in early-onset lung cancer. In: *Origins of Human Cancer: A Comprehensive Review*. New York: Cold Spring Harbor Laboratory Press, 1991:775–80.

88 Akaike H. A new look at the statistical model identification. *IEEE Trans Automatic Control* 1974; **19**: 716–23.

89 Chen PL, Sellers TA, Bailey-Wilson JE, Rothschild H, Elston RC. Segregation analysis of smoking-associated malignancies; Evidence for Mendelian inheritance. *Am J Hum Genet* 1991; **49(Suppl)**:15.

90 Sellers TA, Chen PL, Potter JD, Bailey-Wilson JE, Rothschild H, Elston RC. Segregation analysis of smoking-associated malignancies; evidence for Mendelian inheritance. *Am J Med Genet* 1994; **52**:308–14.

91 Bailey-Wilson JE, Elston RC, Sellers TA, Rothschild H. Segregation analysis of lung cancer using Class A regressive models. *Am J Hum Genet* 1992; **51(Suppl)**:A145.

92 Gauderman WJ, Morrison JL, Carpenter CL, Thomas DC. Analysis of gene-smoking interaction in lung cancer. *Genetic Epidemiol* 1997; **14**:199–214.

93 Yang P, Schwartz AG, McAllister AE, Swanson GM, Aston CE. Lung cancer risk in families of nonsmoking probands: heterogeneity by age at diagnosis. *Genet Epidemiol* 1999; **17(4)**:253–73.

94 Wu PF, Lee CH, Wang MJ *et al.* Cancer aggregation and complex segregation analysis of families with female non-smoking lung cancer probands in Taiwan. *Eur J Cancer* 2004; **40(2)**:260–6.

95 Croce CM. Genetic approaches to the study of the molecular basis of human cancer. *Cancer Res* 1991; **51(Suppl)**:5015s–8s.

96 Thomas RK, Weir B, Meyerson M. Genomic approaches to lung cancer. *Clin Cancer Res* 2006; **12(14, Pt 2)**:4384s–91s.

97 Breuer RH, Postmus PE, Smit EF. Molecular pathology of non-small-cell lung cancer. *Respiration* 2005; **72(3)**:313–30.

98 Bunn PA, Jr. Molecular biology and early diagnosis in lung cancer. *Lung Cancer* 2002; **38(1)**:S5–8.

99 Bailey-Wilson JE, Amos CI, Pinney SM *et al.* A major lung cancer susceptibility locus maps to chromosome 6q23-25. *Am J Hum Genet* 2004; **75(3)**:460–74.

100 Schwartz AG, Prysak GM, Bock CH, Cote ML. The molecular epidemiology of lung cancer. *Carcinogenesis* Dec 20, 2006 [Epub ahead of print].

101 Kiyohara C, Otsu A, Shirakawa T, Fukuda S, Hopkin JM. Genetic polymorphisms and lung cancer susceptibility: a review. *Lung Cancer* 2002; **37(3)**:241–56.

CHAPTER 3

Lung Cancer Susceptibility and Risk Assessment Models

Xifeng Wu, Hushan Yang, Jie Lin, and Margaret R. Spitz

Introduction

In 2007, it is estimated that there will be 213,380 new cases of lung cancer (LC) and 160,390 LC-related deaths in the United States [1]. These deaths represent 31% of total mortality from all cancers in US men and 26% in women. While tobacco smoking is the predominant cause of LC, a variety of other exposures, such as family history of LC, various chronic respiratory diseases, and environmental tobacco smoke (ETS), are also linked to elevated LC risk. Host susceptibility may also be involved in LC risk, since only a fraction of smokers develops LC [2–5]. Because carcinogenesis is a multistep process, multiple molecular events during this process account for the malignant transformation upon initial carcinogenic exposure. Understanding that multiple components contributing to LC can lead to the identification of high-risk subgroups, who may benefit from targeted screening or other interventions. Here, we provide a summary of recent advances in the molecular epidemiology of LC.

Epidemiologic risk factors in LC

Smoking

Cigarette smoking
Cigarette smoke contains >80 carcinogens evaluated by the International Agency for Research on Cancer (IARC) [6] with "sufficient evidence for carcinogenicity" in humans or lab animals. While smokers are at higher risk of LC than those who have never smoked, there is substantial variation in LC risk among smokers [7,8]. Peto *et al.* [7] related UK national trends in smoking, smoking cessation, and LC to the contrasting results from two case–control studies of smoking and LC in the United Kingdom [9]. Results showed large increases in cumulative LC risk among continuing smokers in 1990 data, reflecting prolonged smoking exposure. Among both men and women in 1990, former smokers had lower LC rates than continuing smokers, with the reduction increasing substantially for increased time since quitting. This study stresses the importance of quitting smoking at an earlier age to avoid subsequent risk of LC. The lifetime risk of developing LC remains high for former smokers, no matter how long the period of abstinence; however, longer duration of abstinence is associated with greater reductions in risk [7]. The relationship between ETS exposure and LC has been extensively evaluated in many epidemiologic studies. Results from several meta-analyses report a positive association [10,11].

Family history
There have been a number of published studies showing familial aggregation of LCs in first-degree relatives of probands with LC [12–18]. Schwartz *et al.* [17] showed that the LC risk in a first-degree relative was associated with a 7.2-fold (95%

Lung Cancer, 3rd edition. Edited by Jack A. Roth, James D. Cox, and Waun Ki Hong. © 2008 Blackwell Publishing, ISBN: 978-1-4051-5112-2.

confidence interval (CI), 1.3–39.7) increased risk among nonsmokers with early age at onset (40–59 year old group). The association between an increased risk of LC among first-degree relatives has been confirmed in other studies [19,20]. On the other hand, Kreuzer et al. [21] reported no evidence of familial risk. Familial aggregation only provides indirect evidence for the genetic influence, and could be due to common genetic profiles among the family members, shared smoking patterns, or by a combination of both factors.

Prior respiratory diseases

LC risk may be modified by a prior history of respiratory diseases such as asthma, bronchitis, emphysema, and hay fever. It has been reported that there was a significant protective effect in the association between hay fever and LC (odds ratio (OR) = 0.58; 95% CI, 0.48–0.70), and a significantly increased risk associated with prior physician-diagnosed emphysema (OR = 2.87; 95% CI, 2.20–3.76) [22]. A significantly lower frequency of hay fever was observed among patients with malignancies of lung, colon, bladder, and prostate as compared to controls [23]. It was suggested that the protective effects were attributed to enhanced immune surveillance resulting from better detection and destruction of malignant cells [16,23–27]; also possibly, anti-inflammatory agents used to treat hay fever might contribute to this protection. In contrast, Talbot-Smith et al. [24] and Osann [16] found no association between hay fever and LC risk.

In another large case–control study comprised of 2854 cases and 3116 controls from seven different European countries, a history of eczema was inversely associated with LC risk with an OR of 0.61 (0.5–0.8) [28]. In a meta-analysis, asthma was a significant risk factor for LC among never smokers with a pooled risk ratio (RR) of 1.9 (1.4–2.5) when adjusted for ETS exposure [29]. Currently, there is no consensus on the role of prior respiratory diseases, other than emphysema, in LC and the empirical evidence, which is not entirely consistent, has been largely derived from observational epidemiologic data.

Environmental and occupational exposures

Asbestos, arsenic, bischloromethyl ether, chromium, nickel, polycyclic aromatic compounds, radon, and vinyl chloride have all been implicated in LC etiology, and have been reviewed extensively before.

Nutrition and dietary patterns

Fruits and vegetables

Observational studies strongly suggest that increased vegetable and fruit intake is associated with reduced risk of LC [30–33]. In the European Prospective Investigation into Cancer and Nutrition (EPIC), with data collected from 478,021 subjects, a significant inverse association between LC risk and fruit consumption was observed after adjusting for smoking and other confounders (RR = 0.60; 95% CI, 0.46–0.98 for the highest quintile compared to the lowest); however, there was no such association with vegetable consumption [33]. In a large prospective Danish cohort study comprising 54,158 participants, the incidence rate of LC was highest in the lowest quartile of plant food intake (fruit, vegetable, legumes, and potatoes) [34]. Neuhouser et al. [35] in a pooled analysis of eight prospective studies with a total of 3206 incident LC cases occurring among 430,281 individuals followed for 6–16 years reported that compared to the lowest quintile of consumption, the RRs of the highest quintile consumption for total fruits, total fruits and vegetables, and total vegetables were 0.77 (0.67–0.87; $p < 0.001$), 0.7 (0.69–0.90; $p = 0.001$), and 0.88 (0.78–1.00; $p = 0.12$), respectively. They concluded that elevated fruit and vegetable consumption, mostly due to fruit intake, is associated with a modest reduction in LC risk [35]. Overall, the association between high intake of fruit and vegetables and reduced LC risk appears conclusive but what subtypes of fruits and vegetables and which micronutrients contribute to this protection remain controversial.

Carotenoids

Carotenoids are red and yellow fat-soluble pigments found in many fruits and vegetables. Numerous studies have shown that a diet high in total carotenoids is protectives, but results are inconsistent in the association between individual carotenoids and LC. In a pooled analysis of seven cohort studies in North America and Europe based on a follow-up of 7–16 years with 3155 incident LC cases among 399,765 participants, Mannisto *et al.* [36] reported that only β-cryptoxanthin intake was inversely associated with LC risk with a RR of 0.76 (0.67–0.86) even after controlling for intake of vitamin C, folate, other carotenoids, multivitamin use, and smoking status. In the Alpha-Tocopherol, β-carotene Cancer Prevention Study (ATBC) [37], with 1644 incident LC cases, during 14 years of follow-up, lower risks were observed for the highest versus the lowest quintiles of lycopene (28% reduction), lutein/zeaxanthin (17%), β-cryptoxanthin (15%), total carotenoids (16%), serum β-carotene (19%), and serum retinol (27%), while intakes of β-carotene, α-carotene, and retinol were not associated with significant reduction. In a pooled analysis of the Nurse's Health Study and the Health Professional Follow-up Study (HPFS), Michaud *et al.* [38] reported that only α-carotene and lycopene intakes were significantly associated with lower risk of LC. In overall analyses of all carotenoids combined, LC risk was significantly lower in subjects with high total carotenoid intake with RR of 0.68 (0.49–0.94). Inadequate adjustment for confounding, especially smoking factors, and the lack of consideration of multicollinearity between individual carotenoids may be responsible for inconsistent results across studies.

Data generated by the Beta-Carotene and Retinol Efficacy Trial (CARET) and ATBC trials failed to confirm the protective role of β-carotene in smokers [35,37]. Contrary to the expectation and observational epidemiologic evidence, supplementation of β-carotene resulted in a surprisingly increased overall LC incidence and higher total mortality among current smokers [39–41]. Debate has been focused on dosage, duration of trials, and the difference between dietary intake and supplement use [42]. Preclinical data provide biologic plausibility for this adverse interaction between cigarette smoking and β-carotene [43]. Recently, in a cohort of French Women [44], high intake of β-carotene was significantly protective against LC among never smokers, but was associated with increased LC incidence in ever smokers. Tests for interaction between smoking and β-carotene intake were significant [44].

Folate, isothiocyanates, and phytoestrogens

Folate deficiency is implicated in in vitro studies in alterations in DNA methylation, DNA synthesis, and disruption of DNA repair activities [45]; however, observational studies have yielded inconsistent results [46–49]. In the New York State [46] and Netherland Cohort Studies [48], an inverse association between folate intake and LC risk was reported. Shen *et al.* [49] also reported that dietary folate intake was associated with a 40% reduction in LC risk among former smokers. In contrast, data from the Nurse's Health Study revealed a lack of association [47].

Isothiocyanates (ITCs) are nonnutrient compounds in cruciferous vegetables with anticarcinogenic properties. One possible mechanism for their protective action is through downregulation of cytochrome P-450 biotransformation enzyme levels and induction of phase II enzymes [50,51]. ITCs can also induce apoptosis, cell cycle arrest, and cell differentiation [52]. Brennan *et al.* [53] showed that weekly consumption of cruciferous vegetables protected against LC in those who were *GSTM1* null (OR = 0.67; 95% CI, 0.49–0.91), *GSTT1* null (0.63, 0.37–1.07), or both (0.28, 0.11–0.67). Similar protective results were noted for consumption of specific cruciferous vegetables. However, Spitz *et al.* [54] reported that current smokers with both low ITC dietary intake and the *GSTM1* null genotype or the *GSTT1* null genotype exhibited increased LC risk, with ORs of 2.22 (1.20–4.10) and 3.19 (1.54–6.62), respectively. This association was confirmed by Gao *et al.* [55]. The comparable OR in the presence of both null genotypes was 5.45 (1.72–17.22). Results in former smokers were not statistically significant.

Dietary phytoestrogens are plant-derived nonsteroidal compounds with weak estrogen-like activity. A significant reductions in risk of LC with increased phytoestrogen intake was observed [56]. The highest quartile of intake of total phytoestrogens from food sources was associated with a 46% reduction in risk (OR = 0.54; 95% CI, 0.42–0.70; $p < 0.001$ for trend). Several studies in Asian populations, whose diet contains large quantities of phytoestrogens, also reported reduced risk of LC associated with high intakes of phytoestrogen [57–61].

Genetic variations in LC risk assessment

Individual susceptibility could be modulated by genetic variants in genes involved in many cellular processes such as carcinogen metabolism, DNA repair, cell cycle checkpoint control, apoptosis, telomere integrity and microenvironment control. Numerous molecular epidemiological studies have been conducted to evaluate the associations of common sequence variants of these genes with LC risk but the results are conflicting for most polymorphisms. The following section will focus on some consistent results as well as those contradictory results that merit further investigation.

Carcinogen metabolism

Tobacco carcinogens are metabolized by phase I and phase II xenobiotic enzymes. Phase I enzymes (the cytochrome P450 (CYP) family members) are involved in the activation of carcinogens to form electrophilic metabolites that are further processed by phase II detoxification enzymes through the conjugation of hydrophobic or electrophilic compounds. Several groups of enzymes are involved in these steps.

CYP1A1

CYP1A1 is the most extensively studied phase I carcinogen metabolizing enzyme involved in bioactivation of a wide spectrum of carcinogens including benzo[*a*]pyrene (B[*a*]P), one of the most abundant polycyclic aromatic hydrocarbon (PAH) carcinogens derived from tobacco-smoking. Two *CYP1A1* single nucleotide polymorphisms (SNPs) have been assessed in LC association studies. In a meta-analysis of 22 studies with 1441 Caucasian cases and 1779 controls, when compared to the common homozygotes, the rare homozygote variant T3801C genotype carriers had a 2.28-fold increased LC risk (0.98–5.28) [62]. In a pooled analysis of 11 studies, Le Marchand *et al.* noted a dose–response effect of

increasing risk of LC with increasing number of the variant allele of the *CYP1A1* Ile462Val SNP [63].

CYP1B1

CYP1B1 is an extrahepatic xenobiotic enzyme expressed in the human lung, and is inducible upon exposure to tobacco smoking and B[*a*]P [64]. A nonsynonymous SNP (nsSNP) results in the substitution of leucine by valine in exon 3. Though no significant main effects of this polymorphism and LC risk have been found, subgroup associations have been reported [65,66].

CYP2A6

CYP2A6 transforms nicotine into 3-hydroxycotinine, the primary urinary nicotine metabolite in tobacco smokers. It is also involved in the metabolism of nitrosamine 4-(methylnitrosamino)-1-(3-pyridyl)-1-butanone (NNK), N′-nitrosodimethylamine (NNN), and N-nitrosodiethylamine (NDEA), major nitrosamine carcinogens resulting from tobacco combustion. Considerable interindividual genetic variation exists in the *CYP2A6* gene, many variants of which have been associated with altered carcinogen metabolizing capacity. Particularly interesting, those homozygous for *CYP2A6**4C, a whole-gene deletion polymorphism [67], exhibited lower LC risk only in smokers [68–70], supporting the notion that subjects with reduced activity of phase I metabolism enzymes may have lower cancer risk. It was also suggested that individuals with the variant allele and hence reduced CYP2A6 activity are less likely to become addicted to nicotine, making it is easier to quit smoking and leading to reduced LC risk [71].

CYP2A13

CYP2A13, the primary CYP isoenzyme to activate NNK, is highly expressed in the human respiratory tract [72–74]. Wang *et al.* [75] showed that variant genotypes of the Arg257Cys SNP of *CYP2A13* were associated with substantially decreased LC risk with an OR of 0.41 (0.23–0.71). Furthermore, Zhang *et al.* [76] reported that individuals homozygous for the variant allele exhibited a 2-fold decrease in NNK activation efficiency, and heterozygotes had 37–56% lower metabolic activity.

CYP2C9

CYP2C9 is involved in the activation of PAH and heterocyclic aromatic amines. The *CYP2C9*2* (Arg144Cys) is the most intensively studied SNP, but results have been inconsistent due to small study sizes [77–79].

CYP2D6

CYP2D6 is responsible for the metabolism of NNK. In a meta-analysis of 13 studies, no association was noted with the variant genotype [80]. This was confirmed by studies in different ethnic groups [81,82].

CYP2E1

CYP2E1 metabolizes a wide variety of carcinogens including NNK. There is an Rsa I polymorphism in the 5′ flanking region which has been shown to affect gene transcription [83], and individuals in various populations with the variant allele exhibited a significant reduction in LC risk [84–88]. Phenotypic assays suggest that the variant allele is associated with impaired host capacity to process chlorzoxazone to its active metabolites [89]. However, a few studies reported null results for this polymorphism and LC risk [79]. Similar conflicting results were also reported for the Dra I polymorphism located in intron 6 [83,90–92].

MPO

Myeloperoxidase (MPO) transforms a broad range of tobacco smoking-derived procarcinogens such as B[*a*]P. A promoter SNP (−463G>A) has been associated with reduced gene expression and enzymatic activity, as well as reduced level of tobacco-derived DNA adducts [93,94]. A meta-analysis of 2686 cases and 3325 controls [95] reported a nonsignificantly reduced LC risk associated with the variant allele with an OR of 0.86 (0.67–1.1). This finding is consistent with another study [96].

GST family

GST is a family of soluble detoxification enzymes that mainly catalyzes the conjugation of GSH with intermediate cytotoxic compounds metabolized by phase I enzymes. There are four classes of GST enzymes, namely, GST alpha (GSTA), GST mu (GSTM), GST pi (GSTP), and GST theta (GSTT).

Common variants in the GST family have been extensively investigated but the results have been inconsistent. A recent meta-analysis compiling 119 previous studies with 19,729 cases and 25,921 controls reported a 1.18-fold increased LC risk (1.14–1.23) associated with the null genotype [97]. However, when the analysis was restricted to five large studies (3436 cases and 3897 controls) with >500 cases in each to avoid potential publication bias, only a slight increase in LC risk was identified with an OR of 1.04 (0.95–1.14). For the whole-gene deletion polymorphism of *GSTT1*, a meta-analysis with 9632 cases and 12,322 controls from 44 previous studies reported a 1.09-fold increase in LC risk (1.02–1.16) [97]; however, restricting the analysis to four large studies with >500 cases eliminated this effect with an OR of 0.99 (0.86–1.11). Publication bias and study heterogeneity were not detected in this *GSTT1* meta-analysis, suggesting limited potential of this polymorphism alone as a risk factor for LC. Two SNPs (Ile105Val and Ala114Val) have been commonly studied for the *GSTP1* gene. A reduction in GSTP1 enzyme activity has been reported to be associated with the variant allele of both SNPs [98]. However, a meta-analysis with 6221 cases and 7602 controls from 25 previous studies, and with 1251 cases and 1295 controls from 4 studies did not reveal any significant association with LC risk for either variant [97]. *GSTM3* has a 3bp-deletion polymorphism in intron 6, which has been investigated in different populations but again with mixed results. A meta-analysis of five studies with 1238 cases and 1179 controls did not note any significant association with LC risk with an OR of 1.05 (0.89–1.23) [97].

NAT family

Human N-acetyltransferases (NATs) are generally classified into two categories, slow and fast acetylators, depending on the effect on protein enzymatic activity by the polymorphisms. So far, the studies of LC risk with *NAT* polymorphisms have yielded inconsistent results. For *NAT1*, significant gene–dose effects were observed between slow acetylators and increased risk of LC in one study [99]. Conversely, a German study [100] demonstrated that the *NAT1* fast acetylators had an increased risk of lung adenocarcinoma, but not squamous cell carcinoma, which was consistent with the observation that fast *NAT1* acetylators exhibited a higher level of chromosomal aberrations as well as increased LC risk in smokers [101]. Similarly, discordant conclusions have been noted for *NAT2* polymorphisms with LC risk. A recent meta-analysis of 16 studies with a total of 3865 cases and 6077 controls failed to detect any statistically significant difference in *NAT2* acetylator status and LC risk [102].

UGT family

UDP-glucuronosyltransferase (UGT) superfamily catalyzes the conjugation of a glucuronic acid moiety to the nucleophilic substrate resulting from the phase I bioactivation. A small Japanese study showed that the *UGT1A7*3* polymorphism was associated with a 4.02-fold (1.57–10.30) increased LC risk compared with the wild-type *UGT1A7*1* allele [103].

SULT family

The sulfotransferase (SULT) family catalyzes the sulfonation of a wide spectrum of exogenous and endogenous compounds. *SULT1A1* G638A is the most studied SNP and the variant allele has been associated with reduced sulfotransferase activity [104]. Compared with the wild-type, the variant-containing genotypes exhibited a significantly increased LC risk with an OR of 1.85 (1.44–2.37) in a Chinese population [105], which was in line with a Caucasian study showing a 1.41-fold increased LC risk (1.04–1.91) [106].

NQO1

NAD(P)H:quinono oxidoreductase 1 (NQO1) is a cytosolic protein that metabolizes quinoid compounds and derivatives. In vitro studies demonstrated a significantly reduced enzyme activity associated with the variant allele of a Pro187Ser SNP in a dose-dependent fashion [107,108]. Nonetheless, a meta-analysis of 19 studies with a total of 6980 cases and 8080 controls reported no significant LC risk association [109].

EPHX1

There are two commonly studied SNPs (Try113His and His139Arg) in the microsomal epoxide hydrolase 1 (*EPHX1*) gene that encodes a phase II protein involved in the hydrolysis of reactive aliphatic and arene epoxides derived from PAH and aromatic amines [110]. Mixed results were derived from a number of small case–control studies evaluating their associations with LC risk. A pooled analysis of 986 cases and 1633 controls from eight studies reported a decreased LC risk associated with the variant allele of Try113His polymorphism with OR of 0.70 (0.51–0.96) [111], which was further validated by an Austrian study [112]. In both studies, the rare allele of His139Arg was associated with an increased LC risk that did not reach statistical significance.

GPX1

Glutathione peroxidase I (GPX1) is a selenium-dependent phase II antioxidant enzyme which plays a crucial role in detoxifying organic peroxides and hydrogen peroxides [113]. A nsSNP (Pro198Leu) has been widely assessed for an association with LC risk, but the results appear to be conflicting in different populations [114–116].

DNA damage and repair

The capacity to repair DNA damage from endogenous and exogenous sources is crucial to maintaining genomic integrity. Nucleotide-excision repair (NER), base-excision repair (BER), double-strand-break repair (DSBR), and mismatch repair (MMR) are four key DNA repair pathways that operate on different types of DNA damage. Common genetic variants in genes involved in these repair pathways have been reported in many LC susceptibility studies [117].

Genetic polymorphisms in DNA repair genes
NER
NER is capable of removing a wide class of helix-distorting lesions that interfere with base pairing and generally disrupt transcription and normal replication resulting from tobacco smoking such as benzo[*a*]pyrene diol-epoxide (BPDE) [118]. NER is the most versatile DNA repair pathway and includes ~30 proteins involved in DNA damage recognition,

incision, DNA ligation, and resynthesis [119]. A growing number of studies have examined the association of polymorphisms in NER genes and LC risk.

ERCC2/XPD

Two SNPs in the XPD gene have been particularly well studied: Asp312Asn and Lys751Gln. Manuguerra et al., in a meta-analysis, showed that the two homozygote variant genotypes were associated with increased risk of LC with ORs of 1.25 (1.04–1.51) and 1.24 (1.05–1.47), respectively [120]. Spitz et al. reported that both polymorphisms might modulate NER capacity in LC patients [121]; both cases and controls with the wild-type genotype exhibited the most proficient DNA repair capacity (DRC) as measured by the host cell reactivation assay. A statistically significant difference in allele frequency between different ethnic groups has been observed for these two SNPs [120].

XPA

A polymorphic site (−4A>G) in the 5′ UTR region of the XPA gene has been evaluated in several studies, with most identifying the G allele as being associated with reduced LC risk [122–124]. One study, however, suggested that the A allele had a protective role in LC [125]. Wu et al. reported that control subjects with one or two copies of the G allele demonstrated more efficient DRC than did those with the homozygous A allele as measured by the host cell reactivation assay [122]. This finding is consistent with the putative association reported with reduced LC risk in Caucasians.

XPC

XPC binds to HR23B, and the XPC-HR23B complex functions as an early DNA damage detector in NER [118,119]. Lee et al. studied the association of seven XPC polymorphisms (−449G>C, −371G>A, −27G>C, Ala499Val, PAT −/+, IVS11 −5C>A, and Lys939Gln) with LC risk in a Korean population and found that only the −27C allele was associated with a significantly increased risk for LC with an OR of 1.97 (1.22–3.17) [126]. The PAT−/+ is a biallelic poly (AT) insertion/deletion polymorphism in intron 9. PAT+ homozygotes exhibited significantly

lower DRC than the wild-type homozygotes [127]. PAT+/+ subjects were at significantly increased risk for LC with OR of 1.60 (1.01–2.55) in a Spanish population [128]. Hu et al. showed that the minor Val allele of Ala499Val was associated with increased risk of LC in a Chinese population [129].

ERCC1

ERCC1, a highly conserved enzyme, is required for the incision step of NER [118,119]. Two common polymorphisms, C8092A and Asn118Asn, are associated with altered ERCC1 mRNA stability and mRNA levels [130,131]. Zhou et al. reported no overall association between these two SNPs and LC risk [132]; however, Zienolddiny et al. showed that the rare homozygous genotype of Asn118Asn polymorphism was associated with a significantly increased risk of nonsmall cell LC (NSCLC) (OR = 3.11; 95% CI, 1.82–5.30) [125].

XPG

XPG functions as a structure-specific endonuclease that cleaves the damaged DNA strand in NER [118,119]. Two studies investigating the His1104Asp polymorphism came to the similar conclusion that the rare homozygote genotype had a protective role in LC [133,134].

BER

In parallel with NER proteins which primarily operate on bulky lesions, the BER proteins mainly repair damaged DNA bases arising from endogenous oxidative processes and hydrolytic decay of DNA. OGG1, APE1, and XRCC1 are three key players in BER. OGG1 is a base-specific glycosylase that initiates repair by releasing the modified base, 8-oxoguanine, and creating abasic sites. APE1 is an endonuclease that incises the DNA strand at the abasic site. XRCC1 functions as a scaffold protein in BER by bringing DNA polymerase and ligase together at the site of repair [118]. Genetic polymorphisms in these three genes have also been implicated in LC risk.

OGG1

A high incidence of spontaneous lung adenoma and carcinoma was found in OGG1-knockout mice, which suggested that OGG1 acts as a suppressor of LC [135]. Four studies concluded that the homozygous variant genotype of Ser326Cys was associated with significantly increased risk of LC [125,136–138], while one reported a borderline significance [139]. A meta-analysis also found increased risk among subjects carrying the homozygous variant genotype (OR = 1.24; 95% CI, 1.01–1.53) [140]. These findings are consistent with experimental evidence that this isoform exhibits lower enzyme activity [141].

APE1

Four case–control studies investigated the association between Asp148Glu SNP and LC risk all reporting no significant association [125,142–144]. Subjects who had the rare homozygote of Ile64Val had reduced risk of NSCLC with an OR of 0.10 (0.01–0.81). No significant association was observed for the Gln51His polymorphism [125].

XRCC1

There are three extensively studied SNPs of XRCC1, Arg194Trp, Arg280His, and Arg399Gln. The Arg194Trp variant has been shown to be associated with BPDE sensitivity in vitro [145]. Most studies have reported a trend for reduced risk for the Trp allele in LC [125,139,146,147], as did a meta-analysis of tobacco-related cancers with an OR of 0.86 (0.77–0.95), based on 4895 cases and 5977 controls from 16 studies [140]. The results for the Arg280His polymorphism were contradictory [139,143,146]. Most studies showed no significant association between Arg399Gln and LC risk [125,139,142–144,146,148–151] and this finding has been confirmed by a meta-analysis with 6120 LC cases and 6895 controls [152].

DSB

DSB is considered the most detrimental to cellular DNA damage as both DNA strands are affected. DSBs arise from a number of mechanisms, including ionizing radiation, X-ray, certain chemotherapeutic agents and replication errors [118]. Homologous recombination (HR) and nonhomologous end-joining (NHEJ) are two complementary pathways in DSBR.

ATM

In human cells, ATM is required for the early response to ionizing radiation. ATM senses genomic damage and initiates DNA repair through interacting with the MRN (MRE11, RAD50, and NBS1) complex and subsequently activating a series of downstream signaling mediators [153]. In a Korean study, an SNP in intron 62 (IVS62 +50G>A) exhibited a significantly increased LC risk with an OR of 1.6 (1.1–2.1) [154], and higher risks for haplotypes and diplotypes containing the variant allele with ORs of 7.6 (1.7–33.5) and 13.2 (3.1–56.1), respectively. The close proximity of this SNP to ATM PI3K and FAT domains suggests a potential functional impact on ATM kinase activity.

NBS1

In the HR pathway, the first event is the resection of the DNA to yield single-strand overhangs [118]. NBS1 is part of an exonuclease complex that takes part in this step. Zienolddiny *et al.* and Matullo *et al.* showed no association between the NBS1 Glu185Gln polymorphism and LC risk [125,155], but Lan *et al.* reported that homozygotes for this allele had an increased risk of LC with an OR of 2.53 (1.05–6.08) [156].

XRCC3

XRCC3 is an RAD51-related protein involved in catalyzing the DNA strand exchange reaction during HR [118]. Five epidemiological studies found no association between the thr241Met polymorphism with LC risk [125,143,148,155,157].

LIG4

In the NHEJ pathway, LIG4 has an important role in linking the ends of a double-strand break together [118]. Matullo *et al.* found no association between two LIG4 polymorphisms (Ala3Val and Thr9Ile) and LC risk [155]. Sakiyama *et al.* reported that the variant allele of the Ile658Val polymorphism of LIG4 was associated with a reduced risk of squamous cell carcinoma with an OR of 0.4 (0.1–0.8) [158].

MMR

The MMR system maintains the stability of the genome during repeated duplication, by repairing base–base mismatches, caused not only by errors of DNA polymerases that escape their proofreading function, but also by insertion/deletion loops that result from slippage during replication of repetitive sequences or during recombination [118]. So far, only a few studies have investigated the connection between MMR and LC.

MLH1 –93G>A polymorphism was studied for its association with risk of LC and no overall association was identified [159]; Jung *et al.* investigated the association of *MSH2* –118T>C, IVS1 +9G>C, IVS10 +12A>G, and IVS12 –6T>C genotypes with LC risk [160] and found that the presence of at least one IVS10 +12G allele was associated with a decreased risk of adenocarcinoma as compared with the IVS10 +12AA genotype with OR of 0.59 (0.40–0.88), and the presence of at least one IVS12 –6C allele was associated with an increased risk of adenocarcinoma as compared with the IVS12 –6TT genotype with an OR of 1.52 (1.02–2.27) [160].

DNA damage and repair phenotypic assays

The phenotypic assays for DNA damage and repair include measuring: (a) DNA damage/repair after a chemical or physical mutagen challenge (such as the mutagen sensitivity, comet, and induced adduct assays); (b) unscheduled DNA synthesis; (c) cellular ability to remove DNA lesions from plasmid transfected into lymphocyte cultures in vitro by expression of damaged reporter genes (the host–cell reactivation assay); (d) activity of DNA repair enzyme (repair activity assay for 8-OH-Guanine) [161,162].

Mutagen sensitivity

The mutagen sensitivity assay quantifies chromatid breaks induced by mutagens in cultured lymphocytes in vitro as an indirect measure of DRC [163,164]. Bleomycin is a clastogenic agent that mimics the effects of radiation by generating free oxygen radicals capable of producing DNA single- and double-strand breaks that initiate BER and DSB repair [165]. Wu *et al.* showed that higher BPDE and bleomycin sensitivities were independently significantly associated with increased risks of LC, a finding that has been confirmed by other studies [3–5,166,167].

Comet assay

The comet assay is a single-cell gel electrophoresis method used to measure DNA damage in individual cells. It is a sensitive and versatile method with high throughout potential [168,169]. The alkaline version (pH > 13) of the comet assay can detect DNA damage such as single-strand breaks, double-strand breaks, and alkaline labile sites [170]. Common mutagens used in this assay include BPDE, bleomycin, and γ-radiation. Wu *et al.* found that higher γ-radiation- and BPDE-induced olive tail moments, one of the parameters for measuring DNA damage, were significantly associated with 2.32- and 4.49-fold risks of LC, respectively [171]. Rajaee-Behbahani *et al.* reported lower repair rate of bleomycin-induced DNA damage using the alkaline comet assay in LC patients compared with controls [172].

DNA adducts

Using ^{32}P postlabeling techniques, two studies by the same group indicated a significant association between the level of in vitro BPDE-induced DNA adducts and risk for LC [173,174], suggesting suboptimal ability to remove the BPDE-DNA adduct resulted in increased susceptibility to tobacco carcinogen exposure [174].

Host cell reactivation assay

The host cell reactivation assay measures global NER as a biomarker for LC susceptibility [175–177], by quantifying the activity of a reporter gene (CAT or LUC gene) in undamaged lymphocytes transfected with BPDE-treated plasmids. Because a single unrepaired BPDE-induced DNA adduct can block reporter gene transcription [178], the measured reporter gene activity reflects the ability of the transfected cells to remove the adducts from the plasmid. Reduced capacity to repair adducts is observed in cases compared to controls and is associated with an increased risk of LC with evidence of a significant dose–response association between decreased DRC and risk of LC [175–177].

8-OGG assay

The enzyme 8-oxoguanine DNA N-glycosylase is encoded by the *OGG1* gene and initiates the BER pathway. The OGG activity assay monitors the ability of OGG to remove an 8-oxoguanine residue from a radiolabeled synthetic DNA oligonucleotide, generating two DNA products that can be distinguished on the basis of size [179]. Paz-Elizur *et al.* showed that OGG activity was significantly lower in peripheral blood mononuclear cells from LC patients than in those from controls. Individuals in the lowest tertile of OGG activity exhibited an increased risk of NSCLC compared with those in the highest tertile (OR = 4.8; 95% CI, 1.5–15.9) [179]. Gackowski *et al.* also reported that the repair activity of OGG was significantly higher in blood leukocytes of healthy volunteers than in LC patients [180].

Cell cycle control

The intricate cell cycle regulatory network is essential for cells to undergo replication, division, proliferation, and differentiation. Anomalies of cell cycle regulation genes are frequently observed in a variety of human malignancies including LC, and are considered to be one of the most critical early-stage events in carcinogenesis [181–184].

Genetic polymorphisms in cell cycle-related genes

p53

p53 is the most important tumor suppressor gene of the genome defense system regulating pivotal cellular activities such as DNA damage response, DNA repair, cell cycle control, and apoptosis. Three polymorphisms of the *p53* gene have been commonly studied in cancer susceptibility. Weston *et al.* first reported the association between the Arg72Pro nsSNP in exon 4 and increased LC risk [185], which was confirmed by a number of subsequent studies in various populations [186–191]. Functional assays corroborated this finding by demonstrating the association between the variant allele and increased *p53* mutations in tumor tissues, as well as a reduced rate of apoptosis in white blood cells of LC patients [189,192,193]. Wu *et al.* reported an association with the variant genotype of both the intron 3 16-bp deletion/insertion and the intron 6 polymorphisms [187]. Analyses of haplotypes reconstructed using these three polymorphisms demonstrated an increased LC risk for the variant-harboring haplotypes

compared to the haplotype with wild-type alleles at all three loci. This result was supported by functional studies showing that the variant-harboring haplotypes exhibited a reduced apoptotic index and reduced DNA repair capacity [187]. Moreover, the association with the intron 3 polymorphism was confirmed in a recent large-scale European study, which reported a 2.98-fold [194] increased LC risk for the homozygous variant genotype. Although most studies suggest a positive association between these *p53* polymorphisms and LC risk, disagreements exist including a recent meta-analysis of 13 LC studies showing no LC risk association for any of these polymorphisms [195].

p73

p73 may activate p53 down-stream transcriptional effectors such as p21 to control cell cycle progression and apoptosis [196]. A dinucleotide polymorphism in the 5′UTR of *p73* is associated with an increased risk of LC in a Caucasian population but a protective effect in a Chinese population [197,198], suggesting the possible existence of ethnic-specific risk differentiation. Furthermore, a gene–dosage effect by combining both *p53* and *p73* variant alleles together was demonstrated [199].

MDM2

MDM2, a ubiquitin ligase, negatively regulates p53 activity either by binding to the transactivation domain of p53 protein and inhibiting its transcriptional activation of *p21*, or by targeting p53 protein to ubiquitin-mediated proteasome degradation [200]. A T to G transversion in the intronic promoter region of *MDM2* was associated with increased LC risk in Chinese [190], Koreans [201], and Europeans [202]. Other studies exhibited similarly elevated risk, although not reaching statistical significance [203,204]. The agreement amongst these studies recapitulates the in vivo observation that the variant allele upregulates *MDM2* expression and thus reduces p53 protein level [205].

HRAD9

HRAD9 is a phosphorylation target of ATM kinase that plays a crucial role in DNA repair and cell cycle arrest in response to DNA damage [206]. A nsSNP

(His239Arg) in exon 8 was reported to be over-represented in LC patients in a Japanese population [207]. Moreover, the high homology of the wild-type allele across species and computational predictions that the variant allele might adversely affect protein function support this association [207,208].

CCND1

CCND1 is the most important cyclin that drives the G1-S transition in conjunction with CDK4/CDK6. Overexpression of CCND1 is associated with increased cell proliferation, deviated apoptosis, elevated cancer risk and poor survival [209]. A G807A SNP in exon 4 affects mRNA alternative splicing and the A allele has been shown to be associated with higher nuclear protein level and poor NSCLC patient survival compared with the C allele [210]. Qiuling et al. reported an association of the A allele with early onset and increased LC risk in a Chinese population [211], and Hung et al. noted that individuals with the A allele-containing genotype exhibited an increased LC risk in individuals with prior X-ray exposure [194], confirming the observation that elevated nuclear CCND1 expression might promote carcinogenesis in a milieu of high genomic instability [212].

STK15

STK15 is a serine/threonine protein kinase modulating G2/M cell cycle progression through its regulation of mitotic spindle formation and centrosome duplication [196,213]. Dysfunction of STK15 might result in aberrant chromosome replication and segregation, a potential early event in LC [196,214]. A nsSNP (Phe31Ile) exhibited a protective effect on LC risk [215], a finding discordant with its roles in the carcinogenesis of most other malignancies [216], suggesting that this SNP might modulate tumorigenesis in a cancer type-specific manner.

Cell cycle phenotypic assays

Two types of cell cycle arrest phenotypic assays have been developed to assess LC risk. Using flow cytometry, Zhao et al. showed that when compared to control subjects, LC patients exhibited significantly less γ-radiation-elicited increases in

G2/M cell percentages as well as a lower apoptosis rate [217]. Moreover, the change in p53 protein level correlated with the G2/M delay and chromatid breaks upon gamma exposure, indicating that possible defective cell cycle checkpoint functions in cancer patients might be associated with p53-dependent DNA damage response and DRC. These findings were elaborated in a larger case–control study by Wu et al. reporting that the γ-radiation-induced delay of both S and G2/M phases might also predict LC susceptibility [171]. Similar conclusions were drawn by Zheng et al. [218].

Apoptosis

Genetic polymorphisms in apoptotic pathways

Apoptosis (programmed cell death) is an essential cellular defense mechanism. Two principal signaling pathways, the intrinsic pathway and the extrinsic pathway, are implicated in the coordination of the apoptotic process. In the extrinsic apoptosis pathway, polymorphisms influencing the FASL–FAS interaction might affect LC predisposition. In a Chinese case–control study, two promoter SNPs of FAS (−1377G >A) and FASL (−844T >C) [219] were associated with increased LC risks with ORs of 1.59 (1.21–2.10) and 1.79 (1.26–2.52), respectively, when the rare homozygotes were compared to the common homozygotes. A multiplicative interactive effect was noted. In the intrinsic apoptosis pathway, CASP9 is the only gene that has been assessed for a role in LC development. In a Korean study, Park et al. found that two CASP9 promoter SNPs (−1263A >G and −712C >T) were associated with significantly altered LC risk with OR's of 0.64 (0.42–0.98) and 2.32 (1.09–4.94), respectively, when their homozygous variant genotypes were compared to the homozygous wild-type reference group [220]. Furthermore, the haplotype composed of the G allele of −1263A >G and the C allele of −712C>T was associated with a significantly decreased risk. This was consistent with the results from single SNP analysis and was functionally validated by a promoter-luciferase assay.

Phenotypic assays in apoptotic pathways

Two groups have reported that impaired mutagen-induced apoptotic capacity was associated with increased risk of LC [217] using the TUNEL (Terminal transferase dUTP nick end labeling) method [221]. Biros *et al.* [192] reported that in LC patients, individuals with the variant allele of *p53* Pro72Arg polymorphism exhibited a lower level of apoptotic white blood cells. This finding was consistent with the results from Wu *et al.* [187] who showed that the haplotype containing the wild-type alleles of the three *p53* polymorphisms (intron 3, exon 4, and intron 6) was associated with higher apoptotic index than those with at least one variant allele.

Telomere and telomerase

Telomeres are TTAGGG repeat complexes bound by specialized nucleoproteins at the ends of chromosomes in eukaryotic cells. By capping the ends of chromosomes, telomeres prevent nucleolytic degradation, end-to-end fusion, irregular recombination and other events lethal to cells [222]. Wu *et al.* [223] measured telomere length in the peripheral blood lymphocytes of LC patients and age-matched controls and found significantly shorter telomere length in LC cases.

To date, only two studies have indicated that common sequence variants in the *TERT* genomic region might predispose to LC. TERT is the protein moiety of telomerase, the key enzyme in the maintenance of telomere length by synthesizing TTAGGG nucleotide repeats. In the majority of human cancers, telomerase is activated and cells overcome senescence and become immortalized. Wang *et al.* [224] showed that a polymorphic tandem repeat minisatellite (MNS16A) in the promoter region of an antisense transcript of the *TERT* gene regulates the antisense transcript expression. Cells with short tandem repeats displayed higher promoter activity compared to those with longer tandem repeats. A subsequent case–control study showed that the long tandem repeat variant was associated with a more than 2-fold increase in LC risk in a recessive pattern, supporting the conjecture that the antisense transcript might serve as a tumor suppressor gene inhibiting the expression of *TERT* [224]. Another polymorphism was recently identified in the Ets2 binding site of the *TERT* promoter region [225].

Compared to the common homozygotes, the rare homozygotes exhibited reduced telomerase activity.

Tumor microenvironment

Microenvironmental factors

Matrix metalloproteins (MMPs) degrade a range of extracellular matrix and nonmatrix proteins. Since MMP expression level has been implicated in cancer development, several polymorphisms in the promoter regions of MMPs that might affect gene expression have been evaluated.

MMP1

MMP1 is a highly expressed interstitial collagenase, which degrades fibrillar collagens. *MMP1* is upregulated by tobacco exposure [226] and overexpression of *MMP1* in tumors has been linked to tumor invasion and metastasis [227,228]. A 1G/2G polymorphism in the *MMP1* promoter was associated with altered gene expression [229]. Promoters containing the 2G allele displayed higher transcriptional activity than those with the 1G allele. An increased LC risk was identified with the 2G/2G genotype by Zhu *et al.* [230]. Two other studies, Su *et al.* [231] and Fang *et al.* [232] both noted an increase in LC risk with the 2G allele, but this did not reach statistical significance.

MMP2

MMP2 is a gelatinase whose substrates include gelatins, collagens, and fibronectin. The expression levels of MMP2 have been commonly used to predict cancer prognosis. A promoter SNP ($-1306C>T$) has been associated with reduced activity due to a possible interference with the SP1-binding site [233]. Interestingly, compared to the variant allele associated with lower gene expression, the wild-type allele exhibited an association with LC risk with an OR of 2.18 (1.70–2.79) in a Chinese population [234]. Another promoter SNP ($-735C>T$), which was linked with $-1306C>T$, was also associated with risk for the wild-type allele with an OR of 1.57 (1.27–1.95) [235] which retains the SP1 binding site as well as a higher transcriptional activation efficiency [236]. Moreover, it was noted that an even higher risk was associated with the haplotype containing the wild-type alleles at both loci and this risk showed a multiplicative interaction effect with smoking [235].

MMP3

MMP3 is a stromelysin whose substrates include collagens, gelatin, aggrecan, fibronectin, laminin, and casein. The most commonly studied *MMP3* polymorphism is a promoter variant located at −1171 nucleotide, containing either five or six adenosines that may affect promoter transcription activity [237]. In a Caucasian population, a haplotype containing the 6A allele exhibited a higher LC risk in never smokers [238]. However, in a Chinese study, Fang *et al.* reported that smokers with the *MMP3* 5A allele had a 1.68-fold (1.04–2.70) increased risk to develop NSCLC [232].

MMP7

MMP7 is a matrilysin whose substrates include collagens, aggrecan, decorin, fibronectin, elastin, and casein. *MMP7* is highly expressed in lungs of patients with pulmonary fibrosis and other conditions associated with airway and alveolar injury. The variant allele of a promoter SNP, −181A>G, might lead to higher promoter activity and increased mRNA levels [239]. Consistently, the variant-harboring genotypes, when compared to the common homozygotes, have been proven to predispose to risk of NSCLC [240].

MMP9

MMP9 is a gelatinase and the major structural component of the basement membrane. Hu *et al.* reported that two common nsSNPs, Arg279Gln and Pro574Arg, might confer LC susceptibility in a dose-dependent fashion [241].

MMP12

MMP12 is a metalloelastase required for macrophage-mediated extracellular matrix proteolysis and tissue invasion. A promoter SNP (−82A>G) might regulate *MMP12* expression through modulating the binding affinity of transcription activation protein 1 [242]. Another nsSNP (1082A>G) leads to the substitution of serine for asparagine. Although no significant LC risk associations were identified for either SNP, a haplotype containing the −82A and 1082G alleles

was associated with higher LC risk among never smokers in comparison to haplotypes containing −82G and 1082A [238].

Inflammation

Airway inflammation may promote tumorigenesis through multiple mechanisms such as inducing oxidative stress and lipid peroxidation [243]. To date, only a few polymorphisms in inflammation genes have been evaluated for their roles in lung tumorigenesis and the results have been mostly discrepant.

Anti-inflammatory genes

The major functions of anti-inflammation genes such as *IL4*, *IL10*, *IL13*, and *PPARs* are to resolve the acute inflammatory reactions. Among these, IL10 is produced by monocytes and lymphocytes and exhibits multiple functions in the regulation of cell-mediated immunity, inflammation, and angiogenesis [244]. Three SNPs in the promoter region of *IL10* have been identified (−1082A>G, −819C>T, and −592C>A). In a Chinese study, the variant allele of the −1082A>G SNP was associated with a 5.26-fold (2.65–10.4) increased LC risk [245], which was in agreement with another study in small cell LC [246]. The variant allele has been shown to affect IL10 protein level through regulating gene transcription [247–249].

Proinflammatory genes

Engels *et al.* [250] systematically evaluated a panel of 59 single nucleotide polymorphisms (SNP) in 37 inflammation-related genes among non-Hispanic Caucasian lung cancer cases (N = 1,553) and controls (N = 1,730). They found that Interleukin 1 beta (IL1B) C3954T was associated with increased risk of lung cancer and that one IL1A-IL1B haplotype, containing only the IL1B 3954T allele, was associated with elevated lung cancer risk. These associations were stronger in heavy smokers, particularly for IL 1B C3954T. *IL1B* activates a mixture of inflammatory signaling mediators including NF Kappa B, leading to an amplified proinflammatory effect. A variable number of tandem repeats (VNTR) polymorphism in intron 2 of the *IL1RN* gene [251] influences the expression of both *IL1B* and *IL1RN* [252,253]. Lind *et al.* [251] observed an increased LC risk in individuals with both the *IL1RN**1 and the

IL1B-31T alleles, indicating a possible interacting effect between the two polymorphisms. In addition, compared to *IL1RN**2, the *IL1RN**1 allele carriers exhibited a 2-fold increased level of DNA adducts in normal lung tissues, consistent with its association with elevated cancer risk [251]. *TNFA* stimulates tumor formation through activating multiple pathways leading to an enhanced inflammatory microenvironment [254,255]. In a Chinese study [256], the rare allele of the −308G>A polymorphism, which was associated with increased *TNF* expression [257,258], exhibited a 3.75-fold (2.38–5.92) excess cancer risk compared with the common allele; while the variant allele of the −238G>A polymorphism, which was associated with reduced *TNF* transcription [259], was found to be significantly protective with an OR of 0.26 (0.13–0.50). *IL6* induces the expression of numerous downstream signaling effectors of acute-phase inflammation including COX2 and NFKB [260]. A −634C>G SNP in the promoter region has been associated with increased LC risk only in nonsmoking Chinese women with asthma/atopy [261], suggesting a potential interplay between inflammation polymorphisms and chronic inflammatory conditions. Another *IL6* promoter SNP, −174G>C, which influences the protein levels of IL6 and C-reactive protein, was associated with increased risk of squamous cell but not adenocarcinoma [262]. Cyclooxygenase 2 (COX2) is an essential enzyme in the biosynthesis of inflammation-promoting prostaglandins and is overexpressed in many human cancers including LC [263]. A 3′ UTR SNP (C8473T) was associated with elevated LC risk in a dose-dependent manner [262]. It was suggested that the variant allele might lead to more stabilized *COX2* mRNA and therefore, a stronger inflammatory effect [262].

Growth factor

IGFs

Both insulin growth factors (IFG1 and IGF2) play a major role in fostering cell proliferation, survival, migration and inhibiting apoptosis [264]. The interactions between IGFs and IGFRs are regulated by IGF binding proteins (IGFBPs) functioning in both IGF-dependent and IGF-independent manners to regulate cellular growth [265]. High plasma levels of IGF1 were associated with increased risk of LC in a dose-dependent manner [266]. To date, only two SNPs were reported to predispose to LC. The homozygous variant at the −202 nucleotide position of *IGFBP3* promoter region was reported to be negatively correlated to LC susceptibility in a Korean population [267]. This was supported by the observation that IGFBP3 may have a dual role in the biosynthesis of IGFs [268], and serum-circulating IGFBP3 protein might prolong the half-life of IGF through influencing its interaction with the membrane receptors [269]. A recent study evaluating 1476 nsSNPs of cancer-related genes identified a significantly altered LC risk associated with Trp138Arg of *IGFBP5* [270]. Using the Pathway Assist software, 11 out of 1476 SNPs exhibiting significant LC risk association were mapped to the GH–IGF axis [270], indicating the importance of this pathway in LC development.

EGF

Epidermal growth factor (EGF), a small molecule ligand that activates receptor tyrosine kinase (RTK), mediates signal transduction pathways. An A to G transition in the 5′ UTR of *EGF* gene has been associated with reduced LC risk in a Korean population [271].

VEGF

Vascular endothelial growth factor (VEGF) is a proangiogenesis protein implicated in carcinogenesis and metastasis of many cancers. Three common polymorphisms in the promoter region (−634G>C, −1154G>A, and −2578C>A) regulate VEGF protein level, vascular density, as well as vascularization status of tumor tissues from NSCLC patients [272]. However, no study has assessed their implications in LC risk.

Methylation-related genes

Aberrant methylation of pivotal cell growth-related genes may lead to carcinogenesis through regulating their protein expression and common genetic variants in methylation maintenance genes may also impact cancer susceptibility.

DNMT 3B

DNMT3B is responsible for the generation of genomic methylation patterns. To date, three *DNMT3B* polymorphisms have been evaluated in LC susceptibility. Wang *et al.* reported that a C to T single base substitution in the promoter region was associated with enhanced promoter activity [273]. Genotypes encompassing the variant allele were associated with a 1.88-fold excess of LC risk compared to the common homozygotes in Caucasians [274]. In a Korean population, Lee *et al.* noted that the variant alleles of another two promoter polymorphisms (−283C>T and −579G>T) were both associated with reduced risk for LC [275]. The results of the these studies were in concordance as both reported that the allele leading to enhanced DNMT3B expression was associated with increased cancer risk.

MBD1

MBD1 is a mediator of the DNA methylation-induced gene silencing. Jang *et al.* reported that the wild-type allele of a −634G>A SNP in the promoter region was associated with LC risk with OR of 3.10 (1.24–7.75) in a Korean population [276]. For another two SNPs (−501delT and Pro401Ala), the wild-type alleles were correlated with increased risk of adenocarcinoma but not with other LC subtypes. Luciferase assays demonstrated that the haplotype containing the risk-conferring alleles exhibited higher promoter activity, indicating the presence of a negative correlation between MBD1 expression and LC development.

MTHFR

MTHFR gene encodes an essential enzyme involved in the production of the S-adenosylmethionine intermediate for DNA methylation [277]. Besides a role in DNA methylation, MTHFR is also important in maintaining normal cellular folate levels. So far, two nsSNPs (677C>T and 1298A>C) have been assessed in studies with inconsistent results [278].

SUV39H2

Suppressor of variegation 3–9 homolog 2 (SUV39H2) is a site-specific histone methyltransferase responsible for the methylation of lysine 9 in histone 3. A1624G>C SNP in the 3′ UTR region was associated with a 2.63-fold (1.10–6.29) increased risk of LC in ever smokers when variant-containing genotypes were compared to homozygous wild-types [279]. In vitro assays showed a more than 2-fold higher transcript level for the variant allele, indicating that this SNP might be the causal agent functioning through influencing protein expression.

LC risk assessment models

Statistical models relating multiple risk factors to cancer risk can identify high-risk subsets of smokers. There are three criteria to evaluate the performance of risk assessment models: calibration (reliability), discrimination, and accuracy [280]. Calibration assesses the ability of a model to predict the number of endpoint events in subgroups of the population and is evaluated by using the goodness-of-fit statistic. Discrimination is a measure of a model's ability to distinguish between those who will and will not develop disease, and is quantified by calculating the concordance statistic, or area under a receiver operating characteristic (ROC) curve. Accuracy including positive and negative predictive values refers to the model's ability to categorize specific individuals. The best-known cancer prediction model is the Gail model for breast cancer [281]. It has been validated in several populations [282–285] and appears to give accurate predictions for women undergoing routine mammographic screening but probably overestimates the risk for young women not undergoing routine mammography [286]. The modest discrimination ability of the Gail model calls for the incorporation of promising biological factors [287–290]. Prediction models for other cancers (melanoma [291,292], colorectal cancer [293], and LC [7,8]) have also emerged.

The few published LC risk assessment models mainly focus on smoking behavior and demographic characteristics. Bach *et al.* [8] used data collected from CARET, a large, randomized trial of LC prevention, to derive a LC risk prediction model. The model used the subject's age, sex, asbestos exposure history, and smoking history to predict LC risk and was derived by use of data from five CARET study sites and then validated by assessing the extent it could predict events in the sixth study site. The model was then applied to evaluate the risk of LC among smokers enrolled in a study of LC screening with computed tomography (CT). The model identified smoking variables (duration of smoking, average number of cigarettes smoked per day, duration of abstinence), age, asbestos exposure and the study drug, β-carotene and retinyl palmitate as significant predictors of LC. The model provided strong evidence that LC risk varies greatly among smokers and was internally validated and well calibrated with a cross-validated concordance index of 0.72. Bach's model is most applicable to heavy smokers aged between 50 and 75 years. Recently, Spitz *et al.* [294] developed lung cancer risk models for never, former, and current smokers, respectively. In their models, factors with strong etiological roles, e.g., environmental tobacco smoke, family history of cancer, dust exposure, prior respiratory disease, and smoking history variables were all identified as significant predictors of lung cancer risk. The models were internally validated with cross-validated concordance statistics for the never, former, and current smoker models of 0.57, 0.63, and 0.58, respectively. The computed 1-year absolute risk of lung cancer for a hypothetical male current smoker with an estimated relative risk close to 9 was 8.68%. The ordinal risk index performed well in that true-positive rates in the designated high-risk categories were 69% and 70% for current and former smokers, respectively. When externally validated, this risk assessment procedure could use easily obtained clinical information to identify individuals who may benefit from increased screening surveillance for lung cancer. In summary, current LC risk prediction models have been focused on smoking variables and there is potential to develop more accurate models by collecting more data and incorporating additional risk factors. Moreover, external validation of existing models to independent populations is important.

Concluding remarks

The results of many reported associations of single polymorphism analyses are incongruent and could not be replicated even with key study parameters similar to the original ones. Beyond a possible effect from population heterogeneity, shortcomings in experimental design and statistical methodology such as small sample size, lack of control for confounding, selection bias, and multiple comparisons may account for a large part of these discrepancies. Since cancer is a multistep and multifactorial disease, the influence of individual variants identified from most candidate gene approach studies on overall cancer risk might be minimal. Moreover, many cancer risk-associated genetic variants lack functional validation. To circumvent these caveats, pathway-based approaches have been exploited that simultaneously analyze the impact of multiple variants in the same carcinogenesis-related signaling or function pathway on cancer predisposition. This strategy might amplify the effect from single variants; however, the pathway-based approach also depends on a priori knowledge from basic investigations suggesting the involvement of the pathway in tumorigenesis. A haplotype-based genome scan approach has also been proposed to identify causal variants in the whole-genome scale without any presumption based on prior knowledge, as has been successfully applied to isolate causal polymorphisms in a variety of common human diseases. This approach mandates stringent study designs, adequate sample size, and statistical power. In addition, high-power computational methodologies of data analysis and error shooting should be developed to probe the vast amount of interactions amongst genetic and environmental factors, and molecular function assays should be carried out to determine the genotype–phenotype correlations and validate the biological significance of the identified high risk alleles.

References

1 American Cancer Society: *Cancer Facts & Figures.* Atlanta, GA: American Cancer Society, 2007.

2 Hsu TC, Spitz MR, Schantz SP. Mutagen sensitivity: a biological marker of cancer susceptibility. *Cancer Epidemiol Biomarkers Prev* 1991; **1(1)**:83–9.

3 Spitz MR Hsu TC, Wu X, Fueger JJ, Amos CI, Roth JA. Mutagen sensitivity as a biological marker of lung cancer risk in African Americans. *Cancer Epidemiol Biomarkers Prev* 1995; **4(2)**:99–103.

4 Wu X, Delclos GL, Annegers JF *et al.* A case–control study of wood dust exposure, mutagen sensitivity, and lung cancer risk. *Cancer Epidemiol Biomarkers Prev* 1995; **4(6)**:583–8.

5 Zheng YL, Loffredo CA, Yu Z *et al.* Bleomycin-induced chromosome breaks as a risk marker for lung cancer: a case–control study with population and hospital controls. *Carcinogenesis* 2003; **24(2)**:269–74.

6 Smith-Warner SA, Spiegelman D, Yaun SS *et al.* Fruits, vegetables and lung cancer: a pooled analysis of cohort studies. *Int J Cancer* 2003; **107(6)**:1001–11.

7 Peto R, Darby S, Deo H, Silcocks P, Whitley E, Doll R. Smoking, smoking cessation, and lung cancer in the UK since 1950: combination of national statistics with two case–control studies. *BMJ* 2000; **321(7257)**:323–9.

8 Bach PB, Kattan MW, Thornquist MD *et al.* Variations in lung cancer risk among smokers. *J Natl Cancer Inst* 2003; **95(6)**:470–8.

9 Darby S, Whitley E, Silcocks P *et al.* Risk of lung cancer associated with residential radon exposure in southwest England: a case–control study. *Br J Cancer* 1998; **78(3)**:394–408.

10 Taylor R, Cumming R, Woodward A, Black M. Passive smoking and lung cancer: a cumulative meta-analysis. *Aust N Z J Public Health* 2001; **25(3)**:203–11.

11 Gorlova OY, Zhang Y, Schabath MB *et al.* Never smokers and lung cancer risk: a case–control study of epidemiological factors. *Int J Cancer* 2006; **118(7)**:1798–804.

12 Tokuhata GK, Lilienfeld AM. Familial aggregation of lung cancer in humans. *J Natl Cancer Inst* 1963; **30**:289–312.

13 Ooi WL, Elston RC, Chen VW, Bailey-Wilson JE, Rothschild H. Increased familial risk for lung cancer. *J Natl Cancer Inst* 1986; **76(2)**:217–22.

14 Samet JM, Humble CG, Pathak DR. Personal and family history of respiratory disease and lung cancer risk. *Am Rev Respir Dis* 1986; **134(3)**:466–70.

15 Shaw GL, Falk RT, Pickle LW, Mason TJ, Buffler PA. Lung cancer risk associated with cancer in relatives. *J Clin Epidemiol* 1991; **44(4–5)**:429–37.

16 Osann KE. Lung cancer in women: the importance of smoking, family history of cancer, and medical history of respiratory disease. *Cancer Res* 1991; **51(18)**:4893–7.

17 Schwartz AG, Yang P, Swanson GM. Familial risk of lung cancer among nonsmokers and their relatives. *Am J Epidemiol* 1996; **144(6)**:554–62.

18 Mayne ST, Buenconsejo J, Janerich DT. Previous lung disease and risk of lung cancer among men and women nonsmokers. *Am J Epidemiol* 1999; **149(1)**:13–20.

19 Bromen K, Pohlabeln H, Jahn I, Ahrens W, Jockel KH. Aggregation of lung cancer in families: results from a population-based case–control study in Germany. *Am J Epidemiol* 2000; **152(6)**:497–505.

20 Etzel CJ, Amos CI, Spitz MR. Risk for smoking-related cancer among relatives of lung cancer patients. *Cancer Res* 2003; **63(23)**:8531–5.

21 Kreuzer M, Kreienbrock L, Gerken M *et al.* Risk factors for lung cancer in young adults. *Am J Epidemiol* 1998; **147(11)**:1028–37.

22 Schabath MB, Delclos GL, Martynowicz MM *et al.* Opposing effects of emphysema, hay fever, and select genetic variants on lung cancer risk. *Am J Epidemiol* 2005; **161(5)**:412–22.

23 Cockcroft DW, Klein GJ, Donevan RE, Copland GM. Is there a negative correlation between malignancy and respiratory atopy? *Ann Allergy* 1979; **43(6)**:345–7.

24 Talbot-Smith A, Fritschi L, Divitini ML, Mallon DF, Knuiman MW. Allergy, atopy, and cancer: a prospective study of the 1981 Busselton cohort. *Am J Epidemiol* 2003; **157(7)**:606–12.

25 Vena JE, Bona JR, Byers TE, Middleton E, Jr, Swanson MK, Graham S. Allergy-related diseases and cancer: an inverse association. *Am J Epidemiol* 1985; **122(1)**:66–74.

26 Gabriel R, Dudley BM, Alexander WD. Lung cancer and allergy. *Br J Clin Pract* 1972; **26(5)**:202–4.

27 McDuffie HH. Atopy and primary lung cancer. Histology and sex distribution. *Chest* 1991; **99(2)**:404–7.

28 Castaing M, Youngson J, Zaridze D *et al.* Is the risk of lung cancer reduced among eczema patients? *Am J Epidemiol* 2005; **162(6)**:542–7.

29 Santillan AA, Camargo CA, Jr, Colditz GA. A meta-analysis of asthma and risk of lung cancer (United States). *Cancer Causes Control* 2003; **14(4)**:327–34.

30 Feskanich D, Ziegler RG, Michaud DS *et al.* Prospective study of fruit and vegetable consumption and risk of lung cancer among men and women. *J Natl Cancer Inst* 2000; **92(22)**:1812–23.

31 Voorrips LE, Goldbohm RA, van Poppel G, Sturmans F, Hermus RJ, van den Brandt PA. Vegetable and fruit consumption and risks of colon and rectal cancer in a prospective cohort study: The Netherlands Cohort Study on Diet and Cancer. *Am J Epidemiol* 2000; **152(11)**:1081–92.

32 Brennan P, Fortes C, Butler J *et al.* A multicenter case–control study of diet and lung cancer among non-smokers. *Cancer Causes Control* 2000; **11(1)**:49–58.

33 Miller AB, Atenburg HP, Bueno-de-Mesquita B *et al.* Fruits and vegetables and lung cancer: findings from the European prospective investigation into cancer and nutrition. *Int J Cancer* 2004: **108(2)**:269–76.

34 Skuladottir H, Tjoenneland A, Overvad K *et al.* Does insufficient adjustment for smoking explain the preventive effects of fruit and vegetables on lung cancer? *Lung Cancer* 2004; **45(1)**:1–10.

35 Neuhouser ML, Patterson RE, Thornquist MD, Omenn GS, King IB, Goodman GE. Fruits and vegetables are associated with lower lung cancer risk only in the placebo arm of the beta-carotene and retinol efficacy trial (CARET). *Cancer Epidemiol Biomarkers Prev* 2003; **12(4)**:350–8.

36 Mannisto S, Smith-Warner SA, Spiegelman D *et al.* Dietary carotenoids and risk of lung cancer in a pooled analysis of seven cohort studies. *Cancer Epidemiol Biomarkers Prev* 2004; **13(1)**:40–8.

37 Holick CN, Michaud DS, Stolzenberg-Solomon R *et al.* Dietary carotenoids, serum beta-carotene, and retinol and risk of lung cancer in the alpha-tocopherol, beta-carotene cohort study. *Am J Epidemiol* 2002; **156(6)**:536–47.

38 Michaud DS, Feskanich D, Rimm EB *et al.* Intake of specific carotenoids and risk of lung cancer in 2 prospective US cohorts. *Am J Clin Nutr* 2000; **72(4)**:990–7.

39 The effect of vitamin E and beta carotene on the incidence of lung cancer and other cancers in male smokers. The Alpha-Tocopherol, Beta Carotene Cancer Prevention Study Group. *N Engl J Med* 1994; **330(15)**:1029–35.

40 Hennekens CH, Buring JE, Manson JE *et al.* Lack of effect of long-term supplementation with beta carotene on the incidence of malignant neoplasms and cardiovascular disease. *N Engl J Med* 1996; **334(18)**:1145–9.

41 Omenn GS, Goodman GE, Thornquist MD *et al.* Effects of a combination of beta carotene and vitamin A on lung cancer and cardiovascular disease. *N Engl J Med* 1996; **334(18)**:1150–5.

42 Greenwald P. Beta-carotene and lung cancer: a lesson for future chemoprevention investigations? *J Natl Cancer Inst* 2003; **95(1)**:E1.

43 Palozza P. Prooxidant actions of carotenoids in biologic systems. *Nutr Rev* 1998; **56(9)**:257–65.

44 Touvier M, Kesse E, Clavel-Chapelon F, Boutron-Ruault MC. Dual association of beta-carotene with risk of tobacco-related cancers in a cohort of French women. *J Natl Cancer Inst* 2005; **97(18)**:1338–44.

45 Choi SW, Mason JB. Folate and carcinogenesis: an integrated scheme. *J Nutr* 2000; **130(2)**:129–32.

46 Bandera EV, Freudenheim JL, Marshall JR *et al.* Diet and alcohol consumption and lung cancer risk in the New York State Cohort (United States). *Cancer Causes Control* 1997; **8(6)**:828–40.

47 Speizer FE, Colditz GA, Hunter DJ, Rosner B, Hennekens C. Prospective study of smoking, antioxidant intake, and lung cancer in middle-aged women (USA). *Cancer Causes Control* 1999; **10(5)**:475–82.

48 Voorrips LE, Goldbohm RA, Brants HA *et al.* A prospective cohort study on antioxidant and folate intake and male lung cancer risk. *Cancer Epidemiol Biomarkers Prev* 2000; **9(4)**:357–65.

49 Shen H, Wei Q, Pillow PC, Amos CI, Hong WK, Spitz MR. Dietary folate intake and lung cancer risk in former smokers: a case–control analysis. *Cancer Epidemiol Biomarkers Prev* 2003; **12(10)**:980–6.

50 Zhang Y, Talalay P. Anticarcinogenic activities of organic isothiocyanates: chemistry and mechanisms. *Cancer Res* 1994; **54(Suppl 7)**:1976s–81s.

51 Smith T, Evans K, Lythgoe MF, Anderson PJ, Gordon I. Dosimetry of pediatric radiopharmaceuticals: uniformity of effective dose and a simple aid for its estimation. *J Nucl Med* 1997; **38(12)**:1982–7.

52 Thornalley PJ. Isothiocyanates: mechanism of cancer chemopreventive action. *Anticancer Drugs* 2002; **13(4)**:331–8.

53 Brennan P, Hsu CC, Moullan N *et al.* Effect of cruciferous vegetables on lung cancer in patients stratified by genetic status: a Mendelian randomisation approach. *Lancet* 2005; **366(9496)**:1558–60.

54 Spitz MR, Duphorne CM, Detry MA *et al.* Dietary intake of isothiocyanates: evidence of a joint effect with glutathione S-transferase polymorphisms in lung cancer risk. *Cancer Epidemiol Biomarkers Prev* 2000; **9(10)**:1017–20.

55 Gao CM, Tajima K, Kuroishi T, Hirose K, Inoue M. Protective effects of raw vegetables and fruit against lung cancer among smokers and ex-smokers: a case–control study in the Tokai area of Japan. *Jpn J Cancer Res* 1993; **84(6)**:594–600.

56 Schabath MB, Hernandez LM, Wu X, Pillow PC, Spitz MR. Dietary phytoestrogens and lung cancer risk. *JAMA* 2005; **294(12)**:1493–504.

57 Wakai K, Egami I, Kato K *et al.* Dietary intake and sources of isoflavones among Japanese. *Nutr Cancer* 1999; **33(2)**:139–45.

58 Swanson CA, Mao BL, Li JY *et al.* Dietary determinants of lung-cancer risk: results from a case–control study in Yunnan Province, China. *Int J Cancer* 1992; **50(6)**:876–80.

59 Hu J, Johnson KC, Mao Y *et al.* A case–control study of diet and lung cancer in northeast China. *Int J Cancer* 1997; **71(6)**:924–31.

60 Koo LC. Dietary habits and lung cancer risk among Chinese females in Hong Kong who never smoked. *Nutr Cancer* 1988; **11(3)**:155–72.

61 Seow A, Poh WT, Teh M *et al.* Diet, reproductive factors and lung cancer risk among Chinese women in Singapore: evidence for a protective effect of soy in nonsmokers. *Int J Cancer* 2002; **97(3)**:365–71.

62 Vineis P, Veglia F, Benhamou S *et al.* CYP1A1 T3801 C polymorphism and lung cancer: a pooled analysis of 2451 cases and 3358 controls. *Int J Cancer* 2003; **104(5)**:650–7.

63 Le Marchand L, Guo C, Benhamou S *et al.* Pooled analysis of the CYP1A1 exon 7 polymorphism and lung cancer (United States). *Cancer Causes Control* 2003; **14(4)**:339–46.

64 Spencer DL, Masten SA, Lanier KM *et al.* Quantitative analysis of constitutive and 2,3,7,8-tetrachlorodibenzo-p-dioxin-induced cytochrome P450 1B1 expression in human lymphocytes. *Cancer Epidemiol Biomarkers Prev* 1999; **8(2)**:139–46.

65 Liang G, Pu Y, Yin L. Rapid detection of single nucleotide polymorphisms related with lung cancer susceptibility of Chinese population. *Cancer Lett* 2005; **223(2)**:265–74.

66 Sorensen M, Autrup H, Tjonneland A, Overvad K, Raaschou-Nielsen O. Genetic polymorphisms in CYP1B1, GSTA1, NQO1 and NAT2 and the risk of lung cancer. *Cancer Lett* 2005; **221(2)**:185–90.

67 Nunoya KI, Yokoi T, Kimura K, *et al.* A new CYP2A6 gene deletion responsible for the in vivo polymorphic metabolism of (+)-cis-3,5-dimethyl-2-(3-pyridyl)thiazolidin-4-one hydrochloride in humans. *J Pharmacol Exp Ther* 1999; **289(1)**:437–42.

68 Miyamoto M, Umetsu Y, Dosaka-Akita H *et al.* CYP2A6 gene deletion reduces susceptibility to lung cancer. *Biochem Biophys Res Commun* 1999; **261(3)**:658–60.

69 Ariyoshi N, Miyamoto M, Umetsu Y *et al.* Genetic polymorphism of CYP2A6 gene and tobacco-induced lung cancer risk in male smokers. *Cancer Epidemiol Biomarkers Prev* 2002; **11(9)**:890–4.

70 Fujieda M, Yamazaki H, Saito T *et al.* Evaluation of CYP2A6 genetic polymorphisms as determinants of smoking behavior and tobacco-related lung cancer risk in male Japanese smokers. *Carcinogenesis* 2004; **25(12)**:2451–8.

71 Kubota T, Nakajima-Taniguchi C, Fukuda T *et al.* CYP2A6 polymorphisms are associated with nicotine dependence and influence withdrawal symptoms in smoking cessation. *Pharmacogenomics J* 2006; **6(2)**:115–9.

72 Koskela S, Hakkola J, Hukkanen J *et al.* Expression of CYP2A genes in human liver and extrahepatic tissues. *Biochem Pharmacol* 1999; **57(12)**:1407–13.

73 Gu J, Su T, Chen Y, Zhang QY, Ding X. Expression of biotransformation enzymes in human fetal olfactory mucosa: potential roles in developmental toxicity. *Toxicol Appl Pharmacol* 2000; **165(2)**:158–62.

74 Ding X, Kaminsky LS. Human extrahepatic cytochromes P450: function in xenobiotic metabolism and tissue-selective chemical toxicity in the respiratory and gastrointestinal tracts. *Annu Rev Pharmacol Toxicol* 2003; **43**:149–73.

75 Wang H, Tan W, Hao B *et al.* Substantial reduction in risk of lung adenocarcinoma associated with genetic polymorphism in CYP2A13, the most active cytochrome P450 for the metabolic activation of tobacco-specific carcinogen NNK. *Cancer Res* 2003; **63(22)**:8057–61.

76 Zhang X, Su T, Zhang QY *et al.* Genetic polymorphisms of the human CYP2A13 gene: identification of single-nucleotide polymorphisms and functional characterization of an Arg257Cys variant. *J Pharmacol Exp Ther* 2002; **302(2)**:416–23.

77 Garcia-Martin E, Martinez C, Ladero JM, Gamito FJ, Rodriguez-Lescure A, Agundez JA. Influence of cytochrome P450 CYP2C9 genotypes in lung cancer risk. *Cancer Lett* 2002; **180(1)**:41–6.

78 London SJ, Sullivan-Klose T, Daly AK, Idle JR. Lung cancer risk in relation to the CYP2C9 genetic polymorphism among Caucasians in Los Angeles County. *Pharmacogenetics* 1997; **7(5)**:401–4.

79 London SJ, Daly AK, Leathart JB, Navidi WC, Idle JR. Lung cancer risk in relation to the CYP2C9*1/CYP2C9*2 genetic polymorphism among African-Americans and Caucasians in Los Angeles County, California. *Pharmacogenetics* 1996; **6(6)**:527–33.

80 Christensen PM, Gotzsche PC, Brosen K. The sparteine/debrisoquine (CYP2D6) oxidation polymorphism and the risk of lung cancer: a meta-analysis. *Eur J Clin Pharmacol* 1997; **51(5)**:389–93.

81 Laforest L, Wikman H, Benhamou S *et al.* CYP2D6 gene polymorphism in Caucasian smokers: lung cancer susceptibility and phenotype–genotype relationships. *Eur J Cancer* 2000; **36(14)**:1825–32.

82 Butkiewicz D, Cole KJ, Phillips DH, Harris CC, Chorazy M. GSTM1, GSTP1, CYP1A1 and CYP2D6 polymorphisms in lung cancer patients from an

environmentally polluted region of Poland: correlation with lung DNA adduct levels. *Eur J Cancer Prev* 1999; **8(4)**:315–23.

83 Uematsu F, Kikuchi H, Motomiya M *et al.* Association between restriction fragment length polymorphism of the human cytochrome P450IIE1 gene and susceptibility to lung cancer. *Jpn J Cancer Res* 1991; **82(3)**:254–6.

84 Wang J, Deng Y, Li L *et al.* Association of GSTM1, CYP1A1 and CYP2E1 genetic polymorphisms with susceptibility to lung adenocarcinoma: a case–control study in Chinese population. *Cancer Sci* 2003; **94(5)**:448–52.

85 Persson I, Johansson I, Bergling H *et al.* Genetic polymorphism of cytochrome P4502E1 in a Swedish population. Relationship to incidence of lung cancer. *FEBS Lett* 1993; **319(3)**:207–11.

86 Le Marchand L, Sivaraman L, Pierce L *et al.* Associations of CYP1A1, GSTM1, and CYP2E1 polymorphisms with lung cancer suggest cell type specificities to tobacco carcinogens. *Cancer Res* 1998; **58(21)**:4858–63.

87 Wu X, Shi H, Jiang H *et al.* Associations between cytochrome P4502E1 genotype, mutagen sensitivity, cigarette smoking and susceptibility to lung cancer. *Carcinogenesis* 1997; **18(5)**:967–73.

88 Wang SL, Lee H, Chen KW, Tsai KJ, Chen CY, Lin P. Cytochrome P4502E1 genetic polymorphisms and lung cancer in a Taiwanese population. *Lung Cancer* 1999; **26(1)**:27–34.

89 Marchand LL, Wilkinson GR, Wilkens LR. Genetic and dietary predictors of CYP2E1 activity: a phenotyping study in Hawaii Japanese using chlorzoxazone. *Cancer Epidemiol Biomarkers Prev* 1999; **8(6)**:495–500.

90 Uematsu F, Ikawa S, Kikuchi H *et al.* Restriction fragment length polymorphism of the human CYP2E1 (cytochrome P450IIE1) gene and susceptibility to lung cancer: possible relevance to low smoking exposure. *Pharmacogenetics* 1994; **4(2)**:58–63.

91 Uematsu F, Kikuchi H, Motomiya M *et al.* Human cytochrome P450IIE1 gene: DraI polymorphism and susceptibility to cancer. *Tohoku J Exp Med* 1992; **168(2)**:113–7.

92 Wu X, Amos CI, Kemp BL *et al.* Cytochrome P450 2E1 DraI polymorphisms in lung cancer in minority populations. *Cancer Epidemiol Biomarkers Prev* 1998; **7(1)**:13–8.

93 Piedrafita FJ, Molander RB, Vansant G, Orlova EA, Pfahl M, Reynolds WF. An Alu element in the myeloperoxidase promoter contains a composite SP1-thyroid hormone-retinoic acid response element. *J Biol Chem* 1996; **271(24)**:14412–20.

94 Van Schooten FJ, Boots AW, Knaapen AM *et al.* Myeloperoxidase (MPO) −463G→A reduces MPO activity and DNA adduct levels in bronchoalveolar lavages of smokers. *Cancer Epidemiol Biomarkers Prev* 2004; **13(5)**:828–33.

95 Feyler A, Voho A, Bouchardy C *et al.* Point: myeloperoxidase −463G→ a polymorphism and lung cancer risk. *Cancer Epidemiol Biomarkers Prev* 2002; **11(12)**:1550–4.

96 Schabath MB, Spitz MR, Hong WK *et al.* A myeloperoxidase polymorphism associated with reduced risk of lung cancer. *Lung Cancer* 2002; **37(1)**:35–40.

97 Ye Z, Song H, Higgins JP, Pharoah P, Danesh J. Five glutathione s-transferase gene variants in 23,452 cases of lung cancer and 30,397 controls: meta-analysis of 130 studies. *PLoS Med* 2006; **3(4)**:e91.

98 Ali-Osman F, Akande O, Antoun G, Mao JX, Buolamwini J. Molecular cloning, characterization, and expression in Escherichia coli of full-length cDNAs of three human glutathione S-transferase Pi gene variants. Evidence for differential catalytic activity of the encoded proteins. *J Biol Chem* 1997; **272(15)**:10004–12.

99 Bouchardy C, Mitrunen K, Wikman H *et al.* N-acetyltransferase NAT1 and NAT2 genotypes and lung cancer risk. *Pharmacogenetics* 1998; **8(4)**:291–8.

100 Wikman H, Thiel S, Jager B *et al.* Relevance of N-acetyltransferase 1 and 2 (NAT1, NAT2) genetic polymorphisms in non-small cell lung cancer susceptibility. *Pharmacogenetics* 2001; **11(2)**:157–68.

101 Abdel-Rahman SZ, El-Zein RA, Zwischenberger JB, Au WW. Association of the NAT1*10 genotype with increased chromosome aberrations and higher lung cancer risk in cigarette smokers. *Mutat Res* 1998; **398(1–2)**:43–54.

102 Borlak J, Reamon-Buettner SM. N-acetyltransferase 2 (NAT2) gene polymorphisms in colon and lung cancer patients. *BMC Med Genet* 2006; **7**:58.

103 Araki J, Kobayashi Y, Iwasa M *et al.* Polymorphism of UDP-glucuronosyltransferase 1A7 gene: a possible new risk factor for lung cancer. *Eur J Cancer* 2005; **41(15)**:2360–5.

104 Nowell S, Ambrosone CB, Ozawa S *et al.* Relationship of phenol sulfotransferase activity (SULT1A1) genotype to sulfotransferase phenotype in platelet cytosol. *Pharmacogenetics* 2000; **10(9)**:789–97.

105 Liang G, Miao X, Zhou Y, Tan W, Lin D. A functional polymorphism in the SULT1A1 gene (G638A)

is associated with risk of lung cancer in relation to tobacco smoking. *Carcinogenesis* 2004; **25(5)**:773–8.

106 Wang Y, Spitz MR, Tsou AM, Zhang K, Makan N, Wu X. Sulfotransferase (SULT) 1A1 polymorphism as a predisposition factor for lung cancer: a case–control analysis. *Lung Cancer* 2002; **35(2)**:137–42.

107 Kuehl BL, Paterson JW, Peacock JW, Paterson MC, Rauth AM. Presence of a heterozygous substitution and its relationship to DT-diaphorase activity. *Br J Cancer* 1995; **72(3)**:555–61.

108 Siegel D, McGuinness SM, Winski SL, Ross D. Genotype–phenotype relationships in studies of a polymorphism in NAD(P)H:quinone oxidoreductase 1. *Pharmacogenetics* 1999; **9(1)**:113–21.

109 Chao C, Zhang ZF, Berthiller J, Boffetta P, Hashibe M. NAD(P)H:quinone oxidoreductase 1 (NQO1) Pro187Ser polymorphism and the risk of lung, bladder, and colorectal cancers: a meta-analysis. *Cancer Epidemiol Biomarkers Prev* 2006; **15(5)**: 979–87.

110 Oesch F. Mammalian epoxide hydrases: inducible enzymes catalysing the inactivation of carcinogenic and cytotoxic metabolites derived from aromatic and olefinic compounds. *Xenobiotica* 1973; **3(5)**:305–40.

111 Lee WJ, Brennan P, Boffetta P et al. Microsomal epoxide hydrolase polymorphisms and lung cancer risk: a quantitative review. *Biomarkers* 2002; **7(3)**:230–41.

112 Gsur A, Zidek T, Schnattinger K et al. Association of microsomal epoxide hydrolase polymorphisms and lung cancer risk. *Br J Cancer* 2003; **89(4)**:702–6.

113 Forsberg L, de Faire U, Morgenstern R. Oxidative stress, human genetic variation, and disease. *Arch Biochem Biophys* 2001; **389(1)**:84–93.

114 Ratnasinghe D, Tangrea JA, Andersen MR et al. Glutathione peroxidase codon 198 polymorphism variant increases lung cancer risk. *Cancer Res* 2000; **60(22)**:6381–3.

115 Lee CH, Lee KY, Choe KH et al. Effects of oxidative DNA damage and genetic polymorphism of the glutathione peroxidase 1 (GPX1) and 8-oxoguanine glycosylase 1 (hOGG1) on lung cancer. *J Prev Med Public Health* 2006; **39(2)**:130–4.

116 Raaschou-Nielsen O, Sorensen M, Hansen RD et al. GPX1 Pro198Leu polymorphism, interactions with smoking and alcohol consumption, and risk for lung cancer. *Cancer Lett* 2007; **247(2)**:293–300.

117 Goode EL, Ulrich CM, Potter JD. Polymorphisms in DNA repair genes and associations with cancer risk. *Cancer Epidemiol Biomarkers Prev* 2002; **11(12)**:1513–30.

118 Hoeijmakers JH. Genome maintenance mechanisms for preventing cancer. *Nature* 2001; **411(6835)**:366–74.

119 Friedberg EC. How nucleotide excision repair protects against cancer. *Nat Rev Cancer* 2001; **1(1)**:22–33.

120 Manuguerra M, Saletta F, Karagas MR et al. XRCC3 and XPD/ERCC2 single nucleotide polymorphisms and the risk of cancer: a HuGE review. *Am J Epidemiol* 2006; **164(4)**:297–302.

121 Spitz MR, Wu X, Wang Y et al. Modulation of nucleotide excision repair capacity by XPD polymorphisms in lung cancer patients. *Cancer Res* 2001; **61(4)**:1354–7.

122 Wu X, Zhao H, Wei Q et al. XPA polymorphism associated with reduced lung cancer risk and a modulating effect on nucleotide excision repair capacity. *Carcinogenesis* 2003; **24(3)**:505–9.

123 Park JY, Park SH, Choi JE et al. Polymorphisms of the DNA repair gene xeroderma pigmentosum group A and risk of primary lung cancer. *Cancer Epidemiol Biomarkers Prev* 2002; **11(10, Pt 1)**:993–7.

124 Butkiewicz D, Popanda O, Risch A et al. Association between the risk for lung adenocarcinoma and a (−4) G-to-A polymorphism in the XPA gene. *Cancer Epidemiol Biomarkers Prev* 2004; **13(12)**:2242–6.

125 Zienolddiny S, Campa D, Lind H et al. Polymorphisms of DNA repair genes and risk of non-small cell lung cancer. *Carcinogenesis* 2006; **27(3)**:560–7.

126 Lee GY, Jang JS, Lee SY et al. XPC polymorphisms and lung cancer risk. *Int J Cancer* 2005; **115(5)**:807–13.

127 Qiao Y, Spitz MR, Shen H et al. Modulation of repair of ultraviolet damage in the host-cell reactivation assay by polymorphic XPC and XPD/ERCC2 genotypes. *Carcinogenesis* 2002; **23(2)**:295–9.

128 Marin MS, Lopez-Cima MF, Garcia-Castro L, Pascual T, Marron MG, Tardon A. Poly (AT) polymorphism in intron 11 of the XPC DNA repair gene enhances the risk of lung cancer. *Cancer Epidemiol Biomarkers Prev* 2004; **13(11, Pt 1)**:1788–93.

129 Hu Z, Wang Y, Wang X et al. DNA repair gene XPC genotypes/haplotypes and risk of lung cancer in a Chinese population. *Int J Cancer* 2005; **115(3)**:478–83.

130 Chen P, Wiencke J, Aldape K et al. Association of an ERCC1 polymorphism with adult-onset glioma. *Cancer Epidemiol Biomarkers Prev* 2000; **9(8)**:843–7.

131 Yu JJ, Lee KB, Mu C et al. Comparison of two human ovarian carcinoma cell lines (A2780/CP70 and MCAS) that are equally resistant to platinum, but differ at codon 118 of the ERCC1 gene. *Int J Oncol* 2000; **16(3)**:555–60.

132 Zhou W, Liu G, Park S *et al.* Gene-smoking interaction associations for the ERCC1 polymorphisms in the risk of lung cancer. *Cancer Epidemiol Biomarkers Prev* 2005; **14(2)**:491–6.

133 Jeon HS, Kim KM, Park SH *et al.* Relationship between XPG codon 1104 polymorphism and risk of primary lung cancer. *Carcinogenesis* 2003; **24(10)**:1677–81.

134 Cui Y, Morgenstern H, Greenland S *et al.* Polymorphism of Xeroderma Pigmentosum group G and the risk of lung cancer and squamous cell carcinomas of the oropharynx, larynx and esophagus. *Int J Cancer* 2006; **118(3)**:714–20.

135 Sakumi K, Tominaga Y, Furuichi M *et al.* Ogg1 knockout-associated lung tumorigenesis and its suppression by Mth1 gene disruption. *Cancer Res* 2003; **63(5)**:902–5.

136 Le Marchand L, Donlon T, Lum-Jones A, Seifried A, Wilkens LR. Association of the hOGG1 Ser326Cys polymorphism with lung cancer risk. *Cancer Epidemiol Biomarkers Prev* 2002; **11(4)**:409–12.

137 Park J, Chen L, Tockman MS, Elahi A, Lazarus P. The human 8-oxoguanine DNA N-glycosylase 1 (hOGG1) DNA repair enzyme and its association with lung cancer risk. *Pharmacogenetics* 2004; **14(2)**:103–9.

138 Sugimura H, Kohno T, Wakai K *et al.* hOGG1 Ser326Cys polymorphism and lung cancer susceptibility. *Cancer Epidemiol Biomarkers Prev* 1999; **8(8)**:669–74.

139 Hung RJ, Brennan P, Canzian F *et al.* Large-scale investigation of base excision repair genetic polymorphisms and lung cancer risk in a multicenter study. *J Natl Cancer Inst* 2005; **97(8)**:567–76.

140 Hung RJ, Hall J, Brennan P, Boffetta P. Genetic polymorphisms in the base excision repair pathway and cancer risk: a HuGE review. *Am J Epidemiol* 2005; **162(10)**:925–42.

141 Kohno T, Shinmura K, Tosaka M *et al.* Genetic polymorphisms and alternative splicing of the hOGG1 gene, that is involved in the repair of 8-hydroxyguanine in damaged DNA. *Oncogene* 1998; **16(25)**:3219–25.

142 Popanda O, Schattenberg T, Phong CT *et al.* Specific combinations of DNA repair gene variants and increased risk for non-small cell lung cancer. *Carcinogenesis* 2004; **25(12)**:2433–41.

143 Misra RR, Ratnasinghe D, Tangrea JA *et al.* Polymorphisms in the DNA repair genes XPD, XRCC1, XRCC3, and APE/ref-1, and the risk of lung cancer among male smokers in Finland. *Cancer Lett* 2003; **191(2)**:171–8.

144 Ito H, Matsuo K, Hamajima N *et al.* Gene-environment interactions between the smoking habit and polymorphisms in the DNA repair genes, APE1 Asp148Glu and XRCC1 Arg399Gln, in Japanese lung cancer risk. *Carcinogenesis* 2004; **25(8)**:1395–401.

145 Wang Y, Spitz MR, Zhu Y, Dong Q, Shete S, Wu X. From genotype to phenotype: correlating XRCC1 polymorphisms with mutagen sensitivity. *DNA Repair (Amst)* 2003; **2(8)**:901–8.

146 Ratnasinghe D, Yao SX, Tangrea JA *et al.* Polymorphisms of the DNA repair gene XRCC1 and lung cancer risk. *Cancer Epidemiol Biomarkers Prev* 2001; **10(2)**:119–23.

147 David-Beabes GL, London SJ. Genetic polymorphism of XRCC1 and lung cancer risk among African-Americans and Caucasians. *Lung Cancer* 2001; **34(3)**:333–9.

148 Harms C, Salama SA, Sierra-Torres CH, Cajas-Salazar N, Au WW. Polymorphisms in DNA repair genes, chromosome aberrations, and lung cancer. *Environ Mol Mutagen* 2004; **44(1)**:74–82.

149 Chen S, Tang D, Xue K *et al.* DNA repair gene XRCC1 and XPD polymorphisms and risk of lung cancer in a Chinese population. *Carcinogenesis* 2002; **23(8)**:1321–5.

150 Zhang X, Miao X, Liang G *et al.* Polymorphisms in DNA base excision repair genes ADPRT and XRCC1 and risk of lung cancer. *Cancer Res* 2005; **65(3)**:722–6.

151 Hu Z, Ma H, Lu D *et al.* A promoter polymorphism (−77T>C) of DNA repair gene XRCC1 is associated with risk of lung cancer in relation to tobacco smoking. *Pharmacogenet Genomics* 2005; **15(7)**:457–63.

152 Matullo G, Palli D, Peluso M *et al.* XRCC1, XRCC3, XPD gene polymorphisms, smoking and (32)P-DNA adducts in a sample of healthy subjects. *Carcinogenesis* 2001; **22(9)**:1437–45.

153 Shiloh Y. ATM and related protein kinases: safeguarding genome integrity. *Nat Rev Cancer* 2003; **3(3)**:155–68.

154 Kim JH, Kim H, Lee KY *et al.* Genetic polymorphisms of ataxia telangiectasia mutated affect lung cancer risk. *Hum Mol Genet* 2006; **15(7)**:1181–6.

155 Matullo G, Dunning AM, Guarrera S *et al.* DNA repair polymorphisms and cancer risk in non-smokers in a cohort study. *Carcinogenesis* 2006; **27(5)**:997–1007.

156 Lan Q, Shen M, Berndt SI *et al.* Smoky coal exposure, NBS1 polymorphisms, p53 protein accumulation, and lung cancer risk in Xuan Wei, China. *Lung Cancer* 2005; **49(3)**:317–23.

157 David-Beabes GL, Lunn RM, London SJ. No association between the XPD (Lys751G1n) polymorphism or the XRCC3 (Thr241Met) polymorphism and lung cancer risk. *Cancer Epidemiol Biomarkers Prev* 2001; **10(8)**:911–2.

158 Sakiyama T, Kohno T, Mimaki S *et al.* Association of amino acid substitution polymorphisms in DNA repair genes TP53, POLI, REV1 and LIG4 with lung cancer risk. *Int J Cancer* 2005; **114(5)**:730–7.

159 Park SH, Lee GY, Jeon HS *et al.* −93G→A polymorphism of hMLH1 and risk of primary lung cancer. *Int J Cancer* 2004; **112(4)**:678–82.

160 Jung CY, Choi JE, Park JM *et al.* Polymorphisms in the hMSH2 gene and the risk of primary lung cancer. *Cancer Epidemiol Biomarkers Prev* 2006; **15(4)**:762–8.

161 Potter JD, Goode E, Morimoto L. AACR special conference: the molecular and genetic epidemiology of cancer. *Cancer Epidemiol Biomarkers Prev* 2003; **12(8)**:803–5.

162 Spitz MR, Wei Q, Dong Q, Amos CI, Wu X. Genetic susceptibility to lung cancer: the role of DNA damage and repair. *Cancer Epidemiol Biomarkers Prev* 2003; **12(8)**:689–98.

163 Hsu TC, Johnston DA, Cherry LM *et al.* Sensitivity to genotoxic effects of bleomycin in humans: possible relationship to environmental carcinogenesis. *Int J Cancer* 1989; **43(3)**:403–9.

164 Wu X, Gu J, Amos CI, Jiang H, Hong WK, Spitz MR. A parallel study of in vitro sensitivity to benzo[a]pyrene diol epoxide and bleomycin in lung carcinoma cases and controls. *Cancer* 1998; **83(6)**:1118–27.

165 Burger RM, Peisach J, Horwitz SB. Mechanism of bleomycin action: in vitro studies. *Life Sci* 1981; **28(7)**:715–27.

166 Wei Q, Gu J, Cheng L *et al.* Benzo(a)pyrene diol epoxide-induced chromosomal aberrations and risk of lung cancer. *Cancer Res* 1996; **56(17)**:3975–9.

167 Strom SS, Wu S, Sigurdson AJ *et al.* Lung cancer, smoking patterns, and mutagen sensitivity in Mexican-Americans. *J Natl Cancer Inst Monogr* 1995; **(18)**:29–33.

168 Kassie F, Parzefall W, Knasmuller S. Single cell gel electrophoresis assay: a new technique for human biomonitoring studies. *Mutat Res* 2000; **463(1)**:13–31.

169 Tice RR, Agurell E, Anderson D *et al.* Single cell gel/comet assay: guidelines for in vitro and in vivo genetic toxicology testing. *Environ Mol Mutagen* 2000; **35(3)**:206–21.

170 Moller P, Knudsen LE, Loft S, Wallin H. The comet assay as a rapid test in biomonitoring occupational exposure to DNA-damaging agents and effect of confounding factors. *Cancer Epidemiol Biomarkers Prev* 2000; **9(10)**:1005–15.

171 Wu X, Roth JA, Zhao H *et al.* Cell cycle checkpoints, DNA damage/repair, and lung cancer risk. *Cancer Res* 2005; **65(1)**:349–57.

172 Rajaee-Behbahani N, Schmezer P, Risch A *et al.* Altered DNA repair capacity and bleomycin sensitivity as risk markers for non-small cell lung cancer. *Int J Cancer* 2001; **95(2)**:86–91.

173 Li D, Wang M, Cheng L, Spitz MR, Hittelman WN, Wei Q. In vitro induction of benzo(a)pyrene diol epoxide-DNA adducts in peripheral lymphocytes as a susceptibility marker for human lung cancer. *Cancer Res* 1996; **56(16)**:3638–41.

174 Li D, Firozi PF, Wang LE *et al.* Sensitivity to DNA damage induced by benzo(a)pyrene diol epoxide and risk of lung cancer: a case–control analysis. *Cancer Res* 2001; **61(4)**:1445–50.

175 Shen H, Spitz MR, Qiao Y *et al.* Smoking, DNA repair capacity and risk of nonsmall cell lung cancer. *Int J Cancer* 2003; **107(1)**:84–8.

176 Wei Q, Cheng L, Amos CI *et al.* Repair of tobacco carcinogen-induced DNA adducts and lung cancer risk: a molecular epidemiologic study. *J Natl Cancer Inst* 2000; **92(21)**:1764–72.

177 Wei Q, Cheng L, Hong WK, Spitz MR. Reduced DNA repair capacity in lung cancer patients. *Cancer Res* 1996; **56(18)**:4103–7.

178 Koch KS, Fletcher RG, Grond MP *et al.* Inactivation of plasmid reporter gene expression by one benzo(a)pyrene diol-epoxide DNA adduct in adult rat hepatocytes. *Cancer Res* 1993; **53(Suppl 10)**: 2279–86.

179 Paz-Elizur T, Krupsky M, Blumenstein S, Elinger D, Schechtman E, Livneh Z. DNA repair activity for oxidative damage and risk of lung cancer. *J Natl Cancer Inst* 2003; **95(17)**:1312–9.

180 Gackowski D Speina E, Zielinska M *et al.* Products of oxidative DNA damage and repair as possible biomarkers of susceptibility to lung cancer. *Cancer Res* 2003; **63(16)**:4899–902.

181 Vincenzi B, Schiavon G, Silletta M *et al.* Cell cycle alterations and lung cancer. *Histol Histopathol* 2006; **21(4)**:423–35.

182 Au NH, Cheang M, Huntsman DG *et al.* Evaluation of immunohistochemical markers in non-small cell lung cancer by unsupervised hierarchical clustering analysis: a tissue microarray study of 284 cases and 18 markers. *J Pathol* 2004; **204(1)**:101–9.

183 Singhal S, Vachani A, Antin-Ozerkis D, Kaiser LR, Albelda SM. Prognostic implications of cell cycle, apoptosis, and angiogenesis biomarkers in non-small cell lung cancer: a review. *Clin Cancer Res* 2005; **11(11)**:3974–86.

184 Abdulkader I, Sanchez L, Cameselle-Teijeiro J *et al.* Cell-cycle-associated markers and clinical outcome in human epithelial cancers: a tissue microarray study. *Oncol Rep* 2005; **14(6)**:1527–31.

185 Weston A, Perrin LS, Forrester K *et al.* Allelic frequency of a p53 polymorphism in human lung cancer. *Cancer Epidemiol Biomarkers Prev* 1992; **1(6)**: 481–3.

186 To-Figueras J, Gene M, Gomez-Catalan J *et al.* Glutathione-S-Transferase M1 and codon 72 p53 polymorphisms in a northwestern Mediterranean population and their relation to lung cancer susceptibility. *Cancer Epidemiol Biomarkers Prev* 1996; **5(5)**:337–42.

187 Wu X, Zhao H, Amos CI *et al.* p53 genotypes and haplotypes associated with lung cancer susceptibility and ethnicity. *J Natl Cancer Inst* 2002; **94(9)**:681–90.

188 Liu G, Miller DP, Zhou W *et al.* Differential association of the codon 72 p53 and GSTM1 polymorphisms on histological subtype of non-small cell lung carcinoma. *Cancer Res* 2001; **61(24)**:8718–22.

189 Szymanowska A, Jassem E, Dziadziuszko R *et al.* Increased risk of non-small cell lung cancer and frequency of somatic TP53 gene mutations in Pro72 carriers of TP53 Arg72Pro polymorphism. *Lung Cancer* 2006; **52(1)**:9–14.

190 Zhang X, Miao X, Guo Y *et al.* Genetic polymorphisms in cell cycle regulatory genes MDM2 and TP53 are associated with susceptibility to lung cancer. *Hum Mutat* 2006; **27(1)**:110–7.

191 Irarrazabal CE, Rojas C, Aracena R, Marquez C, Gil L. Chilean pilot study on the risk of lung cancer associated with codon 72 polymorphism in the gene of protein p53. *Toxicol Lett* 2003; **144(1)**:69–76.

192 Biros E, Kohut A, Biros I, Kalina I, Bogyiova E, Stubna J. A link between the p53 germ line polymorphisms and white blood cells apoptosis in lung cancer patients. *Lung Cancer* 2002; **35(3)**:231–5.

193 Hu Y, McDermott MP, Ahrendt SA. The p53 codon 72 proline allele is associated with p53 gene mutations in non-small cell lung cancer. *Clin Cancer Res* 2005; **11(7)**:2502–9.

194 Hung RJ, Boffetta P, Canzian F *et al.* Sequence variants in cell cycle control pathway, X-ray exposure, and lung cancer risk: a multicenter case–control study in central Europe. *Cancer Res* 2006; **66(16)**:8280–6.

195 Matakidou A, Eisen T, Houlston RS. TP53 polymorphisms and lung cancer risk: a systematic review and meta-analysis. *Mutagenesis* 2003; **18(4)**:377–85.

196 Zhu J, Jiang J, Zhou W, Chen X. The potential tumor suppressor p73 differentially regulates cellular p53 target genes. *Cancer Res* 1998; **58(22)**:5061–5.

197 Li G, Wang LE, Chamberlain RM, Amos CI, Spitz MR, Wei Q. p73 G4C14-to-A4T14 polymorphism and risk of lung cancer. *Cancer Res* 2004; **64(19)**:6863–6.

198 Hu Z, Miao X, Ma H *et al.* Dinucleotide polymorphism of p73 gene is associated with a reduced risk of lung cancer in a Chinese population. *Int J Cancer* 2005; **114(3)**:455–60.

199 Schabath MB, Wu X, Wei Q, Li G, Gu J, Spitz MR. Combined effects of the p53 and p73 polymorphisms on lung cancer risk. *Cancer Epidemiol Biomarkers Prev* 2006; **15(1)**:158–61.

200 Brooks CL, Gu W. p53 ubiquitination: Mdm2 and beyond. *Mol Cell* 2006; **21(3)**:307–15.

201 Park SH, Choi JE, Kim EJ *et al.* MDM2 309T>G polymorphism and risk of lung cancer in a Korean population. *Lung Cancer* 2006; **54(1)**:19–24.

202 Lind H, Zienolddiny S, Ekstrom PO, Skaug V, Haugen A. Association of a functional polymorphism in the promoter of the MDM2 gene with risk of nonsmall cell lung cancer. *Int J Cancer* 2006; **119(3)**:718–21.

203 Hu Z, Ma H, Lu D *et al.* Genetic variants in the MDM2 promoter and lung cancer risk in a Chinese population. *Int J Cancer* 2006; **118(5)**:1275–8.

204 Pine SR, Mechanic LE, Bowman ED *et al.* MDM2 SNP309 and SNP354 are not associated with lung cancer risk. *Cancer Epidemiol Biomarkers Prev* 2006; **15(8)**:1559–61.

205 Bond GL, Hu W, Bond EE *et al.* A single nucleotide polymorphism in the MDM2 promoter attenuates the p53 tumor suppressor pathway and accelerates tumor formation in humans. *Cell* 2004; **119(5)**:591–602.

206 Chen MJ, Lin YT, Lieberman HB, Chen G, Lee EY. ATM-dependent phosphorylation of human Rad9 is required for ionizing radiation-induced checkpoint activation. *J Biol Chem* 2001; **276(19)**:16580–6.

207 Maniwa Y, Yoshimura M, Bermudez VP *et al.* His239Arg SNP of HRAD9 is associated with lung adenocarcinoma. *Cancer* 2006; **106(5)**:1117–22.

208 Ng PC, Henikoff S. Accounting for human polymorphisms predicted to affect protein function. *Genome Res* 2002; **12(3)**:436–46.

209 Dobashi Y. Cell cycle regulation and its aberrations in human lung carcinoma. *Pathol Int* 2005; **55(3)**:95–105.

210 Betticher DC, Thatcher N, Altermatt HJ, Hoban P, Ryder WD, Heighway J. Alternate splicing produces a novel cyclin D1 transcript. *Oncogene* 1995; **11(5)**:1005–11.

211 Qiuling S, Yuxin Z, Suhua Z, Cheng X, Shuguang L, Fengsheng H. Cyclin D1 gene polymorphism and susceptibility to lung cancer in a Chinese population. *Carcinogenesis* 2003; **24(9)**:1499–503.

212 Lu F, Gladden AB, Diehl JA. An alternatively spliced cyclin D1 isoform, cyclin D1b, is a nuclear oncogene. *Cancer Res* 2003; **63(21)**:7056–61.

213 Nigg EA. Centrosome aberrations: cause or consequence of cancer progression? *Nat Rev Cancer* 2002; **2(11)**:815–25.

214 Kim TM, Yim SH, Lee JS *et al.* Genome-wide screening of genomic alterations and their clinicopathologic implications in non-small cell lung cancers. *Clin Cancer Res* 2005; **11(23)**:8235–42.

215 Gu J, Gong Y, Huang M, Lu C, Spitz MR, Wu X. Polymorphisms of STK15 (Aurora-A) gene and lung cancer risk in Caucasians. *Carcinogenesis* 2006.

216 Ewart-Toland A, Dai Q, Gao YT *et al.* Aurora-A/STK15 T+91A is a general low penetrance cancer susceptibility gene: a meta-analysis of multiple cancer types. *Carcinogenesis* 2005; **26(8)**:1368–73.

217 Zhao H, Spitz MR, Tomlinson GE, Zhang H, Minna JD, Wu X. Gamma-radiation-induced G2 delay, apoptosis, and p53 response as potential susceptibility markers for lung cancer. *Cancer Res* 2001; **61(21)**:7819–24.

218 Zheng YL, Loffredo CA, Alberg AJ *et al.* Less efficient g2-m checkpoint is associated with an increased risk of lung cancer in African Americans. *Cancer Res* 2005; **65(20)**:9566–73.

219 Zhang X, Miao X, Sun T *et al.* Functional polymorphisms in cell death pathway genes FAS and FASL contribute to risk of lung cancer. *J Med Genet* 2005; **42(6)**:479–84.

220 Park JY, Park JM, Jang JS *et al.* Caspase 9 promoter polymorphisms and risk of primary lung cancer. *Hum Mol Genet* 2006; **15(12)**:1963–71.

221 Gavrieli Y, Sherman Y, Ben-Sasson SA. Identification of programmed cell death in situ via specific labeling of nuclear DNA fragmentation. *J Cell Biol* 1992; **119(3)**:493–501.

222 Rhodes D, Giraldo R. Telomere structure and function. *Curr Opin Struct Biol* 1995; **5(3)**:311–22.

223 Wu X, Amos CI, Zhu Y *et al.* Telomere dysfunction: a potential cancer predisposition factor. *J Natl Cancer Inst* 2003; **95(16)**:1211–8.

224 Wang L, Soria JC, Chang YS, Lee HY, Wei Q, Mao L. Association of a functional tandem repeats in the downstream of human telomerase gene and lung cancer. *Oncogene* 2003; **22(46)**:7123–9.

225 Hsu CP, Hsu NY, Lee LW, Ko JL. Ets2 binding site single nucleotide polymorphism at the hTERT gene promoter—effect on telomerase expression and telomere length maintenance in non-small cell lung cancer. *Eur J Cancer* 2006; **42(10)**:1466–74.

226 Phillips J, Kluss B, Richter A, Massey E. Exposure of bronchial epithelial cells to whole cigarette smoke: assessment of cellular responses. *Altern Lab Anim* 2005; **33(3)**:239–48.

227 Huntington JT, Shields JM, Der CJ *et al.* Overexpression of collagenase 1 (MMP-1) is mediated by the ERK pathway in invasive melanoma cells: role of BRAF mutation and fibroblast growth factor signaling. *J Biol Chem* 2004; **279(32)**:33168–76.

228 Franchi A, Santucci M, Masini E, Sardi I, Paglierani M, Gallo O. Expression of matrix metalloproteinase 1, matrix metalloproteinase 2, and matrix metalloproteinase 9 in carcinoma of the head and neck. *Cancer* 2002; **95(9)**:1902–10.

229 O-charoenrat P, Leksrisakul P, Sangruchi S. A functional polymorphism in the matrix metalloproteinase-1 gene promoter is associated with susceptibility and aggressiveness of head and neck cancer. *Int J Cancer* 2006; **118(10)**:2548–53.

230 Zhu Y, Spitz MR, Lei L, Mills GB, Wu X. A single nucleotide polymorphism in the matrix metalloproteinase-1 promoter enhances lung cancer susceptibility. *Cancer Res* 2001; **61(21)**:7825–9.

231 Su L, Zhou W, Park S *et al.* Matrix metalloproteinase-1 promoter polymorphism and lung cancer risk. *Cancer Epidemiol Biomarkers Prev* 2005; **14(3)**:567–70.

232 Fang S, Jin X, Wang R *et al.* Polymorphisms in the MMP1 and MMP3 promoter and non-small cell lung carcinoma in North China. *Carcinogenesis* 2005; **26(2)**:481–6.

233 Price SJ, Greaves DR, Watkins H. Identification of novel, functional genetic variants in the human matrix metalloproteinase-2 gene: role of Sp1 in allele-specific transcriptional regulation. *J Biol Chem* 2001; **276(10)**:7549–58.

234 Yu C, Pan K, Xing D *et al.* Correlation between a single nucleotide polymorphism in the matrix metalloproteinase-2 promoter and risk of lung cancer. *Cancer Res* 2002; **62(22)**:6430–3.

235 Zhou Y, Yu C, Miao X *et al.* Functional haplotypes in the promoter of matrix metalloproteinase-2 and lung cancer susceptibility. *Carcinogenesis* 2005; **26(6)**:1117–21.

236 Yu C, Zhou Y, Miao X, Xiong P, Tan W, Lin D. Functional haplotypes in the promoter of matrix metalloproteinase-2 predict risk of the occurrence and metastasis of esophageal cancer. *Cancer Res* 2004; **64(20)**:7622–8.

237 Ye S, Eriksson P, Hamsten A, Kurkinen M, Humphries SE, Henney AM. Progression of coronary atherosclerosis is associated with a common genetic variant of the human stromelysin-1 promoter which results in reduced gene expression. *J Biol Chem* 1996; **271(22)**:13055–60.

238 Su L, Zhou W, Asomaning K *et al.* Genotypes and haplotypes of matrix metalloproteinase 1, 3 and 12 genes and the risk of lung cancer. *Carcinogenesis* 2006; **27(5)**:1024–9.

239 Jormsjo S, Whatling C, Walter DH, Zeiher AM, Hamsten A, Eriksson P. Allele-specific regulation of matrix metalloproteinase-7 promoter activity is associated with coronary artery luminal dimensions among hypercholesterolemic patients. *Arterioscler Thromb Vasc Biol* 2001; **21(11)**:1834–9.

240 Zhang J, Jin X, Fang S *et al.* The functional polymorphism in the matrix metalloproteinase-7 promoter increases susceptibility to esophageal squamous cell carcinoma, gastric cardiac adenocarcinoma and non-small cell lung carcinoma. *Carcinogenesis* 2005; **26(10)**:1748–53.

241 Hu Z, Huo X, Lu D *et al.* Functional polymorphisms of matrix metalloproteinase-9 are associated with risk of occurrence and metastasis of lung cancer. *Clin Cancer Res* 2005; **11(15)**:5433–9.

242 Jormsjo S, Ye S, Moritz J *et al.* Allele-specific regulation of matrix metalloproteinase-12 gene activity is associated with coronary artery luminal dimensions in diabetic patients with manifest coronary artery disease. *Circ Res* 2000; **86(9)**:998–1003.

243 Bartsch H, Nair J. Oxidative stress and lipid peroxidation-derived DNA-lesions in inflammation driven carcinogenesis. *Cancer Detect Prev* 2004; **28(6)**:385–91.

244 Blankenstein T. The role of tumor stroma in the interaction between tumor and immune system. *Curr Opin Immunol* 2005; **17(2)**:180–6.

245 Shih CM, Lee YL, Chiou HL *et al.* The involvement of genetic polymorphism of IL-10 promoter in non-small cell lung cancer. *Lung Cancer* 2005; **50(3)**: 291–7.

246 Seifart C, Plagens A, Dempfle A *et al.* TNF-alpha, TNF-beta, IL-6, and IL-10 polymorphisms in patients with lung cancer. *Dis Markers* 2005; **21(3)**:157–65.

247 Reuss E, Fimmers R, Kruger A, Becker C, Rittner C, Hohler T. Differential regulation of interleukin-10 production by genetic and environmental factors—a twin study. *Genes Immun* 2002; **3(7)**:407–13.

248 Suarez A, Castro P, Alonso R, Mozo L, Gutierrez C. Interindividual variations in constitutive interleukin-10 messenger RNA and protein levels and their association with genetic polymorphisms. *Transplantation* 2003; **75(5)**:711–7.

249 Turner DM, Williams DM, Sankaran D, Lazarus M, Sinnott PJ, Hutchinson IV. An investigation of polymorphism in the interleukin-10 gene promoter. *Eur J Immunogenet* 1997; **24(1)**:1–8.

250 Engels E, Wu X, Gu J, Dong Q, Liu J, Spitz M. Systematic evaluation of genetic variants in the inflammation pathway and risk of lung cancer. *Canger Res* 2007; **67(13)**:6520–7.

251 Lind H, Zienolddiny S, Ryberg D, Skaug V, Phillips DH, Haugen A. Interleukin 1 receptor antagonist gene polymorphism and risk of lung cancer: a possible interaction with polymorphisms in the interleukin 1 beta gene. *Lung Cancer* 2005; **50(3)**:285–90.

252 Wilkinson RJ, Patel P, Llewelyn M *et al.* Influence of polymorphism in the genes for the interleukin (IL)-1 receptor antagonist and IL-1beta on tuberculosis. *J Exp Med* 1999; **189(12)**:1863–74.

253 Santtila S, Savinainen K, Hurme M. Presence of the IL-1RA allele 2 (IL1RN*2) is associated with enhanced IL-1beta production in vitro. *Scand J Immunol* 1998; **47(3)**:195–8.

254 Leek RD, Landers R, Fox SB, Ng F, Harris AL, Lewis CE. Association of tumour necrosis factor alpha and its receptors with thymidine phosphorylase expression in invasive breast carcinoma. *Br J Cancer* 1998; **77(12)**:2246–51.

255 Squadrito F, Altavilla D, Ammendolia L *et al.* Improved survival and reversal of endothelial dysfunction by the 21-aminosteroid, U-74389G in splanchnic ischaemia-reperfusion injury in the rat. *Br J Pharmacol* 1995; **115(3)**:395–400.

256 Shih CM, Lee YL, Chiou HL *et al.* Association of TNF-alpha polymorphism with susceptibility to and severity of non-small cell lung cancer. *Lung Cancer* 2006; **52(1)**:15–20.

257 Kroeger KM, Steer JH, Joyce DA, Abraham LJ. Effects of stimulus and cell type on the expression of the -308 tumour necrosis factor promoter polymorphism. *Cytokine* 2000; **12(2)**:110–9.

258 258 Kroeger KM, Carville KS, Abraham LJ. The −308 tumor necrosis factor-alpha promoter polymorphism

effects transcription. *Mol Immunol* 1997; **34(5)**:391–9.

259 Kaluza W, Reuss E, Grossmann S *et al.* Different transcriptional activity and in vitro TNF-alpha production in psoriasis patients carrying the TNF-alpha 238A promoter polymorphism. *J Invest Dermatol* 2000; **114(6)**:1180–3.

260 Coussens LM, Werb Z. Inflammation and cancer. *Nature* 2002; **420(6917)**:860–7.

261 Seow A, Ng DP, Choo S *et al.* Joint effect of asthma/atopy and an IL-6 gene polymorphism on lung cancer risk among lifetime non-smoking Chinese women. *Carcinogenesis* 2006; **27(6)**:1240–4.

262 Campa D, Zienolddiny S, Maggini V, Skaug V, Haugen A, Canzian F. Association of a common polymorphism in the cyclooxygenase 2 gene with risk of non-small cell lung cancer. *Carcinogenesis* 2004; **25(2)**:229–35.

263 Mascaux C, Martin B, Paesmans M *et al.* Has Cox-2 a prognostic role in non-small-cell lung cancer? A systematic review of the literature with meta-analysis of the survival results. *Br J Cancer* 2006; **95(2)**:139–45.

264 Ciampolillo A, De Tullio C, Giorgino F. The IGF-I/IGF-I receptor pathway: implications in the pathophysiology of thyroid cancer. *Curr Med Chem* 2005; **12(24)**:2881–91.

265 Kamangar BB, Gabillard JC, Bobe J. Insulin-like growth factor-binding protein (IGFBP)-1, -2, -3, -4, -5, and -6 and IGFBP-related protein 1 during rainbow trout postvitellogenesis and oocyte maturation: molecular characterization, expression profiles, and hormonal regulation. *Endocrinology* 2006; **147(5)**:2399–410.

266 Yu H, Spitz MR, Mistry J, Gu J, Hong WK, Wu X. Plasma levels of insulin-like growth factor-I and lung cancer risk: a case–control analysis. *J Natl Cancer Inst* 1999; **91(2)**:151–6.

267 Moon JW, Chang YS, Ahn CW *et al.* Promoter −202 A/C polymorphism of insulin-like growth factor binding protein-3 gene and non-small cell lung cancer risk. *Int J Cancer* 2006; **118(2)**:353–6.

268 De Mellow JS, Baxter RC. Growth hormone-dependent insulin-like growth factor (IGF) binding protein both inhibits and potentiates IGF-I-stimulated DNA synthesis in human skin fibroblasts. *Biochem Biophys Res Commun* 1988; **156(1)**:199–204.

269 Stoving RK, Hangaard J, Hagen C, Flyvbjerg A. Low levels of the 150-kD insulin-like growth factor binding protein 3 ternary complex in patients with anorexia nervosa: effect of partial weight recovery. *Horm Res* 2003; **60(1)**:43–8.

270 Rudd MF, Webb EL, Matakidou A *et al.* Variants in the GH-IGF axis confer susceptibility to lung cancer. *Genome Res* 2006; **16(6)**:693–701.

271 Lim YJ, Kim JW, Song JY *et al.* Epidermal growth factor gene polymorphism is different between schizophrenia and lung cancer patients in Korean population. *Neurosci Lett* 2005; **374(3)**:157–60.

272 Koukourakis MI, Papazoglou D, Giatromanolaki A, Bougioukas G, Maltezos E, Sivridis E. VEGF gene sequence variation defines VEGF gene expression status and angiogenic activity in non-small cell lung cancer. *Lung Cancer* 2004; **46(3)**:293–8.

273 Wang L, Wang J, Sun S *et al.* A novel DNMT3B subfamily, DeltaDNMT3B, is the predominant form of DNMT3B in non-small cell lung cancer. *Int J Oncol* 2006; **29(1)**:201–7.

274 Shen H, Wang L, Spitz MR, Hong WK, Mao L, Wei Q. A novel polymorphism in human cytosine DNA-methyltransferase-3B promoter is associated with an increased risk of lung cancer. *Cancer Res* 2002; **62(17)**:4992–5.

275 Lee SJ, Jeon HS, Jang JS *et al.* DNMT3B polymorphisms and risk of primary lung cancer. *Carcinogenesis* 2005; **26(2)**:403–9.

276 Jang JS, Lee SJ, Choi JE *et al.* Methyl-CpG binding domain 1 gene polymorphisms and risk of primary lung cancer. *Cancer Epidemiol Biomarkers Prev* 2005; **14(11, Pt 1)**:2474–80.

277 Castro R, Rivera I, Ravasco P *et al.* 5,10-methylenetetrahydrofolate reductase (MTHFR) 677C→T and 1298A→C mutations are associated with DNA hypomethylation. *J Med Genet* 2004; **41(6)**:454–8.

278 Shi Q, Zhang Z, Li G *et al.* Sex differences in risk of lung cancer associated with methylene-tetrahydrofolate reductase polymorphisms. *Cancer Epidemiol Biomarkers Prev* 2005; **14(6)**:1477–84.

279 Yoon KA, Hwangbo B, Kim IJ *et al.* Novel polymorphisms in the SUV39H2 histone methyltransferase and the risk of lung cancer. *Carcinogenesis* 2006.

280 Freedman AN, Seminara D, Gail MH *et al.* Cancer risk prediction models: a workshop on development, evaluation, and application. *J Natl Cancer Inst* 2005; **97(10)**:715–23.

281 Gail MH, Brinton LA, Byar DP *et al.* Projecting individualized probabilities of developing breast cancer

for white females who are being examined annually. *J Natl Cancer Inst* 1989; **81(24)**:1879–86.

282 Costantino JP, Gail MH, Pee D *et al.* Validation studies for models projecting the risk of invasive and total breast cancer incidence. *J Natl Cancer Inst* 1999; **91(18)**:1541–8.

283 Bondy ML, Lustbader ED, Halabi S, Ross E, Vogel VG. Validation of a breast cancer risk assessment model in women with a positive family history. *J Natl Cancer Inst* 1994; **86(8)**:620–5.

284 Spiegelman D, Colditz GA, Hunter D, Hertzmark E. Validation of the Gail *et al.* model for predicting individual breast cancer risk. *J Natl Cancer Inst* 1994; **86(8)**:600–7.

285 Rockhill B, Spiegelman D, Byrne C, Hunter DJ, Colditz GA. Validation of the Gail *et al.* model of breast cancer risk prediction and implications for chemoprevention. *J Natl Cancer Inst* 2001; **93(5)**:358–66.

286 Armstrong K, Eisen A, Weber B. Assessing the risk of breast cancer. *N Engl J Med* 2000; **342(8)**:564–71.

287 Boyd NF, Byng JW, Jong RA *et al.* Quantitative classification of mammographic densities and breast cancer risk: results from the Canadian National Breast Screening Study. *J Natl Cancer Inst* 1995; **87(9)**:670–5.

288 Byrne C, Schairer C, Wolfe J *et al.* Mammographic features and breast cancer risk: effects with time, age, and menopause status. *J Natl Cancer Inst* 1995; **87(21)**:1622–9.

289 Hankinson SE, Willett WC, Manson JE *et al.* Plasma sex steroid hormone levels and risk of breast cancer in postmenopausal women. *J Natl Cancer Inst* 1998; **90(17)**:1292–9.

290 Palomares MR, Machia JR, Lehman CD, Daling JR, McTiernan A Mammographic density correlation with Gail model breast cancer risk estimates and component risk factors. *Cancer Epidemiol Biomarkers Prev* 2006; **15(7)**:1324–30.

291 Fears TR, Guerry Dt, Pfeiffer RM *et al.* Identifying individuals at high risk of melanoma: a practical predictor of absolute risk. *J Clin Oncol* 2006; **24(22)**:3590–6.

292 Cho E, Rosner BA, Feskanich D, Colditz GA. Risk factors and individual probabilities of melanoma for whites. *J Clin Oncol* 2005; **23(12)**:2669–75.

293 Selvachandran SN, Hodder RJ, Ballal MS, Jones P, Cade D. Prediction of colorectal cancer by a patient consultation questionnaire and scoring system: a prospective study. *Lancet* 2002; **360(9329)**:278–83.

294 Spitz MR, Hong WK, Amos CI *et al.* A risk model for prediction of lung cancer. *J Nati Cancer Inst* 2007; **99(9)**;715–26.

CHAPTER 4

The Molecular Genetics of Lung Cancer

David S. Shames, Mitsuo Sato, and John D. Minna

A brief history of cancer genetics

That cancer is a genetic disease was first understood near the turn of the last century [1]. After the discovery that DNA was the genetic material, cytogenetic studies showed that neoplasms were nearly always clonal with respect to karyotype and chromosomal pattern. These early genetic studies led to the concept of the clonal inheritance of somatically acquired genetic abnormalities in cancer pathogenesis [2].

By the late 1960s, there were two competing hypotheses both of which derived from the observation that retroviral-like sequences of DNA and RNA were frequently found in tumor cells: the idea popularized by Temin involved retrotranscription of viral genes into host cell DNA (this hypothesis eventually led to a Nobel Prize for Temin and his postdoctoral researcher David Baltimore); the other idea developed by Huebner and Todaro led to the concept of the oncogene—genes that promote the development of cancer [3,4]. The distinction between these two ideas was the source of the oncogenic element: in Temin's view, the carcinogen derived from an infectious agent, whereas for Todaro and Huebner, the source was an endogenous, vertically transmitted, retroviral-like gene. Both proposals turned out to partially correct. By directly testing these competing hypotheses, Nobel laureates, Varmus and Bishop were able to show that normal cells contain gene sequences that are homologous to viral oncogenes;

these sequences are "proto-oncogenes" ready to be activated during cancer pathogenesis.

Around the same time Alfred Knudson used statistical inference to devise the complementary concept of recessive anti-oncogenes. In a classic paper, Knudson postulated that if the overall mutation rate between patients with the inherited form of retinoblastoma versus the sporadic version were similar, then the frequent incidence of multifocal or bilateral retinoblastomas in familial cases must occur on the background of a germline mutation in a critical gene [5]. The implication of this study was that, at least in retinoblastoma, two mutations were sufficient for the onset of disease: the so-called "two-hit hypothesis." Several years later, the gene that is responsible for familial retinoblastoma was cloned [6]. In the two decades since retinoblastoma was first cloned and characterized, several hundred genes—either oncogenes or tumor suppressors or their accomplices—have been implicated in cancer pathogenesis [7,8].

The brief overview presented above suggests that there are at least two distinct genetic components to cellular transformation: there are large, clonal chromosome aberrations (aneuploidy) including translocations, amplifications, and deletions, and there are alterations that occur at the level of the gene, which often include point mutations, small amplifications, and deletions. By studying the genetic lesions that frequently occur in primary tumor material, cancer geneticists have made significant inroads into a general understanding of the mechanisms of cancer pathogenesis [9]. Modern molecular biology techniques including cloning, the polymerase chain reaction, and genome-wide DNA

Lung Cancer, 3rd edition. Edited by Jack A. Roth, James D. Cox, and Waun Ki Hong. © 2008 Blackwell Publishing, ISBN: 978-1-4051-5112-2.

microarrays have increased the rate with which new genes are discovered and disease associations determined. The next step in the biotechnology revolution will be to translate our growing understanding of cancer genetics into rational diagnostic and drug development platforms, and ultimately into better treatment strategies. This chapter discusses the genetic basis of lung cancer in light of the ongoing translational and clinical challenges these diseases present to physicians, and describes new approaches to developing molecularly targeted therapies to treating lung cancer.

Overview of lung cancer etiology, incidence, and treatment

Pathologists have described various different histologies of lung cancer. There are two major subtypes: small cell lung cancer (SCLC), and nonsmall cell lung cancer (NSCLC). SCLC accounts for 25% of lung cancer cases in the United States, and NSCLC accounts for the remaining 75%. NSCLCs can be further subdivided into several subtypes: adenocarcinoma (Ad), squamous cell carcinoma (SCC), large cell carcinoma (LCC), bronchioalveolar carcinoma (BAC), and various mixed subtypes. While this classification system is based on histology, there are significant molecular differences between SCLC and NSCLC. Thus, there is an ongoing effort to describe these differences in terms of mRNA expression profiles as well as the acquired genetic and epigenetic changes between the different subtypes. There are significant clinical differences in terms of prognosis and treatment strategies for the different subtypes. Therefore, another effort is directed at determining if specific molecular abnormalities predict stage and prognosis as well as the different responses to chemotherapy and radiation therapy well described in patients.

We need to understand the molecular differences between tumors arising in current smokers, former smokers, and lifetime never smokers. Are there different acquired molecular abnormalities in lung cancers arising in women and men or in persons of different ethnicity or age? Can we use the molecular abnormalities found in lung tissue, sputum, or those shed into the blood as aids for very early diagnosis or learning who is at the highest risk for developing cancer? These patients would be candidates for extensive screening and early detection efforts. Could some of the changes be targets for developing tumor-specific vaccines or targeting drugs to specific molecular abnormalities for therapeutic purposes? A molecular diagnostic platform was recently approved for use in breast cancer, and similar designs must be developed for use in suspected lung cancer cases. Possible targets for these platforms include altered gene expression patterns, serum protein profiles, and aberrantly methylated DNA.

Although it seems intuitive that the large mass of tumor cells that make up the bulk of the tumor should be the target of cancer drugs, recent evidence suggests that this bulk tumor cell population may be less important to tumor progression than a rare cancer stem cell that can self-renew, initiate invasion, and propagate metastases. These cancer stem cells are often less sensitive to cytotoxic chemotherapy than the bulk primary tumor, and evade first-line therapy as a result. The key to targeting these rare cells is the development of molecularly targeted therapies based on the profile of the individual tumors.

Individual tumors exhibit significant phenotypic and epigenetic variation, yet they are normally clonal with respect to crucial genetic alterations. This means that the evolution of a particular tumor is driven, at least in part, by the oncogenic changes it has acquired, and suggests that the continued propagation of the tumor also depends on the activity of the oncogenes it contains. Bernard Weinstein likened this effect of oncogene dependence to an Achilles "heal" for the tumor: he proposed that because tumors are "addicted" to the presence of a particular oncogene, they might be uniquely sensitive to compounds or natural products (antibodies) that specifically target the function of the activated oncogene [10]. Similarly, a given tumor with a mutation in a "gatekeeper" tumor suppressor gene whose loss of function is absolutely required for a particular tumor to develop may be hypersensitive to replacing the activity of that tumor suppressor gene (TSG). These concepts are the basis for rational, or molecularly targeted, therapeutic approaches. Several

Table 4.1 Molecularly targeted therapies that may be of value in lung cancer treatment.

Gene	Type of alteration	Drug or therapeutics targeting abnormalities
EGFR	Mutation and amplification	Tyrosine kinase inhibitors (gefitinib, elrotinib) Chimeric IgG monoclonal antibody (cetuximab)
HER2	Mutation and amplification	Pan-ERBB tyrosine kinase inhibitor (CI-1033) Humanized monoclonal antibody (trastuzumab)
c-KIT	Overexpressed	Tyrosine kinase inhibitor (imatinib)
SRC	Constitutively activated	Src inhibitor (dasatinib)
BRAF	Mutation	Raf kinase inhibitor (sorafenib)
RAS	Mutation	Farnesyl transferase inhibitors (tipifarnib, lonafarnib)
MEK	Constitutively activated	Inhibitor of MEK (CI-1040, PD325901)
PI3K/AKT/mTOR	Constitutively activated	PI3K inhibitor (LY294002) mTOR (rapamycin) and its derivatives (CCI-779, RAD001, AP23576)
BCL2	Overexpressed	Antisense oligonucleotide (oblimersen sodium) Inhibitor of BCL2 (ABT-737)
p53	Mutation and deletion	p53 adenoviral vector (Advexin)
FUS1	Loss of protein expression	FUS1 nanoparticles (DOTAP:Chol-FUS1)
VEGF	Overexpressed	Humanized monoclonal antibody (bevacizumab) VEGFR-2 and EGFR inhibitor (ZD6474)
Telomerase	Overexpressed	Telomerase template antagonist (GRN163L)

EGFR, epidermal growth factor receptor; VEGF, vascular endothelial growth factor.
(Adapted from Ref [11])

examples of this new therapeutic approach are now available and are having a significant impact in the clinic (Table 4.1).

To fully exploit the potential targets in human cancer cells for rational drug design, an understanding of the mutational repertoire of human cancer is necessary. Recently there have been several reports on large-scale sequencing of candidate genes in cancer cells (such as all tyrosine kinases) that have identified mutations in several genes that drug targets such as PI3 kinases [12]. Following this, the NIH, in collaboration with the Broad Institute at MIT and Johns Hopkins University among others, has begun to collect data for The Cancer Genome Atlas (TCGA). Over the next decade, this project will produce a wealth of information that will need to be analyzed and put into biological context to be exploited for pharmaceutical development [13].

Molecular genetics of lung cancer

Tobacco smoke and lung cancer

It is well known that tobacco smoke is the major cause of lung cancer. Smokers are 14-fold more likely to develop lung cancer than nonsmokers [14]. There are more than 60 carcinogens in tobacco smoke, many of which are activated by the p450 enzymes in the cytosol and then interact covalently with DNA, forming DNA adducts [15]. Human cells have evolved specialized mechanisms that repair different types of DNA adducts, as well as a specific DNA polymerase (DNA polymerase) that can bypass the most common types of DNA mutations. Benzopyrene and 5-methylchrysene (as well as other components of tobacco smoke) form large adducts that cannot be bypassed by DNA polymerase eta, and need to be removed by nucleotide excision repair (NER). Enzymes in this DNA repair pathway remove large adducts by cleaving the DNA helix where adducts have formed, replacing the affected base, and then ligat the broken DNA chain. This pathway also repairs inter- and intra-strand DNA cross-links. Another important family of tobacco smoke carcinogens, the *N*-nitrosamines, frequently induce miscoding mutations. The most common type of miscoding mutation involves alkylation of guanine at the ^6O position, and ^6O-methylguanine methyltransferase repairs this particular change.

Several studies have explored the nature of tobacco smoke-induced mutations in lung cancer patients and have found that the most common type of mutation is a G-T transversion. When the profile of tumor-acquired point mutations in the p53 tumor suppressor gene is compared between smokers and nonsmokers with lung cancer, there are clear distinctions in the position and type of mutation that occur. In smokers, the most frequent type of mutation is G:C>T:A transversion, whereas in lung cancer patients with no smoking history, the most common type of mutation is G:C>A:T transition at CpG sites (the cytosine in the CpG dinucleotides is particularly susceptible to spontaneous deamination resulting in a conversion to thymine) [15,16]. Further distinctions are apparent when the positions of G-T transversions are compared between smoking-related lung cancer and other common types of cancer [15].

Chromosomal instability, aneuploidy, and loss of heterozygosity

There are several types of genetic damage that contribute to lung cancer pathogenesis: (i) changes in chromosome number; (ii) changes in chromosome structure; (iii) allelic alterations and loss of heterozygosity (LOH); and (iv) sequence alterations in the form of point mutations or small amplifications or deletions [17]. The first three types of genetic damage fall under the rubric of genomic instability and can occur anywhere in the genome, whereas the final type involves mutations in protein coding sequences. In this section, we will discuss genomic instability in the context of chromosomal instability, aneuploidy, and loss of heterozygosity. In the

next section, we will discuss the genes frequently affected by mutational events in human lung cancer, and how knowledge of their function will translate into novel, effective therapeutics. While we discuss genomic instability and loss or gain of gene function in different sections, it is important to realize that these factors are not mutually exclusive and both contribute to cellular transformation in complex and cooperative ways. The consequences of specific alterations in DNA sequence, be they large-scale translocations or single-point mutations, are rarely binary events; rather, it is the accrued effects of multiple, sequential genetic alterations over time that gives each tumor its idiosyncratic clinical course and outcome.

It has been argued that the term genetic instability properly refers to the rate at which genetic alterations occur [17]. Vogelstein and others correctly argue that the rate of genetic change cannot be inferred from the extant alterations in a given sample, but rather should be determined experimentally. As a result, here we will distinguish between the terms genomic instability and genetic instability, and use the term genomic instability to refer only to the fact of alterations in chromosome number (aneuploidy) or gross alterations in chromosome structure through translocation, amplification, and deletion (chromosomal instability). Genomic instability can involve LOH, particularly in the context of tumor suppressor genes. In this case, one allele has a mutation or epigenetic change inactivating one allele while the other wild-type allele is lost along with many other genes leaving the cell with a completely inactive tumor suppressor gene. This commonly occurs in the case of the well-known TSGs p53, p16, and RB.

LOH refers to the loss of one allele of a given locus, but says nothing about the number of copies of that locus. This distinction is important because tumor cells frequently duplicate their chromosome complement on a background of LOH such that one parental allele of a chromosome is lost, but the other is duplicated. The net effect is that daughter cells are hemizygous for a given allele, but retain a normal karyotype for that particular chromosome. The mechanisms that cause genomic instability include exposure to carcinogens, hypoxia, hypomethylation of heterochromatic DNA, loss of mitotic checkpoint controls, defective DNA repair, and telomere shortening [18–20].

Karyotypic studies were the first to shed light on the genetic complexity of cancer pathogenesis, and one of the first observations was that cancer cells often exhibit significant aneuploidy. Solid tumors frequently undergo genome duplication early in their evolution, and many malignancies exhibit a hypotetraploid genotype. Genome duplication occurs during mitosis, and may involve centrosome amplification and the formation of multipolar spindles prior to cytokinesis [21]. Genome duplication probably occurs in normal cells, but functional mitotic checkpoints and sentinel DNA damage response proteins such as p53 and ATM detect aberrant spindle formation and either induce apoptosis or repair the damage. In preneoplastic cells with mutations in p53 or other crucial genes, this type of damage can go undetected.

Karyotypic studies also yielded the first information about large genetic alterations in lung cancer. A major step to achieve lung cancer chromosome analysis occurred with the ability to grow lung cancer cells in tissue culture, which allowed preparation of cancer cell metaphases for analysis [22]. Indeed, karyotypic studies where the first to demonstrate genetic similarities and differences between NSCLC and SCLC [23]. Frequent sites of chromosomal losses in SCLC include 3p, 5q, 13q, and 17p. These occur together with double minutes associated with amplification of the myelocytomatosis viral oncogene homolog (MYC), particularly the c-Myc, family of genes. In NSCLCs, deletions of 3p, 9q, and 17p; +7, i(5)(p10), and i(8)(q10) are common [23]. Molecular cytogenetic methods including array-based comparative genomic hybridization (CGH), microsatellite marker analysis, and single-nucleotide polymorphism (SNP) studies have confirmed and extended earlier work. CGH analysis incorporates whole genome-scale analyses with relatively high-resolution quantitative information and revealed gains in 5p, 1q24, and Xq26, and deletions in 22q12.1–13.1, 10q26, and 16p11.2 [23].

Comparative genomic studies led to the finding that nearly all SCLCs and many NSCLCs suffer LOH on chromosome 3p, suggesting the presence of one or more tumor suppressor genes in this chromosome region. Although LOH by itself is not sufficient to indicate the presence of a tumor suppressor locus, subsequent, high-resolution analyses showed that in some SCLCs, several genes in the minimally deleted 3p21.3 and 3p14.2 were deleted on both the maternal and paternal alleles and thus completely gone from the cancer cell genome, a so-called homozygous deletion [24]. Homozygous deletions are rare in cancer cell genomes, and are taken as a strong indication that a tumor suppressor gene exists in the affected region. Other homozygous deletions common in lung cancer occur on 9p21 and 17p13. These loci turned out to include the tumor suppressor genes p16 and p53, respectively. Subsequent work showed the 3p14.2 region to include the TSG fragile histidine triad, *FHIT*, while the 3p21.3 region encodes several closely linked TSGs including RASSF1A, FUS1, NPRG2, 101F6, SEMA3B, and SEMA3F [24,25].

Another common type of genomic instability in lung cancer primarily affects short repetitive sequences of DNA, which are called microsatellites. These microsatellites, while polymorphic can undergo tumor-specific (compared to normal DNA from the same patient) alterations in length as a result of insertion or deletion of the repeating units. Tumors vary significantly in the rate of microsatellite instability (MSI), which may be due to differences in extant DNA repair pathways as is the case in colon cancer [17]. MSI can be measured by using a series of microsatellite markers in polymerase chain reaction (PCR)-based assays. The overall frequencies of MSI from 13 studies are 35% for SCLCs and 22% for NSCLCs [26]. However, it remains to be determined whether MSI is a cause or corollary of lung tumorigenesis.

Preneoplasia and the early detection of lung cancer

As discussed above, lung cancer results from the accumulated effects of genetic and epigenetic alterations over time. Strong evidence for this position derives from molecular genetic studies which show that some genetic alterations found in frank tumors can also be identified in preneoplastic lung cells. Using a series of microsatellite markers and precise microdissection of cancer and lung preneoplastic lesions in smoking-damaged lung epithelium as well as primary lung cancers, several groups have shown that as cells progress histologically from hyperplastic epithelium through dysplasia, carcinoma in situ, to invasive carcinomas, they acquire more frequent and extensive genetic alterations [27,28]. The earliest genetic change that has been identified in preneoplastic bronchial epithelial cells often involves the short arm of chromosome 3. The specific region is a 630-kb minimal homozygously deleted portion of cytoband 3p21.3 [24]. This locus encompasses approximately 20 genes, including *RASSF1A*, *FUS1*, and *SEMA3B*, which are discussed in the next section.

The most common genetic alterations and the relative timing of their appearance during lung tumorigenesis are of particular interest because knowledge of their occurrence can be potentially used for risk assessment of who is the most likely to develop lung cancer. However, these changes primarily represent a "full defect" induced by cigarette smoking and only rarely do sites of these changes progress to full-fledged cancer.

In exposure-related cancers such as lung cancer, progenitor epithelial cell clones frequently undergo epigenetic and genetic alterations that expand into "fields" of cells, exacerbating the problem of clonal instances of genetic damage. The presence of specific genetic changes such as a defined mutation can be used to track clonally-related cells. In one such study, a group of pathologists examined 10 widely dispersed sites in the tracheobronchial tree of a patient who died of severe atherosclerosis and found patches of cells with the identical p53 point mutation in seven of these sites [29]. While there was no evidence of cancer in any organ at autopsy, the presence of this mutation indicated that a lung cell with the stem-like properties existed and migrated throughout the lung.

The combination of chronic exposure to cigarette smoke and chromosomal instability lead to LOH in 3p21.3 (several genes), 9p21 (*p16*), and 17p.13 (*p53*) and frequent amplifications in eight (*c-Myc*), which contained defined tumor suppressor genes or oncogenes. Loss of tumor suppressor gene function and activation of oncogenes contribute to the initiation, development, and maintenance of lung cancer by conferring six distinct properties, called the "hallmarks of cancer" [9]. The hallmarks include self-sufficiency in growth signals (activation of oncogenes), insensitivity to growth-inhibitory signals (inactivation of TSGs), evading apoptosis, immortalization, sustained angiogenesis, and tissue invasion and metastases. In the following section, we will discuss the genes involved in conferring these "hallmarks" on lung cancer cells.

Epigenetic basis of lung cancer—DNA methylation and tumor suppressor gene inactivation

Lung cancers turn out to have at least as many epigenetic alterations as genetic changes. Epigenetic phenomena are heritable characteristics (phenotypes) that cannot be explained by differences in the primary structure of DNA. In normal cells, genomic DNA is packaged into chromatin. Chromatin regulates the spatial arrangement and accessibility of DNA to transcription factors in the nucleus. DNA methylation is an important component of epigenetic gene regulation in normal cells and its dysregulation is crucial to cellular transformation on at least two levels: genome-wide hypomethylation and gene-specific promoter hypermethylation. Genome-wide hypomethylation affects heterochromatic regions of the genome, which do not ordinarily code for protein. These regions were believed to be transcriptionally inert, or "junk" DNA, but recent evidence suggests that the transcriptional capacity genome has been underestimated, and thus could encode sequences important for cancer [20].

Genome-wide hypomethylation has several implications in preneoplastic cells, affecting both transcription and genetic integrity. Transcriptional effects include loss of imprinting, re-expression of genes involved in fetal development, and transcriptional activation of repetitive elements [19,30,31]. The genetic effects are indirect and involve larger-scale processes such as overall chromatin architecture, aneuploidy, and DNA replication [20,32,33].

There is overwhelming evidence that tumor-acquired promoter hypermethylation, leading to loss of expression of the associated gene, is a common event during the multistep pathogenesis of human lung cancer [26,34–37]. Over the past decade, nearly 150 genes have been identified that show tumor-specific methylation in primary tumor samples, including many in lung cancer (Table 4.2) [38]. Certain loci are preferentially methylated in certain cancer types [39,40]. Gene-specific promoter hypermethylation is an early event in tumorigenesis and occurs in conjunction with transcriptional silencing of the associated gene. In addition, aberrant promoter hypermethylation often coincides with loss of heterozygosity resulting in complete loss of expression and thus function of the affected locus [16,37]. However, the molecular mechanisms that drive tumor-acquired promoter hypermethylation in cancer progression are not yet known [41].

DNA methylation-dependent transcriptional silencing frequently affects genes that are involved in transcriptional regulation, DNA repair, negative regulation of the cell cycle, as well as growth regulatory signaling pathways (Table 4.2). Similar to genetic changes, promoter hypermethylation increases during tumor progression. However, increasing promoter hypermethylation also occurs with increasing age and with carcinogen exposure-related cancers such as that of the colon and lung [42]. In the lung, a continuum of increasing methylation from hyperplasia through invasive carcinoma is evident [27,28,34,43,44]. Aberrant promoter hypermethylation has been found in a variety of preneoplastic lesions, which supports the hypothesis that this epigenetic alteration is an early event in carcinogenesis. This observation has resulted in substantial interest from the medical community in that detection of methylation in sputum, blood, or bronchial washings may have utility in the early detection of cancer.

Some genes, such as the important TSG *p53*, are never inactivated by promoter hypermethylation because they do not have a promoter region CpG islands. Other genes, such as the tumor suppressor gene *RASSF1A*, which has a prominent CpG island are nearly always inactivated by LOH and promoter hypermethylation in both SCLC and NSCLC. Thus, a curious feature of aberrant promoter hypermethylation is that it does not appear to affect all genes with equal probability. An even more conspicuous example of this phenomenon is evidenced by the difference between *p16* and *RB*; the protein products of these two genes interact directly and inactivation of one or the genes (and thus this regulatory pathway) is nearly universal in tumors. Interestingly in SCLC, *RB* (13q14) is nearly universally inactivated, whereas in NSCLC, it is usually *p16* (9p21) that is lost. Both genes have large CpG islands in their promoter regions, but only *p16* is methylated with significant frequency, whereas inactivation of *RB* almost always occurs through DNA mutations. This suggests tumor-acquired promoter hypermethylation is nonrandom, and that there is something about certain loci that makes them particularly susceptible to aberrant methylation or to mutation [37,45].

Tumor suppressor genes

Several key tumor-suppressor pathways are frequently inactivated in lung cancer. These include the p53 and the p16^{INK4a}—CyclinD1-CDK4-RB pathways.

The p53 pathway

The tumor suppressor gene *p53* is the most frequently mutated gene in human cancer, and *p53* is inactivated by mutation in ∼90% of SCLCs and ∼50% of NSCLCs, respectively [26,46]. Most inactivating mutations in *p53* are caused by point mutations in the DNA-binding domain (missense mutation, 70–80%) of one parental allele and LOH (deletion) of the other. Occasionally homozygous deletions are observed. *p53* is located at chromosome 17p13.1, and codes for a protein that functions as a key transcription factor. The transcriptional targets of p53 include a number of cell cycle regulatory proteins such as p21 and MYC, as well as many proteins involved in apoptosis such as BAX, 14-3-3σ, and GADD45. p53 regulation occurs primarily at

Table 4.2 Genes found to be methylated in primary lung cancers, but not adjacent normal tissue.

Gene	Name	Accession number	Function	Cytoband	Methylated
14-3-3 Sigma	Stratifin	BC023552	p53-regulated inhibitor of g2/m progression	1p36.11	Breast, pancreas, NSCLC, Gyn, GI
ADRB2	Adrenergic, beta-2-, receptor; surface	M15169	G-protein coupled receptor	5q31-q32	NSCLC, GI
ALDH1A3	Aldehyde dehydrogenase 1 family, member A3	AF198444	Recognizes as substrates free retinal and cellular retinol-binding protein-bound retinal	15q26.3	NSCLC, GI, breast, prostate, colon
APC	Adenomatosis polyposis coli	NM.000038	Tumor suppressor. Promotes rapid degradation of β-catenin and participates in wnt signaling	5q21-q22	Colon, gastric, esophegeal, NSCLC
Betaig-h3	Transforming growth factor beta-induced, 68 kDa	NM.000358	Binds to type I, II, and IV collagens. This adhesion protein may play an important role in cell–collagen interactions	5q31	NSCLC
BIK	BCL2-interacting killer (apoptosis-inducing)	AB051441	Accelerates programmed cell death by binding to the apoptosis repressors Bcl-x(l), Bhrf1, Bcl-2 or its adenovirus homolog e1b 19k protein	22q13.31	NSCLC, glioma
BNC1	Basonuclin 1	L03427	Ribosomal transcription factor involved in gametogenesis and squamous cell differentiation	15q25.2	NSCLC, breast, colon, prostate
CALCA	Calcitonin/calcitonin-related polypeptide, alpha	X02330	Regulates calcium levels in plasma	11p15.2-p15.1	Colon, NSCLC, lymphoma, leukemia
CASP8	Caspase 8, apoptosis-related cysteine peptidase	BC017031	Most upstream protease of the activation cascade of caspases in apoptosis	2q33-q34	Pediatric tumors, NSCLC, HCC, leukemia
CAV1	Caveolin 1	NM.001753	May act as a scaffolding protein within caveolar membranes	7q31.1	Breast, NSCLC, prostate, sarcoma
CD24	CD24 molecule	AK057112	Modulates B-cell activation responses	6q21	NSCLC
CDH1	Cadherin 1, type 1, E-cadherin (epithelial)	NM.004360	Cadherins are calcium-dependent cell adhesion proteins. They preferentially interact with themselves in a homophilic manner in connecting cells; cadherins may thus contribute to the sorting of heterogeneous cell types	16q22.1	NSCLC, breast, GI

Gene	Gene name	Accession	Function	Location	Cancer types
CDH13	Cadherin 13, H-cadherin (heart)	BX538273		16q24.2-q24.3	NSCLC, breast, colon, HCC
COX2	Cyclooxygenase 2	NM_000963.1	May have a role as a major mediator of inflammation and/or a role for prostanoid signaling in activity-dependent plasticity	1q25.2-q25.3	Colon, pancreas, prostate, NSCLC
CSPG2	Chondroitin sulfate proteoglycan 2 (versican)	NM_004385	Involved in intercellular signaling and connecting cells with the extracellular matrix	5q14.3	NSCLC, colon
CTSZ	Cathepsin Z	NM_001336	Exhibits carboxy-monopeptidase as well as carboxy-dipeptidase activity	20q13	NSCLC, breast
CX26	Gap junction protein, beta 2, 26 kDa (connexin 26)	NM_004004	Cell to cell communication	13q11-q12	NSCLC, breast
DAPK	Death-associated protein kinase	NM_004938.1	Calcium/calmodulin-dependent serine/threonine kinase which acts as a positive regulator of apoptosis	9q34.1	HCC, head and neck, colon, NSCLC, breast
DCR1	Tumor necrosis factor receptor superfamily, member 10c, decoy without an intracellular domain	NM_003841	Receptor for the cytotoxic ligand TRAIL, but lacks a cytoplasmic death domain and hence is not capable of inducing apoptosis	8p22-p21	NSCLC, breast, leukemia, lymphoma
DCR2	Tumor necrosis factor receptor superfamily, member 10d, decoy with truncated death domain	NM_003840	Receptor for the cytotoxic ligand TRAIL. Contains a truncated death domain and hence is not capable of inducing apoptosis but protects against trail-mediated apoptosis	8p21	NSCLC, breast, leukemia, lymphoma
DIPA	Coiled-coil domain containing 85B	BM558600	Uknown	11q12.1	NSCLC
DUSP1	Dual specificity phosphatase 1	AK127679	Regulates MAPK pathway. Dephosphorylates map kinase ERK2 on both thr-183 and tyr-185	5q34	NSCLC
EDNRB	Endothelian Receptor B	NM_000115	Nonspecific receptor for endothelin 1, 2, and 3. Mediates its action by association with G-proteins that activate a phosphatidylinositol- calcium second messenger system	13q22	Prostate, head and neck, nasopharyngeal, bladder, NSCLC
EPAS1	Endothelial PAS domain protein 1	NM_001430	Transcription factor involved in the induction of oxygen regulated genes. Regulates the VEGF expression	2p21-p16	NSCLC

(cont.)

Table 4.2 (*Continued*)

Gene	Name	Accession number	Function	Cytoband	Methylated
ER	Estrogen receptor	NM_001437	Nuclear hormone receptor. Binds estrogens and activates expression of down stream genes	14q23.2	Colon, CML, NSCLC
GATA-4	GATA-binding protein 4	NM_002052	Transcriptional activator. Binds to the consensus sequence 5'-AGATAG-3'	8p23.1-p22	NSCLC, colon, GI, ovarian
GATA-5	GATA-binding protein 5	BC047790	Binds to CEF-1 nuclear protein binding site in the cardiac-specific slow/cardiac troponin c transcriptional enhancer	20q13.33	Colon, GI, NSCLC
GCAT	Glycine C-acetyltransferase (2-amino-3-ketobutyrate coenzyme A ligase)	AK123190	Amino acid metabolism	22q13.1	NSCLC
GNG11	Guanine nucleotide binding protein (G protein), gamma 11	BF971151	Regulates signalling through G-protein coupled receptors	7q21	NSCLC
GPX1	Glutathione peroxidase 1	BM478682	Protects the hemoglobin in erythrocytes from oxidative breakdown	3p21.3	NSCLC
GREM1	Gremlin 1, cysteine knot superfamily, homolog (Xenopus laevis)	NM_013372	Developmental cytokine required for early limb outgrowth and patterning. Acts as inhibitor of monocyte chemotaxis	15q13-q15	NSCLC, breast, GI
HIC1	Hypermethylated in cancer 1	NM_006497	Transcriptional repressor. Involved in development of head, face, limbs and ventral body wall	17p13.3	Breast, brain, colon, prostate, breast, NSCLC, kidney, leukemia, lymphoma
hMLH1	MutL homolog 1, colon cancer, nonpolyposis type 2 (E. coli)	BX648844	Involved in DNA mismatch repair	3p21.3	Colon, endometrial, GI, NSCLC, breast, lymphoma, leukemia
HS3ST3B1	Heparan sulfate (glucosamine) 3-O-sulfotransferase 3B1	BC063301	Transfers a sulfuryl group to an n-unsubstituted glucosamine linked to a 2-o-sulfo iduronic acid unit on heparan sulfate	17p12-p11.2	NSCLC, breast
IGFBP3	Insulin-like growth factor binding protein 3	NM_001013398	IGF-binding proteins prolong the half-life of the IGF and have been shown to either inhibit or stimulate the growth promoting effects of the IGFs on cell culture	7p13-p12	NSCLC, breast, GI

(cont.)

IGFBP7	Insulin-like growth factor binding protein 7	BX648756	Binds IGF-I and IGF-II with a relatively low affinity. Stimulates prostacyclin (pgi2) production	4q12	NSCLC, GI
IL6R	Interleukin 6 receptor	NM_000565	Low concentration of a soluble form of IL-6 receptor acts as an agonist of IL6 activity	1q21	NSCLC
IMP-3	Insulin-like growth factor 2 mRNA binding protein 3	U97188	Single-stranded nucleic acid binding protein that binds preferentially to oligo dC	7p11	NSCLC
IRF7	Interferon regulatory factor 7	BC021078	Transcriptional activator. Binds to the interferon-stimulated response element in IFN promoters. Functions as a molecular switch for antiviral activity	11p15.5	Astrocytoma, NSCLC, HCC
IRS1	Insulin receptor substrate 1	NM_005544	Mediates the control of various cellular processes by insulin	2q36	NSCLC
IRX4	Iroquois homeobox protein 4	NM_016358	Likely to be an important mediator of ventricular differentiation during cardiac development	5p15.3	NSCLC
JAG1	Jagged 1 (Alagille syndrome)	AF003837	Ligand for multiple NOTCH receptors	20p12.1-p11.23	NSCLC
KRT8	Keratin 8	NM_002273	Together with KRT19, helps to link the contractile apparatus to dystrophin at the costameres of striated muscle	12q13	NSCLC
LHFP	Lipoma HMGIC fusion partner	CR749848	Unknown	13q12	NSCLC
LOX	Lysyl oxidase	NM_002317	Responsible for the posttranslational oxidative deamination of peptidyl lysine residues in precursors to fibrous collagen and elastin, in addition to cross-linking of extracellular matrix proteins	5q23.2	NSCLC, breast, GI
LRCH4	Leucine-rich repeats and calponin homology (CH) domain containing 4	NM_002319	Unknown	7q22	NSCLC
MAD	MAX dimerization protein 1	BC098396	Transcriptional repressor. Antagonizes CMYC transcriptional activity by competing for MAX	2p13-p12	NSCLC
MAF	V-maf musculoaponeurotic fibrosarcoma oncogene homolog (avian)	NM_001031804	Pol II trascription factor activity. Viral oncogene	16q22-q23	NSCLC

Table 4.2 (*Continued*)

Gene	Name	Accession number	Function	Cytoband	Methylated
MGMT	O-6-methylguanine-DNA methyltransferase	AK126049	Repairs alkylated guanine in DNA by stoichiometrically transferring the alkyl group at the O6 position to a cysteine residue in the enzyme	10q26	Brain, colon, NSCLC, breast, lymphoma
MSX1	Msh homeobox homolog 1 (Drosophila)	NM_002448	Transcriptional repressor. Role in limb formation	4p16.3-p16.1	GI, NSCLC, breast, colon, prostate
MYOD1	Myogenic differentiation 1	NM_002478	Involved in muscle differentiation. Induces fibroblasts to differentiate into myoblasts	11p15.4	Colon, breast, bladder, NSCLC, lymphoma, leukemia
NRCAM	Neuronal cell adhesion molecule	NM_001037132	Cell adhesion, ankyrin-binding protein involved in neuron–neuron adhesion	7q31.1-q31.2	NSCLC, breast
p15	Cyclin-dependent kinase inhibitor 2B (p15, inhibits CDK4)	NM_078487		9p21	Colon, NSCLC, breast, AML
p16	Cyclin-dependent kinase inhibitor 2A (melanoma, p16, inhibits CDK4)	NM_000077		9p21	Nearly all
p73	Tumor protein p73	NM_005427	Participates in the apoptotic response to DNA damage. When overproduced, activates transcription from p53-responsive promoters and induces apoptosis	1p36.3	Lymphoma, leukemia, NSCLC, prostate
PCDH20	Protocadherin 20	NM_022843	Potential calcium-dependent cell-adhesion protein	13q21	NSCLC
PGF	Placental growth factor, vascular endothelial growth factor-related protein	AK023843	Growth factor active in angiogenesis, and endothelial cell growth, stimulating their proliferation and migration	14q24-q31	NSCLC
PHLDA1	Pleckstrin homology-like domain, family A, member 1	NM_007350	Regulation of apoptosis. May be involved in detachment-mediated programmed cell death	12q15	NSCLC
PLAGL1	Pleiomorphic adenoma gene-like 1	CR749329	Transcriptional regulator of the type 1 receptor for pituitary adenylate cyclase-activating polypeptide	6q24-q25	GI, NSCLC
RARβ	Retinoic acid receptor, beta	BX640880	Receptor for retinoic acid. This receptor controls cell function by directly regulating gene expression	3p24	Colon, breast, NSCLC

RASSF1A	Ras association (RalGDS/AF-6) domain family 1	NM_170715	Required for full ubiquitin ligase activity of the anaphase promoting complex/cyclosome (apc/c) and may confer substrate specificity upon the complex	3p21.3	All
REPRIMO	Reprimo, TP53 dependent G2 arrest mediator candidate	NM_019845	Involved in p53-dependent cell cycle arrest	2q23.3	GI, lymphomas, colon, esophageal, breast, leukemias, NSCLC
RGC32	Response gene to complement 32	AK095079	May regulate cyclin dependent protein kinase activity	13q14.11	NSCLC
RIS1	Ras-induced senescence 1	CR615050	Unknown	3p21.3	NSCLC, glioma
RNASET2	Ribonuclease T2	AK001769	Unknown	6q27	NSCLC
RUNX3	Runt-related transcription factor 3	NM_004350	Binds to enhancer and promoter elements	1p36	GI, NSCLC, colon, prostate
SFRP1	Secreted frizzled-related protein 1	BC036503	Secreted frizzled-related proteins function as modulators of WNT signaling through direct interaction with WNTs. Regulate cell growth and differentiation in specific cell types	8p12-p11.1	Colon, NSCLC, breast, esophegeal, head and neck
SFRP2	Secreted frizzled-related protein 2	NM_003013		4q31.3	Colon, NSCLC, breast, esophegeal, head and neck
SFRP4	Secreted frizzled-related protein 4	AF026692		7p14.1	Colon, NSCLC, breast, esophegeal, head and neck
SFRP5	Secreted frizzled-related protein 5	AF117758		10q24.1	Colon, NSCLC, breast, esophegeal, head and neck
SLCO3A1	Solute carrier organic anion transporter family, member 3A1	AF205074	Mediates the Na(+)-independent transport of organic anions such as estrone-3-sulfate	15q26	NSCLC
SOCS1	Suppressor of cytokine signaling 1	AK127621	SOCS1 is involved in negative regulation of cytokines that signal through the JAK/STAT3 pathway	16p13.13	NSCLC, breast
SOCS3	Suppressor of cytokine signaling 3	NM_003955	SOCS3 is involved in negative regulation of cytokines that signal through the jak/stat pathway. Inhibits cytokine signal transduction by binding to tyrosine kinase receptors including gp130, LIF, erythropoietin, insulin, IL12, GCSF, and leptin receptors	17q25.3	NSCLC, breast

(cont.)

Table 4.2 (*Continued*)

Gene	Name	Accession number	Function	Cytoband	Methylated
SOX15	SRY (sex determining region Y)-box 15	AB006867	Transcription factor. Binds to the 5'-aacaat-3' sequence	17p13	NSCLC, breast, prostate, colon
SPARC	Secreted protein, acidic, cysteine-rich (osteonectin)	NM_003118	Regulates cell growth through interactions with the extracellular matrix and cytokines	5q31.3-q32	NSCLC, pancreas
TBX1	T-box 1	AF373867	Transcriptional regulator involved in developmental processes	22q11.21	NSCLC
TFPI2	Tissue factor pathway inhibitor 2	AK129833	Regulation of plasmin-mediated matrix remodeling. Inhibits trypsin, plasmin, factor VIIa/tissue factor and weakly factor XA	7q22	NSCLC
TIMP3	TIMP metallopeptidase inhibitor 3 (Sorsby fundus dystrophy, pseudoinflammatory)	AB051444	Complexes with metalloproteinases (such as collagenases) and irreversibly inactivates them	22q12.1-q13.2	Brain, kidney, NSCLC, breast, colon
TJP2	Tight junction protein 2 (zona occludens 2)	AB209630	Plays a role in tight junctions and adherens junctions	9q13-q21	NSCLC, pancreas
TMEFF2	Transmembrane protein with EGF-like and two follistatin-like domains 2	DQ133599	May be a novel survival factor for hippocampal and mesencephalic neurons	2q32.3	Colon, NSCLC, breast, esophegeal
TWIST1	Twist homolog 1 (acrocephalosyndactyly 3; Saethre-Chotzen syndrome) (Drosophila)	NM_000474	Transcription factor involved in the negative regulation of cellular determination and in the differentiation of several lineages including myogenesis, osteogenesis, and neurogenesis. Necessary for breast cancer metastasis	7p21.2	NSCLC, breast, glioma
uPA	Plasminogen activator, urokinase	NM_002658	Potent plasminogen activator	10q24	Breast, NSCLC, prostate
ZNF22	Zinc finger protein 22 (KOX 15)	NM_006963	Binds DNA through the consensus sequence 5'-caatg-3'. May be involved in transcriptional regulation and play a role in tooth formation	10q11	NSCLC

NSCLC, nonsmall cell lung cancer; HCC, hepatocellular carcinoma; Gyn, gynecological tumors including cervical, ovarian, and endometrial cancers; GI, gastrointestinal tumors; AML/CML, acute and chronic myelogenous leukemia; CNS, central nervous system. (Adapted from Shames *et al.* [37].)

the level of protein stability. p53 controls transcription of *MDM2*, an E3 ubiquitin ligase, which in turn regulates p53 stability in a feedback loop. This particular connection in the p53 pathway is a frequent target of dysregulation in tumor cells.

The p53 pathway is activated in response cellular stress and DNA damage induced by gammairradiation, ultraviolet light, DNA damaging drugs, and carcinogens. p53 stabilization results in the expression of downstream genes, which induces either cell cycle arrest to permit DNA repair, or programmed cell death when there is too much damage. Loss of p53 function allows cells to divide in spite of genetic damage, which can result the clonal expansion of premalignant cells. In most cases, only mutant, missense p53 is present because of LOH involving the wild-type p53 allele. However, in some cases, mutant p53 proteins can form heterodimers with wild-type p53 inactivating its tumor suppressive function even before LOH. These "gainof-function" mutations contribute to increased tumorigenicity and invasiveness of several types of cancers [26,46]. However, despite large-scale studies, it is not clear whether NSCLCs with p53 mutations have impaired survival compared to lung cancers with only wild-type p53.

There are two important upstream regulators in the p53 pathway: MDM2 and p14^{ARF}. MDM2 functions as an oncogene by reducing p53 levels through enhancing proteasome-dependent degradation. Amplifications of *MDM2* were reported in ∼7% (2/30) of NSCLCs, resulting in loss of p53 function [46]. *p14*^{ARF} derives from the *p16* locus with an alternatively spliced 5-exon that results in an alternative reading frame for translation. p14 encodes a protein that binds to MDM2 thereby inhibiting its ubiquitination activity, which leads to the stabilization of p53. Immunohistochemistry analyses of p14^{ARF} on lung cancers have shown that p14^{ARF} protein expression was lost in ∼65% of SCLCs and ∼40% of NSCLCs. Thus, through p53 mutation or changes in MDM2 or p14, the p53 pathway is inactivated in the majority of all lung cancers.

Lung cancer cells are addicted to loss of p53 function. When wild-type p53 is re-expressed in lung cancer cells with mutant or deleted p53, the tumor cells undergo apoptosis. These findings have led to clinical trials of p53 gene replacement therapy. The results from preclinical and early-stage clinical trials of p53 gene replacement therapy using a replication incompetent retrovirus p53 expression vector in patients with NSCLCs, show evidence of antitumor activity and the feasibility and safety of gene therapy [47]. INGN 201 (Ad5CMV-p53, Advexin™), a replication-impaired p53 adenoviral vector has been evaluated in clinical trials, and is both safe and effective for the treatment of several different types of cancer [48]. This treatment has been approved in China for the treatment of primary head and neck cancers in combination with radiation therapy and is currently undergoing phase III trials in head and neck cancer in the United States.

The RB pathway

The RB pathway plays a central role in G1/S cell transition. Hypophosphorylated RB exerts its growth suppressive effect by binding to and inhibiting the E2F transcription factor, which promotes cells through the G1/S transition. RB is phosphorylated by the CyclinD1/CDK4 complex. Once these kinases phosphorylate RB, it releases E2F, resulting in transition from G1 to S. Thus, loss of RB function though deletion or mutation leads to loss of the G1/S checkpoint, and is a common event in lung cancer, particularly SCLCs (>90%), while inactivation of RB is found in 15–30% of NSCLCs [26].

The activity of the CDK4/Cyclin D1 complex is regulated by p16. p16 keeps RB hypophosphorylated (and growth suppressing mode) by preventing CDK4 from phosphorylating RB. Thus, loss of p16 function results in loss of function of the RB pathway. By contrast to RB, p16 is more frequently inactivated in NSCLCs (∼70%) than in SCLCs (10%) [26]. Inactivation of p16 is caused by LOH coupled with deletion, intragenic mutations or promoter hypermethylation of the remaining allele. In lung cancer, promoter methylation is the most frequent method of inactivation of p16.

Overexpression of either CDK4 or Cyclin D1 inhibits RB pathway function by saturating the growth suppressive activity of p16. CDK4 is amplified in some cases of NSCLCs, but cyclin D1 is overexpressed in more than 40% of NSCLCs as assessed by immunohistochemistry [26,49]. Recently, overexpression of Cyclin D1 in normal-appearing bronchial epithelial of patients with NSCLCs has been reported to be associated with smoking and to predict shorter survival, suggesting the possible utility of Cyclin D1 as a molecular marker to identify high-risk individuals [50]. Thus through changes in either RB, p16, CDK4, or cyclin D1, this important growth regulatory pathway is inactivated and disrupted in the large majority of lung cancers.

3p tumor suppressor genes

Allele loss in 3p, including LOH and homozygous deletion, occurs in nearly 100% of SCLCs and more than 90% of NSCLCs and is one of the earliest events in lung cancer development. Because of the early changes in chromosome region 3p21.3 (occurring in histologically normal lung epithelium) the presence of 3p allele loss and inactivation of expression of these 3p TSGs can be of use in determining smoking related field effects. Three discreet regions of 3p loss have been identified by allelotyping in lung cancers, including, a 600-kb segment in 3p21.3, the 3p14.2 (*FHIT/FRAB3*), and the 3p12 (*ROBO1/DUTT1*) regions. The 3p21.3 region has been analyzed most extensively and 25 genes were identified from this region.

One of the best studied genes in this region is *RASSF1A*, which is rarely mutated in lung cancer but whose expression is frequently lost by tumor acquired promoter methylation [51,52]. *RASSF1A* is involved in multiple pathways critical to cancer pathogenesis, including cell cycle, apoptosis, and microtubule stability. *RASSF1A* is methylated in ~90% of SCLCs and ~40% of NSCLCs and has the ability to suppress the growth of lung cancer cell lines in tissue culture and as xenografts in nude mice [51,52].

FUS1 is located next to *RASSF1A* and one of the two alleles of the gene is often lost in lung cancers. *FUS1* is rarely mutated in lung cancers, does not undergo promoter hypermethylation, yet the protein product of this gene is frequently lost in lung cancer compared to normal lung tissues [53]. Wild-type FUS1 but not tumor-acquired mutant FUS1 induces G1 growth arrest and apoptosis [53]. Administration of *FUS1* with in DOTAP:cholesterol (DOTAP:Chol) nanoparticles (FUS1-nanoperticles) inhibits cancer cell growth in vitro and in vivo. These preclinical studies provide a basis for *FUS1* gene therapy clinical trials for the treatment of lung tumors using *FUS1*-nanoparticles [54,55].

Two other 3p21.3 candidate tumor suppressor genes, Semaphorin 3B (*SEMA3B*) and a family member SEMA3F, are extracellular secreted members of the semaphorin family, and are important in axonal guidance. Wild-type SEMA3B, but not missense mutant SEMA3B, induces apoptosis when re-expressed in lung cancers or added as a soluble molecule [56,57]. Overexpression of SEMA3F in tissue culture results in inhibition of tumor cell growth and tumor cell invasion. Both SEMA3B and SEMA3F are soluble, secreted proteins, and therefore are promising candidates for drug development.

Two other 3p genes with evidence to support their candidacy as tumor suppressors are *FHIT* and retinoic acid receptor beta (*RARβ*). *FHIT* is located in 3p14.2, one of the most common fragile sites of the human genome. *FHIT* is either homozygously deleted or expresses aberrant transcripts in more than 50% of lung cancers [58]. In addition, *FHIT* overexpression induces apoptosis in lung cancer cells. *RARβ* is located at 3p24 and functions as a receptor for retinoic acid (RA). Although the *RARβ* gene is not mutated in lung cancer, it undergoes methylation in 72% of SCLCs and 41% of NSCLCs, leading to loss of its expression [59]. Re-expression of *RARβ* in lung cancer cell lines suppresses their growth in the culture and nude mice [60].

Oncogenes and the pathways they regulate

While there are multiple components to each of the growth signaling pathways involved in lung cancer, we will focus the discussion on those proteins that are frequently affected by genetic abnormalities in cancer. It has become clear that these mutated proteins, while driving cells toward transformation, also "addict" the cells to their abnormal function. This concept is referred to as "oncogene addiction" and represents a cellular physiologic state where the continued presence of the abnormal function, while oncogenic, also becomes required for the tumor to survive [61]. This means that if the function is removed or inhibited, for example, by a targeted drug, the tumor cells die. By contrast, bystander normal cells, which are not "addicted" to the mutant protein, are much less sensitive to the drug; thus, the targeted drugs have great tumor cell specificity. The most important example of this concept for lung cancer is EGFR. Tumors with mutations in *EGFR* are dependent on survival signals transduced by mutant *EGFR*, and thus are particularly sensitive to tyrosine kinase inhibitors (TKIs) [62]. These findings have led to massive genome-wide sequencing efforts (discussed above) targeting thousands of genes to find additional mutated oncogene targets for rational therapeutics design.

Receptor tyrosine kinases

The *EGFR* family

The *EGFR* family of receptors are transmembrane TK receptors and are composed of *EGFR*, *HER2*, *HER3*, and *HER4* and each has unique properties. For example, *HER2* lacks a functional ligand-binding domain and *HER3* lacks kinase activity [63]. Upon ligand binding, these *EGFR* family members form active homo- and hetero-dimers, leading to autophosphorylation and activation of intracellular signaling cascades. *EGFR* is overexpressed in ~70% of NSCLCs but rarely expressed in SCLCs [64]. There are several drugs targeting *EGFR* or *HER2* currently available including the small molecule TKIs, gefitinib, erlotinib, and the monoclonal antibodies, cetuximab (targeting *EGFR*), and trastuzumab (targeting *HER2*).

Recently, several mutations in the TK domain of *EGFR* have been described, and are not infrequent in NSCLC (10–20%), but never occur in SCLC [65,66]. Of interest is that TK domain mutations are almost exclusive to lung cancer, whereas intracellular region mutations are found in glioblastomas. In lung cancer, these mutations are limited to the first four exons of the TK domain and are categorized into three different types (deletions, insertions, and missense point mutations). Inframe deletions in exon

19 (44% of all mutations) and missense mutations in exon 21 (41% of all mutations) are the most frequent, accounting for more than 80% of all mutations [67]. Importantly, the presence of mutations in TK domain correlates with the drug sensitivity to TKIs [65,66]. An intriguing characteristic of *EGFR* mutations is that they occur in a highly selected subpopulation: female East-Asian never smokers with adenocarcinoma histology [68]. Notably, before EGFR mutations were discovered, all of same clinicopathological factors were found to be associated with tumor responses to TKIs [69,70].

Although several studies have confirmed the relationship between the presence of mutant *EGFR* and the response to TKIs [65,66,71], a subset of NSCLC patients with mutant *EGFRs* do not respond to TKIs. These tumors often (>50%) have a "second" TK domain mutation (T790M) usually found in patients who relapse after TKI treatment, suggesting its contribution to acquired resistance to TKIs [72,73]. However, several examples of the T790M mutations occur in lung tumors not treated with EGFR TKIs, and often the mutation is only in a small subset of the tumor cells. This contrasts with the other *EGFR* TK domain mutations, which are in all tumor cells. Also, a germline EGFR T790M mutation was reported to be associated with familial NSCLC, suggesting that this mutation could predispose people to lung cancer [74]. Fortunately, there are EGFR TKIs that inhibit EGFR with the T790M mutation, and these drugs are currently under clinical evaluation [75].

Some patients without *EGFR* mutation also respond to TKIs, and several predictive markers other than *EGFR* mutation have been reported to correlate with TKI response, including *EGFR* amplification, elevated EGFR protein, *HER2* amplification, *HER3* amplification, and activation of AKT [76–80]. In fact, *KRAS* mutations and EGFR mutations are mutually exclusive. KRAS mutations are associated with cigarette smoking, while EGFR mutations generally occur in never smokers [81]. These studies suggest that other biological features besides *EGFR* mutation status determine TKI response. Among biologic predictors, *EGFR* mutation and amplification by fluorescence in situ hybridization are highly correlated with TKI response while

EGFR protein expression gives conflicting results [65,66,71,76,82]. There is also the possibility that tumors with EGFR mutations are associated with better survival independent of TKI treatment. Thus, all survival studies after TKI treatment need to have molecular analyses for comparison [80,83,84]. Two well-controlled phase III studies were conducted for these drugs. The results of these studies showed that erlotinib prolonged survival of previously treated NSCLC patients by 2 months (BR21 trial), while gefitinib failed to show survival benefit (Iressa Survival Evaluation in Lung Cancer (ISEL)) [86,87]. Despite positive preclinical studies of the combination of TKI and chemotherapy, several phase III studies have failed to show a survival benefit of adding erlotinib or gefitinib to conventional chemotherapy [88,89]. Finally, lung cancers with *EGFR* mutations are more sensitive to ionizing radiation than those without *EGFR* mutations, which potentially provides a molecular basis for combined modality treatment involving TKIs and radiotherapy [90].

While standard criteria for selecting patients with NSCLC for TKI therapy are being developed, in practice, East-Asian female patients with tumors that have *EGFR* mutations or EGFR amplification and that are never smokers often receive TKI therapy. To address this issue, prospective clinical trials designed to incorporate the patient's clinicopathological data as well as molecular biological features (*EGFR* mutation and/or amplification) of the tumors are currently underway.

HER2 mutations occur in 2% of NSCLCs. All reported *HER2* mutations are in-frame insertions in exon 20 and target the corresponding TK domain region as in *EGFR* insertion mutations and occur in the same subpopulation as those with *EGFR* mutations (adenocarcinoma, never smoker, East Asian, and woman) [68,91,92]. So far no small molecule inhibitors show similar potency against *HER2* mutations as seen with *EGFR* TKIs and studies are needed to see if mutant *HER2* lung cancers respond to the anti-HER2 antibody trastuzumab. *HER4* mutations were found in (2.3%) NSCLC tumor samples from Asian patients including male smokers [93].

EGFR mutations occur as preneoplastic lesions occurring in histologically normal bronchial epithe-lial cells adjacent to tumors with *EGFR* mutations. The discovery of *EGFR* mutations could be used as an early detection marker and chemoprevention target [94]. Transgenic mice with either EGFR point mutations or deletion mutations develop lung adenocarcinomas with similar histology to those seen in patients [95,96]. When the mutant gene was "turned-off" in the mice through controlled gene expression the lung tumors all regressed indicating that mutant EGFR is required for both initiation and maintenance of the tumors.

c-KIT

SCLC but not NSCLC frequently express (40–70%) both the receptor c-KIT and its ligand, stem cell factor (SCF) suggesting an autocrine loop may promote the growth of the SCLC cells [97]. However, unlike gastrointestinal stromal tumors which frequently contain c-KIT mutations, activating c-KIT mutations are very rare in lung cancer [98,99]. While imatinib, an inhibitor of c-KIT kinase, inhibits cell growth in some c-KIT expressing SCLC cell lines in vitro, two phase II clinical studies and a mouse xenograft study failed to show tumor regression in SCLC by imatinib monotherapy [100–103].

RAS/RAF/MEK/ERK pathway

The *RAS* family of proto-oncogenes (*HRAS, KRAS,* and *NRAS*) are 21-kD plasma membrane-associated G-proteins that regulate key signal transduction pathways involved in normal cellular differentiation, proliferation, and survival [104]. Multiple studies have shown that oncogenic KRAS (e.g., $KRAS^{V12}$ mutant) activates cell signaling pathways important to cellular transformation [105]. As a result, KRAS abnormalities represent an important therapeutic target. *RAS* mutations (nearly always KRAS mutations in lung cancer) are found in 15–20% of NSCLCs, especially in adenocarcinomas (20–30%), but never in SCLCs [26]. The mutations occur in codons 12, 13, and 61, all of which influence intrinsic GTPase activity [104]. A number of drugs that target different aspects of RAS function and metabolism have been developed and are currently under clinical investigation [104]. These include the farnesyl transferase inhibitors tipifarnib and lonafarnib, which are now being tested in the combination with cytotoxic drugs in phase III clinical trials [106].

BRAF protein serine/threonine kinase is a downstream effecter of the Ras pathway and mutations of *BRAF* occur in ~70% melanoma, but in only 3% of lung cancers [107–109]. However, for those rare lung cancers, mutated BRAF protein is a potentially important and specific therapeutic target. An orally administered Raf kinase inhibitor, BAY 43-9006 (sorafenib), is currently being tested in phase I and phase II trials in lung cancer [110–111].

Activated BRAF phosphorylates and activates MEK1 and MEK2, which in turn phosphorylate and activate ERK1 and ERK2. However, MEK or ERK gene amplification or mutations have not been found in lung cancers. Nevertheless, ERK1/ERK2 are constitutively activated in a subset of lung cancers and MEK and ERK remain therapeutic targets for lung cancer treatment using an oral MEK inhibitor CI-1040 and its derivative PD03255901 [112].

References

1 Mazin B, Qumsiyeh YY. Molecular methods in oncology: cytogenetics. In: Vincent T, Devita SH, Rosenberg SA (eds). *Cancer: Principles and Practice of Oncology*, 7th edn. Philadelphia: Lippincott, Williams & Wilkins, 2005.

2 Nowell PC. The clonal evolution of tumor cell populations. *Science* Oct 1, 1976; **194(4260)**:23–8.

3 Varmus HE. Nobel lecture. Retroviruses and oncogenes. I. *Biosci Rep* Oct 1990; **10(5)**:413–30.

4 Todaro GJ, Huebner RJ. The viral oncogene hypothesis: new evidence. *Proc Natl Acad Sci U S A* 1972; **69**:1009–15.

5 Knudson AG, Jr. Mutation and cancer: statistical study of retinoblastoma. *Proc Natl Acad Sci U S A* Apr 1971; **68(4)**:820–3.

6 Friend SH, Bernards R, Rogelj S *et al.* A human DNA segment with properties of the gene that predisposes to retinoblastoma and osteosarcoma. *Nature* Oct 16–22, 1986; **323(6089)**:643–6.

7 Futreal PA, Coin L, Marshall M *et al.* A census of human cancer genes. *Nat Rev* Mar 2004; **4(3)**:177–83.

8 Sjoblom T, Jones S, Wood LD *et al.* The consensus coding sequences of human breast and colorectal cancers. *Science* Oct 13, 2006; **314(5797)**:268–74.

9 Hanahan D, Weinberg RA. The hallmarks of cancer. *Cell* Jan 7, 2000; **100(1)**:57–70.

10 Weinstein IB. Cancer. addiction to oncogenes—the Achilles heal of cancer. *Science* Jul 5, 2002; **297(5578)**: 63–4.

11 Sato M, Shames DS, Gazdar AF, Minna JD. A Translational View of the Molecular Pathogenesis of Lung Cancer. *J Thorac Oncol* 2007; **2(4)**:327–43.

12 Sjoblom T, Jones S, Wood LD *et al.* The consensus coding sequences of human breast and colorectal cancers. *Science* Oct 13, 2006; **314(5797)**:268–74.

13 Varmus H. The new era in cancer research. *Science* May 26, 2006; **312(5777)**:1162–5.

14 Amos CI, Xu W, Spitz MR. Is there a genetic basis for lung cancer susceptibility? *Recent Results Cancer Res* 1999; **151**:3–12.

15 Pfeifer GP, Denissenko MF, Olivier M, Tretyakova N, Hecht SS, Hainaut P. Tobacco smoke carcinogens, DNA damage and p53 mutations in smoking-associated cancers. *Oncogene* Oct 21, 2002; **21(48)**: 7435–51.

16 Jones PA, Baylin SB. The fundamental role of epigenetic events in cancer. *Nat Rev Genet* Jun 2002; **3(6)**:415–28.

17 Lengauer C, Kinzler KW, Vogelstein B. Genetic instabilities in human cancers. *Nature* Dec 17, 1998; **396(6712)**:643–9.

18 Ma Y, Jacobs SB, Jackson-Grusby L *et al.* DNA CpG hypomethylation induces heterochromatin reorganization involving the histone variant macroH2A. *J Cell Sci* Apr 15, 2005; **118(Pt 8)**:1607–16.

19 Holm TM, Jackson-Grusby L, Brambrink T, Yamada Y, Rideout WM, III, Jaenisch R. Global loss of imprinting leads to widespread tumorigenesis in adult mice. *Cancer Cell* Oct 2005; **8(4)**:275–85.

20 Jaenisch R, Bird A. Epigenetic regulation of gene expression: how the genome integrates intrinsic and environmental signals. *Nat Genet* Mar 2003; **33(Suppl)**:245–54.

21 Fukasawa K. Centrosome amplification, chromosome instability and cancer development. *Cancer Lett* Dec 8, 2005; **230(1)**:6–19.

22 Whang-Peng J, Kao-Shan CS, Lee EC *et al.* Specific chromosome defect associated with human small-cell lung cancer; deletion 3p(14-23). *Science* Jan 8, 1982; **215(4529)**:181–2.

23 Testa JR, Liu Z, Feder M *et al.* Advances in the analysis of chromosome alterations in human lung carcinomas. *Cancer Genet Cytogenet* May 1997; **95(1)**:20–32.

24 Lerman MI, Minna JD. The 630-kb lung cancer homozygous deletion region on human chromosome

3p21.3: identification and evaluation of the resident candidate tumor suppressor genes. The International Lung Cancer Chromosome 3p21.3 Tumor Suppressor Gene Consortium. *Cancer Res* Nov 1, 2000; **60(21)**:6116–33.

25 Ji L, Nishizaki M, Gao B *et al.* Expression of several genes in the human chromosome 3p21.3 homozygous deletion region by an adenovirus vector results in tumor suppressor activities in vitro and in vivo. *Cancer Res* May 1, 2002; **62(9)**:2715–20.

26 Sekido Y, Fong KM, Minna JD. Molecular genetics of lung cancer. *Annu Rev Med* 2003; **54**:73–87.

27 Wistuba II, Gazdar AF. Lung cancer preneoplasia. *Annu Rev Pathol Mech Dis* 2006; **1(1)**:331–48.

28 Wistuba II, Mao L, Gazdar AF. Smoking molecular damage in bronchial epithelium. *Oncogene* Oct 21, 2002; **21(48)**:7298–306.

29 Franklin WA, Gazdar AF, Haney J *et al.* Widely dispersed p53 mutation in respiratory epithelium. A novel mechanism for field carcinogenesis. *J Clin Invest* Oct 15, 1997; **100(8)**:2133–7.

30 Walsh CP, Chaillet JR, Bestor TH. Transcription of IAP endogenous retroviruses is constrained by cytosine methylation. *Nat Genet* Oct 1998; **20(2)**:116–7.

31 Yoder JA, Walsh CP, Bestor TH. Cytosine methylation and the ecology of intragenomic parasites. *Trends Genet* Aug 1997; **13(8)**:335–40.

32 Gaudet F, Hodgson JG, Eden A *et al.* Induction of tumors in mice by genomic hypomethylation. *Science* Apr 18, 2003; **300(5618)**:489–92.

33 Eden A, Gaudet F, Waghmare A, Jaenisch R. Chromosomal instability and tumors promoted by DNA hypomethylation. *Science* Apr 18, 2003; **300(5618)**:455.

34 Zochbauer-Muller S, Lam S, Toyooka S *et al.* Aberrant methylation of multiple genes in the upper aerodigestive tract epithelium of heavy smokers. *Int J Cancer* Nov 20, 2003; **107(4)**:612–6.

35 Zochbauer-Muller S, Fong KM, Virmani AK, Geradts J, Gazdar AF, Minna JD. Aberrant promoter methylation of multiple genes in non-small cell lung cancers. *Cancer Res* Jan 1, 2001; **61(1)**:249–55.

36 Belinsky SA, Liechty KC, Gentry FD *et al.* Promoter hypermethylation of multiple genes in sputum precedes lung cancer incidence in a high-risk cohort. *Cancer Res* Mar 15, 2006; **66(6)**:3338–44.

37 Baylin SB, Ohm JE. Epigenetic gene silencing in cancer—a mechanism for early oncogenic pathway addiction? *Nature Rev* Feb 2006; **6(2)**:107–16.

38 Shames DS, Minna JD, Gazdar AF. DNA methylation in health, disease, and cancer. *Curr Mol Med* Feb 2007; **7(1)**:85–102.

39 Esteller M, Corn PG, Baylin SB, Herman JG. A gene hypermethylation profile of human cancer. *Cancer Res* Apr 15, 2001; **61(8)**:3225–9.

40 Baylin SB, Belinsky SA, Herman JG. Aberrant methylation of gene promoters in cancer—concepts, misconcepts, and promise. *J Natl Cancer Inst* Sep 20, 2000; **92(18)**:1460–1.

41 Bestor TH. Unanswered questions about the role of promoter methylation in carcinogenesis. *Ann NY Acad Sci* Mar 2003; **983**:22–7.

42 Chan AO, Broaddus RR, Houlihan PS, Issa JP, Hamilton SR, Rashid A. CpG island methylation in aberrant crypt foci of the colorectum. *Am J Pathol* May 2002; **160(5)**:1823–30.

43 Shivapurkar N, Stastny V, Suzuki M *et al.* Application of a methylation gene panel by quantitative PCR for lung cancers. *Cancer Lett* Apr 25, 2006; **247(1)**:56–71.

44 Zochbauer-Muller S, Minna JD, Gazdar AF. Aberrant DNA methylation in lung cancer: biological and clinical implications. *Oncologist* 2002; **7(5)**:451–7.

45 Issa JP. CpG island methylator phenotype in cancer. *Nat Rev* Dec 2004; **4(12)**:988–93.

46 Sekido Y, Fong KM, Minna JD. Progress in understanding the molecular pathogenesis of human lung cancer. *Biochim Biophys Acta* Aug 19, 1998; **1378(1)**:F21–59.

47 Roth JA, Nguyen D, Lawrence DD *et al.* Retrovirus-mediated wild-type p53 gene transfer to tumors of patients with lung cancer. *Nat Med* Sep 1996; **2(9)**:985–91.

48 Gabrilovich DI. INGN 201 (Advexin): adenoviral p53 gene therapy for cancer. *Expert Opin Biol Ther* Aug 2006; **6(8)**:823–32.

49 Wikman H, Nymark P, Vayrynen A *et al.* CDK4 is a probable target gene in a novel amplicon at 12q13.3-q14.1 in lung cancer. *Genes Chromosomes Cancer* Feb 2005; **42(2)**:193–9.

50 Ratschiller D, Heighway J, Gugger M *et al.* Cyclin D1 overexpression in bronchial epithelia of patients with lung cancer is associated with smoking and predicts survival. *J Clin Oncol* Jun 1, 2003; **21(11)**:2085–93.

51 Burbee DG, Forgacs E, Zochbauer-Muller S *et al.* Epigenetic inactivation of RASSF1A in lung and breast cancers and malignant phenotype suppression. *J Natl Cancer Inst* May 2, 2001; **93(9)**:691–9.

52 Dammann R, Li C, Yoon JH, Chin PL, Bates S, Pfeifer GP. Epigenetic inactivation of a RAS association domain family protein from the lung tumour suppressor locus 3p21.3. *Nat Genet* Jul 2000; **25(3)**:315–9.

53 Kondo M, Ji L, Kamibayashi C *et al.* Overexpression of candidate tumor suppressor gene FUS1 isolated

from the 3p21.3 homozygous deletion region leads to G1 arrest and growth inhibition of lung cancer cells. *Oncogene* Sep 27, 2001; **20(43)**:6258–62.

54 Ito I, Ji L, Tanaka F *et al.* Liposomal vector mediated delivery of the 3p FUS1 gene demonstrates potent antitumor activity against human lung cancer in vivo. *Cancer Gene Ther* Nov 2004; **11(11)**:733–9.

55 Uno F, Sasaki J, Nishizaki M *et al.* Myristoylation of the fus1 protein is required for tumor suppression in human lung cancer cells. *Cancer Res* May 1, 2004; **64(9)**:2969–76.

56 Castro-Rivera E, Ran S, Thorpe P, Minna JD. Semaphorin 3B (SEMA3B) induces apoptosis in lung and breast cancer, whereas VEGF165 antagonizes this effect. *Proc Natl Acad Sci U S A* Aug 3, 2004; **101(31)**:11432–7.

57 Tomizawa Y, Sekido Y, Kondo M *et al.* Inhibition of lung cancer cell growth and induction of apoptosis after reexpression of 3p21.3 candidate tumor suppressor gene SEMA3B. *Proc Natl Acad Sci U S A* Nov 20, 2001; **98(24)**:13954–9.

58 Sozzi G, Veronese ML, Negrini M *et al.* The FHIT gene 3p14.2 is abnormal in lung cancer. *Cell* Apr 5, 1996; **85(1)**:17–26.

59 Virmani AK, Rathi A, Zochbauer-Muller S *et al.* Promoter methylation and silencing of the retinoic acid receptor-beta gene in lung carcinomas. *J Natl Cancer Inst* Aug 16, 2000; **92(16)**:1303–7.

60 Houle B, Rochette-Egly C, Bradley WE. Tumor-suppressive effect of the retinoic acid receptor beta in human epidermoid lung cancer cells. *Proc Natl Acad Sci U S A* Feb 1, 1993; **90(3)**:985–9.

61 Weinstein IB. Cancer. Addiction to oncogenes—the Achilles heal of cancer. *Science* Jul 5, 2002; **297(5578)**:63–4.

62 Sordella R, Bell DW, Haber DA, Settleman J. Gefitinib-sensitizing EGFR mutations in lung cancer activate anti-apoptotic pathways. *Science* Aug 20, 2004; **305(5687)**:1163–7.

63 Rowinsky EK. The erbB family: targets for therapeutic development against cancer and therapeutic strategies using monoclonal antibodies and tyrosine kinase inhibitors. *Annu Rev Med* 2004; **55**:433–57.

64 Franklin WA, Veve R, Hirsch FR, Helfrich BA, Bunn PA, Jr. Epidermal growth factor receptor family in lung cancer and premalignancy. *Semin Oncol* Feb 2002; **29(1, Suppl 4)**:3–14.

65 Lynch TJ, Bell DW, Sordella R *et al.* Activating mutations in the epidermal growth factor receptor underlying responsiveness of non-small-cell lung cancer to gefitinib. *N Engl J Med* May 20, 2004; **350(21)**:2129–39.

66 Paez JG, Janne PA, Lee JC *et al.* EGFR mutations in lung cancer: correlation with clinical response to gefitinib therapy. *Science* Jun 4, 2004; **304(5676)**:1497–500.

67 Shigematsu H, Gazdar AF. Somatic mutations of epidermal growth factor receptor signaling pathway in lung cancers. *Int J Cancer* Jan 15, 2006; **118(2)**:257–62.

68 Shigematsu H, Lin L, Takahashi T *et al.* Clinical and biological features associated with epidermal growth factor receptor gene mutations in lung cancers. *J Natl Cancer Inst* Mar 2, 2005; **97(5)**:339–46.

69 Fukuoka M, Yano S, Giaccone G *et al.* Multi-institutional randomized phase II trial of gefitinib for previously treated patients with advanced non-small-cell lung cancer (The IDEAL 1 Trial) [corrected]. *J Clin Oncol* Jun 15, 2003; **21(12)**:2237–46.

70 Kris MG, Natale RB, Herbst RS *et al.* Efficacy of gefitinib, an inhibitor of the epidermal growth factor receptor tyrosine kinase, in symptomatic patients with non-small cell lung cancer: a randomized trial. *JAMA* Oct 22, 2003; **290(16)**:2149–58.

71 Pao W, Miller V, Zakowski M *et al.* EGF receptor gene mutations are common in lung cancers from "never smokers" and are associated with sensitivity of tumors to gefitinib and erlotinib. *Proc Natl Acad Sci U S A* Sep 7, 2004; **101(36)**:13306–11.

72 Kobayashi S, Boggon TJ, Dayaram T *et al.* EGFR mutation and resistance of non-small-cell lung cancer to gefitinib. *N Engl J Med* Feb 24, 2005; **352(8)**:786–92.

73 Pao W, Miller VA, Politi KA *et al.* Acquired resistance of lung adenocarcinomas to gefitinib or erlotinib is associated with a second mutation in the EGFR kinase domain. *PLoS Med* Mar 2005; **2(3)**:e73.

74 Bell DW, Gore I, Okimoto RA *et al.* Inherited susceptibility to lung cancer may be associated with the T790M drug resistance mutation in EGFR. *Nat Genet* Dec 2005; **37(12)**:1315–6.

75 Kobayashi S, Ji H, Yuza Y *et al.* An alternative inhibitor overcomes resistance caused by a mutation of the epidermal growth factor receptor. *Cancer Res* Aug 15, 2005; **65(16)**:7096–101.

76 Cappuzzo F, Hirsch FR, Rossi E *et al.* Epidermal growth factor receptor gene and protein and gefitinib sensitivity in non-small-cell lung cancer. *J Natl Cancer Inst* May 4, 2005; **97(9)**:643–55.

77 Cappuzzo F, Magrini E, Ceresoli GL *et al.* Akt phosphorylation and gefitinib efficacy in patients with

advanced non-small-cell lung cancer. *J Natl Cancer Inst* Aug 4, 2004; **96(15)**:1133–41.

78 Cappuzzo F, Toschi L, Domenichini I *et al.* HER3 genomic gain and sensitivity to gefitinib in advanced non-small-cell lung cancer patients. *Br J Cancer* Dec 12, 2005; **93(12)**:1334–40.

79 Cappuzzo F, Varella-Garcia M, Shigematsu H *et al.* Increased HER2 gene copy number is associated with response to gefitinib therapy in epidermal growth factor receptor-positive non-small-cell lung cancer patients. *J Clin Oncol* Aug 1, 2005; **23(22)**:5007–18.

80 Tsao MS, Sakurada A, Cutz JC *et al.* Erlotinib in lung cancer—molecular and clinical predictors of outcome. *N Engl J Med* Jul 14, 2005; **353(2)**:133–44.

81 Pao W, Wang TY, Riely GJ *et al.* KRAS mutations and primary resistance of lung adenocarcinomas to gefitinib or erlotinib. *PLoS Med* Jan 2005; **2(1)**:e17.

82 Cappuzzo F, Gregorc V, Rossi E *et al.* Gefitinib in pretreated non-small-cell lung cancer (NSCLC): analysis of efficacy and correlation with HER2 and epidermal growth factor receptor expression in locally advanced or metastatic NSCLC. *J Clin Oncol* Jul 15, 2003; **21(14)**:2658–63.

83 Bell DW, Lynch TJ, Haserlat SM *et al.* Epidermal growth factor receptor mutations and gene amplification in non-small-cell lung cancer: molecular analysis of the IDEAL/INTACT gefitinib trials. *J Clin Oncol* Nov 1, 2005; **23(31)**:8081–92.

84 Eberhard DA, Johnson BE, Amler LC *et al.* Mutations in the epidermal growth factor receptor and in KRAS are predictive and prognostic indicators in patients with non-small-cell lung cancer treated with chemotherapy alone and in combination with erlotinib. *J Clin Oncol* Sep 1, 2005; **23(25)**:5900–9.

85 Mitsudomi T, Kosaka T, Endoh H *et al.* Mutations of the epidermal growth factor receptor gene predict prolonged survival after gefitinib treatment in patients with non-small-cell lung cancer with postoperative recurrence. *J Clin Oncol* Apr 10, 2005; **23(11)**:2513–20.

86 Shepherd FA, Rodrigues Pereira J, Ciuleanu T *et al.* Erlotinib in previously treated non-small-cell lung cancer. *N Engl J Med* Jul 14, 2005; **353(2)**:123–32.

87 Thatcher N, Chang A, Parikh P *et al.* Gefitinib plus best supportive care in previously treated patients with refractory advanced non-small-cell lung cancer: results from a randomised, placebo-controlled, multicentre study (Iressa Survival Evaluation in Lung Cancer). *Lancet* Oct 29–Nov 4, 2005; **366(9496)**:1527–37.

88 Giaccone G, Herbst RS, Manegold C *et al.* Gefitinib in combination with gemcitabine and cisplatin in advanced non-small-cell lung cancer: a phase III trial—INTACT 1. *J Clin Oncol* Mar 1, 2004; **22(5)**:777–84.

89 Herbst RS, Giaccone G, Schiller JH *et al.* Gefitinib in combination with paclitaxel and carboplatin in advanced non-small-cell lung cancer: a phase III trial—INTACT 2. *J Clin Oncol* Mar 1, 2004; **22(5)**:785–94.

90 Das AK, Sato M, Story MD *et al.* Non-small cell lung cancers with kinase domain mutations in the epidermal growth factor receptor are sensitive to ionizing radiation. *Cancer Res* Oct 1, 2006; **66(19)**:9601–8.

91 Shigematsu H, Takahashi T, Nomura M *et al.* Somatic mutations of the HER2 kinase domain in lung adenocarcinomas. *Cancer Res* Mar 1, 2005; **65(5)**:1642–6.

92 Stephens P, Hunter C, Bignell G *et al.* Lung cancer: intragenic ERBB2 kinase mutations in tumours. *Nature* Sep 30, 2004; **431(7008)**:525–6.

93 Soung YH, Lee JW, Kim SY *et al.* Somatic mutations of the ERBB4 kinase domain in human cancers. *Int J Cancer* Mar 15, 2006; **118(6)**:1426–9.

94 Tang X, Shigematsu H, Bekele BN *et al.* EGFR tyrosine kinase domain mutations are detected in histologically normal respiratory epithelium in lung cancer patients. *Cancer Res* Sep 1, 2005; **65(17)**:7568–72.

95 Ji H, Li D, Chen L *et al.* The impact of human EGFR kinase domain mutations on lung tumorigenesis and in vivo sensitivity to EGFR-targeted therapies. *Cancer Cell* Jun 2006; **9(6)**:485–95.

96 Politi K, Zakowski MF, Fan PD, Schonfeld EA, Pao W, Varmus HE. Lung adenocarcinomas induced in mice by mutant EGF receptors found in human lung cancers respond to a tyrosine kinase inhibitor or to downregulation of the receptors. *Genes Dev* Jun 1, 2006; **20(11)**:1496–510.

97 Sekido Y, Obata Y, Ueda R *et al.* Preferential expression of c-kit protooncogene transcripts in small cell lung cancer. *Cancer Res* May 1, 1991; **51(9)**:2416–9.

98 Boldrini L, Ursino S, Gisfredi S *et al.* Expression and mutational status of c-kit in small-cell lung cancer: prognostic relevance. *Clin Cancer Res* Jun 15, 2004; **10(12, Pt 1)**:4101–8.

99 Hirota S, Isozaki K, Moriyama Y *et al.* Gain-of-function mutations of c-kit in human gastrointestinal stromal tumors. *Science* Jan 23, 1998; **279(5350)**:577–80.

100 Johnson BE, Fischer T, Fischer B *et al.* Phase II study of imatinib in patients with small cell lung cancer. *Clin Cancer Res* Dec 1, 2003; **9(16, Pt 1)**:5880–7.

101 Krug LM, Crapanzano JP, Azzoli CG *et al.* Imatinib mesylate lacks activity in small cell lung carcinoma

expressing c-kit protein: a phase II clinical trial. *Cancer* May 15, 2005; **103(10)**:2128–31.

102 Wolff NC, Randle DE, Egorin MJ, Minna JD, Ilaria RL, Jr. Imatinib mesylate efficiently achieves therapeutic intratumor concentrations in vivo but has limited activity in a xenograft model of small cell lung cancer. *Clin Cancer Res* May 15, 2004; **10(10)**:3528–34.

103 Wang WL, Healy ME, Sattler M *et al.* Growth inhibition and modulation of kinase pathways of small cell lung cancer cell lines by the novel tyrosine kinase inhibitor STI 571. *Oncogene* Jul 20, 2000; **19(31)**:3521–8.

104 Downward J. Targeting RAS signalling pathways in cancer therapy. *Nat Rev Cancer* Jan 2003; **3(1)**:11–22.

105 Stacey DW, Kung HF. Transformation of NIH 3T3 cells by microinjection of Ha-ras p21 protein. *Nature* Aug 9–15, 1984; **310(5977)**:508–11.

106 Isobe T, Herbst RS, Onn A. Current management of advanced non-small cell lung cancer: targeted therapy. *Semin Oncol* Jun 2005; **32(3)**:315–28.

107 Brose MS, Volpe P, Feldman M *et al.* BRAF and RAS mutations in human lung cancer and melanoma. *Cancer Res* Dec 1, 2002; **62(23)**:6997–7000.

108 Davies H, Bignell GR, Cox C *et al.* Mutations of the BRAF gene in human cancer. *Nature* Jun 27, 2002; **417(6892)**:949–54.

109 Naoki K, Chen TH, Richards WG, Sugarbaker DJ, Meyerson M. Missense mutations of the BRAF gene in human lung adenocarcinoma. *Cancer Res* Dec 1, 2002; **62(23)**:7001–3.

110 Liu B, Barrett T, Choyke P *et al.* A phase II study of BAY 43-9006 (Sorafenib) in patients with relapsed non-small cell lung cancer (NSCLC) [Abstract 17119]. *Pro Am Soc Clin Onc* 2005; **24**:18S.

111 Tuveson DA, Weber BL, Herlyn M. BRAF as a potential therapeutic target in melanoma and other malignancies. *Cancer Cell* Aug 2003; **4(2)**:95–8.

112 Hoshino R, Chatani Y, Yamori T *et al.* Constitutive activation of the 41-/43-kDa mitogen-activated protein kinase signaling pathway in human tumors. *Oncogene* Jan 21, 1999; **18(3)**:813–22.

CHAPTER 5

Molecular Biology of Preneoplastic Lesions of the Lung

Ignacio I. Wistuba and Adi F. Gazdar

Introduction

Lung cancer is the leading cause of cancer deaths in the United States and worldwide [1]. The high mortality of this disease is primarily due to the fact that the majority of the lung cancers are diagnosed at advanced stages when the options for treatment are mostly palliative. Experience with other epithelial tumors has shown that if neoplastic lesions can be detected and treated at their intraepithelial stage the chances for survival can be improved significantly. Thus, to reduce the mortality rate of lung cancer, new techniques and approaches must be developed to identify, diagnose, and treat preinvasive lesions. However, the early diagnosis of lung cancer represents an enormous challenge.

From histopathological and biological perspectives, lung cancer is a highly complex set of different but related neoplasms [2], probably having multiple preoplastic pathways. Lung cancer consists of several histological types, including small cell lung carcinoma (SCLC) and nonsmall cell lung carcinoma (NSCLC) types of squamous cell carcinoma, adenocarcinoma (including the noninvasive type of bronchioloalveolar carcinoma, BAC), and large cell carcinoma [3]. Lung cancers may arise from the major bronchi (central tumors) or small bronchi, bronchioles, or alveoli (peripheral tumors)

of the distant airway of the lung. Squamous cell carcinomas and SCLCs usually arise centrally, whereas adenocarcinomas and large cell carcinomas usually arise peripherally [3]. However, the specific respiratory epithelial cell type from which each lung cancer type develops has not been established. As with other epithelial malignancies, it is believed that lung cancers arise after a series of progressive pathological changes, known as preoplastic or premalignant lesions [4,5]. Although the sequential preoplastic changes have been defined for centrally arising squamous carcinomas of the lung [6], they have been poorly documented for the other major forms of lung cancers [4,5].

Although many molecular abnormalities have been described in clinically evident lung cancers [2], relatively little is known about the molecular events preceding the development of lung carcinomas and the underlying genetic basis of lung carcinogenesis. In the past decade, several studies have provided information regarding the molecular characterization of the preoplastic changes involved in the pathogenesis of lung cancer, especially squamous cell carcinoma and adenocarcinoma [7–10]. Many of these molecular changes have been detected in the histologically normal respiratory mucosa of smokers [11,12]. The high-risk population targeted for early detection efforts are heavy smokers and patients who have survived a cancer of the upper aerodigestive tract. However, conventional morphologic methods for the identification of premalignant cell populations in the lung airways have important limitations. This has led to research in

Lung Cancer, 3rd edition. Edited by Jack A. Roth, James D. Cox, and Waun Ki Hong. © 2008 Blackwell Publishing, ISBN: 978-1-4051-5112-2.

biological properties, including molecular and genetic changes, of the respiratory epithelium and its corresponding preneoplastic cells and lesions.

Although several studies have provided relevant information regarding the molecular characterization of the premalignant changes involved in the pathogenesis of lung cancer, especially for squamous cell carcinoma [10], that information is not sufficient to identify with certainty molecular pathogenetic pathways or molecular markers useful for risks assessment, targeted chemoprevention or treatment, and early detection of lung premalignant lesions. Further research in this area may provide new methods for assessing the likelihood of developing invasive lung cancer in smokers and allow for early detection and monitoring of their response to chemopreventive regimens. Attempts to better define the pathogenesis of lung premalignancy have been thwarted by the relative invisibility of the cellular lesions and their random distribution throughout the respiratory airway field, and new methodologies, including computed tomography (CT) imaging [13] and fluorescence bronchoscopy [14], has been introduced to better identify and visualize lung premalignant lesions.

In this chapter we summarize the current information on lung cancer molecular and histopathologic pathogenesis and discuss the complexity of the identification of novel molecular mechanisms involved in the development of the lung premalignant disease, and their relevance to the development of new strategies for early detection and chemoprevention. In addition, we describe the recognized preneoplastic lesions for major types of lung cancers and review the current concepts of early pathogenesis and the progression of the most important histologic types of lung cancer.

Pathology of lung cancer preneoplastic lesions

Lung cancers are believed to arise after a series of progressive pathological changes (preneoplastic or precursor lesions) in the respiratory mucosa. The recent 2004 World Health Organization (WHO) International Association for the Study of Lung Cancer (IASLC) histological classification of preinvasive lesions of the lung lists three main morphologic forms of preneoplastic lesions in the lung [3]: (a) squamous dysplasia and carcinoma in situ (CIS); (b) atypical adenomatous hyperplasia (AAH); and (c) diffuse idiopathic pulmonary neuroendocrine cell hyperplasia (DIPNECH). While the sequential preneoplastic changes have been defined for centrally arising squamous carcinomas, they have been poorly documented for large cell carcinomas, adenocarcinomas and SCLCs [4,5]. Mucosal changes in the large airways that may precede invasive squamous cell carcinoma include squamous dysplasia and CIS [4,5]. Adenocarcinomas may be preceded by morphological changes including AAH in peripheral airway cells [4,15]. While DIPNECH are thought to be precursor lesions for carcinoids of the lung, for SCLC there is no specific preneoplastic change have been identified.

Squamous cell carcinoma preneoplastic lesions

Mucosal changes in the large airways that may precede or accompany invasive squamous cell carcinoma include hyperplasia, squamous metaplasia, squamous dysplasia, and CIS [4,5] (Figure 5.1). There are no squamous cells in the normal airways. The progenitor or stem cells for the squamous metaplastic epithelium of the proximal airway is not known, but it is presumed that the basal cells are pluripotent and can give rise to metaplastic and dysplastic squamous cells, which function as precursors of squamous cell carcinomas.

Dysplastic squamous lesions may be graded in of different intensities (i.e., mild, moderate, and severe); however, these lesions represent a continuum of cytologic and histologic atypical changes that may show some overlapping between categories. Whereas mild squamous dysplasia is characterized by minimal architectural and cytological disturbance, moderate dysplasia exhibits more cytological irregularity, which is even higher in severe dysplasia and is accompanied by considerable cellular polymorphism. In a subset of squamous dysplastic changes, the basal membrane thickens and there is vascular budding in the subepithelial tissue that results in papillary protrusions of the epithelium,

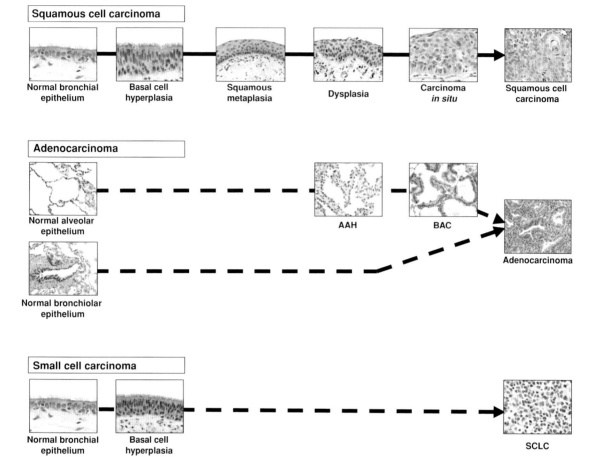

Figure 5.1 Summary of histopathologic changes involved in the pathogenesis of lung cancer. The sequence of preneoplastic lesions involved in the development of squamous cell carcinoma of the lung has been elucidated. For adenocarcinoma histology, the only known preneoplastic lesion is AAH (atypical adenomatous hyperplasia), which seems to be the precursor for a subset of lung adenocarcinomas, those with bronchioloalveolar carcinoma (BAC) features. No preneoplastic lesion has been recognized for SCLC (microphotographs of histology sections stained with hematoxylin and eosin).

lesions that have been termed angiogenic squamous dysplasia (ASD) [16]. These lesions indicate that angiogenesis commences at a relatively early preneoplastic stage. CIS demonstrates extreme cytological aberrations with almost complete architectural disarray, but with an intact basement membrane and absence of stromal invasion. Foci of CIS usually arise near bifurcations in the segmental bronchi, subsequently extending proximally into the adjacent lobar bronchus and distally into subsegmental branches. These lesions are often not detected by conventional white-light bronchoscopy or gross examination. However, the utilization of fluorescent bronchoscopy, such as lung-imaging fluorescent endoscopy (LIFE), greatly increases the sensitivity for detection of squamous dysplastic and CIS lesions [14]. Little is known about the rate and risks of progression from squamous dysplasia to CIS and ultimately to invasive squamous cell carcinoma.

Adenocarcinoma precursor lesions

It has been suggested that peripherally arising adenocarcinomas may be preceded by AAH in peripheral airway cells [4,15]; however, the respiratory structures and the specific epithelia cell types involved in the origin of most lung adenocarcinomas are unknown (Figure 5.1). AAH is considered a putative precursor of adenocarcinoma [4,15]. AAH is a discrete parenchymal lesion arising in the alveoli close to terminal and respiratory bronchioles. Because of their size, AAH are usually incidental histological findings, but they may be detected grossly, especially if they are 0.5 cm or larger. The increasing use of high resolution CT scans for screening purposes has led to an increasing awareness of this entity, as it remains one of the most important differential diagnoses of air filled peripheral lesions (called "ground glass opacities") [17]. AHH maintains an alveolar structure lined by rounded, cuboidal, or low columnar cells.

The postulated progression of AAH to noninvasive BAC adenocarcinoma with, apparent from the increasingly atypical morphology, is supported by morphometric, cytofluorometric, and molecular studies [5,15]. Invasion may follow, especially at the fibrous centers of these lesions, giving rise to adenocarcinomas having mixed features of BAC and tubular or papillary adenocarcinomas. Distinction between highly atypical AAH and nonmucinous BAC is sometimes difficult. However, as these lesions have very high 5-year survival rates after resection provided they are <2 cm in size, the distinction may be academic. Somewhat arbitrarily, BAC are considered generally >10 mm in size, with more cellular atypia than their AAH counterparts. The origin of AAH is still unknown, but the differentiation phenotype derived from immunohistochemical and ultrastructural features suggests an origin from the progenitor cells of the peripheral airways, such Clara cells and type II pneumocytes [18,19].

There is an increasing body of evidence to support the concept of AAH as precursor of at least a subset of adenocarcinomas. AAH is most frequently detected in lung from patients bearing lung cancers (9–20%), especially adenocarcinomas (up to 40%) compared to squamous cell carcinomas (11%) [5,20–22]. By contrast, autopsy studies have reported AAH in ~3% of noncancer patients [23].

Precursor lesions of neuroendocrine tumors

As stated above, the precursor lesions for the most common type of neuroendocrine carcinoma of the lung, the SCLC, are unknown [4,5] (Figure 5.1).

However, a rare lesion called DIPENECH has been associated with the development of other neuroendocrine tumors of the lung, typical and atypical carcinoids [4,24]. DIPENECH lesions include local extraluminal proliferations in the form of tumorlets. Carcinoid tumors are arbitrarily separated from tumorlets if the neuroendocrine proliferation is 0.5 cm or larger.

Molecular pathogenesis of lung cancer

Although our current knowledge of the molecular pathogenesis of lung cancer is still meager, during the last decade, there are several important lessons learnt on the molecular pathogenesis of this tumor, including the following: (a) There are several histopathologic and molecular pathways associated with the development of the major types of NSCLC. (b) Although there is a field effect phenomenon for lung preneoplastic lesions, recent data suggest that there are at least two distinct lung airways compartments (central and peripheral) for lung cancer pathogenesis. (c) Inflammation may play an important role in lung cancer development and it could be an important component of the field effect phenomenon. (d) For lung adenocarcinoma, at least two smoking and nonsmoking-related pathways have been identified. Most of the molecular and histopathologic changes in the respiratory epithelium associated to lung cancer pathogenesis have been related to smoking [10]. However, the recent discovery of frequent *EGFR* gene mutations in lung cancer and adjacent normal epithelium in never or light smokers suggests the presence of at least two distinct molecular pathogenesis for lung cancer, smoking and nonsmoking-related [25,26]. As a relatively small subset of smokers develop lung cancer, attention has been focused in the identification of specific molecular and histopathologic pathways that can predict lung cancer development in high-risk populations. One of those key pathways, currently under intense investigation, is the activation of inflammation-related pathways.

Several studies have revealed that multiple genetic changes are found in clinically evident lung cancers, and involve known and putative tumor suppressor genes as well as several dominant onco-genes [2]. Lung cancers arise after a series of molecular changes that commence in histologically normal epithelium and demonstrate a specific se-quence [7,10]. There is a preferred order of these allele loss changes with 3p allele loss (several 3p sites) followed by 9p ($p16^{INK4a}$ locus) as the earli-est changes occurring in histologically normal ep-ithelium [7,9,27]. Telomerase activation has been also implicated as an early event in lung cancer pathogenesis [28,29]. Telomerase shortening repre-sents an early genetic abnormality in bronchial car-cinogenesis, preceding telomerase expression and p53/Rb inactivation, which predominate in high-grade squamous preinvasive lesions [30]. Precise microscopic-based microdissection of epithelial tis-sue followed by allelotyping of smoking damaged lung from lung cancer patients or current or former smokers without lung cancer revealed multiple le-sions containing clonal abnormalities of allele loss, occurring in both histologically normal as well as mildly abnormal (hyperplasia and squamous meta-plasia) and preneoplastic (dysplasia) respiratory ep-ithelium [31]. While those changes are found in the lungs of current and former smokers without lung cancer they are almost never found in lifetime never smokers [11,12]. Interestingly, these clonal changes persist for decades after smoking cessation [11].

Similar evidence exists for multiple promoter methylation changes in smoking-damaged lung ep-ithelium and sputum specimens [32,33]. Results on methylation analysis of several genes, including $RAR\beta$-2, H-cadherin, APC, $p16^{INK4a}$, and RASFF1A in-dicate that abnormal gene methylation is a relatively frequent (one or more genes in 48%) in oropharyn-geal and bronchial epithelial cells in heavy smokers with evidence of sputum atypia [33]. Methylation in one or more of three genes tested ($p16^{INK4a}$, GSTP1, and DAPK) has been demonstrated in bronchial brush specimens in about one third of smokers [34]. Results from another study indicated that aberrant promoter hypermethylation of the $p16^{INK4a}$ gene occurs frequently in the bronchial epithelium of lung cancer cases and smokers without cancer and persists after smoking cessation [35,36]. Aberrant promoter methylation of $p16^{INK4a}$ was seen in at least one bronchial epithelial site from 44% of lung cancer patients and cancer-free smokers. A recent nested case–control study [37] of incident lung can-cer cases from an extremely high-risk cohort for evaluating promoter methylation of 14 genes in sputum showed that the prevalence for methylation of gene promoters increased as the time to lung can-cer diagnosis decreased. Six ($p16^{INK4a}$, MGMT, DAPK, RASSF1A, PAX5β, and GATA5) of 14 genes were as-sociated with a >50% increased lung cancer risk. In addition, in the same study, the concomitant methy-lation of three or more of these six genes was associ-ated with a 6.5-fold increased risk and a sensitivity and specificity of 64%. Of interest, the methylation patterns of adenocarcinomas arising in smokers and never smokers are different, and may be related to the major genetic changes in these tumors (KRAS and EGFR mutations, respectively) [38].

Considerable attention has been given to the identification of the 3p genes involved in lung can-cer pathogenesis including $RAR\beta$ at 3p24, FHIT at 3p14.2, RASSF1A, BLU, FUS1, and SEMA3B located at 3p21.3, and potentially ROBO1 at 3p12 [9,32,39]. Their expression is frequently lost in lung cancer, usually by promoter methylation [40]. However, specific roles of the genes undergoing activation or inactivation and the order of cumulative molecular changes that lead to the development of each lung tumor histologic type remain to be elucidated.

Profiling studies using high-throughput tech-nologies for the identification of molecular signa-tures associated to the development and progres-sion of lung cancer precursor lesions are extremely difficult to perform because usually they are small size lesions that need histological confirmation by tissue fixation and histopathologic processing. Al-though some profiling studies have been performed using in vitro cultured human normal bronchial ep-ithelial cells [41,42], recently a specific pattern of protein expression using proteomic methodology of the airway epithelium that accurately classified bronchial and alveolar tissue with normal histology from preinvasive bronchial lesions and from inva-sive lung cancer was reported [41]. Although these findings need to be further validated, this represent a first step toward a new proteomic characterization of the human model of lung cancer development.

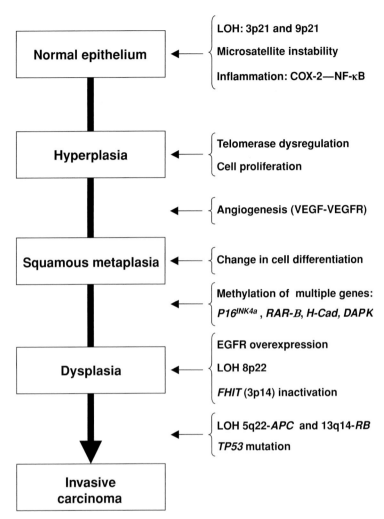

Figure 5.2 Molecular pathogenesis of squamous cell carcinoma of the lung. Several sequential molecular abnormalities have been recognized in the multistep pathogenesis of squamous cell carcinoma of the lung, which have been detected in high-risk individuals.

Pathogenesis of squamous cell carcinoma

The current working model of the sequential molecular abnormalities in the pathogenesis of squamous cell lung carcinoma indicates that: (a) Genetic abnormalities commence in histologically normal epithelium and increase with increasing severity of histologic changes [7] (Figure 5.2). (b) Molecular changes in the respiratory epithelium are extensive and multifocal throughout the bronchial tree of smokers and lung cancer patients, indicating a field effect or field cancerization [7,9,11,12]. (c) Mutations follow a sequence, with progressive allelic losses at multiple 3p (3p21, 3p14, 3p22-24, and 3p12) chromosome sites and 9p21 ($p16^{INK4a}$) as the earliest detected changes. Later changes include 8p21-23, 13q14 (*RB*), and 17p13 (*TP53*) [7,9,27]. $p16^{INK4a}$ methylation has been also detected at an early stage of squamous preinvasive lesions with a frequency that increases during histopathologic progression (24% in squamous metaplasia and 50% in CIS) [35]. (d) Multiple clonal and subclonal patches of molecular abnormalities not much larger in size than the average bronchial biopsy obtained by fluorescent bronchoscopy, estimated to be approximately 40,000–360,000 cells, can be detected in the normal and slightly abnormal bronchial epithelium of patients with lung cancer [31]. Despite encouraging results from isolated studies [37], most of these findings have not been useful for the development of successful strategies for lung cancer risk assessment, early detection, and chemoprevention.

Interestingly, in a subset of squamous metaplastic and dysplastic changes, the basal membrane becomes thickened and there is vascular budding in the subepithelial tissues that results in papillary protrusions of the epithelium, lesions termed ASD [16]. ASD lesions are more frequently detected using fluorescent bronchoscopy compared to white-light conventional bronchoscopy [43]. In the bronchial biopsies with these lesions microvessel density is elevated in comparison to normal mucosa but not in comparison to other forms of hyperplasia or dysplasia. ASD thus represents a qualitatively distinct form of angiogenesis in which there is architectural rearrangement of the capillary microvasculature. Genetic analysis of surface epithelium in a subset of lesions revealed loss of heterozygosity (LOH) at chromosome 3p in 53% of lesions, and compared with normal epithelium, proliferative activity was markedly elevated in ASD lesions. ASD occurs in approximately 19% of high-risk smokers without carcinoma who underwent fluorescence bronchoscopy [44] and was not present in biopsies from 16 normal nonsmoker control subjects [16]. The presence of this lesion in high-risk smokers suggests that aberrant patterns of microvascularization may occur at an early stage of bronchial carcinogenesis. The finding of vascular endothelial growth factor (VEGF) isoforms and VEGF receptors (VEGFR) by semi-quantitative reverse transcriptase-PCR confirmed by immunohistochemistry in bronchial squamous dysplastic compared to normal bronchial epithelia [45] supports the notion that angiogenesis develops early in lung carcinogenesis and that these abnormalities provide rationale for the development of targeted antiangiogenic chemoprevention strategies.

The recent developments in molecular biology have increased our knowledge of critical biological pathways that are deregulated in lung cancer cells and they have provided rationale for the development of targeted therapy in human tumors, including lung. Activation of tyrosine kinases (TK), particularly receptor TK is increasingly recognized as a common cause for deregulation of these pathways, and inhibiting TK has proven to be an effective strategy for a number of malignancies, including lung cancer [46]. Thus, the possible activation of signaling pathways early in the pathogenesis of lung cancer have created an opportunity for the design of targeted chemoprevention strategies [47]. Of interest, most important signaling pathways that are being targeted in lung cancer have been shown to be also deregulated in lung cancer preneoplastic lesions, mostly in the squamous cell carcinoma pathway, including, among others, the inflammation-related polyunsaturated fatty acid metabolic pathways [48], retinoic acid signaling [49], and pathways involving Ras [15,50,51], EGFR [26,52], phosphoinositide 3-kinase (PI3K)/Akt [53,54], insulin-like growth (IGF) factor axis [55], and mTOR [50].

Pathogenesis of lung adenocarcinoma

Several molecular changes frequently present in lung adenocarcinomas are also present in AAH lesions, and they are further evidence that AAH may represent true preneoplastic lesions (Figure 5.3). The most important finding is the presence of *KRAS* (codon 12) mutations in up to 39% of AAHs, which are also a relatively frequent alteration in lung adenocarcinomas [15,56]. Other molecular alterations detected in AAH are overexpression of Cyclin D1 ($\sim$70%), p53 (ranging from 10 to 58%), survivin (48%), and HER2/neu (7%) proteins overexpression [15,57,58]. Some AAH lesions have demonstrated LOH in chromosomes 3p (18%), 9p ($p16^{INK4a}$, 13%), 9q (53%), 17q, and 17p (*TP53*, 6%), changes that are frequently detected in lung adenocarcinomas [59,60]. A study on lung adenocarcinoma with synchronous multiple AAHs showed frequent LOH of tuberous sclerosis complex (TSC)-associated regions (*TSC1* at 9q, 53%, and *TSC2* at 16p, 6%), suggesting that these

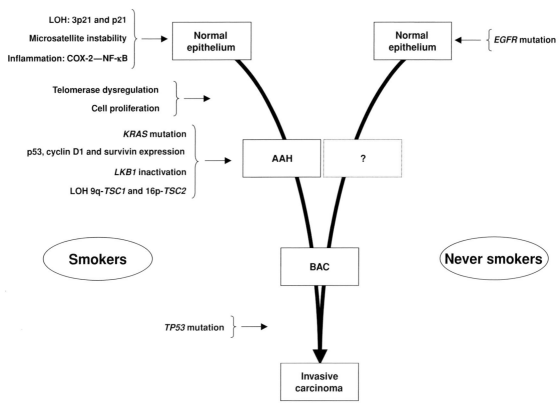

Figure 5.3 Molecular pathogenesis of adenocarcinoma of the lung. At least two molecular pathways have been identified in the development of lung adenocarcinoma, smoking, and nonsmoking-related (AAH, atypical adenomatous hyperplasia; BAC, bronchioloalveolar carcinoma).

are candidate loci for tumor suppressor gene in a subset of adenocarcinomas of the lung [60]. Activation of telomerase expressed by expression of human telomerase RNA component (hTERC) and telomerase reverse transcriptase (hTERT) mRNA, has been detected in 27–78% of AAH lesions, depending in their atypia level [61]. Recently, it has been shown that loss of LKB1, a serine/threonine kinase that functions as a tumor suppressor gene, is frequent in lung adenocarcinomas (25%) and AAH (21%) with severe cytological atypia, while it is rare in mild atypical AAH lesions (5%), suggesting that *LKB1* inactivation may play a role in the AAH progression to malignancy [62].

Several mouse models have been developed to better study various oncogenic molecular signaling pathways and the sequence of molecular events involved in the pathogenesis of peripheral lung

tumors, and to test novel chemopreventive agents [63]. The *KRAS* oncogenic mouse model is characterized for the development of peripheral alveolar type of proliferations, including AAH, adenoma, and adenocarcinoma [63]. Using this mouse model, several important findings that need to be further validated in human tissues have been reported. Kim *et al.* [64] identified the potential stem cell population (expressing Clara cells-specific protein and surfactant protein-C, termed bronchioalveolar stem cell, BASC) that maintains the bronchiolar Clara cells and alveolar cells of the distal respiratory epithelium and which could be considered the precursors of lung *KRAS* neoplastic lesions in mice. Wislez *et al.* [50] provided evidence that the expansion of lung adenocarcinoma precursors induced by oncogenic *KRAS* requires mammalian target of rapamycin (mTOR)-dependent signaling and, most importantly, that inflammation-related host factors, including factors derived from macrophages, play a critical role in mice adenocarcinoma progression. Recent findings reported by Collado *et al.* [65], suggest that *KRAS* oncogene-induced senescence may help to restrict tumor progression of lung peripheral lesions in mice. They discovered that a substantial number of cells in mice premalignant alveolar type of lesions undergo oncogene-induced senescence, but the cells that escape senescence by loss of oncogene-induced senescence effectors, such as p16^{INK4a} or p53, progress to malignancy. Thus, senescence is a defining feature of premalignant lung lesions, but not invasive tumors.

Pathogenesis of SCLC

As stated before, no phenotypically identifiable epithelial lesion has been identified as a precursor for SCLC (Figure 5.1). A study comparing the molecular changes (LOH at several chromosomal sites and microsatellite instability) occurring in histologically normal and mildly abnormal (hyperplastic) centrally located bronchial epithelia accompanying SCLCs and NSCLCs tumors demonstrated a significantly higher incidence of genetic abnormalities in bronchial epithelia accompanying SCLC than those adjacent to NSCLC (squamous cell carcinoma and adenocarcinoma) [8]. These findings indicate that more widespread and more extensive genetic damage is present in bronchial epithelium in patients with SCLC. The finding that some specimens of normal or mildly abnormal epithelia accompanying SCLCs have a high incidence of genetic changes suggests that SCLC may arise directly from histologically normal or mildly abnormal epithelium, without passing through a more complex histologic sequence.

Field defect phenomenon in lung cancer pathogenesis

Current information suggests that lung premalignant lesions are frequently extensive and multifocal throughout the respiratory epithelium, indicating a field effect [66]. This phenomenon is called field defect or field cancerization, by which much of the respiratory epithelium has been mutagenized, presumably from exposure to tobacco-related carcinogenesis [67]. Several studies performed in the respiratory epithelium of lung cancer patients and smokers individuals have demonstrated that multiple molecularly altered foci of bronchial epithelium are present throughout the airway [7,8]. A detailed analysis of premalignant and malignant epithelium from squamous cell carcinoma patients indicated that multiple, sequentially occurring allele-specific chromosomal deletions (LOH) commence in widely dispersed, apparently clonally independent foci, early in the multistage pathogenesis of squamous cell carcinomas of the lung [8]. These observations were extended to former and current smokers [11,12], whose bronchial epithelium demonstrate multiple foci of genetic changes similar to those found in lung cancers and may persist for many years after smoking cessation [11].

Inflammation and lung cancer

Accumulating evidence suggests that tumor progression is governed not only by genetic changes intrinsic to cancer cells but also by epigenetic and environmental factors. Chronic inflammation has been hypothesized as one of the most important epigenetic and environmental factors contributing to epithelial cancer development and tumor progression [68]. A chronic inflammatory process enhances cell proliferation, cell survival, and cell migration in epithelial cells, as well as angiogenesis in the adjacent stroma, thereby promoting epithelial tumor development [68]. In the last decades, inflammation and related pathways have been suggested to play an important role in the pathogenesis of lung cancer, particularly in smoking-damaged respiratory epithelium [69,70]. However, the mechanisms involved are not well understood.

The specific cellular and molecular pathways that link such inflammatory responses to malignant transformation vary depending on the microorganism, target organ, and tumor subtype [68,70]. However, despite these differences, several common features exist, including the release of free radicals that contribute to malignant transformation of epithelial cells by peroxidating lipids and inducing genetic mutations [68]. Such damage to epithelial cells stimulates apoptotic cell death and reactive epithelial hyperproliferation that promotes further mutation. Moreover, inflammation-related carcinogenesis results from the stimulation of angiogenesis and from inflammatory cells and mediators that act directly on epithelial cells and indirectly on stromal cells and extracellular matrix components [68].

The association between chronic inflammatory conditions of the lung and cancer has been studied extensively [70]. As stated above, several studies have found that smoker with chronic obstructive pulmonary disease (COPD) have an increased risk of lung cancer compared to smokers without COPD [70]. In COPD, at the level of the alveoli, inflammation leads to protease release and oxidative inactivation of antiproteases by inflammatory cells contributing to degradation of the extracellular matrix [71,72]. At the level of the conducting airways, there is metaplasia of the airway epithelium to a mucus-secreting phenotype, thickening of the airway wall from the increased deposition of matrix molecules and the proliferation of mesenchymal cells, and narrowing from fibrosis [71,72]. These changes are also present in the lungs of smokers without COPD but they are not as severe [73]. COPD patients with 40 or more pack-years of smoking history have demonstrated a high prevalence of premalignant dysplasia (24% severe and CIS) detectable through sputum cytology [74]. Compared with men, women smokers have a lower prevalence of high-grade preinvasive lesions in the observed airways (14% versus 31%), and women with preinvasive lesions had fewer such lesions. The prevalence of preinvasive lesions did not change substantially for more than 10 years after cessation of smoking. Lung function was associated with the prevalence of preinvasive lesions, but the association was weaker in women than in men [75].

A number of lines of evidence suggest that chronic inflammation contributes to the process of lung carcinogenesis through activation of a number of molecular pathways, including the nuclear factor kappa B (NF-κB) [69,70]. In NSCLC cell lines, it has been demonstrated that tobacco components stimulate NF-κB-dependent survival [76]. It has been recently demonstrated that NF-κB p65 protein nuclear overexpression is an early and frequent

phenomenon in the pathogenesis of lung cancer, being frequently detected in bronchial squamous dysplastic changes and peripheral lung AAH lesions in lung cancer patients [77], and in a limited number of squamous dysplasias obtained from smokers without cancer [78]. NF-κB has recently identified as a molecular link between chronic inflammation and cancer [79,80], suggesting that NF-κB exerts its oncogenic effects in both the tumor and the microenvironment, promoting the survival of premalignant epithelial cells [81]. NF-κB has shown to suppress apoptosis and induce expression of proto-oncogenes such as c-myc and cyclin D1, which directly stimulate cell proliferation [82]. In addition, NF-κB regulates the expression of various molecules important in tumorigenesis, such as matrix metalloproteinases, COX-2, inducible nitric oxide synthase, chemokines, and inflammatory cytokines, all of which promote tumor cell invasion and angiogenesis [83].

The eicosanoid pathway, specifically COX-2, has been involved in the pathogenesis of lung cancer. COX-2, an intermediate early response gene induced by growth factors, oncogenes, carcinogens, and tumor-promoter phorbol esters [84], has been shown to be overexpressed in lung adenocarcinoma and squamous cell carcinoma [85]. Cyclooxygenase catalyzes the synthesis of prostaglandins from arachidonic acid, and both arachidonic acid and eicosanoids are potent inflammatory and growth agents. Both preclinical and clinical trials of the effect of celecoxib on lung cancer prevention have shown a marked reduction in PGE2 production [86]. COX-2 immunohistochemical expression has shown to be highly expressed in bronchial squamous dysplasias, especially those having high-grade histology (severe dysplasia and CIS) [87]. Recent findings suggest that the COX-2 inhibitor celecoxib may be capable of modulating the proliferation indices and apoptotic balance in bronchial tissue of active smokers [88].

However, it is currently unknown whether NF-κB or COX-2 activity itself plays a causal role in the initiation event leading to lung cancer or whether it may participate in tumor promotion and progression. Clearly, despite recent advances, the role of inflammation in lung cancer pathogenesis still remains an open question.

Nonsmoking-related pathways

Although most lung cancers are smoking-related tumors, a subset of NSCLCs arises in never smoker patients. Adenocarcinoma histology is the tumor type most frequently detected in never smoker population. Recently, somatic mutations of *EGFR and HER-2/NEU*, TK members of the ErbB family, have been reported in a subset of lung adenocarcinoma patients having never or light smoker status, female gender and East Asian ethnicity [89–96]. The *EGFR* mutations are clinically relevant because most of them have been associated with sensitivity of lung adenocarcinoma to small molecule TK inhibitors (gefitinib and erlotinib) [89–91,97]. Over 80% of the mutations detected in *EGFR* are in-frame deletions in exon 19 and a single missense mutation in exon 21 (L858R) [89–92,94,95]. It has been proposed that lung cancer cells with mutant *EGFR* might become physiologically dependent on the continued activity of the gene for the maintenance of their malignant phenotype, leading to accelerated development of lung adenocarcinoma [25]. Recent studies have demonstrated that tumor cell high *EGFR* copy number, identified by fluorescent in situ hybridization (FISH) technique, may also be predictor for response to EGFR TK inhibitors [98–100] and may involved in the pathogenesis of lung adenocarcinoma.

To better understand the pathogenesis of *EGFR* mutant lung adenocarcinomas, the presence of *EGFR* mutations in the normal bronchial and bronchiolar epithelium adjacent to mutant tumors has been investigated. *EGFR* mutations have been detected in normal appearing peripheral respiratory epithelium in 9 out 21 (44%) adenocarcinoma patients, but not in patients without mutations in the tumors [26]. The findings of more frequent *EGFR* mutations in normal epithelium within the tumor (43%) than in adjacent sites (24%) suggest a localized field effect phenomenon, probably affecting preferentially the peripheral lung airway compartment, for this abnormality in the respiratory epithelium of the lung. Although the cell type having those mutations is unknown, it has been hypothesized that stem or progenitor cells of the bronchial and bronchiolar epithelium are the cell type bearing such mutations. The finding of relatively infrequent *EGFR* mutations in AAH lesions (3 out of 40 examined) [101,102], and the finding of no mutation [95] or relatively low frequency of mutation in true BACs of the lung, support the concept that genetic abnormalities of *EGFR* are no relevant in the pathogenesis of alveolar-type lung neoplasia. Thus, two different molecular pathways have been identified in the pathogenesis of lung adenocarcinoma, a smoking-associated activation of KRAS signaling, and nonsmoking-associated activation of EGFR signaling, the latter detected in histologically normal bronchial and bronchiolar epithelium (Figure 5.3).

Summary

Lung cancer results from the accumulation of multiple genetic and epigenetic changes and different patterns of molecular alterations have been detected among the major lung cancer histology types. There are three main morphologic forms of preneoplastic lesions recognized in the lung: squamous dysplasias, AAH, and DIPENECH. However, these lesions account for the development of only a subset of lung cancers. For squamous cell carcinoma of the lung, the current working model indicates a stepwise sequence of molecular and histopathological changes, with the molecular abnormalities starting in histologically normal and mildly abnormal epithelia. AAH is considered a putative precursor of a subset of lung adenocarcinoma, and they demonstrate similar molecular changes than invasive tumors. At least, two different molecular pathways have been detected in lung adenocarcinoma pathogenesis: smoking-related pathways associated with *KRAS* mutations and nonsmoking-related pathways associated with *EGFR* mutations; the latter are detected in histologically normal respiratory epithelium. Molecular changes detected in lung tumors and associated preneoplastic lesions have been detected in smoking-damaged epithelium of smokers, including histologically normal bronchial epithelium. A number of lines of evidence suggest that chronic inflammation contributes to the process of lung carcinogenesis through activation of a number of molecular pathways. Molecular and histopathological changes in the respiratory epithelium are extensive and multifocal throughout the bronchial tree of smokers and lung cancer patients, indicating a field effect phenomenon.

References

1 Jemal A, Murray T, Ward E *et al.* Cancer statistics, 2005. *CA Cancer J Clin* Jan–Feb 2005; **55(1)**:10–30.

2 Minna JD, Gazdar A. Focus on lung cancer. *Cancer Cell* 2002; **1**:49–52.

3 Travis WD, Brambilla E, Muller-Hermelink HK, Harris CC. Tumours of the lung. In: Travis WD, Brambilla E, Muller-Hermelink HK, Harris CC (eds). *Pathology and Genetics: Tumours of the Lung, Pleura, Thymus and Heart.* Lyon: International Agency for Research on Cancer (IARC), 2004:9–124.

4 Colby TV, Wistuba II, Gazdar A. Precursors to pulmonary neoplasia. *Adv Anat Pathol* 1998; **5(4)**:205–15.

5 Kerr KM. Pulmonary preinvasive neoplasia. *J Clin Pathol* 2001; **54**:257–71.

6 Franklin W, Wistuba I, Geisinger K *et al.* Squamous dysplasia and carcinoma in situ. In: Travis W, Brambilla E, Muller-Hermelink HK, Harris CC (eds). *Pathology and Genetics Tumors of the Lung, Pleura, Thymus and Heart.* Lyon: International Agency for Research on Cancer (IARC), 2004:68–72.

7 Wistuba II, Behrens C, Milchgrub S *et al.* Sequential molecular abnormalities are involved in the multistage development of squamous cell lung carcinoma. *Oncogene* 1999; **18**:643–50.

8 Wistuba II, Berry J, Behrens C *et al.* Molecular changes in the bronchial epithelium of patients with small cell lung cancer. *Clin Cancer Res* 2000; **6**:2604–10.

9 Wistuba II, Behrens C, Virmani AK *et al.* High resolution chromosome 3p allelotyping of human lung cancer and preneoplastic/preinvasive bronchial epithelium reveals multiple, discontinuous sites of 3p allele loss and three regions of frequent breakpoints. *Cancer Res* 2000; **60(7)**:1949–60.

10 Wistuba II, Mao L, Gazdar AF. Smoking molecular damage in bronchial epithelium. *Oncogene* Oct 21, 2002; **21(48)**:7298–306.

11 Wistuba II, Lam S, Behrens C *et al.* Molecular damage in the bronchial epithelium of current and former smokers. *J Natl Cancer Inst* 1997; **89**:1366–73.

12 Mao L, Lee JS, Kurie JM *et al.* Clonal genetic alterations in the lungs of current and former smokers. *J Natl Cancer Inst* 1997; **89**:857–62.

13 Mulshine JL. Current issues in lung cancer screening. *Oncology (Williston Park)* Nov 2005; **19(13)**:1724–30; discussion 30–1.

14 Lam S, MacAulay C, leRiche JC, Palcic B. Detection and localization of early lung cancer by fluorescence bronchoscopy. *Cancer* Dec 1, 2000; **89(Suppl 11)**: 2468–73.

15 Westra WH. Early glandular neoplasia of the lung. *Respir Med* 2000; **1**:163–9.

16 Keith RL, Miller YE, Gemmill RM *et al.* Angiogenic squamous dysplasia in bronchi of individuals at high risk for lung cancer. *Clin Cancer Res* 2000; **6(5)**:1616–25.

17 Ohtsuka T, Watanabe K, Kaji M, Naruke T, Suemasu K. A clinicopathological study of resected pulmonary nodules with focal pure ground-glass opacity. *Eur J Cardiothorac Surg* Jul 2006; **30(1)**:160–3.

18 Kitamura H, Kameda Y, Ito T, Hayashi H. Atypical adenomatous hyperplasia of the lung. Implications for the pathogenesis of peripheral lung adenocarcinoma [see comments]. *Am J Clin Pathol* 1999; **111(5)**:610–22.

19 Osanai M, Igarashi T, Yoshida Y. Unique cellular features in atypical adenomatous hyperplasia of the lung: ultrastructural evidence of its cytodifferentiation. *Ultrastruct Pathol* 2001; **25**:367–73.

20 Nakanishi K. Alveolar epithelial hyperplasia and adenocarcinoma of the lung. *Arch Pathol Lab Med* 1990; **114(4)**:363–8.

21 Chapman AD, Kerr KM. The association between atypical adenomatous hyperplasia and primary lung cancer. *Br J Cancer* 2000; **83**:632–6.

22 Koga T, Hashimoto S, Sugio K *et al.* Lung adenocarcinoma with bronchioloalveolar carcinoma component is frequently associated with foci of high-grade atypical adenomatous hyperplasia. *Am J Clin Pathol* 2002; **117**:464–70.

23 Yokose T, Doi M, Tanno K, Yamazaki K, Ochiai A. Atypical adenomatous hyperplasia of the lung in autopsy cases. *Lung Cancer* 2001; **33**:155–61.

24 Armas OA, White DA, Erlanson RA, Rosai J. Diffuse idiopathic pulmonary neuroendocrine cell proliferation presenting as interstitial lung disease. *Am J Surg Pathol* 1995; **19**:963–70.

25 Gazdar AF, Shigematsu H, Herz J, Minna JD. Mutations and addiction to EGFR: the Achilles "heal" of lung cancers? *Trends Mol Med* Oct 2004; **10(10)**:481–6.

26 Tang X, Shigematsu H, Bekele BN *et al.* EGFR tyrosine kinase domain mutations are detected in histologically normal respiratory epithelium in lung

cancer patients. *Cancer Res* Sep 1, 2005; **65(17)**:7568–72.

27 Wistuba II, Behrens C, Virmani AK *et al.* Allelic losses at chromosome 8p21-23 are early and frequent events in the pathogenesis of lung cancer. *Cancer Res* 1999; **59(8)**:1973–9.

28 Yashima K, Milchgrub S, Gollahon LS *et al.* Telomerase enzyme activity and RNA expression during the multistage pathogenesis of breast carcinoma. *Clin Cancer Res* 1998; **4(1)**:229–34.

29 Miyazu YM, Miyazawa T, Hiyama K *et al.* Telomerase expression in noncancerous bronchial epithelia is a possible marker of early development of lung cancer. *Cancer Res* Nov 1, 2005; **65(21)**:9623–7.

30 Lantuejoul S, Soria JC, Morat L *et al.* Telomere shortening and telomerase reverse transcriptase expression in preinvasive bronchial lesions. *Clin Cancer Res* Mar 1, 2005; **11(5)**:2074–82.

31 Park IW, Wistuba II, Maitra A *et al.* Multiple clonal abnormalities in the bronchial epithelium of patients with lung cancer [in process citation]. *J Natl Cancer Inst* 1999; **91(21)**:1863–8.

32 Zochbauer-Muller S, Fong KM, Maitra A *et al.* 5′ CpG island methylation of the FHIT gene is correlated with loss of gene expression in lung and breast cancer. *Cancer Res* 2001; **61(9)**:3581–5.

33 Zochbauer-Muller S, Lam S, Toyooka S *et al.* Aberrant methylation of multiple genes in the upper aerodigestive tract epithelium of heavy smokers. *Int J Cancer* Nov 20, 2003; **107(4)**:612–6.

34 Soria JC, Rodriguez M, Liu DD, Lee JJ, Hong WK, Mao L. Aberrant promoter methylation of multiple genes in bronchial brush samples from former cigarette smokers. *Cancer Res* Jan 15, 2002; **62(2)**:351–5.

35 Belinsky SA, Nikula KJ, Palmisano WA *et al.* Aberrant methylation of p16(INK4a) is an early event in lung cancer and a potential biomarker for early diagnosis. *Proc Natl Acad Sci U S A* 1998; **95(20)**:11891–6.

36 Belinsky SA, Palmisano WA, Gilliland FD *et al.* Aberrant promoter methylation in bronchial epithelium and sputum from current and former smokers. *Cancer Res* Apr 15, 2002; **62(8)**:2370–7.

37 Belinsky SA, Liechty KC, Gentry FD *et al.* Promoter hypermethylation of multiple genes in sputum precedes lung cancer incidence in a high-risk cohort. *Cancer Res* Mar 15, 2006; **66(6)**:3338–44.

38 Toyooka S, Tokumo M, Shigematsu H *et al.* Mutational and epigenetic evidence for independent pathways for lung adenocarcinomas arising in smokers and never smokers. *Cancer Res* Feb 1, 2006; **66(3)**:1371–5.

39 Lerman MI, Minna JD. The 630-kb lung cancer homozygous deletion region on human chromosome 3p21.3: identification and evaluation of the resident candidate tumor suppressor genes. The International Lung Cancer Chromosome 3p21.3 Tumor Suppressor Gene Consortium. *Cancer Res* 2000; **60(21)**:6116–33.

40 Zabarovsky ER, Lerman MI, Minna JD. Tumor suppressor genes on chromosome 3p involved in the pathogenesis of lung and other cancers. *Oncogene* Oct 7, 2002; **21(45)**:6915–35.

41 Rahman SM, Shyr Y, Yildiz PB *et al.* Proteomic patterns of preinvasive bronchial lesions. *Am J Respir Crit Care Med* Dec 15, 2005; **172(12)**:1556–62.

42 Jorgensen ED, Dozmorov I, Frank MB, Centola M, Albino AP. Global gene expression analysis of human bronchial epithelial cells treated with tobacco condensates. *Cell Cycle* Sep 2004; **3(9)**:1154–68.

43 Hirsch FR, Franklin WA, Gazdar AF, Bunn PA, Jr. Early detection of lung cancer: clinical perspectives of recent advances in biology and radiology. *Clin Cancer Res* Jan 2001; **7(1)**:5–22.

44 Hirsch FR, Prindiville SA, Miller YE *et al.* Fluorescence versus white-light bronchoscopy for detection of preneoplastic lesions: a randomized study. *J Natl Cancer Inst* Sep 19, 2001; **93(18)**:1385–91.

45 Merrick DT, Haney J, Petrunich S *et al.* Overexpression of vascular endothelial growth factor and its receptors in bronchial dysplasia demonstrated by quantitative RT-PCR analysis. *Lung Cancer* Apr 2005; **48(1)**:31–45.

46 Santarpia M, Altavilla G, Salazar F, Taron M, Rosell R. From the bench to the bed: individualizing treatment in non-small-cell lung cancer. *Clin Transl Oncol* Feb 2006; **8(2)**:71–6.

47 Abbruzzese JL, Lippman SM. The convergence of cancer prevention and therapy in early-phase clinical drug development. *Cancer Cell* Oct 2004; **6(4)**:321–6.

48 Hirsch FR, Lippman SM. Advances in the biology of lung cancer chemoprevention. *J Clin Oncol* May 10, 2005; **23(14)**:3186–97.

49 Khuri FR, Cohen V. Molecularly targeted approaches to the chemoprevention of lung cancer. *Clin Cancer Res* Jun 15, 2004; **10(12, Pt 2)**:4249s–53s.

50 Wislez M, Spencer ML, Izzo JG *et al.* Inhibition of mammalian target of rapamycin reverses alveolar epithelial neoplasia induced by oncogenic K-ras. *Cancer Res* Apr 15, 2005; **65(8)**:3226–35.

51 Wislez M, Fujimoto N, Izzo JG *et al.* High expression of ligands for chemokine receptor CXCR2 in alveolar epithelial neoplasia induced by oncogenic KRAS. *Cancer Res* Apr 15, 2006; **66(8)**:4198–207.

52 Merrick DT, Kittelson J, Winterhalder R *et al.* Analysis of c-ErbB1/epidermal growth factor receptor and c-ErbB2/HER-2 expression in bronchial dysplasia: evaluation of potential targets for chemoprevention of lung cancer. *Clin Cancer Res* Apr 1, 2006; **12(7, Pt 1)**:2281–8.

53 Tsao AS, McDonnell T, Lam S *et al.* Increased phospho-AKT (Ser(473)) expression in bronchial dysplasia: implications for lung cancer prevention studies. *Cancer Epidemiol Biomarkers Prev* Jul 2003; **12(7)**:660–4.

54 Lee HY, Oh SH, Woo JK *et al.* Chemopreventive effects of deguelin, a novel Akt inhibitor, on tobacco-induced lung tumorigenesis. *J Natl Cancer Inst* Nov 16, 2005; **97(22)**:1695–9.

55 Lee HY, Moon H, Chun KH *et al.* Effects of insulin-like growth factor binding protein-3 and farnesyltransferase inhibitor SCH66336 on Akt expression and apoptosis in non-small-cell lung cancer cells. *J Natl Cancer Inst* Oct 20, 2004; **96(20)**:1536–48.

56 Westra WH, Baas IO, Hruban RH *et al.* K-ras oncogene activation in atypical alveolar hyperplasias of the human lung. *Cancer Res* 1996; **56**:2224–8.

57 Tominaga M, Sueoka N, Irie K *et al.* Detection and discrimination of preneoplastic and early stages of lung adenocarcinoma using hmRNP B1, combined with the cell cycle-related markers p16, cyclin D1, and Ki-67. *Lung Cancer* 2003; **40**:45–53.

58 Nakanishi K, Kawai T, Kumaki F, Hiroi S, Mukai M, Ikeda E. Survivin expression in atypical adenomatous hyperplasia of the lung. *Am J Clin Pathol* 2003; **120**:712–9.

59 Kitaguchi S, Takeshima Y, Nishisaka T, Inai K. Proliferative activity, p53 expressin and loss of heterozygosity on 3p, 9 and 17p in atypical adenomatous hyperplasia of the lung. *Hiroshima J Med Sci* 1998; **47**:17–25.

60 Takamochi K, Ogura T, Suzuki K *et al.* Loss of heterozygosity on chromosome 9q and 16p in atypical adenomatous hyperplasia concomitant with adenocarcinoma of the lung. *Am J Pathol* 2001; **159**:1941–8.

61 Nakanishi K, Kawai T, Kumaki F, Hirot S, Mukai M, Ikeda E. Expression of human telomerase RNA component and telomerase reverse transcriptase mRNA in atypical adenomatous hyperplasia of the lung. *Hum Pathol* 2002; **33**:697–702.

62 Ghaffar H, Sahin F, Sanchez-Cespedes M *et al.* LKB1 protein expression in the evolution of glandular neoplasia of the lung. *Clin Cancer Res* 2003; **9**:2998–3003.

63 Nikitin AY, Alcaraz A, Anver MR *et al.* Classification of proliferative pulmonary lesions of the mouse: recommendations of the mouse models of human cancers consortium. *Cancer Res* Apr 1, 2004; **64(7)**:2307–16.

64 Kim CF, Jackson EL, Woolfenden AE *et al.* Identification of bronchioalveolar stem cells in normal lung and lung cancer. *Cell* Jun 17, 2005; **121(6)**:823–35.

65 Collado M, Gil J, Efeyan A *et al.* Tumour biology: senescence in premalignant tumours. *Nature* Aug 4, 2005; **436(7051)**:642.

66 Auerbach O, Stout AP, Hammond EC, Garfinkel L. Changes in bronchial epithelium in relation to smoking and cancer of the lung. *N Engl J Med* 1961; **265**:253–67.

67 Slaughter DP, Southwick HW, Smejkal W. "Field cancerization" in oral stratified squamous epithelium: clinical implications of multicentric origin. *Cancer* 1954; **6(963)**:963–8.

68 Coussens LM, Werb Z. Inflammation and cancer. *Nature* Dec 19–26, 2002; **420(6917)**:860–7.

69 Ballaz S, Mulshine JL. The potential contributions of chronic inflammation to lung carcinogenesis. *Clin Lung Cancer* Jul 2003; **5(1)**:46–62.

70 Anderson GP, Bozinovski S. Acquired somatic mutations in the molecular pathogenesis of COPD. *Trends Pharmacol Sci* Feb 2003; **24(2)**:71–6.

71 Hogg JC. Pathophysiology of airflow limitation in chronic obstructive pulmonary disease. *Lancet* Aug 21–27, 2004; **364(9435)**:709–21.

72 Barnes PJ. Chronic obstructive pulmonary disease. *N Engl J Med* Jul 27, 2000; **343(4)**:269–80.

73 Hida T, Kozaki K, Muramatsu H *et al.* Cyclooxygenase-2 inhibitor induces apoptosis and enhances cytotoxicity of various anticancer agents in non-small cell lung cancer cell lines. *Clin Cancer Res* May 2000; **6(5)**:2006–11.

74 Kennedy TC, Proudfoot SP, Franklin WA *et al.* Cytopathological analysis of sputum in patients with airflow obstruction and significant smoking histories. *Cancer Res* 1996; **56(20)**:4673–8.

75 Lam S, leRiche JC, Zheng Y *et al.* Sex-related differences in bronchial epithelial changes associated with tobacco smoking. *J Natl Cancer Inst* 1999; **91(8)**:691–6.

76 Tsurutani J, Castillo SS, Brognard J *et al.* Tobacco components stimulate Akt-dependent proliferation and NFκB-dependent survival in lung cancer cells. *Carcinogenesis* Jul 2005; **26(7)**:1182–95.

77 Tang X, Liu D, Shishodia S *et al.* Nuclear factor-kB (NF-kB) is frequently activated in lung cancer and preneoplastic lesions. *Cancer* Dec 1, 2006; **107(11)**:2637–46.

78 Tichelaar JW, Zhang Y, leRiche JC, Biddinger PW, Lam S, Anderson MW. Increased staining for phospho-Akt, p65/RELA and cIAP-2 in

pre-neoplastic human bronchial biopsies. *BMC Cancer* 2005; **5**:155.

79 Aggarwal BB. Nuclear factor-kappaB: the enemy within. *Cancer Cell* Sep 2004; **6(3)**:203–8.

80 Karin M, Greten FR. NF-kappaB: linking inflammation and immunity to cancer development and progression. *Nat Rev Immunol* Oct 2005; **5(10)**:749–59.

81 Pikarsky E, Porat RM, Stein I *et al.* NF-kappaB functions as a tumour promoter in inflammation-associated cancer. *Nature* Sep 23, 2004; **431 (7007)**:461–6.

82 Kumar A, Takada Y, Boriek AM, Aggarwal BB. Nuclear factor-kappaB: its role in health and disease. *J Mol Med* Jul 2004; **82(7)**:434–48.

83 Shishodia S, Aggarwal BB. Nuclear factor-kappaB: a friend or a foe in cancer? *Biochem Pharmacol* Sep 15, 2004; **68(6)**:1071–80.

84 Dannenberg AJ, Altorki NK, Boyle JO *et al.* Cyclooxygenase 2: a pharmacological target for the prevention of cancer. *Lancet Oncol* Sep 2001; **2(9)**:544–51.

85 Hasturk S, Kemp B, Kalapurakal SK, Kurie JM, Hong WK, Lee JS. Expression of cyclooxygenase-1 and cyclooxygenase-2 in bronchial epithelium and nonsmall cell lung carcinoma. *Cancer* Feb 15, 2002; **94(4)**:1023–31.

86 Mao JT, Cui X, Reckamp K *et al.* Chemoprevention strategies with cyclooxygenase-2 inhibitors for lung cancer. *Clin Lung Cancer* Jul 2005; **7(1)**:30–9.

87 Mascaux C, Martin B, Verdebout JM, Ninane V, Sculier JP. COX-2 expression during early lung squamous cell carcinoma oncogenesis. *Eur Respir J* Aug 2005; **26(2)**:198–203.

88 Mao JT, Fishbein MC, Adams B *et al.* Celecoxib decreases Ki-67 proliferative index in active smokers. *Clin Cancer Res* Jan 1, 2006; **12(1)**:314–20.

89 Paez JG, Janne PA, Lee JC *et al.* EGFR mutations in lung cancer: correlation with clinical response to gefitinib therapy. *Science* Jun 4, 2004; **304(5676)**:1497–500.

90 Lynch TJ, Bell DW, Sordella R *et al.* Activating mutations in the epidermal growth factor receptor underlying responsiveness of non-small-cell lung cancer to gefitinib. *N Engl J Med* May 20, 2004; **350(21)**:2129–39.

91 Pao W, Miller V, Zakowski M *et al.* EGF receptor gene mutations are common in lung cancers from "never smokers" and are associated with sensitivity of tumors to gefitinib and erlotinib. *Proc Natl Acad Sci U S A* Sep 7, 2004; **101(36)**:13306–11.

92 Huang SF, Liu HP, Li LH *et al.* High frequency of epidermal growth factor receptor mutations with complex patterns in non-small cell lung cancers related to gefitinib responsiveness in Taiwan. *Clin Cancer Res* Dec 15, 2004; **10(24)**:8195–203.

93 Kosaka T, Yatabe Y, Endoh H, Kuwano H, Takahashi T, Mitsudomi T. Mutations of the epidermal growth factor receptor gene in lung cancer: biological and clinical implications. *Cancer Res* Dec 15, 2004; **64(24)**:8919–23.

94 Tokumo M, Toyooka S, Kiura K *et al.* The relationship between epidermal growth factor receptor mutations and clinicopathologic features in non-small cell lung cancers. *Clin Cancer Res* Feb 1, 2005; **11(3)**:1167–73.

95 Shigematsu H, Lin L, Takahashi T *et al.* Clinical and biological features associated with epidermal growth factor receptor gene mutations in lung cancers. *J Natl Cancer Inst* Mar 2, 2005; **97(5)**:339–46.

96 Shigematsu H, Takahashi T, Nomura M *et al.* Somatic mutations of the HER2 kinase domain in lung adenocarcinomas. *Cancer Res* Mar 1, 2005; **65(5)**:1642–6.

97 Amann J, Kalyankrishna S, Massion PP *et al.* Aberrant epidermal growth factor receptor signaling and enhanced sensitivity to EGFR inhibitors in lung cancer. *Cancer Res* Jan 1, 2005; **65(1)**:226–35.

98 Cappuzzo F, Hirsch FR, Rossi E *et al.* Epidermal growth factor receptor gene and protein and gefitinib sensitivity in non-small-cell lung cancer. *J Natl Cancer Inst* May 4, 2005; **97(9)**:643–55.

99 Hirsch FR, Varella-Garcia M, McCoy J *et al.* Increased epidermal growth factor receptor gene copy number detected by fluorescence in situ hybridization associates with increased sensitivity to gefitinib in patients with bronchioloalveolar carcinoma subtypes: a Southwest Oncology Group Study. *J Clin Oncol* Oct 1, 2005; **23(28)**:6838–45.

100 Tsao MS, Sakurada A, Cutz JC *et al.* Erlotinib in lung cancer—molecular and clinical predictors of outcome. *N Engl J Med* Jul 14, 2005; **353(2)**:133–44.

101 Yatabe Y, Kosaka T, Takahashi T, Mitsudomi T. EGFR mutation is specific for terminal respiratory unit type adenocarcinoma. *Am J Surg Pathol* May 2005; **29(5)**:633–9.

102 Yoshida Y, Shibata T, Kokubu A *et al.* Mutations of the epidermal growth factor receptor gene in atypical adenomatous hyperplasia and bronchioloalveolar carcinoma of the lung. *Lung Cancer* Oct 2005; **50(1)**:1–8.

CHAPTER 6

Detection of Preneoplastic Lesions

Stephen Lam

Introduction

Currently, lung cancer survival is poor with only 15% of patients surviving 5 years after diagnosis [1]. While new chemotherapy agents and radiotherapy have improved survival and quality of life of patients, the overall impact in the last decade has been mainly on palliation rather than cure (reduction in mortality). Lung cancer survival is strongly associated with stage, and the 5-year survival statistics reflect the stage distribution. The surveillance epidemiology and end results (SEER) data indicate that only 16% of lung cancer patients present with localized disease while the remaining presents with either regional or distant metastasis [2]. Improving cure rates involves diagnosing patients at an earlier stage, when the cancer is still localized. Despite more optimistic reports from tertiary care or academic centers, population-based statistics from the SEER cancer registry (1988–2002) indicate that for localized disease, 5-year survival is only 49.1% [2]. Thus, approximately half of the individuals diagnosed with localized disease will die within 5 years, with the vast majority of them dying from recurrence and progression of their disease. Clearly, strategies to improve outcome by detecting and treating the disease in the preinvasive stage is needed.

There are unique challenges to localize preneoplastic lesions in the lung. In contrast to other epithelial organs, the lung is an internal organ con-

sisting of a complex branching system of conducting airways leading to peripheral gas exchange units with a surface area of the size of a tennis court. In addition, instead of a single cell type, lung cancer consists of several cell types and they are preferentially located in different parts of the tracheobronchial tree. There is no single method that can scan the entire bronchial epithelium for preneoplastic lesions and allow tissue sampling for pathological diagnosis and molecular profiling. Several biophotonic imaging methods have been developed such as autofluorescence bronchoscopy and optical coherence tomography (OCT) for localization of preneoplastic lesions in areas accessible by fiberoptic probes. Multidetector spiral CT is a sensitive tool to detect preneoplastic lesions in the peripheral lung. CT can serve as a virtual map to enable biopsy of peripheral lung lesions using navigational systems. In this chapter, current evidence supporting the use of these methods and direction for future research is discussed.

Detection of preneoplastic lesions in central airways

Principles of biophotonic imaging

When the bronchial surface is illuminated by light, the light can be absorbed, reflected, back scattered, or induce fluorescence [3]. These optical properties can be used for determining the structural features as well as the biochemical composition and functional changes in normal and abnormal bronchial tissues. White-light bronchoscopy (WLB) makes use of differences in specular reflection, back

Lung Cancer, 3rd edition. Edited by Jack A. Roth, James D. Cox, and Waun Ki Hong. © 2008 Blackwell Publishing, ISBN: 978-1-4051-5112-2.

scattering, and absorption properties of broadband visible light to define the structural features of the bronchial surface to discriminate between normal and abnormal tissues. Although it is the simplest imaging technique, less than 40% of carcinoma in situ is detectable by standard WLB [4]. Autofluorescence bronchoscopy makes use of fluorescence and absorption properties to provide information about the biochemical composition and metabolic state of bronchial tissues. Most endogenous fluorophores are associated with the tissue matrix or are involved in cellular metabolic processes. Collagen and elastin are the most important structural fluorophores and their composition involves cross-linking between fluorescing amino acids. Fluorophores involved in cellular metabolism include nicotinamide adenine dinucleotide (NADH) and flavins. Other fluorophores include the aromatic amino acids (e.g., tryptophan, tyrosine, phenylalanine), various porphyrins, and lipopigments (e.g., ceroids, lipofuscin). The fluorescence properties of bronchial tissue is determined by the concentration of these fluorophores, the distinct excitation and emission spectrum of each fluorophore, distribution of various fluorophores in the tissue, the metabolic state of the fluorophores, the tissue architecture and the wavelength-dependent light attenuation due to the concentration as well as distribution of nonfluorescent chromophores such as hemoglobin [3]. Upon illumination by violet or blue light, normal bronchial tissues fluoresce strongly in the green. As the bronchial epithelium changes from normal to dysplasia, and then to carcinoma in situ and invasive cancer, there is a progressive decrease in green autofluorescence but proportionately less decrease in red fluorescence intensity [5]. This change is due to a combination of several factors. The autofluorescence yield in the submucosa is approximately 10 times higher than the epithelium [3,5–7]. There is a decrease in extracellular matrix in the submucosa such as collagen and elastin in dysplasia and cancer. Secondly, the increase in the number of cell layers associated with dysplasia or cancer decreases the fluorescence measured in the bronchial surface due to reabsorption of light by the thickened epithelium [6,7]. Thirdly, the microvascular density is increased in dysplastic and malignant tissues. The presence of an increased concentration and distribution of hemoglobin results in increased absorption of the blue excitation light and reduced fluorescence. For example, angiogenic squamous dysplasia was found to have decreased autofluorescence [8]. Fourthly, there is a reduction in the amount of flavins and NADH in premalignant and malignant cells. Other factors such as pH and oxygenation may also alter the fluorescence quantum yield [9,10]. The extent to which these metabolic and morphologic changes will alter the fluorescence signal depends on the excitation and emission wavelengths used for illumination and detection in fluorescence imaging devices used clinically. In bronchoscopy, the excitation wavelengths producing the highest tumor to normal tissue contrasts are between 400 and 480 nm with a peak at 405 nm [5,11]. The spectral differences between 500 and 700 nm in normal, premalignant and malignant tissues serve as the basis for the design of several autofluorescence endoscopic imaging devices for localization of early lung cancer in the bronchial tree [3,12,13]. Recent versions of these devices usually use a combination of reflectance and fluorescence for imaging to make use of all the optical properties to optimize detection of subtle preneoplastic lesions [14–16].

Autofluorescence bronchoscopy

Autofluorescence bronchoscopic (AFB) imaging was initially developed in the early 1990s at the British Columbia Cancer Research Centre in Vancouver, British Columbia, as a method to localizing high-grade dysplasia (moderate and severe dysplasia), carcinoma in situ (CIS), and microinvasive squamous cell carcinoma [17]. Prior efforts at imaging these lesions used porphyrin products which, while allowing better imaging, was limited by skin photosensitivity reactions, high false-positive rates as well as added costs related to the drug. These methods did not gain significant acceptance by clinicians [3].

The first FDA-approved autofluorescence bronchoscopy device—LIFE-Lung (Novadaq Inc., Richmond, BC)—was made commercially available in 1998 [12]. This system used a 442 nm light from a helium–cadmium laser for illumination. The red and green autofluorescent light emitted from the airways are captured by two image-intensified charge-coupled device (CCD) cameras. A combined color image of the relative red–green fluorescence intensity is generated in real-time by a computer. The image is displayed green in normal areas and reddish-brown in abnormal areas, due to reduced green autofluorescence in preneoplastic and neoplastic lesions.

Improvements in sensor technology, light source and filters make it possible to use nonimage intensified CCDs for detection. Two second-generation devices approved by FDA make use of a combination of fluorescence and reflectance to enhance contrast between normal and abnormal tissues. The D-Light system (Karl Storz Endoscopy of America, Culver City, California, USA) consists of an RGB CCD camera and a filtered Xe lamp (380–460 nm). It combines an autofluorescence image from wavelengths >480 nm with a blue reflectance image [14]. The lesions appear purple against a bluish-green background. Frame averaging is used to amplify the weak autofluorescence signal.

The Onco-LIFE system (Novadaq Inc., Richmond, Canada) utilizes a combination of reflectance and fluorescence imaging. Blue light (395–445 nm) and small amount of red light (675–720 nm) from a filtered mercury arc lamp is used for illumination. A red reflectance image is captured in combination with the green autofluorescence image to enhance the contrast between premalignant, malignant, and normal tissues as well as to correct for differences in light intensities from changes in angle and distance of the bronchoscope from the bronchial surface [18]. Using reflected infrared red light as a reference has the theoretical advantage over reflected blue light in that it is less absorbed by hemoglobin and hence less influenced by changes in vascularity associated with inflammation.

Outside of the United States and Canada, other systems are available for clinical use. The Pentax SAFE-3000 system (Pentax Corp., Tokyo, Japan) uses a semiconductor laser diode that emits 408 nm wavelength light for illumination and detects autofluorescence using a single high sensitivity color CCD sensor in the fluorescence spectrum 430–700 nm. Reflected blue light is used to generate a fluorescence–reflectance image. The white-light and fluorescence images can also be made displayed simultaneously [16].

The Olympus autofluorescence imaging bronchovideoscope (AFI) system (Olympus Corp., Tokyo, Japan) uses blue light (395–445 nm) for illumination. An autofluorescence image (490–700 nm) as well as two reflectance images, one green (550 nm) and other red (610 nm), are captured sequentially and integrated by a videoprocessor to produce a composite image [15]. Normal tissue appears green, abnormal tissues appear blue or magenta.

Clinical trial results

In addition to a number of single center studies [19–28], three multicenter clinical trials [12,18,29] and two randomized studies [30,31] using different devices that are based on the same optical properties principles showed that autofluorescence bronchoscopy improves the detection rate of high-grade dysplasia, carcinoma in situ and microinvasive cancers compared to WLB by 1.4–6.3 times (Table 6.1).

A multi-institutional trial involving 173 subjects and 700 biopsies acquired after white-light examination followed by autofluorescence examination using the LIFE-Lung device showed that fluorescence examination provided a 2.7 times increase in relative sensitivity compared to white-light examination alone for localization of moderate/severe dysplasia, CIS, and invasive carcinoma [12]. When invasive carcinoma was excluded, the relative sensitivity rose to 6.3. A second multicenter trial using the D-Light device involving 293 subjects and 821 biopsies showed a sixfold improvement in relative sensitivity using autofluorescence examination [29]. A third multicenter trial using the Onco-LIFE device showed a fourfold improvement using autofluorescence examination [18].

There are two randomized trials. One study using the LIFE-Lung device randomized the order of the examination and randomized the operators blinded as to the results of the other observer [30]. In this study the relative sensitivity was 3.1. A second large, randomized, controlled multicenter trial in Europe examined subjects who were current smokers over 40 years of age with at least 20 pack-years of

Table 6.1 Results of multicenter clinical trials and randomized studies.

Reference	Device	Number of subjects	Sensitivity (%)		Specificity (%)	
			WLB	AFB	WLB	AFB
Lam et al.[12][*]	LIFE-Lung	173	9	66	90	66
Ernst et al. [29][*]	D-Light	293	11	66	95	73
Edell et al. [18][*]	Onco-LIFE	170	10	44	94	75
Hirsch et al. [30][†]	LIFE-Lung	55	18	73	78	46
Haussinger et al. [31][†]	D-Light	1173	58	82	62	58

[*]Multicenter clinical trial.
[†]Randomized trial.

smoking and had either symptoms suspicious for lung cancer or radiological abnormality suspicious for cancer [31]. The study randomized 1173 subjects to white light (WLB) only, or to WLB + ABF examination. The D-Light system was used. The authors reported a lower overall yield of high-grade dysplasia or CIS (3.9%) compared to other studies but reaffirmed the increased sensitivity of AFB + WLB compared to WLB alone (82% versus 58%).

A direct comparative study between WLB using fiberoptic bronchoscopes versus CCD-tipped video-bronchoscopes has not been performed. A recent study showed that AFB using the LIFE-Lung system was more sensitive than WLB using state-of-the-art videobronchoscope in the detection of high-grade dysplasia and carcinoma in situ (96% versus 72%, respectively) [25]. Studies using videobronchoscope for both white-light and fluorescence examinations instead of fiberoptic bronchoscopes showed similar improvements in detection rates with AFB [15,16].

Several general observations can be made from the published clinical trials. A high sensitivity in either WLB or AFB is associated with a lower specificity (Figure 6.1). In other words, if a bronchoscopist considers any bifurcation that is thickened or erythematous as being abnormal, the detection rate would be higher than another bronchoscopist who would only score areas that are irregular or granular in addition to thickening. The same bronchoscopist is also more likely to score lesser degree of abnormal fluorescence as being suspicious for high-grade dysplasia or cancer. One way to overcome the interobserver variation is to quantitate the red to green fluorescence intensities. An example of this approach is illustrated by the ROC curve in Figure 6.1. It is possible to set a threshold for the red to green fluorescence intensity ratios for more consistent scoring to reduce interobserver variation.

In addition to interobserver variation, the relative sensitivity between WLB and AFB is also influenced by the type of subjects included in the study and the mode of referral. Studies involving patients who are referred for endobronchial therapy after diagnosis of CIS under WLB could not expect to have any change in the diagnosis with AFB for obvious reason. Participants who were examined because of abnormal sputum based on conventional sputum cytology and those with known or suspected cancer in the upper aerodigestive tract tend to have a higher yield of high-grade dysplasia or CIS as well as a higher detection rate under WLB [19,23,24,26,32] compared to screening studies of heavy smokers without a history of cancer in the upper aerodigestive tract [13]. The detected lesions in clinical cases are probably larger and hence more obvious under WLB than those discovered in screening studies.

All studies appear to show a lower specificity with AFB compare to WLB. False-positive fluorescence can occur due to the presence of inflammation, suction, or contact trauma of the bronchial surface by the bronchoscope or coughing. Recent data on lesions that are positive on AFB but negative on pathology (mild dysplasia or lower grade) suggests that these lesions are not entirely normal. These

Figure 6.1 Receiver operating curve of quantitative fluorescence imaging using red to green intensity ratios of areas that showed moderate dysplasia ($N = 50$), severe dysplasia ($N = 8$) or carcinoma in situ ($N = 15$) versus those that were normal ($N = 462$), hyperplasia ($N = 1581$), metaplasia ($N = 455$) or mild dysplasia ($N = 549$) on biopsy. The sensitivity and specificity of six reported clinical trials using the LIFE-Lung device in the white-light examination mode (WLB) or the autofluorescence examination (LIFE-Lung) mode are represented by • or ■ respectively. Subjective scorings paralleled the objective measurements with higher sensitivities associated with lower specificities and vice versa.

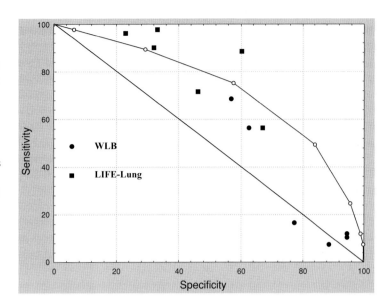

lesions show more genetic alterations than those with normal fluorescence suggesting they may have a higher potential for progression [33]. The presence of multiple areas of abnormal autofluorescence, notwithstanding the histopathology grade, appears to be a risk factor for subsequent development of lung cancer. Pasic *et al.* evaluated a group of 46 subjects with either previous aerodigestive cancer or sputum atypia and reported that the presence of two or more areas of abnormal autofluorescence increased the risk of developing subsequent lung cancer over the next 4 years compared to subjects with only one suspicious area (50% versus 8%) [34]. Therefore, the presence of autofluorescence abnormalities in some cases may be an indicator of field cancerization and increased cancer risk.

False-positive fluorescence can be minimized by the use of OCT. In principle, OCT is similar to endoscopic ultrasound. Instead of sound waves, OCT uses infrared light. Back scattered light from different layers of the bronchial wall is captured to form an image [35,36]. High-grade dysplasia and CIS appears as a multilayer structure compare to normal, hyperplasia or metaplasia. An example of OCT imaging is shown in Figure 6.2. The ability to visualize structures below the bronchial surface is a distinct improvement. Another approach that has

been used to improve the specificity of AFB is by adding optical spectroscopy [37,38]. Further studies are required to determine the practicality of performing spectroscopy during a standard bronchoscopic procedure.

Indications for autofluorescence bronchoscopy

Evaluation of patients with high-grade sputum atypia

There is no controversy that a finding of cells suspicious or diagnostic of malignancy on sputum cytology examination requires further investigation, usually bronchoscopy and CT scanning. Sato *et al.* reported a marked improvement in survival of patients with a sputum diagnosis of squamous cell carcinoma and negative chest radiographs who were treated following bronchoscopic localization of the cancer compared to a group with the same diagnosis but declined treatment. The treated group had a 94.9% survival at 10 years and the untreated group had a 33.5% survival in the same time period [26].

Severe atypia on sputum cytology examination has been reported in several studies to have a risk of developing lung cancer within 2 years of approximately 45% [39,40]. In the Johns Hopkins Early

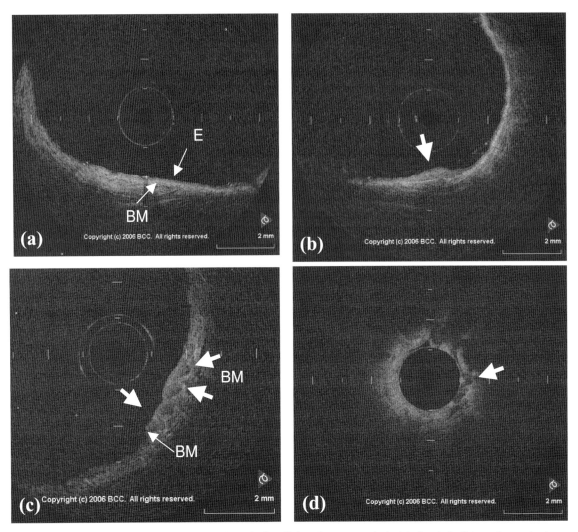

Figure 6.2 Optical coherence tomography of bronchial wall that shows metaplasia (a), dysplasia (b), carcinoma in situ (c), or invasive cancer (d). BM, basement membrane; E, epithelial surface. The invasive cancer has invaded through the basement membrane.

Lung Cancer Detection Project, moderate atypia was also found to have an increased risk of the subsequent development of lung cancer. Fourteen percent of the participants with moderate atypia developed lung cancer on long-term follow-up, compared to 3% of participants without atypia [39]. In the Colorado SPORE cohort of high-risk smokers and ex-smokers with airflow obstruction, the relative risks of developing lung cancer, adjusted for age, gender, recruitment year, pack-years, and smoking

status, was found to increase from 1.10 for mild atypia, 1.68 for moderate atypia, 3.18 for moderate atypia or worse, and 31.4 for severe atypia or worse [41]. Sputum cytology of severe atypia or worse clearly carries a risk of lung cancer that is high enough to warrant an aggressive diagnostic approach with combined white-light and fluorescence bronchoscopy.

A case may also be made for bronchoscopic examination of patients with moderate atypia although the evidence is not as strong as patients with severe atypia. In a series of 79 subjects with moderate sputum atypia with chest radiographs negative for cancer, lung cancer was found at bronchoscopy in 5 (6.3%; 95% CI, 0.7–11%) [32]. Two of the cancers were carcinoma in situ lesions and three were invasive. This rate of discovery of cancer at bronchoscopy exceeds the rate of discovery of colon cancer when colonoscopy is performed for a positive fecal occult blood test.

Evaluation of patients with suspected, known or previous lung cancer

Autofluorescence bronchoscopy can play a useful role in both the delineation of tumor margins and to assess the presence of synchronous lesions in patients with early lung cancer who are being assessed for curative surgical resection [32–35,42,43]. A careful clinical–pathological study by Ikeda *et al.* in 30 patients with NSCLC who had preoperative AFB examination and subsequently surgical resection showed more accurate delineation of the tumor extent as well as finding other sites of dysplasia with AFB compared to WLB [17,44].

Synchronous cancer can be found on autofluorescence bronchoscopy in up to 15% of these patients and up to 44% of patients may also have other moderate/severe dysplastic lesions that will require bronchoscopic follow-up [19,43,45,46]. For example, Pierard *et al.* found that in 43 preoperative lung, 9.3% had a synchronous occult CIS, and 19% had high-grade dysplasia [45]. Lam *et al.* reported synchronous site of CIS in 15% of 53 subjects with lung cancer [19]. van Rens *et al.* reported the preoperative evaluation of 72 NSCLC patients and found 3 synchronous NSCLC lesions in 3 patients (4.2%) and 13 high-grade dysplasia in 10 patients (14%) [43]. Venmans *et al.* detected other sites of moderate dysplasia or worse in 44% subjects with a known site of CIS referred for endobronchial therapy [46]. The discovery of these synchronous lesions altered the therapeutic plan in these patients.

Following successful curative resection of nonsmall cell carcinoma, a high rate (1–3% per year) of second primary (metachronous) tumors is reported [47]. In the subset of patients with prior early central squamous cell carcinoma, the reported rate of metachronous lesions appears even higher with up to nearly 30% develop a second central carcinoma within 4 years [40–43,47–49]. Postoperative surveillance white-light and fluorescence bronchoscopy was performed in patients with completely resected NSCLC [34,49,50]. In 25 patients, Weigel *et al.* found 12% of the patients subsequently developed three lesions of moderate/severe dysplasia and one microinvasive cancer over an average of 20.5 months of follow-up [48]. Pasic *et al.*, found that 28% of patients with a previous lung cancer developed metachronous central squamous cell carcinoma within a median of 47 months of follow-up [34]. The predominance of metachronous lesions in the central airways in patients with previous squamous cell carcinoma versus those with peripheral adenocarcinoma is suggested by a study that showed 30% of the patients with a previously resected squamous cell carcinoma had high-grade dysplasia or worse compared to only 4% with a previously resected adenocarcinoma [51]. Patients with a previous curative resection for lung cancer are at high risk of developing second primary lung cancers. Surveillance AFB may be useful in those with previous squamous cell carcinoma who have good performance status and no significant comorbidities.

Patients with early central lung cancer eligible for curative endobronchial therapy

When considering an early central carcinoma for curative endobronchial therapy, autofluorescence examination plays an important role in determining the extent of the lesion. Complete response after endobronchial therapy such as photodynamic therapy is influenced by the surface area of the lesion and whether all margins can be visualized [52]. These factors have an important impact on the success of endobronchial treatment, and cannot be accurately assessed with white-light bronchoscopy. Sutedja *et al.* performed AFB on 23 patients referred for intraluminal therapy of NSCLC following WLB [53]. In four, CT scans showed the lesions too extensive for intraluminal therapy. In the remaining 19 patients, 13 patients (68%) were found to have lesions too extensive for intraluminal therapy by AFB examination.

Follow-up of high-grade bronchial intraepithelial neoplasia

In an attempt to clarify the natural history of premalignant lesions and CIS, longitudinal study using serial bronchoscopy and biopsy were performed in patients with dysplasia or CIS [46,49,51,54]. These studies were small (~50 patients or less). The duration of follow-up was short (<5 yr). A significant proportion of the subjects were patients with lung or head and neck cancer. Overall, <2% of lesions with moderate dysplasia and 11–50% of lesions with severe dysplasia progressed to CIS/invasive cancer. As high as 9% of lesions with metaplasia/mild dysplasia had been reported to progress to CIS/invasive cancer [55], but the number is likely to be falsely high. The color ratio threshold in the LIFE-Lung device is optimized to detect moderate dysplasia or worse. Therefore, the denominator for the progression rate of low-grade lesions such as metaplasia/mild dysplasia was probably grossly underestimated.

As part of several chemoprevention trials, 1881 heavy volunteer smokers above 45 years of age with ≥20 pack-years smoking history without previous cancer in the upper aerodigestive tract were screened by AFB (S. Lam, unpublished data). In a total of 5060 random and fluorescence bronchoscopy directed biopsies, normal/hyperplasia were found in 2925 sites, metaplasia/mild dysplasia in 1922, moderate dysplasia in 164, and severe dysplasia in 49 of the biopsies. During an average follow-up of 4.4 years (range 1.3–12.4 yr), progression to CIS/invasive cancer was found in the same site where the initial biopsy was taken in 8.2% of severe dysplasia, 1.2% of moderate dysplasia, 0.26% of metaplasia/mild dysplasia, and 0.58% of areas that were normal/hyperplasia. Although some lesions appear to progress from normal/hyperplasia to CIS/invasive cancer within 2–3 years—much shorter than the traditional thinking of 10–20 years, in general, the progression rate appears to correlate with the initial pathological change.

The progression rate of CIS to invasive cancer is difficult to evaluate as most centers treat these lesions at the time of diagnosis or when the lesion persists on repeat bronchoscopy and biopsy within 3 months. Overall, 39–84% of CIS were found to persist or progress to invasive cancer [46,54–56]. There is only one study where patients with severe dysplasia or CIS were not treated until development of invasive cancer. George *et al.* recently reported the results of observation in 22 patients [57]. Forty-one percent of these patients had previous lung cancer. High-grade lesions included 7 severe dysplasia and 29 CIS were found in 16 patients. The remaining patients had mild/moderate dysplasia. None of the lesions with mild or moderate dysplasia progressed during the period of follow-up. Among 18 high-grade lesions that were evaluable without the influence of treatment to synchronous lesion in the same area, 6 lesions (33%) progressed to invasive cancer within 17 months; all of these were previous sites of CIS. Another 5 lesions (28%) persisted during follow-up. Three of the five patients with 6 CIS who developed invasive cancer had progressive disease despite radical radiotherapy or photodynamic therapy. Distinguishing between severe dysplasia versus carcinoma in situ was found to be difficult due to intra- and interobserver variation in the pathological classification highlighting some of the problems comparing studies or trying to pool data from different series. Repeatedly biopsies of the same site may also remove the lesion mechanically leading to falsely high regression rates.

The studies reviewed showed that the risk of progression is very high for severe dysplasia and CIS. The presence of high-grade dysplasia is also a risk marker for lung cancer developing elsewhere in the lung. Therefore, close follow-up with AFB and radiological imaging are indicated in patients with these lesions. Carcinoma in situ, when allowed to progress to invasive cancer can become incurable by local therapy. Since endobronchial therapy such as electrocautery treatment and cryotherapy is quick, low cost and safe [58–60], treatment is preferable for CIS lesions instead of observation with repeated bronchoscopies and biopsies.

Detection of preneoplastic lesions in peripheral lung

Atypical adenomatous hyperplasia (AAH) is considered to be the preinvasive lesion of adenocarcinoma [61,62]. These lesions are usually less than 7 mm in diameter and are detectable on CT scan as small, "ground glass" densities [63–66]. In resected lungs, the incidence of AAH was estimated to be 9–21% in patients with primary lung cancer and 4–10% in patients without lung cancer [61]. Laboratory investigations demonstrate that AAH cells have the ultrastructural features of Clara cells or Type II pneumocytes [67,68] and that many of the molecular changes present in lung adenocarcinomas are present in these lesions supporting the concept that AAH lesions are precursor lesions of peripheral adenocarcinoma. Tumors with a predominant ground glass CT appearance showed a growth pattern involving replacement of alveolar lining cells, and a better prognosis. As tumors appeared more solid on CT, they were associated with central fibrosis, alveolar collapse, and eventually a solid mass, and a less favorable outcome. The theory is that there is progression from the earlier lepidic growth with ground glass appearance to more solid tumors.

Unfortunately, the finding of ground glass densities or small noncalcified nodules in the lung is not specific for AAH, bronchioloalveolar carcinoma (BAC) or adenocarcinoma. The majority of these small lung densities are not preneoplastic or neoplastic [64,65]. Transthoracic needle aspiration biopsy of small lung densities ≤7 mm in size is difficult to perform even under CT guidance. It also carries a significant risk for pneumothorax. A promising approach is to use either endoscopic ultrasound [69], or an electromagnetic guidance system to navigate a small sensor tipped catheter to the peripheral lung density using virtual CT as a road map [70–72]. Early experience of this approach showed improved diagnostic accuracy but the average size of the lung nodules detected are ≥2 cm in diameter. Further improvement in the technology with better co-registration of the bronchoscopic image and the virtual CT is needed to biopsy subcentimeter lesions. Coupling the navigation system with OCT may allow better localization and characterization of small lung densities to separate preneoplastic lesions and early adenocarcinoma from benign lesions.

Summary

Rapid advances in optical imaging such as autofluorescence bronchoscopy, optical coherent tomography, and computerized tomography as well as an image-guided navigation biopsy devices provide unprecedented opportunity to localize preneoplastic lesions in the lung, allow biopsy to characterize these lesions better and to study their natural history. Localization of these lesions also enables minimally invasive endobronchial treatment without removing adjacent normal lung tissue.

References

1 Jemal A, Siegel R, Ward E *et al*. Cancer statistics, 2006. *CA Cancer J Clin* 2006; **56**:106–30.

2 Surveillance, Epidemiology, and End Results (SEER) Program (www.seer.cancer.gov) SEER*Stat Database: Incidence—SEER 17 Regs Public-Use, Nov 2005 Sub (1973–2003 varying), National Cancer Institute, DC-CPS, Surveillance Research Program, Cancer Statistics Branch, released April 2006, based on the November 2005 submission.

3 Wagnieres G, McWilliams A, Lam S. Lung cancer imaging with fluorescence endoscopy. In: Mycek M, Pogue B (eds). *Handbook of Biomedical Fluorescence*. New York: Marcel Dekker, 2003:361–96.

4 Woolner L. Pathology of cancer detected cytologically. In: *Atlas of Early Lung Cancer*, National Institutes of Health, US Department of Health and Human Services. Tokyo: Igaku-Shoin, 1983:107–213.

5 Hung J, Lam S, leRiche J, Palcic B. Autofluorescence of normal and malignant bronchial tissue. *Laser Surg Med* 1991; **11**:99–105.

6 Qu J, MacAulay C, Lam S, Palcic B. Laser-induced fluorescence spectroscopy at endoscopy: tissue optics, Monte Carlo modeling, and in vivo measurements. *Opt Eng* 1995; **34**:3334–43.

7 Qu J, MacAulay C, Lam S, Palcic B. Optical properties of normal and carcinoma bronchial tissue. *Appl Opt* 1994; **33(31)**:7397–405.

8 Keith R, Miller Y, Gemmill R *et al*. Angiogenic squamous dysplasia in bronchi of individuals at high risk for lung cancer. *Clin Cancer Res* 2000; **6**:1616–25.

9 Gardner C, Jacques S, Welch A. Fluorescence spectroscopy of tissue: recovery of intrinsic fluorescence

from measured fluorescence. *Appl Opt* 1996; **35(10)**:1780–92.

10 Wolfbeis O. Fluorescence of organic natural products. In: Schulman SG (ed). *Molecular Luminescence Spectroscopy*, Vol. 1. New York: John Wiley and Sons, 1973:167–370.

11 Zellweger M, Grosjean P, Goujon D, Monnier P, Van Den Bergh H, Wagnières G. Autofluorescence spectroscopy to characterize the histopathological status of bronchial tissue in vivo. *J Biomed Opt* 2001; **6(1)**: 41–52.

12 Lam S, Kennedy T, Unger M *et al.* Localization of bronchial intraepithelial neoplastic lesions by fluorescence bronchoscopy. *Chest* 1998; **113**:696–702.

13 Lam S, MacAulay C, leRiche J, Palcic B. Detection and localization of early lung cancer by fluorescence bronchoscopy. *Cancer* 2000; **89(Suppl 11)**:2468–73.

14 Häussinger K, Pichler J, Stanzel F *et al.* Autofluorescence bronchoscopy: the D-light system. *Intervent Bronchosc* 2000; **30**:243–52.

15 Chiyo M, Shibuya K, Hoshino H *et al.* Effective detection of bronchial preinvasive lesions by a new autofluorescence imaging bronchovideoscope system. *Lung Cancer* 2005; **48**:307–13.

16 Ikeda N, Honda H, Hayashi A *et al.* Early detection of bronchial lesions using newly developed videoendoscopy-based autofluorescence bronchoscopy. *Lung Cancer* 2006; **52**:21–7.

17 Lam S, MacAulay C, Hung J, leRiche J, Profio A, Palcic B. Detection of dysplasia and carcinoma in situ with a lung imaging fluorescence endoscope device. *J Thorac Cardiovasc Surg* 1993; **105**:1035–40.

18 Onco-LIFE endoscopic light source and camera. P950043/S003. June 30, 2005. Available from http://www.fda.gov/cdrh/pmapage/html.

19 Lam S, MacAulay C, leRiche J, Ikeda N, Palcic B. Early localization of bronchogenic carcinoma. *Diagn Ther Endosc* 1994; **1**:75–8.

20 Venmans BJW, van Boxem AJM, Smit EF *et al.* Early detection of preinvasive lesions in high-risk patients. A comparison of conventional flexible and fluorescence bronchoscopy. *J Bronchol* 1998; **5**:280–3.

21 Vermylen P, Pierard P, Roufosse C *et al.* Detection of bronchial preneoplastic lesions and early lung cancer with fluorescence bronchoscopy: a study about its ambulatory feasibility under local anesthesis. *Lung Cancer* 1999; **25(3)**:161–8.

22 Horvath T, Horvathova M, Salajka F *et al.* Detection of bronchial neoplasia in uranium miners by autofluorescence bronchoscopy. *Diagn Ther Endosc* 1999; **5**:91–8.

23 Kusunoki Y, Imamura F, Uda H, Mano M, Horai T. Early detection of lung cancer with laser-induced fluorescence endoscopy and spectrofluorometry. *Chest* 2000; **118(6)**:1776–82.

24 Shibuya K, Fujisawa T, Hoshino H *et al.* Fluorescence bronchoscopy in the detection of preinvasive bronchial lesions in patients with sputum cytology suspicious or positive for malignancy. *Lung Cancer* 2001; **32(1)**:19–25.

25 Chhajed PN, Shibuya K, Hoshino H *et al.* A comparison of video and autofluorescence bronchoscopy in patients at high risk of lung cancer. *Eur Respir J* 2005; **25(6)**: 951–5.

26 Sato M, Sakurada A, Sagawa M *et al.* Diagnostic results before and after introduction of autofluorescence bronchoscopy in patients suspected of having lung cancer detected by sputum cytology in lung cancer mass screening. *Lung Cancer* 2001; **32(3)**:247–53.

27 Goujon D, Zellweger M, Radu A *et al.* In vivo autofluorescence imaging of early cancers in the human tracheobronchial tree with a spectrally optimized system. *Biomed Opt J* 2003; **8(1)**:17–25.

28 Fielding D. Practical issues in autofluorescence bronchoscopy with Storz D Light bronchoscope. *Photodiagn Photodynam Ther* 2004; **1(3)**:247–51.

29 Ernst A, Simoff MJ, Mathur PN, Yung RC, Beamis JF, Jr. D-light autofluorescence in the detection of premalignant airway changes: a multicenter trial. *J Bronchol* 2005; **12(3)**:133–8.

30 Hirsch FR, Prindiville SA, Miller YE *et al.* Fluorescence versus white-light bronchoscopy for detection of preneoplastic lesions: a randomized study. *J Natl Cancer Inst* 2001; **93(18)**:1385–91.

31 Haussinger K, Becker H, Stanzel F *et al.* Autofluorescence bronchoscopy with white light bronchoscopy compared with white light bronchoscopy alone for the detection of precancerous lesions: a European randomised controlled multicentre trial. *Thorax* 2005; **60(6)**:496–503.

32 Kennedy TC, Franklin WA, Prindiville SA *et al.* High prevalence of occult endobronchial malignancy in high risk patients with moderate sputum atypia. *Lung Cancer* 2005; **49(2)**:187–91.

33 Helfritzsch H, Junker K, Bartel M, Scheele J. Differentiation of positive autofluorescence bronchoscopy findings by comparative genomic hybridization. *Oncol Rep* 2002; **9(4)**:697–701.

34 Pasic A, Vonk-Noordegraaf A, Risse EK, Postmus PE, Sutedja TG. Multiple suspicious lesions detected by autofluorescence bronchoscopy predict malignant

development in the bronchial mucosa in high risk patients. *Lung Cancer* 2003; **41(3)**:295–301.

35 Aguirre A, Hsiung P, Ko T, Hartl I, Fujimoto J. High-resolution optical coherence microscopy for high-speed, in vivo cellular imaging. *Opt Lett* 2003; **28(21)**: 2064–6.

36 Tsuboi M, Hayashi A, Ikeda N *et al.* Optical coherence tomography in the diagnosis of bronchial lesions. *Lung Cancer* 2005; **49**:387–94.

37 Bard MPL, Amelink A, Skurichina M *et al.* Improving the specificity of fluorescence bronchoscopy for the analysis of neoplastic lesions of the bronchial tree by combination with optical spectroscopy: preliminary communication. *Lung Cancer* 2005; **47(1)**:41–7.

38 Zeng H, Petek M, Zorman MT, McWilliams A, Palcic B, Lam S. Integrated endoscopy system for simultaneous imaging and spectroscopy for early lung cancer detection. *Opt Lett* 2004; **29**:587–9.

39 Frost JK, Ball WC, Jr, Levin ML *et al.* Sputum cytopathology: use and potential in monitoring the workplace environment by screening for biological effects of exposure. *J Occup Med* 1986; **28(8)**:692–703.

40 Risse EK, Vooijs GP, van't Hof MA. Diagnostic significance of "severe dysplasia" in sputum cytology. *Acta Cytol* 1988; **32**:629–34.

41 Prindiville SA, Byers T, Hirsch FR *et al.* Sputum cytological atypia as a predictor of incident lung cancer in a cohort of heavy smokers with airflow obstruction. *Cancer Epidemiol Biomarkers Prev* 2003; **12**:987–93.

42 Pierard P, Faber J, Hutsebaut J *et al.* Synchronous lesions detected by autofluorescence bronchoscopy in patients with high-grade preinvasive lesions and occult invasive squamous cell carcinoma of the proximal airways. *Lung Cancer* 2004; **46(3)**:341–7.

43 van Rens MT, Schramel FM, Elbers JR, Lammers JW. The clinical value of lung imaging fluorescence endoscopy for detecting synchronous lung cancer. *Lung Cancer* 2001; **32(1)**:13–8.

44 Ikeda N, Hiyoshi T, Kakihana M *et al.* Histopathological evaluation of fluorescence bronchoscopy using resected lungs in cases of lung cancer. *Lung Cancer* 2003; **41(3)**:303–9.

45 Pierard P, Vermylen P, Bosschaerts T *et al.* Synchronous roentgenographically occult lung carcinoma in patients with resectable primary lung cancer. *Chest* 2000; **117(3)**:779–85.

46 Venmans B, vanBoxem A, Smit E, Postmus P, Sutedja T. Outcome of bronchial carcinoma in-situ. *Chest* 2000; **117**:1572–6.

47 Johnson B. Second lung cancers in patients after treatment for an initial lung cancer. *J Natl Cancer Inst* 1998; **90(18)**:1335–45.

48 Nakamura H, Kawasaki N, Hagiwara M *et al.* Early hilar lung cancer—risk for multiple lung cancers and clinical outcome. *Lung Cancer* 2001; **33(1)**:51–7.

49 Weigel TL, Yousem S, Dacic S, Kosco PJ, Siegfried J, Luketich JD. Fluorescence bronchoscopic surveillance after curative surgical resection for non-small-cell lung cancer. *Ann Surg Oncol* 2000; **7(3)**:176–80.

50 Weigel TL, Kosco PJ, Dacic S, Rusch VW, Ginsberg RJ, Luketich JD. Postoperative fluorescence bronchoscopic surveillance in non-small cell lung cancer patients [see comment]. *Ann Thorac Surg* 2001; **71(3)**:967–70.

51 Moro-Sibilot D, Fievet F, Jeanmart M *et al.* Clinical prognostic indicators of high-grade pre-invasive bronchial lesions. *Eur Respirol J* 2004; **24**:24–9.

52 Kato H, Okunaka T, Shimatani H. Photodynamic therapy for early stage bronchogenic carcinoma. *J Clin Laser Med Surg* Oct 1996; **14(5)**:235–8.

53 Sutedja TG, Codrington H, Risse EK *et al.* Autofluorescence bronchoscopy improves staging of radiographically occult lung cancer and has an impact on therapeutic strategy. *Chest* 2001; **120(4)**:1327–32.

54 Hoshino H, Shibuya K, Chiyo M *et al.* Biological features of bronchial squamous dysplasia followed up by autofluorescence bronchoscopy. *Lung Cancer* 2004; **46**:187–96.

55 Breuer RH, Pasic A, Smit EF *et al.* The natural course of pre-neoplastic lesions in bronchial epithelium. *Clin Cancer Res* 2005; **11(2, Pt 1)**:537–43.

56 Bota S, Auliac JB, Paris C *et al.* Follow-up of bronchial precancerous lesions and carcinoma in situ using fluorescence endoscopy. *Am J Respir Crit Care Med* 2001; **164(9)**:1688–93.

57 George P, Banerjee A, Read C *et al.* Surveillance for the detection of early lung cancer in patients with bronchial dysplasia. *Thorax* 2007; **63**:43–50.

58 Deygas N, Froudarakis M, Ozenne G, Vergnon JM. Cryotherapy in early superficial bronchogenic carcinoma. *Chest* 2001; **120**:26–31.

59 Sutedja G, Postmus PE. Bronchoscopic treatment of lung tumors. Review article. *Lung Cancer* 1994; **11**:1–17.

60 Pasic A, Brokx HAP, Nooregraaf AV *et al.* Cost-effectiveness of early interventions: comparison between intraluminal bronchoscopic treatment and surgical resection for T1N0 lung cancer patients. *Respiration* 2004; **71**:391–6.

61 Miller R. Bronchoalveolar cell adenomas. *Am J Surg Pathol* 1990; **14**:904–12.

62 Mori M, Chiba R, Takahashi T. Atypical adenomatous hyperplasia of the lung and its differentiation. Characterization of atypical cells by morphometry ad multivariate cluster analysis. *Cancer* 1993; **72**:2331–40.

63 Henschke C, McCauley D, Yankelevitz D *et al.* Early lung cancer action project: overall design and findings from baseline screening. *Lancet* 1999; **354**:99–105.

64 McWilliams AM, Mayo JR, Ahn MI, MacDonald SLS, Lam S. Lung cancer screening using multi-slice thin-section computed tomography and autofluorescence bronchoscopy. *J Thorac Oncol* 2006; **1(1)**:61–8.

65 Swensen SJ, Jett JR, Hartman TE *et al.* CT screening for lung cancer: five-year prospective experience. *Radiology* 2005; **235**:259–65.

66 Vazquez M, Flieder D. Small peripheral glandular lesions detected by screening CT for lung cancer. A diagnostic dilemma for the pathologist. *Radiol Clin North Am* 2000; **38(3)**:1–11.

67 Mori M, Kaji M, Tezuka F, Takahasi T. Comparative ultrastructural study of atypical adenomatous hyperplasia and adenocarcinoma of the human lung. *Ultrastruct Pathol* 1998; **22**:459–66.

68 Kerr K. Adenomatous hyperplasia and the origin of peripheral adenocarcinoma of the lung. In: Corrin B (ed). *Pathology of Lung Tumours*. New York: Churchill Livingstone, 1997:119–33.

69 Herth FJ, Everhardt R, Becker HD, Ernst A. Endobronchial ultrasound-guided transbronchial lung biopsy in fluoroscopically invisible solitary pulmonary nodules: a prospective trial. *Chest* 2006; **129**:147–50.

70 Hautmann H, Schneider A, Pinkau T, Peltz F, Feussner H. Electromagnetic catheter navigation during bronchoscopy validation of a novel method by a conventional fluoroscopy. *Chest* 2005; **128**:382–7.

71 Schwarz Y, Greif J, Becker HD, Ernst A, Mehta A. Real-time electromagnetic navigation bronchoscopy to peripheral lung lesions using overlaid CT images: the first human study. *Chest* 2006; **129**:988–94.

72 Gildea TR, Mazzone PJ, Karnak D, Meziane M, Mehta AC. Electromagnetic navigation diagnostic bronchoscopy: a prospective study. *Am J Respir Crit Care Med* 2006; **174**:982–9.

CHAPTER 7

Treatment of Preneoplastic Lesions of the Lung

Annette McWilliams

Introduction

Localization of intraepithelial neoplasia (IEN) (moderate/severe dysplasia, and carcinoma in situ (CIS)) has been made possible by the development of autofluorescence imaging of the bronchial mucosa as these lesions are difficult to detect with white-light examination even with the new generation of videoendoscopes [1]. Information about the natural history of IEN is now emerging but considerable controversy still exists regarding prognosis and indications for treatment. Currently, histopathology is the only available tool to predict the biological behavior of IEN and it remains the gold standard for assessment of lesions that are abnormal on autofluorescence examination. Interobserver variation in reporting the presence or degree of IEN has been an important issue but the recent development of new WHO classification will act to reduce this problem [2]. The development of endobronchial carcinoma has been proposed to occur through progressive premalignant changes and higher degrees of dysplasia are associated with increased risk for subsequent invasive cancer [3]. However, some lesions may persist without progression, show nonstepwise progression or spontaneous regression [4]. Interpretation of regression rates may be confounded by the removal of part or the entire lesion by bronchial

biopsy. Angiogenic squamous dysplasia is a recently described histopathological change in the bronchial epithelium of heavy smokers that is felt to be a possible intermediate biomarker in bronchial carcinogenesis [5]. This lesion is detected by autofluorescence bronchoscopy and is a collection of capillary-sized blood vessels closely juxtaposed to dysplastic epithelial cells. The capillary loops project upward into the bronchial mucosa and the lesion is associated with increased expression of proliferative markers. Although the long-term prognostic significance is unknown, short-term follow-up at 1 year shows persistence of 45% of these lesions and they were more common in subjects with a concurrent lung cancer, particularly squamous cell carcinoma.

In association with its improved ability to detect IEN, autofluorescence bronchoscopy has been shown to have reduced specificity due to the identification of multiple false-positive lesions. However, this has been challenged by recent data showing that false-positive lesions (abnormal autofluorescence but benign pathology) have increased chromosomal aberrations [6]. The presence of autofluorescence abnormalities may be a marker of field carcinogenesis and overall cancer risk. Patients harboring high-grade lesions appear to be at risk for developing lung cancers at remote sites [7]. The presence of two areas or more of abnormal autofluorescence in high-risk patients, despite histopathological grade, has been shown to be associated with a significantly increased risk of developing subsequent lung cancer [8].

Lung Cancer, 3rd edition. Edited by Jack A. Roth, James D. Cox, and Waun Ki Hong. © 2008 Blackwell Publishing, ISBN: 978-1-4051-5112-2.

Table 7.1 Longitudinal outcome of intraepithelial neoplasia.

	Number of patients	Number of lesions	Median follow-up (months)	Moderate dysplasia Progression to cancer	Severe dysplasia Progression to cancer	Carcinoma in situ Persistance	Carcinoma in situ Progression to invasive cancer
Venmans et al. [14]	9	9	22	–	–	–	67%*
Deygas et al. [15]	35	41	NR	–	–	–	20%[†]
Bota et al. [16]	104	228	24	0%[‡]	11%	75%[§]	–
George et al. [7]	22	53	23	0%[‡]	0%	64%	21%
Lam et al. [17]	566	208	21	1.3%	6%	–	–
Breuer et al. [4]	52	89	17.5	9%[‡]	32%	–	–
Hoshino et al. [11]	50	66	6.9[‖]	1.8%	18%	–	–

*Progression occurred despite initial endobronchial treatment in 67% lesions.
[†]Progression occurred despite initial cryotherapy in all lesions.
[‡]Mild and moderate dysplasia reported together.
[§]Persisted at 3 months and were treated.
[‖]Only mean followup duration reported.
NR, not reported.

There are presently no molecular markers to reliably predict the biological behavior of IEN although work in this area is progressing. Suprabasal p53 staining has been shown to be predictive of subsequent development of bronchial cancer in the same lobe or bronchial spur, and may be a useful tool in combination with histopathology [9]. Telomerase expression in nonmalignant epithelium in high-risk patients with treated lung cancer is associated with an increased subsequent development of second bronchial malignancies [10]. In addition, high telomerase activity, increased Ki-67 expression and p53 positivity in IEN have been found to be associated with persistence or progression of the lesion on longitudinal observation [11].

The natural history of high-grade bronchial intraepithelial neoplasia

Autopsy data has revealed that some patients harbor radiographically occult lung cancer at the time of their death from another cause [12]. This finding has raised the possibility of overdiagnosis and

stimulated discussion regarding the need to treat CIS when it is diagnosed in the bronchus. However, this approach does not yield information about the development or progression of the disease. Retrospective analysis of untreated patients with radiologically occult lung cancer has revealed much lower 5-year survival rates compared to surgically treated cases who can achieve >90% survival at 5 years [13]. Certainly some subjects with significant comorbidities may succumb to cardiopulmonary or other disease before their lung cancer, but in healthier or younger patients who have longer expected survival, ignoring the presence of carcinoma at an early curable stage is likely to be detrimental.

Longitudinal observational data using serial autofluorescence bronchoscopy and biopsy in patients with IEN has now been reported by a number of centers (Table 7.1) [4,7,11,14–17]. The observed rate of progression to carcinoma of moderate dysplasia is up to 9% and severe dysplasia is up to 32%. CIS is seen to either persist in >60% cases on short- to medium-term follow-up or progress to invasive cancer in more than 20–60% cases despite initial treatment in some instances. Carcinoma has also been seen to develop from nondysplastic areas supporting the field carcinogenesis theory. Lam *et al.* found carcinoma arising from areas of hyperplasia (0.3%) and metaplasia (0.4%), and Breuer *et al.* found the rate of progression to carcinoma from metaplasia of 9% [4,17]. Breuer *et al.* also observed that many sites showed nonstepwise progression and erratic fluctuations between histologic grades [4]. Bota *et al.* also reported carcinoma arising from areas of hyperplasia/metaplasia at a rate of 2% [16].

The variable rates in progression of these lesions may be due to the different patient populations evaluated and variation in histopathological interpretation. Patients with a diagnosis of lung cancer or other aerodigestive cancers are at risk of developing metachronous lung cancers, and this subset represents a very high-risk group who are likely to have greater observed rates of progression. In Lam *et al.*'s reported series, with lower rates of progression of moderate/severe dysplasia to carcinoma, the subjects were smokers with no clinical suspicion of cancer or previous history of aerodigestive cancer [17]. In the series reported by George *et al.*, who also documented lower rates of progression of IEN, only 40% of study subjects had previous lung cancer and subjects were excluded if they had a clinical suspicion of lung cancer [7]. The remainder had other risk factors such as significant smoking history, airflow limitation or asbestos exposure. Venmans *et al.*, Deygas *et al.*, Breuer *et al.*, and Hoshino *et al.* published series where the majority of the subject population included those with prior or current aerodigestive cancers or a clinical suspicion of lung cancer (Table 7.1) [4,11,14,15].

There are no published guidelines for the follow-up or treatment of moderate and severe dysplasia. Most centers that perform autofluorescence bronchoscopy keep these lesions under periodic surveillance with autofluorescence examination although treatment of large areas of severe dysplasia may be performed. There is also considerable controversy regarding the appropriate management of CIS. Carcinoma in situ is difficult to detect without autofluorescence bronchoscopy and therefore large observational series of long-term behavior do not exist as the imaging technique has only been developed in the last decade. In addition, some centers treat CIS immediately upon diagnosis rather than continue observation. Reported spontaneous regression of CIS is likely influenced by diagnostic biopsy that may remove small lesions completely, thereby falsely increasing the rate of regression. Historically, variation in histopathological reporting and differentiation between severe dysplasia and CIS may also have influenced reported outcomes. These factors have stimulated much debate as to whether these lesions should be observed or treated at initial detection. However, reported data from small published prospective series is helpful in this situation (Table 7.1). These series have shown that the majority of CIS persists on short- to medium-term follow-up and a significant proportion (21–67%) will progress to invasive cancer. In the series where CIS lesions were observed without treatment, only half of the lesions that progressed to invasive cancer were successfully treated, raising concerns that delay in treatment may have resulted in a poorer outcome for the patients [7].

There are no present biological or histopathological markers to assist in the assessment of these lesions and to predict future progression or stability. Therefore, although some lesions of CIS may be indolent in the short- to medium-term, a significant proportion is likely to eventually progress to invasive cancer. The clinical relevance will vary according to individual patient characteristics and life expectancy, e.g., an elderly patient with severe airflow limitation compared to a 50-year-old patient with no significant comorbidities. The risk of continued observation may be the lost opportunity to treat an early-stage lesion and a worse final outcome due to bronchial wall invasion and lymph node metastasis.

Treatment of CIS

Surgery remains the mainstay of treatment of CIS as the traditional and proven therapy, and results in >80–90% 5-year survival rate [18–21]. However, up to 30% may require bilobectomy or pneumonectomy to achieve cure, and the remaining 70% usually require lobectomy [18,20,21]. Segmentectomy has only been used in small series of selected patients with good 5-year survival rates (>90%) [19]. The risk of metachronous lung cancer in patients with central squamous cell carcinoma is significant, ranging from 14 to 30% and synchronous lesions can be detected in up to 20% of patients [13,15, 18–27]. In addition, surgery is not without risk in these patients due to comorbidities associated with their smoking history and some patients will be inoperable due to limited pulmonary reserves. Therefore, tissue-sparing methods to conserve pulmonary parenchyma need to be considered in the management of selected small CIS, reserving surgical resection for lesions that are ineligible or have failed endobronchial therapy.

There are no prospective, randomized studies comparing surgery to endobronchial therapy for CIS and they are unlikely to be performed in the near future, in part due to the difficulty in obtaining sufficient number of cases without a very large multicenter study [28]. However, outcomes of similar cases of early central lung cancer treated with endobronchial therapy or surgery are comparable [20,21,29]. In one cost-effectiveness analysis, the total cost of treatment and follow-up of bronchoscopically treated small stage 1A cancers in inoperable patients was 30% of the cost of standard surgery in matched operable patients [29].

Endobronchial therapy is not curative for lesions that have invaded into the bronchial cartilage or wall and is therefore limited to ≤3 mm thickness [22,30]. Information gained from surgical series have been helpful in identifying lesions that have a low risk of bronchial wall invasion and lymph node metastasis that may be amenable to curative endobronchial therapy [19,21,31]. Bronchial wall invasion and lymph node involvement were seen to be associated a number of features including: extension of the lesion beyond endoscopic visibility; greater longitudinal dimension of the lesion (>10 mm length); and greater nodularity of the tumor. Clinical trials with photodynamic therapy in the treatment of small central cancers have confirmed that a maximum diameter of 10 mm is an important predictor of response to therapy [32,33].

Assessment of eligibility for curative endobronchial therapy

Features predictive of response to endobronchial therapy include surface appearance, depth of in-

vasion and lymph node involvement. All margins of the lesion must be visualized endoscopically, the maximum diameter should be ≤10 mm and the whole lesion must be bronchoscopically accessible. Flat superficial lesions are more appropriate than those with a nodular or polypoid appearance. There should be no invasion into or beyond the cartilage layer of the bronchial wall and lymph nodes should be of normal appearance and size [33]. Lesions that do not fit these criteria should be referred directly for curative surgery if the patient is an operable candidate.

Multiple technologies should be used in combination to accurately assess these lesions and assist in the choice of the most suitable treatment option. These include autofluorescence bronchoscopy, endobronchial ultrasound, and computed tomography (CT), in addition to the clinical assessment of the patient and their comorbidities that may influence management.

Surface characteristics

Autofluorescence bronchoscopy is the best modality to evaluate surface features such as extent and size of the lesion and to accurately visualize all margins [34,35]. These features cannot be accurately assessed with white-light imaging alone. In one series, 70% of CIS cases diagnosed with white-light bronchoscopy and referred for therapy were not eligible for endobronchial therapy with curative intent when assessed by autofluorescence imaging, thereby resulting in a change in clinical management [35]. In addition, autofluorescence bronchoscopy has the added benefit of detecting other synchronous sites of IEN that may require surveillance or treatment. These are particularly common with central squamous cell carcinoma where up to ~20% patients have a synchronous carcinoma and up to ~45% patients have other lesions of moderate or severe dysplasia [24–26,36,37].

Depth of invasion and lymph node assessment

Although the endoscopic features of CIS are useful in predicting bronchial wall invasion and lymph node involvement, a more detailed assessment is required. Imaging modalities to consider are endobronchial ultrasound (EBUS), CT scan, and positron emission tomography (PET). Thoracic CT and PET are useful techniques for the evaluation of hilar and mediastinal lymph nodes and also to exclude synchronous peripheral tumors. Positive lymph nodes either on CT or PET imaging should be investigated to exclude metastases before curative endobronchial treatment is performed.

Although true CIS is not visible with EBUS or CT scan, as it is only cell layers thick, unexpected deeper invasion is visible and would correctly exclude these lesions from endobronchial treatment [38–40]. CT scan can detect bronchial wall thickening, peribronchial extension, and lymph node enlargement and has been shown to alter clinical management in 22–35% of cases being considered for curative therapy after bronchoscopy [38,39].

Endobronchial ultrasonography has been evaluated prospectively in the assessment of cases of small central squamous cell carcinoma for curative endobronchial treatment [39,41,42]. The sensitivity for cartilaginous involvement has been reported as 86% with a specificity of 67% [42]. Results have confirmed that the ultrasound images correlate well with surgical resection findings and lesions that appear intracartilaginous on EBUS have excellent long-term results after endobronchial therapy. EBUS resulted in a change in management in 36% of tumors thought to be curable by endobronchial therapy after white-light bronchoscopy and thoracic CT [39].

CIS lesions were not generally thought to be visible with PET scan as the lesion size is often below the resolution threshold, but one center has reported 73% sensitivity and 80% specificity with PET in CT occult CIS/microinvasive carcinoma of ≤10 mm diameter [43]. The development of new combined CT/PET imaging is interesting and may provide further advances in imaging these small lesions.

Endobronchial therapies

There are a number of well-described techniques that have been developed to treat endoluminal disease. These include photodynamic therapy (PDT), electrocautery, argon plasma coagulation (APC), cryotherapy, brachytherapy, and Nd-YAG laser therapy [44–47]. Despite some promising findings in the

treatment of a series of CIS, Nd-YAG laser therapy is not generally considered appropriate for curative therapy due to the increased risk of perforation and hemorrhage with the treatment of these flat lesions and the availability of safer techniques [48]. All the techniques can be used with flexible bronchoscopy under conscious sedation as the CIS lesions are small and easily treated compared to bulkier obstructive endoluminal disease that may require rigid bronchoscopy.

Photodynamic therapy has the most worldwide clinical experience, mainly in Japan, but there are issues of cost and photosensitivity. Electrocautery/APC and cryotherapy are cheaper and easier alternatives to PDT but large studies are not available. There have been no prospective, randomized studies comparing these methods for curative treatment of CIS. There is one reported prospective series comparing the side effects of electrocautery, PDT or Nd-YAG laser in patients with similar small, intraluminal tumors treated with curative intent [30]. Significant airway scarring with/without stenosis was more common with PDT or Nd-YAG laser therapy than with electrocautery. This is not surprising considering the deeper penetrative properties of PDT and Nd-YAG laser compared to electrocautery. As CIS is limited to the epithelium and only cell layers thick it is likely that the technique itself is not the determinant of cure but that correct staging and selection of lesions are the most important factors in achieving a good outcome. It is important to limit tissue damage in order to avoid stenosis that could cause further complications for the patient.

Many of the published studies included both stage 1A as well as stage 0 (CIS) disease in both surgically operable and inoperable patients and the size of the lesion was not always reported. Definitions of complete response and duration of follow-up vary between reports. These factors are important to consider when assessing treatment outcomes and therefore this review focused, where possible, on results of treatment of either CIS or microinvasive disease ≤10 mm diameter with long-term follow-up.

Photodynamic therapy

Photodynamic therapy uses the interaction of a photosensitizing drug and light of a specific wavelength in the presence of oxygen to produce a

Table 7.2 Outcome of photodynamic therapy in CIS/microinvasive disease ≤10 mm diameter.

	Number of treated lesions	Lesion type	Initial response	Long-term response
Furukawa *et al.* [33]	83	CIS/microinvasive <10 mm	93%	82%
Imamura *et al.* [50]	19	CIS ≤10 mm²	79%	42%
Radu *et al.* [51]	20	CIS (size NR)	—	90%
Cortese *et al.* [28]	15	Superficial squamous cancer <10 mm	87%	73%

NR, not reported.

photochemical reaction to destroy the tumor by a number of different mechanisms including tumor cell apoptosis, vascular damage, and inflammatory/immune reaction. The main limitations of its use are the cost and size of the laser equipment, cost of drug and skin photosensitization, but the development of new diode laser systems and photosensitizers will help to reduce these issues [32,49].

The majority of clinical data has emerged from Japan and 5-year follow-up data of the largest, most well-described series of squamous cell carcinoma <10 mm diameter has recently been published [33]. In this report, 83 CIS/microinvasive lesions treated with PDT between 1980 and 2001 achieved an initial bronchoscopic cure rate of 93% that fell to 82% over the follow-up duration due to recurrences at or near the treated site within 3–18 months after treatment (8/9 occurring within 12 mo) (Table 7.2) [33]. The recurrences were thought to be due to inappropriate estimation of the peripheral margin, inadequate laser irradiation or unsuspected intracartilaginous invasion. A smaller Japanese series of 19 CIS lesions ≤10 mm² achieved initial bronchoscopic eradication in 79% lesions, but on longer follow-up some cases showed local recurrence and the final cure rate was only 42% [50]. It is uncertain as to why the results in this study are much lower than other series (Table 7.2).

Other studies have been performed in North America and Europe (Table 7.2). A European study reported the treatment of 20 bronchial CIS as part of a larger series of aerodigestive cancers achieving bronchoscopic eradication in 90% cases over a mean follow-up of 27 months [51]. The Mayo Clinic

included 15 superficial carcinoma ≤10 mm diameter in their series evaluating the role of PDT as a surgical alternative and achieved an initial response of 87% and a long-term response of 73%. A second treatment to achieve cure was needed in 13% of these lesions [28].

Electrocautery

Endobronchial electrocautery uses a high-frequency alternating current that is converted to heat when passing through tissue. A small probe is used to focus the heat at the point of contact and achieve tissue destruction. It is an inexpensive technique with rapid and easy application and low complication rates. There is one report of a series of 13 patients with 15 small intraluminal lesions ≤10 mm² with normal CT scans. The majority of these lesions were stage 1A (13/15) and the remaining two lesions were CIS (stage 0). No residual disease was seen at a median follow-up of 22 months in 80% lesions. The failures were found to be due to more extensive disease on surgical resection, i.e., diameter >10 mm and deeper invasion [52].

A further subsequent report by the same group evaluating curative endobronchial treatment of small intraluminal, microinvasive stage 1A disease (CIS excluded) in 32 inoperable patients achieved bronchoscopic eradication in >95% of treated cases. Lesions were ≤10 mm in diameter and were assessed to be appropriate for endobronchial therapy by autofluorescence imaging and CT scan. Most patients were treated with electrocautery (75%) and the remainder with APC, PDT, or Nd-YAG laser. A second treatment to achieve cure was required in 9% subjects. Half the patients died in the mean follow-up of 5 years due to other disease or cancers, but only one death was attributable to the failure of treatment of achieve cure. The remainder of patients is alive without recurrent disease at the treated site after mean follow-up of 5 years [23].

Argon plasma coagulation is a more recent development that delivers electrocautery by a noncontact method using ionized argon gas to conduct electricity between the active electrode and the tissue. It has excellent coagulative properties and is a cheap and easy technique [44,47]. There is little published data of its use in treatment of bronchial CIS but due to its superficial coagulation properties it would also be a useful technique [53].

Cryotherapy

Cryotherapy is an inexpensive and safe technique where tissue is destroyed by freezing and is particularly useful for CIS situated on the membranous portion of the trachea or main bronchi where the risk of perforation is greater than the cartilaginous portion. Nitrous oxide is the most commonly used agent in bronchoscopic cryotherapy. There are limited reports of its use for curative therapy of CIS but no adverse events have been reported [15]. Deygas *et al.* reported the largest series of 35 patients with CIS/microinvasive disease detected by white-light bronchoscopy and achieved 91% cure at 12 months follow-up. Initial size of the lesions was not reported. A second cryotherapy treatment was required in 8.6% patients to achieve cure. The overall long-term cure rate was 80% as 7/35 patients (20%) subsequently developed invasive disease at the previously treated sites. It is uncertain from the reported data whether the invasive disease occurred at the sites of CIS or microinvasive disease. The lesions were only assessed with white-light bronchoscopy and thoracic CT scan and therefore it is likely that some lesions may not have been eligible for curative endobronchial therapy according to the aforementioned criteria that has been subsequently developed [15].

Brachytherapy

Brachytherapy involves the insertion of a radioactive source (usually Iridium[192]) near an endo-

bronchial malignancy to deliver local irradiation and requires the placement of an afterloading polyurethane catheter into the airway during flexible bronchoscopy. This technique is not usually used as first-line endobronchial therapy for cure of CIS or small microinvasive disease, but as second-line therapy or for bulkier disease in an inoperable patient. Brachytherapy has been evaluated as a sole modality in a study of high dose iridium in 18 inoperable patients with endobronchial cancers ≤10 mm and normal CT scan, achieving 83% initial response rates that fell to 72% at 1 year follow-up [54]. Intraluminal dosage ranged between 21 and 35 Gy. However, 55% subjects developed asymptomatic partial bronchial stenosis and 16.5% developed bronchial wall necrosis and/or fatal hemoptysis [54]. A similar study in 34 patients with endobronchial cancer and normal CT scan was subsequently published but the lesion size was not reported although it included six CIS lesions. Similar results were obtained with 85% eradication at 2 years and 73% at 3 years follow-up with similar intraluminal dosages. Hemoptysis was only seen in 2.9% cases [55].

Therefore, PDT, electrocautery, and cryotherapy are effective in treating small CIS/microinvasive lesions ≤10 mm diameter and achieving long-term cure rates of between 73 and 90% in most studies. Brachytherapy appears similarly effective but has higher complication rates and requires repeat treatment fractions. Response rates may be further improved in the future by the incorporation of newer technologies such as autofluorescence imaging and EBUS to improve eligibility assessment.

Follow-up after endobronchial treatment

Careful surveillance with repeat biopsies after the initial therapy is required as up to 10–15% of patients may require a second treatment to achieve cure [15,23,28]. However, this may be an overestimate of the true need for repeat treatment of CIS as it arises from series that include microinvasive disease and lesions not assessed with autofluorescence imaging or EBUS. In surgically operable patients, if cure is not achieved with endobronchial therapy, then prompt referral for surgery is required to avoid progressive disease. In addition, longer-term surveillance is recommended after curative therapy as up to 30% subjects will develop metachronous disease at other sites. Follow-up bronchoscopy and biopsy are generally performed at 4–6 weeks after the initial treatment, 3–6 monthly for the first 1–2 years, and then 6–12 monthly for up to 5 years.

Conclusion

The detection of moderate or severe dysplasia requires the consideration of longitudinal surveillance as patients harboring these lesions are at increased risk of developing malignancy either at the detected dysplastic site or at another site in the lungs. Future development of biological markers may assist in the task of risk prediction in these patients. CIS should be considered for curative therapy in patients with good life expectancy as there are high rates of persistence or progression to invasive carcinoma. Information from surgical series and prospective data from clinical trials have enabled the development of clear guidelines in the assessment of lesions for curative endobronchial therapy. There are a number of available tools that can be used for endobronchial treatment that are safe and easy to use with flexible bronchoscopy under conscious sedation. Eligible lesions include flat, bronchoscopically accessible lesions ≤10 mm diameter with visible margins on autofluorescence imaging, no invasion on endobronchial ultrasound or CT scan and normal lymph nodes. If the patient is a surgical candidate, curative endobronchial therapy could be discussed with the patient as a possible surgical alternative and parenchymal sparing measure in light of the high risk of metachronous disease. If the patient is not a surgical candidate, endobronchial treatment could be considered as first-line therapy if appropriate or in combination with radiation therapy [50,56].

References

1 Chhajed P, Shibuya K, Hoshino H *et al.* A comparison of video and autofluorescence bronchoscopy in patients at high risk of lung cancer. *Eur Respir J* 2005; **25(6)**:951–5.

2 Brambilla E, Travis WD, Colby TV, Corrin B, Shimosato Y. The New World Health Organization classification of lung tumors. *Eur Respir J* 2001; **18**:1059–68.

3 McWilliams A, MacAulay C, Gazdar AF, Lam S. Innovative molecular and imaging approaches for the detection of lung cancer and its precursor lesions. *Oncogene* 2002; **21(45)**:6949–59.

4 Breuer R, Pasic A, Smit E *et al.* The natural course of preneoplastic lesions in bronchial epithelium. *Clin Cancer Res* 2005; **15**:537–43.

5 Keith R, Miller Y, Gemmill R *et al.* Angiogenic squamous dysplasia in bronchi of individuals at high risk for lung cancer. *Clin Cancer Res* 2000; **6**:1616–25.

6 Helfritzsch H, Junker K, Bartel M, Scheele J. Differentiation of positive autofluorescence bronchoscopy findings by comparative genomic hybridization. *Oncol Rep* 2002; **9(4)**:697–701.

7 George P, Banerjee A, Read C *et al.* Surveillance for the detection of early lung cancer in patients with bronchial dysplasia. *Thorax* 2007; **62**:43–50.

8 Pasic A, Vonk-Noordegraaf A, Risse E, Postmus P, Sutedja T. Multiple suspicious lesions detected by autofluorescence bronchoscopy predict malignant development in the bronchial mucosa in high risk patients. *Lung Cancer* 2003; **41(3)**:295–301.

9 Breuer R, Snijders P, Sutedja T *et al.* Suprabasal p53 immunostaining in premalignant endobronchial lesions in combination with histology is associated with bronchial cancer. *Lung Cancer* 2003; **40(2)**:165–72.

10 Miyazu Y, Miyazawa T, Hiyama K *et al.* Telomerase expression in noncancerous bronchial epithelia is a possible marker of early development of lung cancer. *Cancer Res* 2005; **65(21)**:9623–7.

11 Hoshino H, Shibuya K, Chiyo M *et al.* Biological features of bronchial squamous dysplasia followed up by autofluorescence bronchoscopy. *Lung Cancer* 2004; **46**:187–96.

12 Manser R, Dodd M, Byrnes G, Irving L, Campbell DA. Incidental lung cancers identified at coronial autopsy: implications for overdiagnosis of lung cancer by screening. *Respir Med* 2005; **99(4)**:501–7.

13 Sato M, Saito Y, Endo C *et al.* The natural history of radiographically occult bronchogenic squamous cell carcinoma: a retrospective study of overdiagnosis bias. *Chest* 2004; **126(1)**:108–13.

14 Venmans B, van Boxem T, Smit E, Postmus P, Sutedja T. Outcome of bronchial carcinoma in situ. *Chest* 2000; **117(6)**:1572–6.

15 Deygas N, Froudarakis M, Ozenne G, Vergnon JM. Cryotherapy in early superficial bronchogenic carcinoma. *Chest* 2001; **120(1)**:26–31.

16 Bota S, Auliac J, Paris C *et al*. Follow-up of bronchial precancerous lesions and carcinoma in situ using fluorescence endoscopy. *Am J Respir Crit Care Med* 2001; **164(9)**:1688–93.

17 Lam S, Slivinskas J, McWilliams A *et al*. Natural history of premalignant bronchial lesions: implications for chemoprevention. *Am Assoc Cancer Res* 2002.

18 Cortese D, Pairolero P, Bergstralh E *et al*. Roentgenographically occult lung cancer. A ten-year experience. *J Thorac Cardiovasc Surg* 1983; **86(3)**:373–80.

19 Fujimura S, Sagawa M, Saito Y *et al*. A therapeutic approach to roentgenographically occult squamous cell carcinoma of the lung. *Cancer* 2000; **89(Suppl 11)**:2445–8.

20 Nakamura H, Kawasaki N, Hagiwara M *et al*. Early hilar lung cancer-risk for multiple lung cancers and clinical outcome. *Lung Cancer* 2001; **33(1)**:51–7.

21 Nakamura H, Kawasaki N, Haigwara M, Ogata A, Kato H. Endoscopic evaluation of centrally located early squamous cell carcinoma of the lung. *Cancer* 2001; **91**:1142–7.

22 Woolner L, Fontana R, Cortese D *et al*. Roentgenographically occult lung cancer; pathologic findings and frequency of multicentricity during a 10-year period. *Mayo Clin Proc* 1984; **59**:453–66.

23 Vonk-Noordegraaf A, Postmus P, Sutedja T. Bronchoscopic treatment of patients with intraluminal microinvasive radiographically occult lung cancer not eligible for surgical resection: a follow-up study. *Lung Cancer* 2003; **39(1)**:49–53.

24 Lam S, MacAulay C, Hung J, LeRiche J, Profio A, Palcic B. Detection of dysplasia and carcinoma in situ with a lung imaging fluorescence endoscope device. *J Thorac Cardiovasc Surg* 1993; **105(6)**:1035–40.

25 Pierard P, Vermylen P, Bosschaerts T *et al*. Synchronous roentgenographically occult lung carcinoma in patients with resectable primary lung cancer. *Chest* 2000; **117(3)**:779–85.

26 Pierard P, Faber J, Hutsebaut J *et al*. Synchronous lesions detected by autofluorescence bronchoscopy in patients with high-grade preinvasive lesions and occult invasive squamous cell carcinoma of the proximal airways. *Lung Cancer* 2004; **46(3)**:341–7.

27 van Rens M, Schramel F, Elbers J, Lammers J. The clinical value of lung imaging fluorescence endoscopy for detecting synchronous lung cancer. *Lung Cancer* 2001; **32(1)**:13–8.

28 Cortese D, Edell E, Kinsey J. Photodynamic therapy for early stage squamous cell carcinoma of the lung. *Mayo Clin Proc* 1997; **72(7)**:595–602.

29 Pasic A, Brokx H, Vonk Noordegraaf A, Paul R, Postmus P, Sutedja T. Cost-effectiveness of early intervention: comparison between intraluminal bronchoscopic treatment and surgical resection for T1N0 lung cancer patients. *Respiration* 2004; **71**:391–6.

30 van Boxem A, Westerga J, Venmans B, Postmus P, Sutedja G. Photodynamic therapy, Nd-YAG laser and electrocautery for treating early-stage intraluminal cancer: which to choose? *Lung Cancer* 2001; **31**:31–6.

31 Konaka C, Hirano T, Kato H *et al*. Comparison of endoscopic features of early-stage squamous cell lung cancer and histological findings. *Br J Cancer* 1999; **80**:1435–9.

32 Furuse K, Fukuoka M, Kato H *et al*. A prospective phase II study on photodynamic therapy for centrally located early-stage lung cancer. *J Clin Oncol* 1993; **11(10)**:1852–7.

33 Furukawa K, Kato H, Konaka C, Okunaka T, Usuda J, Ebihara Y. Locally recurrent central-type early stage lung cancer <1.0 cm in diameter after complete remission by photodynamic therapy. *Chest* 2005; **128**:3269–75.

34 Ikeda N, Hiyoshi T, Kakihana M *et al*. Histopathological evaluation of fluorescence bronchoscopy using resected lungs in cases of lung cancer. *Lung Cancer* 2003; **41(3)**:303–9.

35 Sutedja T, Codrington H, Risse E *et al*. Autofluorescence bronchoscopy improves staging of radiographically occult lung cancer and has an impact on therapeutic strategy. *Chest* 2001; **120(4)**:1327–32.

36 Lam S, MacAulay C, LeRiche J, Ikeda N, Palcic B. Early localization of bronchogenic carcinoma. *Diagn Ther Endosc* 1994; **1**:75–8.

37 Pierard P, Martin B, Verdebout JM *et al*. Fluorescence bronchoscopy in high-risk patients comparison of LIFE and pentax systems. *J Bronchol* 2001; **8**:254–9.

38 Sutedja G, Golding R, Postmus P. High resolution computed tomography in patients referred for intraluminal bronchoscopic therapy with curative intent. *Eur Respir J* 1996; **9(5)**:1020–3.

39 Miyazu Y, Miyazawa T, Kurimoto N, Iwamoto Y, Kanoh K, Kohno N. Endobronchial ultrasonography in the assessment of centrally located early-stage lung cancer before photodynamic therapy. *Am J Respir Crit Care Med* 2002; **165**:832–7.

40 McWilliams A, Mayo J, Ahn MI, MacDonald S, Lam S. Lung cancer screening using multi-slice thin-section computed tomography and autofluorescence bronchoscopy. *J Thorac Oncol* 2006; **1(1)**:61–8.

41 Kurimoto N, Murayama M, Yoshioka S, Nishisaka T, Inai K, Dohi K. Assessment of usefulness of

endobronchial ultrasonography in determination of depth of tracheobronchial tumor invasion. *Chest* 1999; **115**:1500–6.

42 Takahasi H, Sagawa M, Sato M *et al.* A prospective evaluation of transbronchial ultrasonography for assessment of depth of invasion in early bronchogenic squamous cell carcinoma. *Lung Cancer* 2003; **42**: 43–9.

43 Pasic A, Brokx H, Comans E *et al.* Detection and staging of preinvasive lesions and occult lung cancer in the central airways with [18] F-Fluorodeoxyglucose positron emission tomography: a pilot study. *Clin Cancer Res* 2005; **11(17)**:6186–9.

44 Sutedja G, Bolliger C. Endobronchial electrocautery and argon plasma coagulation. Interventional bronchoscopy. *Prog Respir Res* 2000; **30**:120–32.

45 Lee P, Kupeli E, Mehta A. Therapeutic bronchoscopy in lung cancer. *Clin Chest Med* 2002; **23(1)**:241–56.

46 Sheski F, Mathur P. Endoscopic treatment of early-stage lung cancer. *Cancer Control* 2000; **7(1)**:35–44.

47 Beamis J. Interventional pulmonology techniques for treating malignant large airway obstruction. *Curr Opin Pulm Med* 2005; **11**:292–5.

48 Cavaliere S, Foccoli P, Toninelli C. Curative bronchoscopic laser therapy for surgically resectable tracheobronchial tumors. *J Bronchol* 2002; **9**:90–5.

49 Kato H, Furukawa K, Sato M *et al.* Phase II clinical study of photodynamic therapy using mono-L-aspartyl chlorine e6 and diode laser for early superficial squamous cell carcinoma of the lung. *Lung Cancer* 2003; **42**: 103–11.

50 Imamura S, Kusunoki Y, Takifuji N *et al.* Photodynamic therapy and/or external beam radiation therapy for roentgenologically occult lung cancer. *Cancer* 1994; **73(6)**:1608–14.

51 Radu A, Grosjean P, Fontolliet C *et al.* Photodynamic therapy for 101 early cancers of the upper aerodigestive tract, the esophagus, and the bronchi: a single-institution experience. *Diagn Ther Endosc* 1999; **5**:145–54.

52 van Boxem T, Venmans B, Schramel F *et al.* Radiographically occult lung cancer treated with fibreoptic bronchoscopic electrocautery: a pilot study of a simple and inexpensive technique. *Eur Respir J* 1998; **11(1)**:169–72.

53 Schuurman B, Postmus P, van Mourik J, Risse E, Sutedja T. Combined use of autofluorescence bronchoscopy and argon plasma coagulation enables less extensive resection of radiographically occult lung cancer. *Respiration* 2004; **71**:410–1.

54 Perol M, Caliandro R, Pommier P *et al.* Curtive irradiation of limited endobronchial carcinomas with high dose brachytherapy: results of a pilot study. *Chest* 1997; **111(5)**:1417–23.

55 Marsiglia H, Baldeyrou P, Lartigau E *et al.* High-dose-rate brachytherapy as sole modality for early-stage endobronchial carcinoma. *Int J Radiat Oncol Biol Phys* 2000; **47(3)**:665–72.

56 Freitag L, Ernst A, Thomas M, Prenzel R, Whalers B, Macha HN. Sequential photodynamic therapy (PDT) and high dose brachytherapy for endobronchial tumour control in patients with limited bronchogenic carcinoma. *Thorax* 2004; **59**:790–3.

CHAPTER 8

The Pathology and Pathogenesis of Peripheral Lung Adenocarcinoma Including Bronchioloalveolar Carcinoma

Wilbur A. Franklin

Introduction

The histopathological classification of adenocarcinoma of lung has received extraordinary scrutiny during the past several years for several reasons. First, improved sensitivity of thoracic imaging methods has resulted in resection of increasingly smaller peripheral lung lesions, more than 70% of which are adenocarcinomas [1–3]. Second, high throughput gene expression methods and molecular models have changed molecular understanding of adenocarcinoma. Finally, new targeted therapeutic agents have provided tools that are effective in subsets of adenocarcinomas and challenge pathologists to account for selective drug sensitivity. This chapter will review the historical development of the current histopathological classification pulmonary adenocarcinoma and how this classification is being affected by changing concepts of pathogenesis and molecular properties of this increasingly common tumor.

Lung Cancer, 3rd edition. Edited by Jack A. Roth, James D. Cox, and Waun Ki Hong. © 2008 Blackwell Publishing, ISBN: 978-1-4051-5112-2.

Adenocarcinoma and the anatomy of the peripheral airway

Adenocarcinoma is the most common tumor of the peripheral airway, an anatomic region that is not easily accessible for tissue sampling. In this region the bronchioles terminate in microscopic alveolar sacs where gas exchange occurs. The transition from bronchus to alveolus is accompanied by a transition from the pseudostratified mucociliary epithelium of the distal bronchi and proximal bronchioles to nonmucinous epithelium in the distal bronchiole that contains a mixture of ciliated and nonciliated cells, including the Clara cells [4]. Clara cells synthesize numerous proteins specific for this region including surfactant apoproteins A, B and D, tryptase, β-galactoside-binding lectin, a specific phospholipase, and a 10 kD protein, CC10 [5]. These proteins are stored in secretory granules and are released into lower airway fluid. The most abundant protein in airway fluid is CC10, a uteroglobin-like protein whose function has not been conclusively established but may be to protect the lung from environmental toxins [6,7]. It serves as a marker for distal bronchial epithelial differentiation.

At the bronchiolar terminus where the bronchiole merges with the alveolar septum, a short segment of the airway is surfaced by a simple agranular, nonciliated cuboidal epithelium. The nondescript cuboidal cells give way distally to the flattened and thin alveolar cells that line the alveolar sacs. Alveolar cells are of two types, the thin plate-like type I cells that cover more than 90% of the alveolar septa and through which gas exchange occurs and the type II cells which are more numerous than type I cell but cover only a small fraction of the alveolar surface. Type I cells are only 0.1–0.2 microns in thickness and may not be visible by light microscopy, but are consistently detected by electron microscopy as a continuous lining of alveolar surfaces. Type II cells are more easily identified as cuboidal cells protruding into the alveolar space. These cells have several functions including secretion of surfactant, absorption of ions and fluid from the alveolar space, and repair of alveolar injury [4]. The molecular apparatus that permits the type II cell to accomplish these functions is evident in many pulmonary adenocarcinomas [8] (see below).

In addition to mimicking normal adult tissue, lung tumors may recapitulate cellular and molecular properties of the embryonic lung. Lung anatomy develops rapidly and continuously during embryonic life through five more or less distinct anatomic stages (reviewed in [9]) beginning with the formation of the lung bud from the foregut endoderm in the embryonic stage (gestational age 9–12 days). During the succeeding stages, pseudoglandular, canalicular and saccular structures, and finally alveoli develop under the strictly timed regulation of transcription factors [9–11]. Distinct patterns of gene expression correspond to each stage of development [12]. Similarities between gene expression profiles of developing lung and tumor have been described in mouse models [13] and these findings have been extrapolated to human tumors. One study suggests that adenocarcinomas recapitulate gene expression patterns that correspond to the saccular and alveolar developmental stages of the lung while large cell and squamous carcinomas exhibit profiles that more closely match the earlier pseudoglandular and canalicular stages of development [14]. Overall comparisons of gene expression profiles suggest that tumors re-express genes that are associated with embryonic development

and support the analogy between fetal development and lung tumor differentiation. An incompletely exploited consequence of this analogy is the revelation of new biomarkers and possible targets for early detection and therapeutic intervention as discussed below.

Classification of pulmonary adenocarcinoma

The classification of lung cancer in general and adenocarcinoma in particular remains grounded in the careful microscopic study of human tumors in hematoxylin and eosin-stained sections. This basic information has been buttressed in recent years by new immunohistochemical and molecular data, but histological diagnosis remains the *sina qua non* of treatment and evaluation of outcome. At the most basic level, adenocarcinoma is defined in the most recent WHO monograph on lung cancer as "a malignant epithelial tumour with glandular differentiation or mucin production..." [15]. This recent edition, published in 2004, includes 13 types and subtypes of adenocarcinoma, the most common of which is the adenocarcinoma, mixed subtype. A detailed histological description is provided for each of the major subtypes of adenocarcinoma as well as for some of the more unusual subtypes in order to illustrate the diversity of histological appearances in adenocarcinoma of the lung and to provide information on their differential diagnosis. The defining features of each subtype are listed in Table 8.1.

The current classification is the result of a long historical process in which definitions and terminology have been refined to accommodate observations regarding cellular structure and clinical outcome. Adenocarcinoma has been a recognized tumor type since the first codified histological classifications of lung cancer were introduced in the early twentieth century when lung cancer was still a rare disease. In 1924, Marchesani produced one of the first widely adopted histological classifications of lung and included "zylinderzellige adenokarzinome" (cylindrical cell adenocarcinoma) as one of four main histological types of lung carcinoma. The Marchesani classification was used widely without

Table 8.1 Pathological features of adenocarcinomas.

Tumors of the lung	ICD-O codes	Defining features
Adenocarcinoma group	8140/3	Malignant epithelial tumors with glandular differentiation or mucin production.
Adenocarcinoma mixed subtype	8255/3	Invasive adenocarcinoma with acinar, papillary, bronchioloalveolar or solid components. Representing approximately 80% of resected adenocarcinomas.
Acinar adenocarcinoma subtype	8550/3	Invasive tumor with tissue destruction and composed of cuboidal or columnar cells.
Papillary adenocarcinoma subtype	8260/3	Invasive carcinoma with >75% of tumor forming papillae with secondary and tertiary papillary structures that replace the underlying lung architecture.
Bronchioloalveolar adenocarcinoma subtype	8250/3	Growth along pre-existing alveolar structures (lepidic growth) without evidence of stromal, vascular, or pleural invasion.
Solid adenocarcinoma subtype	8230/3	Sheets of polygonal cells lacking acini, tubules, and papillae but with mucin production in at least five tumor cells in each of two high power fields.
Fetal adenocarcinoma subtype	8333/3	Glandular elements composed of tubules of glycogen-rich, nonciliated cells that resemble fetal lung tubules with focal rounded morules of polygonal cells.
Mucinous ("colloid") adenocarcinoma subtype	8480/3	Dissecting pools of mucin containing islands of neoplastic epithelium. Tumor cells are well differentiated and sometimes tumor cells float within the pools of mucin.
Mucinous cystadenocarcinoma subtype	8470/3	A circumscribed tumor that may have a partial fibrous tissue capsule. Centrally there is cystic change with mucin pooling. Neoplastic mucinous epithelium grows along alveolar walls.
Signet ring adenocarcinoma subtype	8490/3	Usually a focal pattern associated with other histologic subtypes of adenocarcinoma. Large mucin vacuoles displace nuclei in tumor cells.
Clear cell adenocarcinoma subtype	8310/3	Most often a focal pattern, but rarely it may be the major component of the tumor (clear cell adenocarcinoma). Tumor cells have clear, featureless cytoplasm due to mucin or glycogen accumulation.
Adenosquamous carcinoma	8560/3	A carcinoma showing components of both squamous cell carcinoma and adenocarcinoma with each comprising at least 10% of the tumor.
Atypical adenomatous hyperplasia		Small (<5 mm) localized proliferation of atypical cells lining involved alveoli. Generally occurs in the absence of underlying interstitial inflammation and fibrosis.

Summary of defining histological features along with ICD-O codes. The table includes features defining the entire group of tumors as well as specific subtypes.

change for the next 25 years as the frequency of lung cancer increased. Following World War II, the prevalence of lung cancer grew into a major public health problem and a universally applicable revised classification was needed. In 1967, the first WHO lung cancer classification was published, representing the consensus of an expert panel of pathologists. The classification included three subtypes of adenocarcinoma, acinar, papillary, and bronchioloalveolar. Over the succeeding 40 years, WHO-sponsored panels have convened periodically to revise the original classification. The most notable trend in the revisions has been the increase in the number of tumor subtypes. The increase in diagnostic categories has been engendered largely by the recognition of histologically distinct categories that have clinical or biological significance. The prototypical pulmonary adenocarcinoma is bronchioloalveolar carcinoma (BAC), a tumor that uniquely reflects the macroscopic and microscopic organization of the lung as discussed below.

Bronchioloalveolar carcinoma

BAC is a well-differentiated adenocarcinoma originating in the peripheral lung that spreads through the airways. Its defining histological feature is its nondestructive growth along the alveolar septae, a feature that has been referred to as "lepidic" spread. The cells that exhibit this pattern of growth are of two types, nonmucinous (Plate 8.1a) and mucinous (Plate 8.1b). Mucinous tumors have vacuoles, usually in the upper cytoplasm, that are large enough to compress and deform the nuclei of the cell. Large amounts of mucin may be present in the alveoli adjacent to tumor cells. The nonmucinous cells resemble Clara cells or type II pneumocytes. The Clara cell-type tumors are composed of columnar cells with eosinophilic cytoplasm and apical cytoplasmic projections ("snouts"). Type II cell tumors are more cuboidal with foamy, vacuolated cytoplasm. Nuclei of all types of BAC are usually low grade with mitotic figures few in number. In a small percentage of BAC mixtures of cell types may occur. In such cases mucin stains may be useful in confirming the mucinous or mixed mucinous/nonmucinous subtype.

Current definitions permit no evidence of stromal invasion in BAC. To understand the rationale for this definition, it is necessary to understand the evolution of the concept of BAC.

The evolving definition of BAC

Although the hypothesis that lung tumors may originate in the alveoli was proposed as early as the mid-nineteenth century [16], it was not until 1953 that the thin layer of pneumocytes along the surface of the alveolar septae was discovered by electron microscopy [17]. By 1960, the observation that some well-differentiated lung cancers resembled bronchiolar or alveolar epithelium and could spread along the alveolar surfaces led to the introduction and general acceptance of the designation "bronchioloalveolar" carcinoma by Leibow in 1960. These tumors were described as " . . . well-differentiated adenocarcinomas primary in the periphery of the lung beyond a grossly recognizable bronchus, with a tendency to spread chiefly within the confines of the lung by aerogenous and lymphatic routes . . . " [18]. According to this definition, BAC could be invasive or noninvasive carcinoma. The WHO classifications accepted this definition until 1999, when BAC was reclassified strictly as an in situ tumor.

The change in classification was based on evidence that began to accumulate in the late 1970s and early 1980s. Shimosato *et al.* reported in 1980 that peripheral adenocarcinomas <3 cm without fibrosis had a significantly better prognosis than tumors of the same size with central scarring [19]. Noguchi *et al.* later reported that tumors <2 cm had a 100% 5-year survival while the presence of fibrosis indicating stromal invasion reduced 5-year survival to 75% [20]. Fibrosis was strictly defined in this study as an active fibroblastic focus and was distinguished from "collapse" in which compressed alveoli are admixed with elastic tissue. These studies highlighted the importance of fibrosis in small solitary nodules and it has been subsequently shown that not only is the presence of fibrosis important but the size of the fibroblastic focus also affects prognosis. Tumors with areas of scarring <5–10 mm in maximum diameter have a significantly worse outcome that those without fibrosis [21,22]. Tumors

<2.0 cm with invasion at the center of a fibroblastic focus have 60% 5-year survival while tumors with more minimal fibrotic foci have 100% survival at 5 years [23].

The prognostic importance of a fibroblastic stromal response prompted a reassessment of BAC that is reflected in the 1999 [24] and 2004 [15] WHO classifications. In the revised classifications, BAC is considered to be a purely in situ lesion that can spread through alveolar spaces but exhibits no stromal invasion and does not metastasis to distant sites through blood or lymphatics. Since most tumors have a component of stromal invasion, a possible effect of changing the definition of BAC could be to reduce its frequency. By exactly how much is not known. In Japanese studies in which the invasion exclusion was first applied, 28 of 236 solitary tumors (12%) were classified as noninvasive [20]. In a more recent CT screening study in the United States, where the in situ only criterion was applied, 20 of 348 tumors (6%) were classified as BAC [1]. These figures are similar to older figures to which the in situ criterion was not applied (reviewed in [25]). These preliminary numbers suggest that the frequency of BAC is not likely to drastically change as a result of changes in the criteria for the diagnosis of BAC. The overwhelming majority of lung adenocarcinomas will continue to be classified as invasive, either of the acinar type or the mixed subtype (mixed acinar and bronchioloalveolar subtype).

Invasive adenocarcinoma: acinar and mixed subtype

Invasive pulmonary adenocarcinoma is characterized by the formation of tubules or acini in a fibrous stroma with the destruction of the underlying lung architecture (Plate 8.2). This pattern of growth may occur without an associated BAC component (acinar adenocarcinoma) or as an epicenter adjacent to a BAC component (adenocarcinoma mixed subtype). Invasive adenocarcinoma cells are columnar or cuboidal and may produce mucin. The production of mucin is a useful diagnostic feature and may be demonstrated by mucin or PAS stains. These stains help to distinguish true mucus production from nonmucinous vacuolation that can occur as

a result of fat or glycogen production or fixation artifact. Nonadenocarcinomas may produce small amounts of mucin and by convention, 10% tumor cells producing mucin is a requirement for the diagnosis of invasive adenocarcinoma.

Adenocarcinoma is graded on the basis of level of cellular size and deformity, variation of nuclear size and shape, chromatin configuration, nuclear/cytoplasmic ration, and mitotic activity. In the better-differentiated tumors, cells have finely granular chromatin that is evenly dispersed. At the more poorly differentiated end of the spectrum, adenocarcinoma may resemble large cell carcinoma with only a few tubular structures in a background of sheets of tumor cells. In more poorly differentiated, higher-grade tumors nuclear chromatin is coarse, clumped, and irregular. Nuclear membranes are well defined and may be folded and angulated. Nucleoli are prominent and may be single or multiple and rounded or irregularly shaped.

Precise grading criteria are not widely employed nor are they well defined at the present time. Generally the closer to recapitulation of normal lung tissue, the lower the grade. Histological grade, nuclear grade, necrosis, and the presence of lymphatic invasion or a greater than 25% papillary growth component have been associated with more aggressive behavior. However, the predictive accuracy of any of these features is low and generally not sufficient for extrapolation to individual cases. Even small, well-differentiated adenocarcinomas have an 8% frequency of metastasis at the time of surgery. There is little evidence that grade of invasive tumor is of prognostic importance, the major determinant of prognosis being stage.

Necrosis may be pronounced in untreated invasive adenocarcinomas. This feature may hinder efforts to microscopically assess chemotherapeutic intervention following drug administration. Levels of both necrosis pretreatment and posttreatment should be taken into account when protocols designed to assess the effect of chemotherapy are implemented.

In some tumors, a recently described pattern of differentiation referred to as micropapillary and consisting of tufts of tumor cells without vascular cores, may be present in variable numbers of tumor cells [26]. Metastases from these tumors are more frequent and the metastatic tumor deposits are more frequently micropapillary than in conventional adenocarcinomas [26]. Most studies to date have suggested that this micropapillary pattern of tumor growth is associated with considerably worse survival, particularly in early-stage tumors [26–29], although at least one study has found no increase in survival risk for this pattern of tumor growth. More data will be needed from larger cohorts to resolve this issue but for the moment the micropapillary pattern of tumor cell growth is best regarded carcinoma patients as a feature of lung adenocarcinoma that may predict an aggressive clinical course.

The hallmark of invasive carcinoma is stromal invasion, which is characterized by the presence of active appearing fibroblasts in association with tumor cells. The significance of the fibrosis has been debated for many years. Fibrotic scars may occur as a result of inflammatory conditions such as tuberculosis, infarction, pneumoconiosis, and many other conditions. In some cases, these postinflammatory scars may predate adenocarcinoma and it has been suggested that scarring may play a causative role in adenocarcinoma of the lung, often in the apex of the lung [30]. Tumors associated with scarring were referred to as "lung scar cancers" [31] or simply "scar carcinoma." However, by the 1980s, it was becoming evident that tumor itself could induce scar formation [19,32] and that the cellular and molecular composition of tumor-associated scars was different than that of post-inflammatory scars with the former containing considerably greater numbers of myofibroblasts [33] and larger quantities of types I [34] and V [33,34] collagen. The presence of scarring in adenocarcinoma is now considered to be largely a host response to tumor rather than an active carcinogenic process. Those cases in which scar precedes tumor are now attributed to coincidental occurrence of separate disease processes in the same anatomic location.

Recently, tumor–stromal relationships in adenocarcinoma have been approached from an entirely different perspective. It has been observed that carcinoma cells, which are epithelium-derived, begin to express cellular and molecular properties that are more characteristic of stromal or mesenchymal cells than their cells of origin. This phenomenon is referred to as an epithelial–mesenchymal transition (EMT). EMT is accompanied by loss of epithelial intercellular junctions and changes in the pattern of growth from the characteristic sheet-like epithelial monolayer to a single cell infiltrating pattern, characteristic of mesenchymal cells [35]. Morphological change is accompanied by changes in patterns of gene expression. Tumor cells express mesenchyme-associated genes such as vimentin and zeb1 at a high level and epithelium-associated genes such as E-cadherin and snail at a low level [36]. Cell lines with mesenchymal patterns of gene expression are less sensitive to EGFR blockade than those with a more characteristically epithelial phenotype [37]. How far this line of reasoning will take us is not evident at the present time but the predictive edifice provided by the EMT hypothesis may provide a theoretical rationale for drug sensitivity and early detection algorithms that may be clinically applicable in the future.

The stromal reaction in pulmonary adenocarcinoma also includes leukocytic infiltrates and in some cases dramatic lymphocytic responses accompanied by mononuclear dendritic cells and eosinophils. Whether this infiltrate represents an active immunological response directed against tumor cell antigens or an epiphenomenon mediated by cytokines produced by tumor cells is currently being debated. A detailed discussion of immunological response to tumor is beyond the scope of this chapter but the presence of an inflammatory infiltrate, particularly the presence of tumor infiltrating lymphocytes (TIL) in adenocarcinoma (Plate 8.3), raises hope that enhancing an immunological response to tumor may be a feasible treatment. TIL concentrations estimated by simple microscopic inspection of sections of nonsmall cell lung carcinoma (NSCLC) stained for the T cell receptor CD3 [38,39] or dendritic cells [38], have shown a modest survival advantage in those subjects with relatively high concentrations of these cells. Recent preliminary data suggests that the subset of lymphocytes may predict outcome. It has been reported that CD8 cells infiltrating tumor may be inactive [40] and the stimulation of TIL may activate CD8 cells [39,41] and thus have an antitumor effect. Whether it will be possible to translate these descriptive studies into clinical advance remains to be determined. What is clear is that the stromal and immunological response to tumor is complex and that enhancement of specific responses to tumor may not only elicit an antitumor response but stimulate tumor growth as well. Possible stimulatory effects from the cytokine-rich stromal environment of lung NSCLC [42,43] (including adenocarcinoma) must be accounted for in immunological approaches to lung cancer treatment.

Unusual lung cancers and differential diagnosis

In addition to the relatively common types of BAC and invasive adenocarcinoma, several less common histological patterns are encountered in pulmonary adenocarcinoma that may present diagnostic difficulties. Many of these tumors resemble metastatic carcinoma with which they are prone to be confused. However, careful histological examination supplemented by appropriate immunohistochemical profiling will usually permit precise histological classification.

Papillary adenocarcinoma

Papillary carcinomas are tumors in which the predominant pattern is one in which papillary structures supported by central fibrovascular cores form secondary and tertiary branches (Plate 8.4). By current WHO definition, this is an invasive tumor that replaces the underlying architecture of the lung [44]. Tumor cells exhibit marked nuclear atypia. Papillary adenocarcinoma may contain psammoma bodies and areas of necrosis. This tumor is sometimes difficult to distinguish from BAC in which there may be simple papillary structures but in BAC there is underlying preservation of the alveolar architecture. Papillary adenocarcinoma occurs in an older population (mean age 65) and most patients (86%) are smokers [45]. It is important to recognize this subtype of adenocarcinoma since survival is poor (3.4 yr for stage I tumors) [45].

Tumors with abnormal mucin production—mucinous (colloid) adenocarcinoma, mucinous cystadenocarcinoma, and signet ring adenocarcinoma

These tumors are discussed together since they share the common feature of strikingly aberrant production of mucin. In colloid adenocarcinoma, tumor cells are suspended in large mucinous pools and may partially line fibrous septae within the tumor (Plate 8.5). Mucinous cystadenocarcinoma is usually well circumscribed with tumor cells lining cyst-like, mucin-containing spaces. Finally, signet ring adenocarcinoma is composed of clusters and singly infiltrating tumor cells that contain large intracellular mucin vacuoles [46]. They may be part of a more copious acinar tumor [47]. All of these tumors are invasive tumors and resemble their counterparts in other organs including breast and gastrointestinal tract. Immunohistochemical stains may help to distinguish tumors originating in lung from those of GI origin. Pulmonary signet ring tumors express cytokeratin 7 and TTF-1 but not cytokeratin 20, MUC2 or the intestine-specific homeobox gene CDX-2 [46,48–50], an immunohistochemical profile typical of primary lung carcinoma. However, a proportion of mucinous tumor in which lung is the only detectable site may not have immunohistochemical findings that are typical of lung cancer [50] and in these cases diagnosis of lung primary can only be made by exclusion.

Clear cell adenocarcinoma

In this tumor, cytoplasmic contents do not stain giving the cells an empty or "clear" appearance under the microscope. The cytoplasmic clearing may be due to the accumulation of lipid or glycogen, which is dissolved during conventional histological processing. Clear cell differentiation may occur in any of the pulmonary adenocarcinoma subtypes [51]. Tumors with this morphological appearance must be distinguished from renal cell carcinoma, which is typically TTF-1 negative, and from the so-called "sugar tumor," a benign neoplasm that is thought to arise from perivascular epithelioid cells that contains copious glycogen and strongly express the HMB45 immunohistochemical marker (reviewed in [52]).

Fetal adenocarcinoma

Low-grade tumors resembling fetal lung have been distinguished in recent decades from higher-grade pulmonary blastoma [53–57]. These tumors have a peak incidence in the fourth decade and more often occur in females than males. They typically occur in smokers. The characteristic feature of this tumor is the formation of tubules by glycogen-rich cells that resemble fetal bronchial tubes at 10–15 weeks gestational age (Plate 8.6). The tubules contain numerous neuroendocrine cells and frequently form squamous morules. The stroma is composed of myofibroblastic cells but is not a prominent feature of this tumor, distinguishing it from the more aggressive pulmonary blastoma. It is important to recognize this tumor because of its excellent prognosis with surgery alone, and to avoid overtreatment.

Sclerosing hemangioma

Pulmonary sclerosing hemangioma is a generally benign tumor that has a prominent epithelial component and may be mistaken for adenocarcinoma. Typically, it is a well-circumscribed lesion that is hemorrhagic and sclerotic (Plate 8.7a) but contains a mixture of cells arranged in papillary structures in which the surface cells are strongly positive for epithelial immunohistochemical markers including pancytokeratin, EMA, and surfactant proteins. The central round cells at the center of papillary structures (Plate 8.7b) are less distinctly epithelial and are negative for pancytokeratin, EMA, and surfactant proteins. Both types of cells are TTF-1 positive [58]. This immunophenotype profile suggests that sclerosing hemangioma is actually a tumor of pulmonary progenitor cells. The clinical importance of the lesion is its benign clinical course.

Macroscopic patterns of peripheral lung adenocarcinoma and correlation with high-resolution imaging

The most sensitive current method for the detection of BAC is computed tomography since PET scans may miss heavily mucinous or small lesions [59,60]. Tumor cells are often arrayed along the alveolar septum as a single cell or multicell layer that can create a characteristic CT image, the so-called "ground glass opacity" [61] (Plate 8.8) [62,63]. The small peripheral ground glass opacity is often a presenting feature of BAC and is one of three major patterns of spread recognizable on CT scans described below and reviewed in [64].

1 *Solitary mass or nodule.* Nodules may be "solid," obscuring of the underlying lung markings, or non-solid ("ground glass opacity") in which the underlying lung architecture remains visible. The latter appearance is due to the preservation of alveolar air spaces and is characteristic of BAC but may also be observed in non-BAC tumors and inflammatory conditions. It might be expected that all BAC would have a ground glass appearance but the phenomenon of collapse causes partial or complete opacification of tumor tissue so that histological confirmation of BAC diagnosis is required for definitive diagnosis.

2 *Pneumonic form.* In this form, there is a pneumonia-like consolidation of a segment, lobe or entire lung that may be difficult to distinguish from benign peripheral airway disease [65]. This pattern is due to lepidic spread of tumor in the affected lung and partial filling of the alveoli with tumor cells, mucous, or inflammatory cells.

3 *Diffuse BAC.* Diffuse BAC appears as nodular solid or ground glass opacities throughout the lungs. This form of the disease is rare.

In general, while imaging studies may be suggestive of BAC, definitive diagnosis continues to depend on histological confirmation.

Cytology of BAC

BAC, because of its peripheral location, is rarely detected during early stages in sputum. The main application for cytology in the diagnosis of BAC is in fine needle aspiration. Because of its relatively low morbidity, fine needle aspiration is often used to access cells from peripheral lung nodules and other intrathoracic sites difficult to reach by other means. Aspirates of BAC contain epithelial tumor cell clusters arranged in spheres, papillary clusters or sheets of uniform cells with round pale-staining nuclei containing grooves in the usually prominent nuclear membranes [66,67]. Aspirates usually contain

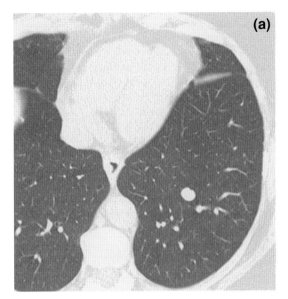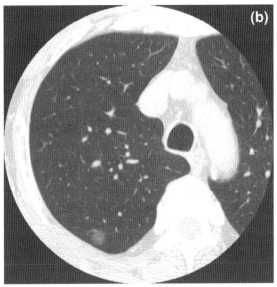

Figure 8.1 Helical CT image showing (a) solid nodule in the left lower lobe; (b) nonsolid nodule (ground glass opacity [GGO]) in the posterior right upper lobe. Although the GGO has been associated with BAC, some BAC exhibit central collapse and can appear solid. (Provided by Dr Kavita Garg of the Department of Radiology, University of Colorado, Denver, and Health Sciences Center.)

minimal inflammatory infiltrate [68]. In mucinous tumor, mucin may be visible in the aspirate [69]. Well-differentiated invasive adenocarcinoma of the lung may have cytological features similar to BAC. Because it is not possible to evaluate stromal invasion by cytological examination, it is also not possible to distinguish early invasive adenocarcinoma from BAC, an exclusively in situ lesion, by fine needle aspiration alone [70]. It may also be difficult to unequivocally distinguish adenocarcinoma from reactive processes. A recent online survey has uncovered a high degree of diagnostic inaccuracy among even experienced cytologists in the diagnosis of lung cancer by fine needle aspiration (FNA) [71], an observation that suggests ancillary tests such as FISH (fluorescence in situ hybridization) [72] may ultimately prove useful in diagnosing carcinoma by FNA.

Origins of adenocarcinoma and atypical adenomatous hyperplasia

The application of computed tomography to the detection of early lung cancers during the past 20 years has provided an opportunity to examine small lung cancers and premalignant lesions in the earliest stages of neoplastic transformation. Currently, the most likely candidate progenitor lesion for adenocarcinoma is atypical adenomatous hyperplasia (AAH) (also referred to as atypical alveolar hyperplasia, bronchial adenoma). This is a small (<5 mm) proliferation of alveolar or terminal bronchial cells. In histological sections it appears as a well-circumscribed cluster of alveoli that are lined by a single layer of type II pneumocytes or "hobnail" Clara-type cells without scarring or significant inflammation (Figure 8.1). Involved alveoli are sometimes clustered around terminal bronchioles. The cells of AAH are sparsely distributed along the alveolar surfaces. More densely cellular lesions may be difficult to distinguish from BAC, leading to the suggestion that lesions under 5 mm be considered AAH with larger lesions classified as BAC [70].

AAH was originally discovered incidentally in lungs resected for invasive adenocarcinoma [73]. Since the original description of AAH, many studies have consistently document its presence in lung cancer with reported frequency varying from 14 to 57% in adenocarcinoma [74–80] and 3–30% in squamous carcinoma [75,77–80]. This variability may be in part due to the difficulty in identifying the lesions. Because of their small size they are best found in lungs inflated with formalin and thinly sectioned. Even with these precautions, AAH is often macroscopically invisible and is discovered only incidentally on microscopic examination [78]. AAH may also be found without associated lung cancer. In an autopsy study, 2.8% of an elderly Japanese population without carcinoma had AAH [81].

The frequent association of AAH with adenocarcinoma and BAC has suggested that AAH is a precursor of these types of tumors. The strong morphological similarity to adenocarcinoma, particularly to BAC, has led to the suggestion that a stepwise sequence of premalignant changes occurs in lung similar to the well-established stepwise changes that occur in the colon [75]. The precursor roll of AAH is supported by a large and growing body of morphometric and molecular evidence. Cells of AAH have been found to be aneuploid by both morphometric analysis [82–84] and flow cytometry [84,85]. Molecular changes frequently present in carcinoma have also been found in AAH including Ki-ras mutation [86] and loss of heterozygosity in chromosomal regions thought to harbor tumor suppressor including 3p and 9p [87,88], 9q [89,90], 16p [89], and 17q [90]. Finally, genomic and chromosomal imbalance has been demonstrated in AAH by comparative genomic hybridization [91].

Despite this evidence, crucial longitudinal studies confirming the precursor roll of AAH in human adenocarcinogenesis have not been possible to date. Current CT screening algorithms exclude nodules <5 mm, the size of most AAH, from study [1]. Chemopreventive agents that could reduce the malignant potential of AAH have not been tested because of the difficulty of localizing these tiny lesions in the lungs of patients at risk and because of the lack of practical means to confirm the diagnosis. A high-resolution imaging or molecular signature of AAH may help to resolve this problem but these are not currently available. Until this confirmatory data is available, it seems reasonable to regard AAH as part of a continuous spectrum of neoplastic change in the peripheral lung with AAH an early noninvasive lesion, the histologically similar BAC a further step in malignant progression and invasive tumors with mixed bronchioloalveolar and acinar subtype or purely invasive acinar carcinomas a final step in malignant progression.

Molecular correlates of BAC and invasive adenocarcinoma

Molecular correlates have conventionally been used to verify the anatomical diagnosis of adenocarcinoma, its types and subtypes as alluded to above. Recently, as agents targeting specific signaling pathways have been introduced, information regarding the status of those pathways has become more than a diagnostic tool. Protein expression, gene copy number, and mutational status have become important predictors of response to treatment and are being considered for use in selection of treatment, much as *HER2/neu* status, is used to select treatment in breast cancer. Finally, molecular studies of early lesions have been applied on a limited basis to early adenocarcinoma and premalignant lesions in an attempt to reconstruct the molecular changes that lead to pulmonary adenocarcinoma. All these applications employ tissue biomarkers in specific contexts and for specific purposes that are listed in Table 8.2 and discussed below. The information provided by these studies has changed and will continue to affect the approach to patients with lung cancer and has in turn changed our understanding of the pathology and pathogenesis of adenocarcinoma.

Diagnostic molecular studies

Immunohistochemistry
Immunohistochemical tests have most commonly been applied to pulmonary adenocarcinoma in the context of distinguishing lung from nonlung origin.

Table 8.2 Tissue biomarkers in adenocarcinoma.

Biomarker	Common abbreviation	Gene/RNA/protein	Abnormality/property	Testing method	Context
Thyroid transcription factor	TTF-1	Protein	Overexpression	Immunohistochemistry	Diagnostic
Cytokeratin 7	CK7	Protein	Overexpression	Immunohistochemistry	Diagnostic
Cytokeratin 20	CK20	Protein	Overexpression	Immunohistochemistry	Diagnostic
CDX2	CDX2	Protein	Overexpression	Immunohistochemistry	Diagnostic
Carcinoembryonic antigen	CEA	Protein	Overexpression	Immunohistochemistry	Diagnostic
Cluster of differentiation 15	CD15	Protein	Overexpression	Immunohistochemistry	Diagnostic
Tumor-associated glycoprotein 72	TAG72	Protein	Overexpression	Immunohistochemistry	Diagnostic
Calretinin	NA	Protein	Underexpression	Immunohistochemistry	Diagnostic
Wilm's Tumor 1	WT1	Protein	Underexpression	Immunohistochemistry	Diagnostic
E-cadherin	E-cad	Protein	Overexpression	Immunohistochemistry	Prognostic
Microarray gene expression profiling	NA	RNA	Over-/underexpression	Oligonucleotide microarray (multiple platforms)	Prognostic/predictive?
Multigene probe sets	NA	DNA probe	Aneuploidy	Multi-color FISH	Diagnostic
Zinc finger E-box binding homeobox 1	zeb1	Protein/RNA	E-cadherin regulation	Immunohistochemistry	Predictive
Epidermal growth factor receptor	EGFR	Protein	Overexpression	Immunohistochemistry	Predictive
Epidermal growth factor receptor	EGFR	Gene copy number	Aneusomy	FISH	Predictive
Epidermal growth factor receptor	EGFR	Gene	Deletion/point mutation	Sequencing	Predictive
HER2/neu	HER2/neu	Protein	Overexpression	Immunohistochemistry	Predictive
HER2/neu	HER2/neu	Gene copy number	Aneusomy	FISH	Predictive
HER2/neu	HER2/neu	Gene	Deletion/point mutation	Sequencing	Predictive
Ki-ras	Ki-ras	Gene	Point mutation	Sequencing	Mechanistic/prognostic
p53	p53	Protein	Overexpression	Immunohistochemistry	Mechanistic/prognostic
p53	p53	Gene	Point mutation	Sequencing	Mechanistic/prognostic
Excision repair cross-complementation group-1	ERCC1	RNA/protein	Underexpression	Immunohistochemistry/qRT-PCR	Prognostic/predictive?
Regulatory subunit of ribonucleotide reductase	RRM1	RNA/protein	Underexpression	Immunohistochemistry/qRT-PCR	Prognostic/predictive?
Notch3	Notch3	Gene	Translocation/overexpression	Cytogenetics	Mechanistic

Molecular biomarkers assessed in tissue including glossary, specimen tested, methods, and major application. *Diagnostic* refers to biomarkers that are primarily useful in the pathological diagnosis. *Prognostic* refers to biomarkers that are significant associated with outcome. *Predictive* refers to biomarkers that can be used to evaluate specific pathways targeted by therapeutic drugs. *Mechanistic* refers to markers that are involve in pulmonary adenocarcinogenesis but whose clinical roll is not yet established.

Table 8.3 Immunohistochemical markers useful for differential diagnosis.

	CK7	CK20	TTF-1	CDX2	Calretinin
Bronchioloalveolar	+++	−	++	−	+
Acinar and mixed subtype	+++	−	++	−	+
Mucinous ("colloid," etc.)	+++	+	+++	+	+
Metastatic	++	++	−	+++	+
Mesothelioma	++	+++	−	NA	+++

Immunohistochemical biomarkers useful in the differential diagnosis of lung cancer. The reactivity scale refers to the percentage of cases reported positive with for the marker as − (<1%), + (1–25%), ++ (25–70%), and +++ (>70%).

Results of these tests reflect a unique molecular configuration in lung tumors that differs from that of histologically similar adenocarcinomas originating at other sites. The expected results of diagnostic immunohistochemical stains for BAC and invasive carcinoma are compared to expected results for tumors of other types and origins in Table 8.3. Perhaps the most useful immunohistochemical marker that has become available in recent years is thyroid transcription factor 1 (TTF-1, Nkx2.1). TTF-1 is necessary for branching morphogenesis in the developing lung [10,92] and is first expressed early in embryonic development and in the normal adult alveolar and thyroid cells. With the exception of the thyroid tumors and occasional nonpulmonary small carcinomas [93], its expression is confined to lung cancer. More than three quarters of pulmonary adenocarcinomas express TTF-1 [94]. A high proportion of pulmonary adenocarcinomas also express a specific pattern of cytokeratin isotypes and are positive for CK7 but not CD20. The TTF-1 positive, CK7 positive, and CK20 negative phenotype has become established as standard procedure in distinguishing histologically similar pulmonary from nonpulmonary adenocarcinomas and can greatly assist in guiding diagnosis, staging, and treatment of adenocarcinoma.

Less helpful have been immunohistochemical stains for surfactant proteins. Although the expression of these proteins is regulated by TTF-1 [10], immunohistochemical stains for these proteins has been relatively insensitive and unspecific with approximately half of all pulmonary carcinomas and approximately the same proportion of metastatic tumors positive for these proteins [94–96]. An even smaller proportion of lung adenocarcinomas are positive so that expression of TTF-1 appears to be a better marker of lung origin than the surfactant proteins.

A frequent clinical problem is the distinction between adenocarcinoma and mesothelioma. Several markers have been identified empirically that address this problem. BAC and adenocarcinoma are positive for CEA, CD-15, and TAG72 but are negative for calretinin and WT1 distinguishing them from mesothelioma. This immunohistochemical panel or modifications are now almost uniformly applied to address the differential diagnosis of mesothelioma versus adenocarcinoma.

Finally, several immunohistochemical biomarkers are prognostically important. The most prominent of these is E-cadherin. E-cadherin forms a complex with β-catenin and other molecules at the cell surface that is critical for intercellular adhesion and intracellular signaling (reviewed in [97]). Loss of E-cadherin expression may reduce intercellular adhesion among tumor cells and render them more discohesive and prone to disperse into the circulation. In a tissue microarray study, E-cadherin has been shown to be an independent prognostic indicator in NSCLC including adenocarcinoma [98]. Also, there may be crosstalk between the E-cadherin pathway and EGFR in adenocarcinoma and other lung tumors so that intact E-cadherin signaling may be necessary for response to EGFR blockade [37]. Expression of E-cadherin may ultimately prove useful as a predictor of response to treatment, as discussed below.

High throughput gene expression profiling

Oligonucleotide microarrays have been used to comprehensively assess gene expression in adenocarcinoma and to relate these patterns to outcome. Based on patterns of gene expression tumors were found to segregate into groups that are not predictable by conventional morphological classification schemes with some tumors expressing profiles of neuroendocrine, pneumocyte, or squamoid differentiation [8,99]. The prognoses of tumors that are defined by these classifier groups are statistically different [8,100]. Although specific genes in the classifiers may vary somewhat, raw data from across institutions is similar and can be harmonized mathematically to arrive at a common informative gene list [101,102]. There is considerable overlap in tumor-associated gene expression between human and mouse tumors [103], supporting the notion that the animal tumors are driven by some of the same molecular mechanisms as human tumors.

While these studies are of biological interest and illustrate the power of microarray analyses, the technology involved remains complicated and expensive and to date most studies have been used primarily to supplement existing morphological lung cancer categorizations. Recently, an approach that addresses changes in gene expression profiles engendered by molecular pathology that is frequently present in adenocarcinoma. This has been accomplished by examining changes in gene expression in cell lines into which genes regulating specific cell signaling pathways are introduced using recombinant adenoviral constructs [104]. The resulting gene expression profiles correlate with clinical outcome in NSCLC so that it is now possible to relate outcome with underlying molecular pathology without reference to histology. The implications of this work for assessment of outcome and selection therapy are discussed below.

Fluorescence in situ hybridization

Structural chromosomal abnormalities abound in pulmonary adenocarcinomas and include whole or partial chromosomal losses, gains, translocations, and amplifications [105,106]. However, because of the high frequency of chromosome imbalance (aneuploidy), multicolor FISH probes have been developed [107] with the aim of using aneuploidy as a diagnostic tool. In equivocal cases, FISH can be helpful to confirm diagnosis and may enhance the sensitivity of cytological procedures [72,107–109]. It may also be useful as a predictive tool in assessing risk for future carcinoma in high-risk patients [110]. FISH may be employed more broadly in the future as significance of aneuploidy becomes evident and better probes are developed. Finally, FISH for specific genetic imbalances has shown promise as a predictor of response to EGFR blockade as described below.

Predictors of response to treatment

NSCLC has long been known to strongly express EGFR (reviewed in [111]) but the molecular mechanism behind this overexpression has only recently been addressed. Nonmucinous and some mucinous BAC are among the NSCLC that strongly express EGFR protein [112], either with or without coexpression of the ErbB partner, HER2/neu. In 2003, it was reported that 21% of NSCLC contain high copy number (>3) or amplification of chromosomal loci containing the *EGFR1* gene [113]. Tumors with either true amplification consisting of clustered signals or high polysomy behaved similarly in statistical analyses and tumors with either abnormality were therefore considered together as high copy number tumors or "FISH positive." FISH-positive NSCLC with high-level protein expression generally had a worse prognosis than FISH-negative NSCLC but adenocarcinomas were not considered separately in this study and the overall numbers of tumors were small.

In 2004, point mutations in exon 18 and 21 and deletions in exon 19, all in the ATP-binding region of the EGFR tyrosine kinase domain were reported almost simultaneously in lung tumors by two separate groups [114]. In one reported series [78], 16 mutations were found in 119 tumors and all but one of these tumors were adenocarcinomas. Slightly less than half (49%) of the tumors were from Japanese patients and all but one of the mutations was found in the Japanese cohort. Several of the patients tested in this study had been treated by EGFR blockade with gefitinib. Four of five responders to this treatment had mutated EGFR but none of the nonresponding tumors were mutant. In the second study [115], eight of nine carcinomas including three BAC and five adenocarcinomas contained a mutation. These tumors were selected for testing because of their responsiveness to EGFR blockade from a cohort of 275 patients treated with gefitinib. All the responsive mutant tumors were from never or former smokers. Since these original observations, mutational data on a large series of tumors from Japan, Taiwan, Australia, and the United States has been published confirming the mutations are more common in never smokers, adenocarcinoma, Asian ethnicity, and females [116]. The association with BAC was questioned [117], since, using the strict noninvasive criteria for BAC, none of the BAC from the United States that were available for review were mutant [116]. It therefore appears that mutation is associated with peripheral airway tumors, usually of mixed subtype, but not necessarily with pure BAC.

Following the discovery of EGFR mutations in adenocarcinoma, it was reported at two different institutions that, while mutation correlates with response to EGFR blockade in NSCLC including adenocarcinoma, it does not predict survival [118–121]. Protein overexpression (Plate 8.9a) and high gene copy number (Plate 8.9b) were reported to correlate survival in adenocarcinoma [120] as well as in NSCLC in general [119,121]. Moreover, virtually all available EGFR-mutated cell lines are amplified at the EGFR locus. These data suggest that the combination of high gene copy number and protein expression may be the most potent predictor of response to treatment and appears to identify a subset of NSCLC, mostly adenocarcinomas, that are EGFR dependent for growth and malignant properties [122]. Whether single or multiple marker testing of the EGFR pathway can be used to select patients who would respond to EGFR blockade is currently under active investigation.

Pathological alteration of specific signaling pathways generates specific gene expression profiles that may correlate with response to treatment [123]. Signatures of pathologically altered signaling pathways have been generated in order to predict response to therapy by two different approaches. One is to simply evaluate gene expression profiles of tumors and cell lines known to harbor an abnormality associated with a pathway altered in carcinoma such as EGFR [124]. A second approach (mentioned above) is to create a specific lesion in order to observe the effect on gene expression using high throughput oligonucleotide microarrays [104]. Both methods have generated gene lists of biological significance. The predictive power of these lists is still under investigation. The former approach has identified E-cadherin as a gene of interest and detailed studies have revealed a reciprocal relationship between E-cadherin expression and the status of the zinc finger transcriptional repressor, zeb1 [37]. Downregulation of E-cadherin through zeb1 reduces sensitivity to EGFR, suggesting new targets for prediction of response to treatment and for intervention in adenocarcinoma.

Most BACs occur in smokers. Several studies have indicated that *Ki-ras* mutations in adenocarcinoma are highly associated with smoking [125,126]. There is little overlap between those tumors with EGFR mutations and those with *Ki-ras* mutations [127,128]. Thus, mutations in separate EGFR pathway genes caused by different mutagens all activate signaling and result in the single BAC/adenocarcinoma phenotype. *Ki-ras* mutations are reported to be resistant to EGFR blockade [118,122].

Several other mutational abnormalities have been reported in adenocarcinoma that are thought to be smoking induced. The most frequent of these is *p53*. *P53* mutation is uncommon in pure BAC but may be found in 11% of mixed adenocarcinoma/BAC and in 48% of tumors that are strictly invasive adenocarcinomas [129]. This suggests a role for *p53* in progression to aggressive forms of invasive peripheral lung cancer. That *p53* mutation may precede other mutations and chromosomal rearrangements illustrated by the Li-Fraumeni patient is discussed below.

Finally, DNA repair systems may be of practical importance in predicting response to DNA damaging agents such as platinum-based drugs used to treat adenocarcinoma. *Untreated* early-stage patients with high levels of the repair enzymes ERCC1 and RRM1 measured by a simple immunohistochemical test [130], have a better prognosis than patients with low levels. The opposite is true for *treated* patients; those with low levels of the same enzymes survive significantly longer than patients with high levels [131,132]. The likely explanation for these seemingly contradictory findings is that *untreated* tumors with low ability to repair DNA damage may be prone to rapid accumulation of the genetic alterations and malignant progression while *treated* tumors with low DNA repair capacity are likely to be damaged or destroyed by chemotherapy with resulting improved patient survival. The gene encoding the excision repair enzyme, ERCC1, contains a common polymorphism at codon 118 (AAC→AAT, exon 4) [133], which is silent (both alleles encode arginine). However, the homozygous AAC codon is associated with lower expression levels of ERCC1 [134]. These data offer the prospect of predicting response to proven chemotherapeutic agents by simple testing of tumor tissue or blood, resulting better response and survival rates and reduced morbidity from futile treatment of this common lung tumor type.

Molecular pathogenesis of peripheral adenocarcinoma

The molecular and biological mechanisms involved in adenocarcinogenesis are not as well understood as those involved in central airway carcinogenesis due to the inaccessibility of the peripheral lung for sequential analysis. Recently, however, improved understanding of genetic and gene expression changes in adenocarcinoma have provided insight into the molecular processes that lead to lung cancer. These insights have come from evaluation of large cohorts of subjects as well as from careful study of individual cases. The conclusions of these studies can be divided into the two broad categories of structural genetic and chromosomal changes that are thought to represent stages in multistep carcinogenesis in the peripheral lung.

The status of genes involved in several signaling pathways has been intensively evaluated because of the availability of targeted agents that can interfere with or block those pathways. Most notable of these targets is EGFR. Despite the large amount of information regarding the EGFR pathway gene status in fully developed carcinoma (discussed above), information regarding the status of this pathway in premalignancy is limited. Tang *et al.* have found the same EGFR mutations in nonmalignant epithelium adjacent tumor from 24% of patients with EGFR mutant adenocarcinoma, suggesting that *EGFR* mutation may precede frank carcinoma [135]. Possible synergism between separate mutations was recently reported in a patient with Li-Fraumeni syndrome. This patient had a germline mutation in *p53* codon 273 and developed a breast tumor at age 30 that was amplified for *HER2/neu*. At age 34, the patient was diagnosed with a second carcinoma, this time an adenocarcinoma of lung with the characteristic deletion in *EGFR* exon 19 encompassing bases 2413–2428 (codon 746–750) and high copy number for both EGFR and HER2/*neu*. This unusual case suggests that mutation in the *p53* mitotic checkpoint gene may induce a sufficient level of genetic and chromosomal instability over time to induce *EGFR* pathway mutation and gene dosage imbalance. This study also suggests that the sequence in which mutation occurs may not be as important as the number of mutations that occur during the carcinogenic process.

A considerably simple somatic genetic alteration leading to adenocarcinoma in a 34-year-old female nonsmoker has been described. In this case, a single translocation [t(15;19) (q11;p13)], was detected in tumor cells mapped to a region 50 kb upstream of the notch3 gene on chromosome 19p and resulted in an increase in notch3 expression. Examination of several cell lines indicated that *notch3* was involved in several different translocations involving many different reciprocal chromosome partners. Notch3 is involved in differentiation, apoptosis and regulation of the cell cycle and is therefore a candidate oncogene. This translocation and the Li-Fraumeni case described above indicate that a wide diversity of molecular mechanisms may be at play in adenocarcinogenesis and that targeting a single gene or pathway may not be successful as a means of early detection or treatment.

In addition to analysis of existing malignancy, several studies have evaluated the molecular changes in AAH as a window on peripheral airway carcinogenesis. The most striking molecular change is the high frequency of *Ki-ras* mutation with one study showing 39% of AAH with mutations [86]. *Ki-ras* mutation thus is likely to be a major event in early lung carcinogenesis but appears to require a second event to progress to invasive carcinoma. That silencing of other tumor suppressor genes may be present in AAH is suggested by the finding of loss of heterozygosity at chromosomal sites of putative tumor suppressor genes including 3p and 9p [87,88], 9q [89,90], 16p [89], and 17q [90]. These molecular changes are also frequent in BAC, suggesting that these lesions are related and perhaps the result of action of similar carcinogens.

Finally, AAH is frequently aneuploid [82–85] indicating significant chromosomal instability and missegregation. Chromosomal imbalance has been demonstrated by comparative genomic hybridization suggesting that AAH may represent a morphological change that is late in the multistep sequence of molecular events that ends in carcinoma.

Experimental models

Animal models for human lung adenocarcinoma have been available for many decades and have recently provided increasingly comprehensive understanding of pulmonary adenocarcinogenesis. In the early twentieth century, an endemic infectious disease (jagziekte) was described in South African sheep [136] that produced multicentric alveolar epithelial proliferation similar to BAC in man [137]. This disease, now referred to as ovine pulmonary adenocarcinoma (OPA) has more recently been shown to be the result of infection with a retrovirus, jaagsiekte sheep retrovirus (JSRV) [138–141]. This retrovirus is unique in its tropism for differentiated pulmonary epithelial cells and to date is the only known naturally occurring viral cause of pulmonary adenocarcinoma [142]. However, the virus does appear to be confined to sheep and has not been demonstrated in human pulmonary tumors [143]. Whether this reflects an inability of present methods to detect the virus or that the virus is simply absent from human tumor is not completely resolved but it appears at the moment that models more analogous to the clinicoepidemiological setting in the human might be insightful.

One animal model has become predominant in recent years and that is the mouse model of pulmonary adenocarcinoma. Mice have several obvious advantages as experimental models including the small size of the host animal, affordability of housing, and short life span. In addition, the ability to genetically engineer this animal has provided recently improved understanding of lung carcinogenesis in the mouse as well as in man.

While wild mice are relatively resistant to the development of lung tumors, certain inbred stains have a high frequency of lung tumors and can be induced to develop tumors by exposure to tobacco smoke itself [144] and to the potent carcinogens that are present in tobacco smoke including urethane, nitrosamines, and polyaromatic hydrocarbons (reviewed in [145]).

Detailed review of mouse lung carcinogenesis is beyond the scope of this review. However, several new insights into the cellular origin and composition of adenocarcinoma have been provided by recent mouse experiments that are important to the current understanding of human lung tumor pathology. In these experiments putative stem cells for peripheral lung and for adenocarcinoma have been identified. Stem cells have the ability to regenerate themselves, to form multiple cell lineages and to proliferate [146]. They are important since genetic lesions in stem cells may be replicated and passed on to large populations of cells that may increase the probability of tumor development in premalignant cells or resistance to treatment in fully developed tumors.

Until recently, models testing for the presence of stem cells have focused on separate local cellular compartments of the lung including tracheal mucociliary epithelium, bronchial glands, Clara cells, and alveolar cells. These experiments have identified progenitor cells that can repopulate local compartments after injury but not resident multipotential stem cells that can repopulate any lung epithelium [147]. Recently, cells capable of self-renewal, able to regenerate both Clara cells and alveolar pneumocytes in injured lungs have been enriched by flow cytometry from whole mouse lung preparations and thus have properties of stem cells [148]. These cells reside at the bronchoalveolar junction and have consistently expressed both surfactant protein C and CC10. In a genetically engineered mouse adenocarcinoma model in which cells are transformed by conditional expression of mutant Ki-ras [149], cells with stem cell properties can be found early in neoplastic transformation and are proposed as the cell of origin of adenocarcinoma. This hypothesis has yet to be confirmed in human adenocarcinoma but provides a model that in many respects is analogous if not to invasive lung carcinoma, then to AAH and BAC, well-differentiated tumors with frequent Ki-ras mutation (discussed above).

Conclusions and predictions

Advances in technology and the availability of a large armamentarium of targeted agents pose new challenges for pathological classifications of lung cancer and premalignancy. It is unlikely that lung cancer will respond uniformly to the new agents. The heterogeneity of lung cancer and the diversity of its morphological appearances and molecular properties evident from the data presented above imply that molecular targets will be applicable to an increasingly narrow range of lung cancers in the future and that treatments will have to be tailored to the molecular as well as to the cellular characteristics of individual tumors. Pathologists will continue to play a large and increasing role in tissue management and molecular testing for which strong grounding in both the detailed anatomical analysis and molecular testing will continue to be essential.

References

1 Henschke CI, Yankelevitz DF, Libby DM, Pasmantier MW, Smith JP, Miettinen OS. Survival of patients with stage I lung cancer detected on CT screening. *N Engl J Med* 2006; **355**:1763–71.

2 Flieder DB, Vazquez M, Carter D *et al*. Pathologic findings of lung tumors diagnosed on baseline CT screening. *Am J Surg Pathol* 2006; **30**:606–13.

3 Carter D, Vazquez M, Flieder DB *et al*. Comparison of pathologic findings of baseline and annual repeat cancers diagnosed on CT screening. *Lung Cancer* 2007; **56**:193–9.

4 Kuhn C, Wright JL. The normal lung. In: Churg AM, Myers JL, Tazelaar HD, Wright JL (eds). *Thurlbeck's Pathology of the Lung*, 3rd edn. New York: Thieme Medical Publications, 2005:1–37.

5 Singh G, Katyal SL. Clara cell proteins. *Ann N Y Acad Sci* 2000; **923**:43–58.

6 Linnoila RI, Szabo E, DeMayo F, Witschi H, Sabourin C, Malkinson A. The role of CC10 in pulmonary carcinogenesis: from a marker to tumor suppression. *Ann N Y Acad Sci* 2000; **923**:249–67.

7 Stripp BR, Reynolds SD, Plopper CG, Boe IM, Lund J. Pulmonary phenotype of CCSP/UG deficient mice: a consequence of CCSP deficiency or altered Clara cell function? *Ann N Y Acad Sci* 2000; **923**:202–9.

8 Bhattacharjee A, Richards WG, Staunton J *et al*. Classification of human lung carcinomas by mRNA expression profiling reveals distinct adenocarcinoma subclasses. *Proc Natl Acad Sci U S A* 2001; **98**: 13790–5.

9 Whitsett JA, Wert SE, Trapnell BC. Genetic disorders influencing lung formation and function at birth. *Hum Mol Genet* 2004; **13(2)**:R207–15.

10 Warburton D, Zhao J, Berberich MA, Bernfield M. Molecular embryology of the lung: then, now, and in the future. *Am J Physiol* 1999; **276**:L697–704.

11 Mendelson CR. Role of transcription factors in fetal lung development and surfactant protein gene expression. *Annu Rev Physiol* 2000; **62**:875–915.

12 Bonner AE, Lemon WJ, You M. Gene expression signatures identify novel regulatory pathways during murine lung development: implications for lung tumorigenesis. *J Med Genet* 2003; **40**:408–17.

13 Bonner AE, Lemon WJ, Devereux TR, Lubet RA, You M. Molecular profiling of mouse lung tumors: association with tumor progression, lung development, and human lung adenocarcinomas. *Oncogene* 2004; **23**:1166–76.

14 Borczuk AC, Gorenstein L, Walter KL, Assaad AA, Wang L, Powell CA. Non-small-cell lung cancer molecular signatures recapitulate lung developmental pathways. *Am J Pathol* 2003; **163**:1949–60.

15 Colby TV, Noguchi M, Henschke C *et al*. Adenocarcinoma. In: Travis WD, Brambilla E, Muller-Hermelink HK, Harris CC (eds). *Pathology and Genetics of Tumours*

of the Lung, Pleura, Thymus and Heart, 1st edn. Lyon: IARC Press, 2004:35–44.

16 Malassez L. Examen histologique d'un cas de cancer encephaloide du poumon (epithelioma). *Arch Phys Norm Pathol* 1876; **3**:353.

17 Low FN. The pulmonary alveolar epithelium of laboratory mammals and man. *Anat Rec* 1953; **117**:241.

18 Liebow AA. Bronchiolo-alveolar carcinoma. *Adv Intern Med* 1960; **10**:329–58.

19 Shimosato Y, Suzuki A, Hashimoto T *et al*. Prognostic implications of fibrotic focus (scar) in small peripheral lung cancers. *Am J Surg Pathol* 1980; **4**:365–73.

20 Noguchi M, Morikawa A, Kawasaki M *et al*. Small adenocarcinoma of the lung. Histologic characteristics and prognosis. *Cancer* 1995; **75**:2844–52.

21 Suzuki K, Yokose T, Yoshida J *et al*. Prognostic significance of the size of central fibrosis in peripheral adenocarcinoma of the lung. *Ann Thorac Surg* 2000; **69**:893–7.

22 Maeshima AM, Niki T, Maeshima A, Yamada T, Kondo H, Matsuno Y. Modified scar grade: a prognostic indicator in small peripheral lung adenocarcinoma. *Cancer* 2002; **95**:2546–54.

23 Sakurai H, Maeshima A, Watanabe S *et al*. Grade of stromal invasion in small adenocarcinoma of the lung: histopathological minimal invasion and prognosis. *Am J Surg Pathol* 2004; **28**:198–206.

24 Travis WD, Colby TV, Corrin B *et al*. Adenocarcinoma. In: *Histological Typing of Lung and Pleural Tumours*, 3rd edn. Berlin: Springer, 1999:34–8.

25 Barkley JE, Green MR. Bronchioloalveolar carcinoma. *J Clin Oncol* 1996; **14**:2377–86.

26 Amin MB, Tamboli P, Merchant SH *et al*. Micropapillary component in lung adenocarcinoma: a distinctive histologic feature with possible prognostic significance. *Am J Surg Pathol* 2002; **26**:358–64.

27 Makimoto Y, Nabeshima K, Iwasaki H *et al*. Micropapillary pattern: a distinct pathological marker to subclassify tumours with a significantly poor prognosis within small peripheral lung adenocarcinoma (</= 20 mm) with mixed bronchioloalveolar and invasive subtypes (Noguchi's type C tumours). *Histopathology* 2005; **46**:677–84.

28 Hoshi R, Tsuzuku M, Horai T, Ishikawa Y, Satoh Y. Micropapillary clusters in early-stage lung adenocarcinomas: a distinct cytologic sign of significantly poor prognosis. *Cancer* 2004; **102**:81–6.

29 Miyoshi T, Satoh Y, Okumura S *et al*. Early-stage lung adenocarcinomas with a micropapillary pattern, a distinct pathologic marker for a significantly poor prognosis. *Am J Surg Pathol* 2003; **27**:101–9.

30 Raeburn C, Spencer H. A study of the origin and development of lung cancer. *Thorax* 1953; **8**:1–10.

31 Raeburn B, Spencer H. Lung scar cancers. *Br J Tuberc Dis Chest* 1957; **51**:237–45.

32 Kung IT, Lui IO, Loke SL *et al*. Pulmonary scar cancer. A pathologic reappraisal. *Am J Surg Pathol* 1985; **9**:391–400.

33 Barsky SH, Huang SJ, Bhuta S. The extracellular matrix of pulmonary scar carcinomas is suggestive of a desmoplastic origin. *Am J Pathol* 1986; **124**:412–9.

34 el-Torkey M, Giltman LI, Dabbous M. Collagens in scar carcinoma of the lung. *Am J Pathol* 1985; **121**:322–6.

35 Lee JM, Dedhar S, Kalluri R, Thompson EW. The epithelial–mesenchymal transition: new insights in signaling, development, and disease. *J Cell Biol* 2006; **172**:973–81.

36 Thomson S, Buck E, Petti F *et al*. Epithelial to mesenchymal transition is a determinant of sensitivity of non-small-cell lung carcinoma cell lines and xenografts to epidermal growth factor receptor inhibition. *Cancer Res* 2005; **65**:9455–62.

37 Witta SE, Gemmill RM, Hirsch FR *et al*. Restoring E-cadherin expression increases sensitivity to epidermal growth factor receptor inhibitors in lung cancer cell lines. *Cancer Res* 2006; **66**:944–50.

38 Johnson SK, Kerr KM, Chapman AD *et al*. Immune cell infiltrates and prognosis in primary carcinoma of the lung. *Lung Cancer* 2000; **27**:27–35.

39 Petersen RP, Campa MJ, Sperlazza J *et al*. Tumor infiltrating Foxp3(+) regulatory T-cells are associated with recurrence in pathologic stage I NSCLC patients. *Cancer* 2006; **107**:2866–72.

40 Trojan A, Urosevic M, Dummer R, Giger R, Weder W, Stahel RA. Immune activation status of CD8+ T cells infiltrating non-small cell lung cancer. *Lung Cancer* 2004; **44**:143–7.

41 Woo EY, Chu CS, Goletz TJ *et al*. Regulatory CD4(+)CD25(+) T cells in tumors from patients with early-stage non-small cell lung cancer and late-stage ovarian cancer. *Cancer Res* 2001; **61**:4766–72.

42 Strieter RM, Belperio JA, Burdick MD, Sharma S, Dubinett SM, Keane MP. CXC chemokines: angiogenesis, immunoangiostasis, and metastases in lung cancer. *Ann N Y Acad Sci* 2004; **1028**:351–60.

43 Wislez M, Fujimoto N, Izzo JG *et al*. High expression of ligands for chemokine receptor CXCR2 in alveolar epithelial neoplasia induced by oncogenic kras. *Cancer Res* 2006; **66**:4198–207.

44 Colby TV, Noguchi M, Henschke C *et al*. Adenocarcinoma. In: Travis WD, Brambilla E, Muller-Hermelink

HK, Harris CC (eds). *Tumors of the Lung, Pleura, Thymus and Heart.* Lyon: IARC Press, 2004:35–44.

45 Silver SA, Askin FB. True papillary carcinoma of the lung: a distinct clinicopathologic entity. *Am J Surg Pathol* 1997; **21**:43–51.

46 Castro CY, Moran CA, Flieder DG, Suster S. Primary signet ring cell adenocarcinomas of the lung: a clinicopathological study of 15 cases. *Histopathology* 2001; **39**:397–401.

47 Tsuta K, Ishii G, Yoh K *et al.* Primary lung carcinoma with signet-ring cell carcinoma components: clinicopathological analysis of 39 cases. *Am J Surg Pathol* 2004; **28**:868–74.

48 Yousem SA. Pulmonary intestinal-type adenocarcinoma does not show enteric differentiation by immunohistochemical study. *Mod Pathol* 2005; **18**:816–21.

49 Merchant SH, Amin MB, Tamboli P *et al.* Primary signet-ring cell carcinoma of lung: immunohistochemical study and comparison with non-pulmonary signet-ring cell carcinomas. *Am J Surg Pathol* 2001; **25**:1515–9.

50 Rossi G, Murer B, Cavazza A *et al.* Primary mucinous (so-called colloid) carcinomas of the lung: a clinicopathologic and immunohistochemical study with special reference to CDX-2 homeobox gene and MUC2 expression. *Am J Surg Pathol* 2004; **28**:442–52.

51 Gaffey MJ, Mills SE, Ritter JH. Clear cell tumors of the lower respiratory tract. *Semin Diagn Pathol* 1997; **14**:222–32.

52 Nicholson AG. Clear cell tumour. In: Travis WD, Brambilla E, Muller-Hermelink HK, Harris CC (eds). *Tumours of the Lung, Pleura, Thymus and Heart.* Lyon: IARC Press, 2004:118.

53 Kradin RL, Young RH, Dickersin GR, Kirkham SE, Mark EJ. Pulmonary blastoma with argyrophil cells and lacking sarcomatous features (pulmonary endodermal tumor resembling fetal lung). *Am J Surg Pathol* 1982; **6**:165–72.

54 Kodama T, Shimosato Y, Watanabe S, Koide T, Naruke T, Shimase J. Six cases of well-differentiated adenocarcinoma simulating fetal lung tubules in pseudoglandular stage. Comparison with pulmonary blastoma. *Am J Surg Pathol* 1984; **8**:735–44.

55 Nakatani Y, Kitamura H, Inayama Y *et al.* Pulmonary adenocarcinomas of the fetal lung type: a clinicopathologic study indicating differences in histology, epidemiology, and natural history of low-grade and high-grade forms. *Am J Surg Pathol* 1998; **22**:399–411.

56 Nakatani Y, Dickersin GR, Mark EJ. Pulmonary endodermal tumor resembling fetal lung: a clinicopatho-

logic study of five cases with immunohistochemical and ultrastructural characterization. *Hum Pathol* 1990; **21**:1097–107.

57 Koss MN, Hochholzer L, O'Leary T. Pulmonary blastomas. *Cancer* 1991; **67**:2368–81.

58 Devouassoux-Shisheboran M, Hayashi T, Linnoila RI, Koss MN, Travis WD. A clinicopathologic study of 100 cases of pulmonary sclerosing hemangioma with immunohistochemical studies: TTF-1 is expressed in both round and surface cells, suggesting an origin from primitive respiratory epithelium. *Am J Surg Pathol* 2000; **24**:906–16.

59 Heyneman LE, Patz EF. PET imaging in patients with bronchioloalveolar cell carcinoma. *Lung Cancer* 2002; **38**:261–6.

60 Yap CS, Schiepers C, Fishbein MC, Phelps ME, Czernin J. FDG-PET imaging in lung cancer: how sensitive is it for bronchioloalveolar carcinoma? *Eur J Nucl Med Mol Imaging* 2002; **29**:1166–73.

61 Wislez M, Massiani MA, Milleron B *et al.* Clinical characteristics of pneumonic-type adenocarcinoma of the lung. *Chest* 2003; **123**:1868–77.

62 Kakinuma R, Ohmatsu H, Kaneko M *et al.* Progression of focal pure ground-glass opacity detected by low-dose helical computed tomography screening for lung cancer. *J Comput Assist Tomogr* 2004; **28**:17–23.

63 Gaeta M, Caruso R, Barone M, Volta S, Casablanca G, La Spada F. Ground-glass attenuation in nodular bronchioloalveolar carcinoma: CT patterns and prognostic value. *J Comput Assist Tomogr* 1998; **22**:215–9.

64 Garfield DH, Cadranel JL, Wislez M, Franklin WA, Hirsch FR. The bronchioloalveolar carcinoma and peripheral adenocarcinoma spectrum of diseases. *J Thorac Oncol* 2006; **1**:344–59.

65 Akata S, Fukushima A, Kakizaki D, Abe K, Amino S. CT scanning of bronchioloalveolar carcinoma: specific appearances. *Lung Cancer* 1995; **12**:221–30.

66 Tao LC, Weisbrod GL, Pearson FG, Sanders DE, Donat EE, Filipetto L. Cytologic diagnosis of bronchioloalveolar carcinoma by fine-needle aspiration biopsy. *Cancer* 1986; **57**:1565–70.

67 Auger M, Katz RL, Johnston DA. Differentiating cytological features of bronchioloalveolar carcinoma from adenocarcinoma of the lung in fine-needle aspirations: a statistical analysis of 27 cases. *Diagn Cytopathol* 1997; **16**:253–7.

68 Elson CE, Moore SP, Johnston WW. Morphologic and immunocytochemical studies of bronchioloalveolar carcinoma at Duke University Medical Center, 1968–1986. *Anal Quant Cytol Histol* 1989; **11**:261–74.

69 MacDonald LL, Yazdi HM. Fine-needle aspiration biopsy of bronchioloalveolar carcinoma. *Cancer* 2001; **93**:29–34.

70 Flieder DB. Screen-detected adenocarcinoma of the lung. Practical points for surgical pathologists. *Am J Clin Pathol* 2003; **119(Suppl)**:S39–57.

71 Glatz K, Savic S, Glatz D *et al*. An online quiz uncovers limitations of morphology in equivocal lung cytology. *Cancer* 2006; **108**:480–7.

72 Savic S, Glatz K, Schoenegg R *et al*. Multitarget fluorescence in situ hybridization elucidates equivocal lung cytology. *Chest* 2006; **129**:1629–35.

73 Shimosato Y, Kodama T, Kameya T. Morphogenesis of peripheral type adenocarcinoma of the lung. In: Shimosato Y, Melamed MR, Nettesheim P (eds). *Morphogenesis of Lung Cancer*, Vol. 1. Boca Raton, FL: CRC Press, 1982:65–89.

74 Kodama T, Nishiyama H, Nishiwaki Y *et al*. Histopathological study of adenocarcinoma and hyperplastic epithelial lesions of the lung. *Jpn J Lung Cancer (Haigan)* 1988; **28**:325–33.

75 Miller RR. Bronchioloalveolar cell adenomas. *Am J Surg Pathol* 1990; **14**:904–12.

76 Nakanishi K. Alveolar epithelial hyperplasia and adenocarcinoma of the lung. *Arch Pathol Lab Med* 1990; **114**:363–8.

77 Weng SY, Tsuchiya E, Kasuga T, Sugano H. Incidence of atypical bronchioloalveolar cell hyperplasia of the lung: relation to histological subtypes of lung cancer. *Virchows Arch A Pathol Anat Histopathol* 1992; **420**:463–71.

78 Chapman AD, Kerr KM. The association between atypical adenomatous hyperplasia and primary lung cancer. *Br J Cancer* 2000; **83**:632–6.

79 Nakahara R, Yokose T, Nagai K, Nishiwaki Y, Ochiai A. Atypical adenomatous hyperplasia of the lung: a clinicopathological study of 118 cases including cases with multiple atypical adenomatous hyperplasia. *Thorax* 2001; **56**:302–5.

80 Koga T, Hashimoto S, Sugio K *et al*. Lung adenocarcinoma with bronchioloalveolar carcinoma component is frequently associated with foci of high-grade atypical adenomatous hyperplasia. *Am J Clin Pathol* 2002; **117**:464–70.

81 Yokose T, Ito Y, Ochiai A. High prevalence of atypical adenomatous hyperplasia of the lung in autopsy specimens from elderly patients with malignant neoplasms. *Lung Cancer* 2000; **29**:125–30.

82 Kodama T, Biyajima S, Watanabe S, Shimosato Y. Morphometric study of adenocarcinomas and hyperplastic epithelial lesions in the peripheral lung. *Am J Clin Pathol* 1986; **85**:146–51.

83 Mori M, Chiba R, Takahashi T. Atypical adenomatous hyperplasia of the lung and its differentiation from adenocarcinoma. Characterization of atypical cells by morphometry and multivariate cluster analysis. *Cancer* 1993; **72**:2331–40.

84 Kitamura H, Kameda Y, Nakamura N *et al*. Atypical adenomatous hyperplasia and bronchoalveolar lung carcinoma. Analysis by morphometry and the expressions of p53 and carcinoembryonic antigen. *Am J Surg Pathol* 1996; **20**:553–62.

85 Nakayama H, Noguchi M, Tsuchiya R, Kodama T, Shimosato Y. Clonal growth of atypical adenomatous hyperplasia of the lung: cytofluorometric analysis of nuclear DNA content. *Mod Pathol* 1990; **3**:314–20.

86 Westra WH, Baas IO, Hruban RH *et al*. K-ras oncogene activation in atypical alveolar hyperplasias of the human lung. *Cancer Res* 1996; **56**:2224–8.

87 Kohno H, Hiroshima K, Toyozaki T, Fujisawa T, Ohwada H. p53 mutation and allelic loss of chromosome 3p, 9p of preneoplastic lesions in patients with nonsmall cell lung carcinoma. *Cancer* 1999; **85**:341–7.

88 Yamasaki M, Takeshima Y, Fujii S *et al*. Correlation between genetic alterations and histopathological subtypes in bronchiolo-alveolar carcinoma and atypical adenomatous hyperplasia of the lung. *Pathol Int* 2000; **50**:778–85.

89 Takamochi K, Ogura T, Suzuki K *et al*. Loss of heterozygosity on chromosomes 9q and 16p in atypical adenomatous hyperplasia concomitant with adenocarcinoma of the lung. *Am J Pathol* 2001; **159**:1941–8.

90 Anami Y, Matsuno Y, Yamada T *et al*. A case of double primary adenocarcinoma of the lung with multiple atypical adenomatous hyperplasia. *Pathol Int* 1998; **48**:634–40.

91 Ullmann R, Bongiovanni M, Halbwedl I *et al*. Is highgrade adenomatous hyperplasia an early bronchioloalveolar adenocarcinoma? *J Pathol* 2003; **201**:371–6.

92 Minoo P, Hamdan H, Bu D, Warburton D, Stepanik P, deLemos R. TTF-1 regulates lung epithelial morphogenesis. *Dev Biol* 1995; **172**:694–8.

93 Ordonez NG. Value of thyroid transcription factor-1 immunostaining in distinguishing small cell lung carcinomas from other small cell carcinomas. *Am J Surg Pathol* 2000; **24**:1217–23.

94 Bejarano PA, Baughman RP, Biddinger PW *et al*. Surfactant proteins and thyroid transcription factor-1 in

pulmonary and breast carcinomas. *Mod Pathol* 1996; **9**:445–52.

95 Noguchi M, Nakajima T, Hirohashi S, Akiba T, Shimosato Y. Immunohistochemical distinction of malignant mesothelioma from pulmonary adenocarcinoma with anti-surfactant apoprotein, anti-Lewisa, and anti-Tn antibodies. *Hum Pathol* 1989; **20**:53–7.

96 Kaufmann O, Dietel M. Thyroid transcription factor-1 is the superior immunohistochemical marker for pulmonary adenocarcinomas and large cell carcinomas compared to surfactant proteins A and B. *Histopathology* 2000; **36**:8–16.

97 Bremnes RM, Veve R, Hirsch FR, Franklin WA. The E-cadherin cell-cell adhesion complex and lung cancer invasion, metastasis, and prognosis. *Lung Cancer* 2002; **36**:115–24.

98 Bremnes RM, Veve R, Gabrielson E *et al.* High-throughput tissue microarray analysis used to evaluate biology and prognostic significance of the e-cadherin pathway in non-small-cell lung cancer. *J Clin Oncol* 2002; **20**:2417–28.

99 Garber ME, Troyanskaya OG, Schluens K *et al.* Diversity of gene expression in adenocarcinoma of the lung. *Proc Natl Acad Sci U S A* 2001; **98**:13784–9.

100 Beer DG, Kardia SL, Huang CC *et al.* Gene-expression profiles predict survival of patients with lung adenocarcinoma. *Nat Med* 2002; **8**:816–24.

101 Barash Y, Dehan E, Krupsky M *et al.* Comparative analysis of algorithms for signal quantitation from oligonucleotide microarrays. *Bioinformatics* 2004; **20**:839–46.

102 Chen G, Gharib TG, Wang H *et al.* Protein profiles associated with survival in lung adenocarcinoma. *Proc Natl Acad Sci U S A* 2003; **100**:13537–42.

103 Stearman RS, Dwyer-Nield L, Zerbe L *et al.* Analysis of orthologous gene expression between human pulmonary adenocarcinoma and a carcinogen-induced murine model. *Am J Pathol* 2005; **167**:1763–75.

104 Bild AH, Yao G, Chang JT *et al.* Oncogenic pathway signatures in human cancers as a guide to targeted therapies. *Nature* 2006; **439**:353–7.

105 Sy SM, Wong N, Lee TW *et al.* Distinct patterns of genetic alterations in adenocarcinoma and squamous cell carcinoma of the lung. *Eur J Cancer* 2004; **40**:1082–94.

106 Luk C, Tsao MS, Bayani J, Shepherd F, Squire JA. Molecular cytogenetic analysis of non-small cell lung carcinoma by spectral karyotyping and comparative genomic hybridization. *Cancer Genet Cytogenet* 2001; **125**:87–99.

107 Bubendorf L, Muller P, Joos L *et al.* Multitarget FISH analysis in the diagnosis of lung cancer. *Am J Clin Pathol* 2005; **123**:516–23.

108 Halling KC, Rickman OB, Kipp BR, Harwood AR, Doerr CH, Jett JR. A comparison of cytology and fluorescence in situ hybridization for the detection of lung cancer in bronchoscopic specimens. *Chest* 2006; **130**:694–701.

109 Barkan GA, Caraway NP, Jiang F *et al.* Comparison of molecular abnormalities in bronchial brushings and tumor touch preparations. *Cancer* 2005; **105**:35–43.

110 Romeo MS, Sokolova IA, Morrison LE *et al.* Chromosomal abnormalities in non-small cell lung carcinomas and in bronchial epithelia of high-risk smokers detected by multi-target interphase fluorescence in situ hybridization. *J Mol Diagn* 2003; **5**:103–12.

111 Franklin WA, Veve R, Hirsch FR, Helfrich BA, Bunn PA, Jr. Epidermal growth factor receptor family in lung cancer and premalignancy. *Semin Oncol* 2002; **29**:3–14.

112 Gandara DR, West H, Chansky K *et al.* Bronchioloalveolar carcinoma: a model for investigating the biology of epidermal growth factor receptor inhibition. *Clin Cancer Res* 2004; **10**:4205S–9S.

113 Hirsch FR, Varella-Garcia M, Bunn PA, Jr. *et al.* Epidermal growth factor receptor in non-small-cell lung carcinomas: correlation between gene copy number and protein expression and impact on prognosis. *J Clin Oncol* 2003; **21**:3798–807.

114 Paez JG, Janne PA, Lee JC *et al.* EGFR mutations in lung cancer: correlation with clinical response to gefitinib therapy. *Science* 2004; **304**:1497–500.

115 Lynch TJ, Bell DW, Sordella R *et al.* Activating mutations in the epidermal growth factor receptor underlying responsiveness of non-small-cell lung cancer to gefitinib. *N Engl J Med* 2004; **350**:2129–39.

116 Shigematsu H, Lin L, Takahashi T *et al.* Clinical and biological features associated with epidermal growth factor receptor gene mutations in lung cancers. *J Natl Cancer Inst* 2005; **97**:339–46.

117 Shigematsu H, Gazdar AF. Somatic mutations of epidermal growth factor receptor signaling pathway in lung cancers. *Int J Cancer* 2006; **118**:257–62.

118 Eberhard DA, Johnson BE, Amler LC *et al.* Mutations in the epidermal growth factor receptor and in KRAS are predictive and prognostic indicators in patients with non-small-cell lung cancer treated with chemotherapy alone and in combination with erlotinib. *J Clin Oncol* 2005; **23**:5900–9.

119 Cappuzzo F, Hirsch FR, Rossi E *et al*. Epidermal growth factor receptor gene and protein and gefitinib sensitivity in non-small-cell lung cancer. *J Natl Cancer Inst* 2005; **97**:643–55.

120 Hirsch FR, Varella-Garcia M, McCoy J *et al*. Increased epidermal growth factor receptor gene copy number detected by fluorescence in situ hybridization associates with increased sensitivity to gefitinib in patients with bronchioloalveolar carcinoma subtypes: a Southwest Oncology Group Study. *J Clin Oncol* 2005; **23**:6838–45.

121 Tsao MS, Sakurada A, Cutz JC *et al*. Erlotinib in lung cancer—molecular and clinical predictors of outcome. *N Engl J Med* 2005; **353**:133–44.

122 Hirsch F, Varella-Garcia M, Cappuzzo F *et al*. Combination of EGFR gene copy number and protein expression predicts outcome for advanced non-small-cell lung cancer patients treated with gefitinib. *Ann Oncol* 2007; **18**:752–60.

123 Potti A, Mukherjee S, Petersen R *et al*. A genomic strategy to refine prognosis in early-stage non-small-cell lung cancer. *N Engl J Med* 2006; **355**:570–80.

124 Coldren CD, Helfrich BA, Witta SE *et al*. Baseline gene expression predicts sensitivity to gefitinib in non-small cell lung cancer cell lines. *Mol Cancer Res* 2006; **4**:521–8.

125 Ahrendt SA, Decker PA, Alawi EA *et al*. Cigarette smoking is strongly associated with mutation of the K-ras gene in patients with primary adenocarcinoma of the lung. *Cancer* 2001; **92**:1525–30.

126 Le Calvez F, Mukeria A, Hunt JD *et al*. TP53 and KRAS mutation load and types in lung cancers in relation to tobacco smoke: distinct patterns in never, former, and current smokers. *Cancer Res* 2005; **65**:5076–83.

127 Kosaka T, Yatabe Y, Endoh H, Kuwano H, Takahashi T, Mitsudomi T. Mutations of the epidermal growth factor receptor gene in lung cancer: biological and clinical implications. *Cancer Res* 2004; **64**:8919–23.

128 Tam IY, Chung LP, Suen WS *et al*. Distinct epidermal growth factor receptor and KRAS mutation patterns in non-small cell lung cancer patients with different tobacco exposure and clinicopathologic features. *Clin Cancer Res* 2006; **12**:1647–53.

129 Koga T, Hashimoto S, Sugio K *et al*. Clinicopathological and molecular evidence indicating the independence of bronchioloalveolar components from other subtypes of human peripheral lung adenocarcinoma. *Clin Cancer Res* 2001; **7**:1730–8.

130 Zheng Z, Chen T, Li X, Haura E, Sharma A, Bepler G. DNA synthesis and repair genes RRM1 and ERCC1 in lung cancer. *N Engl J Med* 2007; **356**:800–8.

131 Lord RV, Brabender J, Gandara D *et al*. Low ERCC1 expression correlates with prolonged survival after cisplatin plus gemcitabine chemotherapy in non-small cell lung cancer. *Clin Cancer Res* 2002; **8**:2286–91.

132 Ceppi P, Volante M, Novello S *et al*. ERCC1 and RRM1 gene expressions but not EGFR are predictive of shorter survival in advanced non-small-cell lung cancer treated with cisplatin and gemcitabine. *Ann Oncol* 2006; **17**:1818–25.

133 Yu JJ, Mu C, Lee KB *et al*. A nucleotide polymorphism in ERCC1 in human ovarian cancer cell lines and tumor tissues. *Mutat Res* 1997; **382**:13–20.

134 Yu JJ, Lee KB, Mu C *et al*. Comparison of two human ovarian carcinoma cell lines (A2780/CP70 and MCAS) that are equally resistant to platinum, but differ at codon 118 of the ERCC1 gene. *Int J Oncol* 2000; **16**:555–60.

135 Tang X, Shigematsu H, Bekele BN *et al*. EGFR tyrosine kinase domain mutations are detected in histologically normal respiratory epithelium in lung cancer patients. *Cancer Res* 2005; **65**:7568–72.

136 Cowdry EV. Studies on the etiology of Jagziekte: origin of the epithelial proliferations and subsequent changes. *J Exp Med* 1925; **42**:335.

137 Bonne C. Morphological resemblance of pulmonary adenomatosis (jaagseikte) in sheep and certain cases of cancer of the lung in man. *Am J Cancer* 1939; **35**:491–501.

138 York DF, Vigne R, Verwoerd DW, Querat G. Isolation, identification, and partial cDNA cloning of genomic RNA of jaagsiekte retrovirus, the etiological agent of sheep pulmonary adenomatosis. *J Virol* 1991; **65**:5061–7.

139 Palmarini M, Cousens C, Dalziel RG *et al*. The exogenous form of Jaagsiekte retrovirus is specifically associated with a contagious lung cancer of sheep. *J Virol* 1996; **70**:1618–23.

140 Cousens C, Minguijon E, Garcia M *et al*. PCR-based detection and partial characterization of a retrovirus associated with contagious intranasal tumors of sheep and goats. *J Virol* 1996; **70**:7580–3.

141 Palmarini M, Sharp JM, de las Heras M, Fan H. Jaagsiekte sheep retrovirus is necessary and sufficient to induce a contagious lung cancer in sheep. *J Virol* 1999; **73**:6964–72.

142 Palmarini M, Fan H. Retrovirus-induced ovine pulmonary adenocarcinoma, an animal model for lung cancer. *J Natl Cancer Inst* 2001; **93**:1603–14.

143 Yousem SA, Finkelstein SD, Swalsky PA, Bakker A, Ohori NP. Absence of jaagsiekte sheep retrovirus DNA and RNA in bronchioloalveolar and conventional human pulmonary adenocarcinoma by PCR and RT-PCR analysis. *Hum Pathol* 2001; **32**:1039–42.

144 Witschi H. Tobacco smoke as a mouse lung carcinogen. *Exp Lung Res* 1998; **24**:385–94.

145 Malkinson AM. Primary lung tumors in mice as an aid for understanding, preventing, and treating human adenocarcinoma of the lung. *Lung Cancer* 2001; **32**:265–79.

146 Jordan CT, Guzman ML, Noble M. Cancer stem cells. *N Engl J Med* 2006; **355**:1253–61.

147 Otto WR. Lung epithelial stem cells. *J Pathol* 2002; **197**:527–35.

148 Kim CF, Jackson EL, Woolfenden AE *et al.* Identification of bronchioalveolar stem cells in normal lung and lung cancer. *Cell* 2005; **121**:823–35.

149 Jackson EL, Willis N, Mercer K *et al.* Analysis of lung tumor initiation and progression using conditional expression of oncogenic K-ras. *Genes Dev* 2001; **15**:3243–8.

CHAPTER 9

Treatment of Bronchioloalveolar Carcinoma

Ji-Youn Han, Dae Ho Lee, and Jin Soo Lee

Introduction

The latest World Health Organization (WHO) classification divides lung adenocarcinoma mainly into adenocarcinoma mixed subtype, acinar adenocarcinoma, papillary adenocarcinoma, bronchioloalveolar carcinoma (BAC), and solid adenocarcinoma with mucin production [1]. BAC is characterized by distinct clinical presentation, radiographic appearance, tumor biology, response to therapy, and prognosis. It disproportionately affects women, never smokers, and Asians and tends to be younger at diagnosis. These differences raise the question of whether BAC represents a separate biologic entity [2,3]. Although pure BAC accounts for approximately 4% of lung cancers, tumors with histologically mixed BAC and adenocarcinoma account for >20% of all lung cancers, and the incidence of BAC might be increasing [3–5]. In a recent report of 278 lung resections for adenocarcinoma between 1992 and 2001, the proportion of BAC rose from 6.9% of adenocarcinoma in 1992 to 46.9% in 2001 [6]. The increasing numbers of BAC cases suggest that there might be a change in the etiologic factors of lung cancer. Although smoking remains a very important factor of lung cancer, the higher proportion of BAC in never smoker postulates that BAC can develop in a previously scarred area of the lung parenchyma. A

Lung Cancer, 3rd edition. Edited by Jack A. Roth, James D. Cox, and Waun Ki Hong. © 2008 Blackwell Publishing, ISBN: 978-1-4051-5112-2.

scar of previous inflammation, such as tuberculosis, could be the bed of BAC [7].

It is generally observed that the prognosis for BAC is better than those for other types of lung cancer [6,8–12]. Previously, Noguchi *et al.* pointed out that small (3 cm or less) peripheral lung adenocarcinoma with a pure BAC pattern and no invasion had 5-year survival rate of 100%, and patients with mixed BAC and invasive components had a survival of 75% in contrast to those with a purely invasive growth pattern who had a survival of 52% [13]. These findings greatly influenced the 1999 WHO/the International Association for the Study of Lung Cancer (IASLC) panel, which strictly redefined BAC as a subtype of pulmonary adenocarcinoma with growth of neoplastic cells along pre-existing alveolar structures (lepidic growth) without evidence of stromal, vascular, or pleural invasion [14]. BACs are formally classified into three subtypes, nonmucinous, mucinous, and mixed mucinous and nonmucinous type [1,14]. They have been recognized as a solitary peripheral nodule, multiple nodules, and lobar consolidation and characterized by a higher incidence of intrathoracic recurrence and second primary lung cancers, and less frequent distant metastasis compared to other type of nonsmall cell lung cancer (NSCLC) [9,11,14]. The mucinous BAC, which accounts for 20% of BACs, has worse outcome than the nonmucinous BACs. While nonmucinous BACs most commonly present as small peripheral nodules, mucinous BACs tend to spread aerogenously and develop multifocal lesions and frequently masquerade as pneumonia often resulting in a delay in diagnosis [15]. As with other subsets of NSCLC, surgical resection is the only potentially curative treatment. Patients with unresectable BAC are more likely to respond to the epidermal growth factor receptor (EGFR) tyrosine kinase inhibitors (TKIs) gefitinib and erlotinib than patients with other subtypes of NSCLC [16,17].

Surgery

Surgery in a curative intent

BAC is most commonly found in small peripheral lesions, and it is subjected to surgery in an early stage [18]. While only 15–25% of all lung cancers are in stage I, the proportion of stage I in BAC is 68%, suggesting the growth of BAC is slower than other types of NSCLC [6,12,18–21]. BAC usually spreads by the aerogenous route, and lymph node metastasis is rare, reported in less than 10% [18,19]. After curative resection, 92% of patients display intrathoracic recurrence, while 29% of resected cases display extrathoracic recurrence. For example, brain metastasis is frequently occurred in non-BAC lung cancer, for about 20%, it is rarely seen in BAC, for only about 8% [9,11]. Thus, surgical resection appears to have a pivotal role in the treatment of BAC [9].

Localized BAC is treated like other NSCLCs with lobar lung resection and ipsilateral mediastinal lymphadenectomy [20,22]. Although lobectomy is the most commonly performed surgical procedure, the extent of resection has been somewhat controversial. Some investigators have suggested that patients treated with less than a lobectomy have higher recurrence rates and a worse prognosis [18,23]. Given the propensity of the disease to occur in a multifocal fashion, others have advocated lung-sparing procedures (wedge or segmentectomy) [9,24,25]. Sometimes bilobectomy and pneumonectomy are required for complete resection of the diffuse or multifocal BAC. However, the extent of resection never remained significant in multivariate analysis maybe because the surgical procedure is closely linked to the tumor node metastasis (TNM) stage [22].

Completely resected BAC is associated with better disease-free (DFS) and overall survival (OS) rate than those of other types of lung cancer [11–13]. In stage I disease, both 5-year DFS and OS were significantly higher in patients with pure BAC than adenocarcinoma (DFS, 81% versus 51%; OS, 86% versus 71%; $p = 0.005$) [11]. In addition, 76–95% of patients with recurrence initially recur locally, which is higher than other types of lung cancer [11–13]. Early stage, nonmucinous type, and the absence of vascular or lymphatic invasion are associated with better survival after surgical resection [6,11,20,22,26]. Apart from the fact that advanced stage is generally associated with a worse prognosis, the management of patients with multiple nodules is controversial and the presence of multiple or satellite nodule is not an adverse prognostic factor in BAC [20,27]. Thus, surgery should not be denied for patients with multiple nodules who are younger than 60 years of age and without lymph node involvement. In the absence of mediastinal involvement or distant metastasis, possible multifocal BACs should be treated as separate primary tumors [17,27].

Palliative surgery for BAC

In a highly selected subgroup of patients who present with bilateral BAC, palliative pneumonectomy or lobectomy could be considered because of the unequal involvement of the lungs and major hypoxemia in relation to a severe intrapulmonary shunting. Both symptoms and respiratory function could be quickly improved postoperatively with tolerable morbidity [28]. However, palliative surgery should be considered exclusively for very highly selected patients and further discussion in a multidisciplinary manner would be needed [22,29].

Transplantation

Because of the theoretical risk of rapid cancer dissemination with posttransplant immunosuppression, bronchogenic carcinoma has been considered a strict contraindication to lung transplantation [30]. BAC can present as a localized discrete lesion or with a diffuse multifocal pattern involving one or both lungs [14]. Pulmonary recurrence without systemic dissemination is often observed after lung resection for multifocal BAC, and survival beyond 2 years is uncommon [9,11]. Death usually occurs as

Table 9.1 Paclitaxel chemotherapy trials in advanced BAC or NSCLC.

Study	Histology	Phase	Patients no.	Schedule	Response rate	Median survival
SWOG 9714 [35]	BAC	II	58	35 mg/m^2/24 h CI over 96 h	8/58 (14%)	12 M
EORTC 08956 [36]	BAC	II	19	200 mg/m^2 IV for 3 h	2/18 (11%)	8.6 M
Ranson et al. [37]	NSCLC	III	79	200 mg/m^2 IV for 3 h	12/76 (16%)	6.8 M

BAC, bronchioloalveolar carcinoma; NSCLC, nonsmall cell lung cancer; CI, continuous infusion; IV, intravenously; M, month; BST, best supportive care.

a result of pulmonary failure secondary to tumor replacement of the functioning lung [19]. Despite case reports and small case series on lung transplantation for multifocal BAC, the role of lung transplantation in the treatment of patients with bronchogenic carcinoma and end-stage lung disease remains unresolved [31,32].

A recent international survey determined the outcome of patients who presented with bronchogenic carcinoma in the explanted lung at the time of transplantation [33]. This survey demonstrates that the 5-year actuarial survival rate was 51% in patients with stage I bronchogenic carcinomas, which was significantly better than for patients with stage II and III bronchogenic carcinomas (survival of 14%) or with incidental multifocal BAC (survival of 23%). Time from transplantation to recurrence and from recurrence to death was significantly longer in patients with multifocal BAC than in patients with other types of bronchogenic carcinoma. In addition, the site of recurrence was limited to the transplanted lung in 88% of the patients with multifocal BAC, whereas it was always widespread in patients with other types of bronchogenic carcinoma. Thus, although rarely curative, lung transplantation remains a valuable procedure for patients with impending respiratory failure secondary to advanced multifocal BAC [33].

Chemotherapy

Despite the slow growth kinetics and prolonged survival after repeated surgical resection of multifocal lesions, advanced bilateral multifocal BAC remains incurable. There is no optimal established therapy for unresectable multifocal BAC. Multifocal BAC may be indolent enough to follow asymptomatic patients without any systemic therapy if patients are comfortable with this approach. It is because the rate of disease progression may be slow enough to warrant no therapy for many months or even years. For patients with symptoms and/or clear evidence of disease progression over a short interval, standard chemotherapy is appropriate [17].

Advanced multifocal BAC has been considered to be relatively resistant to chemotherapy based on limited retrospective data [27]. However, all BAC chemotherapy studies are limited by their sample size and the use of old regimens. In addition, analysis of the response of BAC to chemotherapy is complicated by the classification of most patients with mixed BAC as adenocarcinoma, and also by misclassification of histologic type when the diagnosis is made by cytology and by the absence of independent pathologic review in most chemotherapy trials [2]. Moreover, retrospective reviews have suggested that patients with BAC survive longer than those with other types of NSCLC after chemotherapy [8,34]. Thus, little can be said about the chemosensitivity of these tumors based on the limited retrospective data.

Recently, two clinical trials of chemotherapy in advanced BAC have been reported (Table 9.1). In the Southwest Oncology Group (SWOG) trial 9714 [35], 58 chemonaïve patients with advanced BAC received a 96-hour infusion of paclitaxel (35 mg/m^2 for 24 h). The overall response rate was 14% with the time to progression of 5 months, median survival of 12 months, and 3-year overall survival rate of 10%. However, the toxicity of the infusional paclitaxel dissuaded the general use of this regimen.

Table 9.2 Phase II trials of EGFR-TKIs in patients with previously treated NSCLC.

Study	Agent	Dose	Patients no.*	Response rate	Median survival	1-year survival
IDEAL 1 [39]	Gefitinib	250 vs. 500 mg/day	216	12/102 (12%) vs. 10/114 (9%)	7 M vs. 6 M	27% vs. 24%
IDEAL 2 [40][†]	Gefitinib	250 vs. 500 mg/day	208	18/103 (17.5%) vs. 19/105 (18.1%)	7.6 M vs. 8 M	35% vs. 29%
Perez-Soler *et al.* [41][‡]	Erlotinib	150 mg/day	55	7/55 (12.7%, 2CR, 5PR)	8.4 M	40%

*Evaluable patients.
[†]The response rate was higher for Japanese patients than non-Japanese patients (27.5% vs. 10.4%; odds ratio = 3.27; $p = 0.0023$).
[‡]NSCLC with EGFR expression.

A similar study was conducted by the European Organisation for Research and Treatment of Cancer; EORTC trial 08956 [36]. In this study, a 3-hour infusion of paclitaxel (200 mg/m^2 on day 1 every 3 weeks) was used to treat chemonaïve patients with advanced BAC. The overall response rate was 11%, time to progression was 2.2 months, median survival was 8.6 months, and 1-year overall survival was 35%. These results are comparable to the single-agent paclitaxel activity in advanced NSCLC [37]. It is generally accepted that patients with BAC should not be excluded from the clinical trials evaluating efficacy of chemotherapy and new targeted agents. Particularly in the absence of an optimal standard therapy, clinical trials should remain as a viable treatment option for these patients.

Epidermal growth factor receptor-tyrosine kinase inhibitors

Although patients with advanced NSCLC are commonly treated with chemotherapy, there is a general consensus in that the benefits of traditional chemotherapy have reached a plateau. In the past few years, several agents that are more specific for cancer cell targets have shown significant antitumor activity in NSCLC. The EGFR-TKI is the first class of molecular-targeted agent approved in the United States and other countries for the treatment of advanced NSCLC that progressed after both platinum- and docetaxel-containing regimens [38]. Belonged to this class of agents are gefitinib (Iressa®, AstraZeneca, Wilmington, DE) and erlotinib (Tarceva®, OSI Pharmaceuticals Inc, Melville, NY). Both agents are small molecules that belong to the quinazolinamine class and inhibit the tyrosine kinase (TK) activity of the EGFR by competing ATP for the ATP-binding site. Single agent trials of gefitinib or erlotinib in patients with previously treated advanced NSCLC have reported response rates in approximately 10% of Caucasian patients and 28% of Japanese patients (Table 9.2) [39–41].

Accumulating evidence from these trials of gefitinib or erlotinib suggest that such patient characteristics as never smoker, female gender, East Asian origin, adenocarcinoma histology, and bronchioloalveolar carcinoma subtype, are associated with a grater benefit from treatment with these TKIs [16,34,42,43]. In light of these observations, two prospective phase II trials were undertaken in patients with advanced BAC or adenocarcinoma with BAC features (Table 9.3). In SWOG S0126 trial [44], 136 (101 chemonaïve, 35 previously treated) patients with advanced BAC received gefitinib single treatment. The response rates were 17 and 9% for chemonaïve and previously treated patients, respectively. Median survival was 13 months for both chemonaïve and previously treated patients. These results are similar to that achieved in SWOG S9714 trial with 96-hour paclitaxel infusion. However,

Table 9.3 Clinical trials of EGFR-TKIs in BAC.

Study	Agent	Dose	Patients no.*	Response rate	Median survival	1-year survival
SWOG S0126 [44]	Gefitinib	500 mg/day	Previously untreated-69	17% (12/69, 4CR, 8PR)	13 M	51%
			Previously treated-22	9% (2/22, 2PR)	12 M	51%
Kris *et al.* [45]	Erlotinib	150 mg/day	59	25% (15/59)	NR	58%

*Evaluable patients.
CR, completer response; PR, partial response.

survival at 2 and 3 years in S0126 (chemonaïve patents) is 39% and 23% versus 29% and 13% in S9714, respectively. Kris *et al.* [45] also conducted a similar study of erlotinib in 69 patients with adenocarcinoma with any BAC features. The preliminary data also showed encouraging results of erlotinib single treatment in these patients. These long-term survival results observed in EGFR-TKI trials in advanced BAC support the preferred treatment of these agents as the first-line or second-line for patients with BAC feature. However, whether the results of EGFR-TKIs in BAC are superior to those achieved with platinum-based chemotherapy remains unclear.

The discovery of *EGFR* gene mutations in the receptor TK domain and their association with high response rate to EGFR-TKIs has had a profound impact on understanding the role of these agents in NSCLC. A recent comprehensive review on EGFR somatic mutations provided detailed information on clinicopathologic features in lung cancer that are associated with these mutations. A total of over 2000 NSCLC samples have been analyzed, and a total of 477 mutations were detected. A significantly higher frequency of *EGFR* kinase domain mutations found in patients with adenocarcinoma (30% versus 2%; $p < 0.001$), never smoker (45% versus 7%; $p < 0.001$), female (38% versus 10%; $p < 0.001$), and East Asian individuals (33% versus 6%; $p < 0.001$), which matches the profile of NSCLC patients who likely to respond to EGFR-TKIs [46]. In a study of EGFR tyrosine kinase domain mutations in 860 lung cancers, Marchetti *et al.* [47] found that there were no EGFR mutations in 454 squamous cell carcinomas and 31 large cell carci-

nomas investigated. A total of 39 mutations were found in a series of 375 adenocarcinomas. Among them, 22 (26%) were found in 86 BACs, which is very similar to the response rates of BAC to EGFR-TKIs (Table 9.3). These findings suggest that about one fourth of BACs may respond to EGFR-TKIs because mutations affecting the gene.

Nevertheless, it is unclear whether all BACs respond better than conventional adenocarcinoma to EGFR-TKIs. Although it is preliminary, Kris *et al.* [45] reported that patients with adenocarcinoma with BAC features showed higher response to erlotinib compared to pure BAC (30% versus 7%, respectively). Marchetti *et al.* [47] reported that all the EGFR mutations found in BAC were seen in the nonmucinous type. Eighteen (35%) of 52 nonmucinous BACs had EGFR mutations. Conversely, mucinous BACs were always negative for EGFR mutations. They also investigated for K-ras mutations at codon 12 and all of the tumors affected by EGFR were found to be negative for K-ras mutations, whereas, tumors negative for EGFR mutations showed a K-ras mutation in 32% of cases ($p = 0.000001$). The prevalence of K-ras mutations was 29% in conventional lung adenocarcinoma and 27% in BAC. Fourteen percent of nonmucinous BACs carried K-ras mutations, while 76% of mucinous BACs showed K-ras mutations ($p = 0.00002$) [47]. K-ras mutations are strongly associated with smoking status and more common in nonresponders to EGFR-TKIs [48]. These findings suggest that *EGFR* and *K-ras* genes seem to be related to the development of different BAC types and resulting different effects on responding to EGFR-TKIs. However, due to the limited number of BAC cases, additional studies are required to confirm these data. Prospective trials evaluating response to EGFR-TKIs including EGFR and K-ras sequencing are under way to help shed more light on this intriguing finding.

Other molecular target agents in BAC

Eastern Cooperative Oncology Group (ECOG) has conducted a study evaluating the role of adenovirus p53 administered by bronchoalveolar lavage to patients with BAC (ECOG 6597). The rationale for this study included the fact that NSCLCs have a high frequency of p53 mutations and that BAC tends to spread as a thin layer of cells along the airways rather than developing into a solid tumor mass. Some previous gene therapy studies have used injections into the tumor mass, but success is often limited because the gene-carrying viruses cannot reach most of the cancer cells in the solid tumor. In BAC, on the other hand, it may be possible to deliver gene therapy directly through the air passages. Thus, adequate dissemination of adenovirus p53 might be obtained in this locoregional setting. Of 27 patients enrolled, 25 were treated and one partial response and 17 stable diseases were observed of 24 evaluable patients. Three patients had more than 20% improvement in the diffusion capacity of carbon monoxide, and subjectively improved breathing was noted in many patients [49].

Therapeutic cancer vaccines derived from whole tumor cells have also been tested in patients with resected early-stage NSCLC, which demonstrated immunologic activity and the suggestion of survival advantage [50,51]. G8123 (GVAX) is a genetically engineered autologous anticancer vaccine to secrete granulocyte-macrophage colony-stimulating factor (GM-CSF). In head-to-head comparison, genetically engineered anticancer vaccines secreting GM-CSF have shown greater activity than vaccines using other cytokines in murine tumor models including the Lewis lung carcinoma [52,53]. In a phase I/II trial of this vaccine, complete responses were seen in three of 33 previously treated patients with advanced NSCLC with a median duration of response

of 17.8 months. Notably, two of these responders had BAC. Responses in the two BAC patients were durable and complete and the response duration measured 18 months in one patient and exceeded 22 months in the other patient. The median survival of all 33 patients was 11.6 months, which compares favorably to the approved second-line docetaxel chemotherapy for such patients [54]. An ongoing phase II CG8123 (GVAX) trial (SWOG 0310) will treat nearly 100 patients with advanced BAC both untreated and previously treated [34].

Another agent of interest is a proteasome inhibitor. The proteasome plays a critical role in the degradation of proteins involved in the regulation of cell cycle, apoptosis, and angiogenesis [55]. Bortezomib (VELCADE, Vc, Millennium Pharmaceuticals) is a reversible novel proteasome inhibitor approved for the treatment of relapsed multiple myeloma [56]. In the initial phase I study of bortezomib in advanced solid tumors, one of 43 patients, a patient with heavily pretreated BAC, achieved a PR [57]. Recent studies in patients with advanced NSCLC as a single agent or in combination with other chemotherapy have demonstrated encouraging results (Table 9.4) [58–60]. In addition, there are anecdotal reports of objective responses of bortezomib in BAC [61]. Currently, the California–Pittsburgh Cancer Consortium is conducting a phase II study to evaluate the activity and safety of bortezomib in patients with advanced BAC or adenocarcinoma with BAC features.

Summary

BAC is previously considered an uncommon subset of NSCLC with unique epidemiology, pathology, clinical features, radiographic presentation, and natural history compared with other subtypes of NSCLC. However, recent data suggest that the incidence of BAC is increasing. Despite reports of prolonged survival after repeated surgical resection of multifocal lesions and slow growth kinetics, advanced bilateral or recurrent diffuse BAC remains incurable, with the vast majority of patients dying of respiratory failure or intercurrent pneumonia within 5 years. Most of the clinical information

Table 9.4 Clinical trials of Bortezomib in NSCLC.

Author	Phase	Patients no.*	Prior chemotherapy	Regimen	Efficacy	Median TTP
Davies *et al.* [58]	I	10	0	Bortezomib + gemcitabine + carboplatin	PR 40% (4/10) SD 50% (5/10)	NR
Stevenson *et al.* [59]	II	22	≤ 1	Bortezomib	PR 5% (1/22) SD 41% (9/22)	NR
Fanucchi *et al.* [60]	II	155	1	Bortezomib vs. Bortezomib + docetaxel	PR 8% (6/75) vs. PR 9% (7/80)	1.5 mo vs. 4 mo

*Evaluable patients.
PR, partial response; SD, stable disease; TTP, time to progression; NR, not reported.

on BAC comes from retrospective institutional reviews. Recent studies of molecular-targeted therapies, however, have focused more specifically on BAC. In particular, clinical trials of EGFR-TKIs have led to a deeper understanding of the distinct features of this cancer and suggest that BAC may require a new therapeutic paradigm different from that of other NSCLCs. The limited utility of chemotherapy necessitates the investigation of novel agents and combinations for the treatment of BAC. Identification of molecular pathways unique to BAC would enable faster the development of more efficacious therapy for this unique subset of NSCLC.

References

1 Travis WD, Brambilla E, Muller-Hermelink HK, Harris CC. World Health Organization classification. In: *Tumors of the Lung, Pleura, Thymus, and Heart*. Lyon, France: IARC Press, 2004.

2 Laskin JJ, Sandler AB, Johnson DH. Redefining bronchioloalveolar carcinoma. *Semin Oncol* 2005; **32**:329–35.

3 Zell JA, Ou SH, Ziogas A, Anton-Culver H. Epidemiology of bronchioloalveolar carcinoma: improvement in survival after release of the 1999 WHO classification of lung tumors. *J Clin Oncol* 2005; **23**:8396–405.

4 Barsky SH, Cameron R, Osann KE, Tomita D, Holmes EC. Rising incidence of bronchioloalveolar lung carcinoma and its unique clinicopathologic features. *Cancer* 1994; **73**:1163–70.

5 Auerbach O, Garfinkel L. The changing pattern of lung carcinoma. *Cancer* 1991; **68**:1973–7.

6 Furak J, Trojan I, Szoke T *et al.* Bronchioloalveolar lung cancer: occurrence, surgical treatment and survival. *Eur J Cardiothorac Surg* 2003; **23**:818–23.

7 Barkley JE, Green MR. Bronchioloalveolar carcinoma. *J Clin Oncol* 1996; **14**:2377–86.

8 Breathnach OS, Ishibe N, Williams J, Linnoila RI, Caporaso N, Johnson BE. Clinical features of patients with stage IIIB and IV bronchioloalveolar carcinoma of the lung. *Cancer* 1999; **86**:1165–73.

9 Breathnach OS, Kwiatkowski DJ, Finkelstein DM *et al.* Bronchioloalveolar carcinoma of the lung: recurrences and survival in patients with stage I disease. *J Thorac Cardiovasc Surg* 2001; **121**:42–7.

10 Grover FL, Piantadosi S. Recurrence and survival following resection of bronchioloalveolar carcinoma of the lung—The Lung Cancer Study Group experience. *Ann Surg* 1989; **209**:779–90.

11 Rena O, Papalia E, Ruffini E *et al.* Stage I pure bronchioloalveolar carcinoma: recurrences, survival and comparison with adenocarcinoma of the lung. *Eur J Cardiothorac Surg* 2003; **23**:409–14.

12 Sakurai H, Dobashi Y, Mizutani E *et al.* Bronchioloalveolar carcinoma of the lung 3 centimeters or less in diameter: a prognostic assessment. *Ann Thorac Surg* 2004; **78**:1728–33.

13 Noguchi M, Morikawa A, Kawasaki M *et al.* Small adenocarcinoma of the lung. Histologic characteristics and prognosis. *Cancer* 1995; **75**:2844–52.

14 Travis WD, Garg K, Franklin WA *et al.* Evolving concepts in the pathology and computed tomography imaging of lung adenocarcinoma and bronchioloalveolar carcinoma. *J Clin Oncol* 2005; **23**:3279–87.

15 Raz DJ, He B, Rosell R, Jablons DM. Current concepts in bronchioloalveolar carcinoma biology. *Clin Cancer Res* 2006; **12**:3698–704.

16 Miller VA, Kris MG, Shah N *et al.* Bronchioloalveolar pathologic subtype and smoking history predict sensitivity to gefitinib in advanced non-small-cell lung cancer. *J Clin Oncol* 2004; **22**:1103–9.

17 West H. Emerging approaches to advanced bronchioloalveolar carcinoma. *Curr Treat Options Oncol* 2006; **7**:69–76.

18 Liu YY, Chen YM, Huang MH, Perng RP. Prognosis and recurrent patterns in bronchioloalveolar carcinoma. *Chest* 2000; **118**:940–7.

19 Okubo K, Mark EJ, Flieder D *et al.* Bronchoalveolar carcinoma: clinical, radiologic and pathologic factors and survival. *J Thorac Cardiovasc Surg* 1999; **118**:702–9.

20 Dumont P, Gasser B, Rougé C, Massard G, Wihlm JM. Bronchoalveolar carcinoma. Histopathologic study of evolution in a series of 105 surgically treated patients. *Chest* 1998; **113**:391–5.

21 Kwiatkowski DJ, Harpole DH, Godleski J *et al.* Molecular pathologic substaging in 244 stage I non-small-cell lung cancer patients: clinical implication. *J Clin Oncol* 1998; **16**:2468–77.

22 Barlesi F, Doddoli C, Gimenez C *et al.* Bronchioloalveolar carcinoma: myths and realities in the surgical management. *Eur J Cardiothorac Surg* 2003; **24(l)**:159–64.

23 Miller DL, Rowland CM, Deschamps C, Allen MS, Trastek VF, Pairolero PC. Surgical treatment of non-small cell lung cancer 1 cm or less in diameter. *Ann Thorac Surg* 2002; **73**:1545–50.

24 Harpole DH, Bigelow C, Young WG, Wolfe WG, Sabiston DC. Alveolar cell carcinoma of the lung: a retrospective analysis of 205 patients. *Ann Thorac Surg* 1988; **46**:502–7.

25 Yamato Y, Tsuchida M, Watanabe T *et al.* Early results of a prospective study of limited resection for bronchioloalveolar adenocarcinoma of the lung. *Ann Thorac Surg* 2001; **71**:971–4.

26 Ebright MI, Zakowski MF, Martin J *et al.* Clinical pattern and pathologic stage but not histologic features predict outcome for bronchioloalveolar carcinoma. *Ann Thorac Surg* 2002; **74**:1640–7.

27 Donker R, Stewart DJ, Dahrouge S *et al.* Clinical characteristics and the impact of surgery and chemotherapy on survival of patients with advanced and metastatic bronchioloalveolar carcinoma: a retrospective study. *Clin Lung Cancer* 2000; **1**:211–6.

28 Barlesi F, Doddoli C, Thomas P, Kleisbauer JP, Giudicelli R, Fuentes P. Bilateral bronchioloalveolar lung carcinoma: is there a place for palliative pneumonectomy? *Eur J Cardiothorac Surg* 2001; **20**:1113–6.

29 Chetty KG, Dick C, McGovern J, Conroy RM, Mahutte CK. Refractory hypoxemia due to intrapulmonary shunting associated with bronchioloalveolar carcinoma. *Chest* 1997; **111**:1120–1.

30 Maurer JR, Frost AE, Estenne M, Higenbottam T, Glanville AR. International guidelines for the selection of lung transplant candidates. *J Heart Lung Transplant* 1998; **17**:703–9.

31 Etienne B, Bertocchi M, Gamondes JP, Wiesendanger T, Brune J, Mornex JF. Successful double-lung transplantation for bronchioalveolar carcinoma. *Chest* 1997; **112**:1423–4.

32 de Perrot M, Fischer S, Waddell TK *et al.* Management of lung transplant recipients with bronchogenic carcinoma in the native lung. *J Heart Lung Transplant* 2003; **22**:87–9.

33 de Perrot M, Chernenko S, Waddell TK *et al.* Role of lung transplantation in the treatment of bronchogenic carcinomas for patients with end-stage pulmonary disease. *J Clin Oncol* 2004; **22**:4351–6.

34 Miller VA, Hirsch FR, Johnson DH. Systemic therapy of advanced bronchioloalveolar cell carcinoma: challenges and opportunities. *J Clin Oncol* 2005; **23**:3288–93.

35 West HL, Crowley JJ, Vance RB *et al.* Advanced bronchioloalveolar carcinoma: a phase II trial of paclitaxel by 96-hour infusion (SWOG 9714): a Southwest Oncology Group study. *Ann Oncol* 2005; **16**:1076–80.

36 Scagliotti GV, Smit E, Bosquee L *et al.* A phase II study of paclitaxel in advanced bronchioloalveolar carcinoma (EORTC trial 08956). *Lung Cancer* 2005; **50**:91–6.

37 Ranson M, Davidson N, Nicolson M *et al.* Randomized trial of paclitaxel plus supportive care versus supportive care for patients with advanced non-small-cell lung cancer. *J Natl Cancer Inst* 2000; **92**:1074–80.

38 Giaccone G, Rodriguez JA. EGFR inhibitors: what have we learned from the treatment of lung cancer? *Nat Clin Pract Oncol* 2005; **2**:554–61.

39 Kris MG, Natale RB, Herbst RS *et al.* Efficacy of gefitinib, an inhibitor of the epidermal growth factor receptor tyrosine kinase, in symptomatic patients with non-small cell lung cancer: a randomized trial. *JAMA* 2003; **290**:2149–58.

40 Fukuoka M, Yano S, Giaccone G *et al.* Multi-institutional randomized phase II trial of gefitinib for

previously treated patients with advanced non-small-cell lung cancer. *J Clin Oncol* 2003; **21**:2237–46.

41 Perez-Soler R, Chachoua A, Hammond LA *et al.* Determinants of tumor response and survival with erlotinib in patients with non-small-cell lung cancer. *J Clin Oncol* 2004; **22**:3238–47.

42 Blackhall F, Ranson M, Thatcher N. Where next for gefitinib in patients with lung cancer? *Lancet Oncol* 2006; **7**:499–507.

43 Calvo E, Baselga J. Ethnic differences in response to epidermal growth factor receptor tyrosine kinase inhibitors. *J Clin Oncol* 2006; **24**:2158–63.

44 West HL, Franklin WA, McCoy J *et al.* Gefitinib therapy in advanced bronchioloalveolar carcinoma: Southwest Oncology Group Study S0126. *J Clin Oncol* 2006; **24**:1807–13.

45 Kris MG, Sandler A, Miller V *et al.* Cigarette smoking history predicts sensitivity to erlotinib: results of a phase II trial in patients with bronchioloalveolar carcinoma (BAC) [Abstract 7062]. *Proc Am Soc Clin Oncol* 2004; **22**:14S.

46 Shigematsu H, Gazdar AF. Somatic mutations of epidermal growth factor receptor signaling pathway in lung cancers. *Int J Cancer* 2006; **118**:257–62.

47 Marchetti A, Martella C, Felicioni L *et al.* EGFR mutations in non-small-cell lung cancer: analysis of a large series of cases and development of a rapid and sensitive method for diagnostic screening with potential implications on pharmacologic treatment. *J Clin Oncol* 2005; **23**:857–65.

48 Janne PA, Engelman JA, Johnson BE. Epidermal growth factor receptor mutations in non-small-cell lung cancer: implications for treatment and tumor biology. *J Clin Oncol* 2005; **23**:3227–34.

49 Carbone DP, Adak S, Schiller J *et al.* Adenovirus p53 administered by bronchoalveolar lavage in patients with bronchioalveolar cell lung carcinoma (BAC) [Abstract 2492]. *Proc Am Soc Clin Oncol* 2003; **22**: 620.

50 Schulof R, Mai D, Nelson M *et al.* Active specific immunotherapy with an autologous tumor cell vaccine in patients with resected non-small cell lung cancer. *Mol Biother* 1988; **1**:30–6.

51 Stack BH, McSwan N, Stirling JM *et al.* Autologous x-irradiated tumour cells and percutaneous BCG in operable lung cancer. *Thorax* 1982; **37**:588–93.

52 Dranoff G, Jaffee E, Lazenby A *et al.* Vaccination with irradiated tumor cells engineered to secrete murine granulocyte-macrophage colony-stimulating factor stimulates potent, specific, and long-lasting anti-tumor immunity. *Proc Natl Acad Sci U S A* 1993; **90**:3539–43.

53 Lee CT, Wu S, Ciernik IF *et al.* Genetic immunotherapy of established tumors with adenovirus-murine granulocyte-macrophage colony-stimulating factor. *Hum Gene Ther* 1997; **8**:187–93.

54 Nemunaitis J, Sterman D, Jablons D *et al.* Granulocyte-macrophage colony-stimulating factor gene-modified autologous tumor vaccines in non-small-cell lung cancer. *J Natl Cancer Inst* 2004; **96**:326–31.

55 Mitchell BS. The proteasome—an emerging therapeutic target in cancer. *N Engl J Med* 2003; **348**:2597–8.

56 San Miguel J, Blade J, Boccadoro M *et al.* A practical update on the use of bortezomib in the management of multiple myeloma. *Oncologist* 2006; **11**:51–61.

57 Aghajanian C, Soignet S, Dizon DS *et al.* A phase I trial of the novel proteasome inhibitor PS341 in advanced solid tumor malignancies. *Clin Cancer Res* 2002; **8**:2505–11.

58 Davies M, Lara PN, Lau DH *et al.* The proteasome inhibitor, bortezomib, in combination with gemcitabine (Gem) and carboplatin (Carbo) in advanced non-small cell lung cancer (NSCLC): final results of a phase I California Cancer Consortium study [Abstract 7106]. *Proc Am Soc Clin Oncol* 2004; **22**:14S.

59 Stevenson JP, Nho CW, Johnson SW *et al.* Effects of bortezomib (PS-341) on NF-κB activation in peripheral blood mononuclear cells (PBMCs) of advanced non-small lung cancer (NSCLC) patients: a phase II/pharmacodynamic trial [Abstract 7145]. *Proc Am Soc Clin Oncol* 2004; **22**:14S.

60 Fanucchi MP, Fossella FV, Belt R *et al.* Randomized phase II study of bortezomib alone and bortezomib in combination with docetaxel in previously treated advanced non-small-cell lung cancer. *J Clin Oncol* 2006; **24**:5025–33.

61 Subramanian J, Pillot G, Narra V, Govindan R. Response to bortezomib (velcade) in a case of advanced bronchiolo-alveolar carcinoma (BAC). A case report. *Lung Cancer* 2006; **51**:257–9.

CHAPTER 10

Molecular Profiling for Early Detection and Prediction of Response in Lung Cancer

Jacob M. Kaufman and David P. Carbone

Introduction

Patterns of gene and protein expression determine the biologic behavior of all cells, normal and malignant, and it is now well accepted that aberrant gene expression underlies all aspects of the malignant phenotype, including uncontrolled cell proliferation, faulty apoptosis, local invasion, and metastasis. Three decades of molecular and cellular research have led to a complex picture of the cancer cell, with disruptions of normal controls of cellular homeostasis at every level, from the outer and inner cell membranes, to cytoplasmic signaling cascades, to nuclear transcription factors; these processes result from as well as lead to abnormalities in regulation of transcription, DNA replication and cell division, DNA repair, energy utilization, and cellular waste management. It is clear that abnormal expression of not just a few, but potentially dozens or hundreds of genes and proteins may be detectable in biopsy specimens or in serum or other body fluids. With the sequencing of the entire human genome and the development of technologies for simultaneously assaying the expression of thousands of mRNA species or proteins from a single biological sample, the emerging field of molecular profiling will provide a more comprehensive understanding of the biology and clinical behavior of cancer in general, and, in particular for the purposes of this review, lung cancer.

Investigations of the expression of single genes and proteins, particularly oncogenes and tumor suppressor genes—e.g., membrane tyrosine kinases, ras family signaling proteins, p53, and bcl-2 [1–4]—have identified important correlations with certain clinical variables, such as survival. Unfortunately, these correlations generally lack the predictive power to affect clinical decision-making. Molecular profiling, on the other hand, because of the very large numbers of genes simultaneously analyzed, may yield more statistically powerful correlations and, thus, clinically important diagnostics and treatment planning.

Molecular profiling techniques of either mRNA or proteins have potential use for earlier and more accurate detection and diagnosis of cancer, as an adjunct to traditional pathological diagnosis and subclassification, for assigning prognostic categories, and for guiding the inclusion of chemotherapy, radiation or surgery or for selecting agents for use with conventional or targeted chemotherapy. Additionally, molecular profiling can enrich the information obtained from molecular biology to give a greater understanding of lung cancer and to generate hypotheses about lung cancer that can guide further in depth basic laboratory investigations of lung cancer.

Lung Cancer, 3rd edition. Edited by Jack A. Roth, James D. Cox, and Waun Ki Hong. © 2008 Blackwell Publishing, ISBN: 978-1-4051-5112-2.

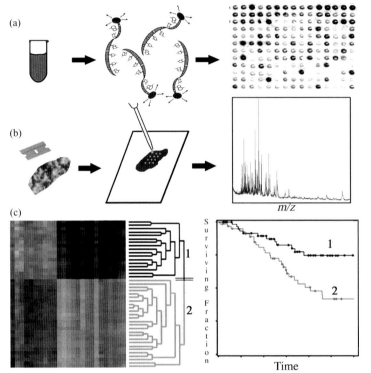

Figure 10.1 In a microarray gene profiling experiment (a), RNA isolated from homogenized tumor tissue is labeled with a fluorescent dye and hybridized with an array of oligomers representing thousands of individual genes. The expression level of any gene in the sample is estimated by the intensity of fluorescence at the gene's position in the array. In one type of MALDI protein profiling experiment (b), thinly sliced sections from a frozen tumor specimen are fixed to a conductive instrument probe, and spotted with an organic acid solution that dries to form a thin crystalline layer. A laser irradiates the sample in a mass spectrometer, producing intact protein ions that are detected according to their molecular weight-to-charge (m/z) ratio. Statistical analysis (c), e.g., with hierarchical clustering of the resulting data can define patient subgroups and relationships between clinical and molecular variables.

Molecular profiling encompasses experiments in which expression of hundreds or thousands of unique molecules (e.g., mRNA, genomic DNA, proteins, phosphorylated peptides, etc.) are measured from a single sample (Figure 10.1). The resulting sets of measurements are compared over a large collection of patient samples, using a variety of statistical techniques, to clinical and biological parameters of interest to identify molecular features that underlie specific disease behavior. A certain relationship between the expression pattern and the disease behavior is first posited based on analysis of a "training set" of samples, which might have been obtained and analyzed years before the clinical data are fully available. The training set conclusions are then validated in one or more "testing set" cohorts to determine whether the posited relationship holds in an independent set of samples. Molecular profiling is a dynamic concept—theoretically it can be used to investigate and define unknown relationships between any measurable set of analytes and any phenotype associated with a pathological

or normal state with any organism—provided each is adequately described and reliably measurable.

Here, we will first briefly review the available profiling technologies and then some clinical applications and data.

Techniques used in molecular profiling

Molecular profiling experiments can be used to investigate relationships between any clinical variable and any type of analyte. Thus, any technique that measures a large number of distinct molecules from a sample could find application for particular clinical questions. For example, lipid and carbohydrate profiling have each begun to identify interesting patterns associated with cellular phenotypes and processes. However, partially due to the diverse actions of proteins in the regulation of all cellular processes and the dependence of protein translation on the transcription and processing of mRNA, and partially due to key enabling technological developments, the profiling of proteins (proteomics), and of mRNA and DNA (genomics) are best developed, and perhaps hold the most potential for the understanding of human disease. Hence, this chapter will focus on the reported and potential future applications of genomics and proteomics in lung cancer.

Genomics and proteomics are complementary modes of investigation. Genomics is currently more widely used and more developmentally mature than proteomics. The physical properties of DNA and RNA that allow complementary base pairing simplify their analysis. Proteins are, by virtue of their heterogeneity, more difficult to characterize. However, proteins have more direct impact on pathological behavior, and many complexities of their regulation and function are not captured by studies of gene expression levels. Studies that compare genomic and proteomic data show that the correlation between gene and protein levels is quite low, and changes in expression level often occur discordantly [5–7]. Thus, although it is easier to assay mRNA levels, they may provide a rougher surrogate of biologic activity than knowledge of protein expression and modifications.

Genomics

Genomics can be defined as the study of the genes and their expression in normal or diseased cells and tissues, to determine correlations with growth, development and disease states. Technologies that have enabled the efficient detection of patterns of altered expression of many genes in a single experiment, coupled with powerful statistical techniques correlating the expression pattern with the biologic phenotype, afford a deeper understanding of the phenotype and offer the possibility to predict biological or clinical behavior in subsequent unknown analytes. Genomics has already yielded clinically useful results in oncology, particularly breast cancer, lymphomas, and leukemias.

The predominant technology currently employed is the DNA microarray chip, which has rapidly evolved into a highly versatile, standardized research tool and is poised to have an important impact clinically. A chip is composed of short synthetic oligomer probes, corresponding to each of the genes of interest, up to all possible expressed genes, attached to an inert platform. A microarray chip can then simultaneously assay thousands of expressed genes by measuring hybridization of sample mRNA to RNA oligomers fixed to an inert substrate in a two-dimensional array. Hybridization of complementary strands of RNA or DNA occurs with extremely high affinity allowing very sensitive and specific detection of low-level species with the ability to distinguish between sequences differing by only a single nucleotide.

Messenger RNA is isolated from a homogenized biological sample and a fluorescent dye is bound to the mRNA. The labeled RNA is then applied to the gene chip and allowed to hybridize with the pre-fixed oligomers, each of which represents a short sequence usually selected from the exon region of a particular gene. After hybridization and washing to remove unhybridized species, a scanner measures at each position in the array the level of fluorescence that corresponds to the measure of expression for each gene represented on the chip. The fluorescence measurements for each of the thousands of genes across each of the samples are stored in a database. Quackenbush offers an excellent review of the use of microarrays for tumor analysis [8].

Early microarray studies used fewer than 10,000 oligomer probes mounted on in-house produced chips. The potential power of microarray technology was readily apparent, and the technique was featured on the cover of the journal *Science* in 1991 3 years after the first prototype was manufactured. As interest and use increased dramatically, chips are now commercially manufactured and the number of oligomer probes represented on a chip has also greatly increased, recently culminating in the Affymetrix Human Exon chip, which contains ~1.4 million probes that cover each exon in the human genome, allowing alternate splicing to be investigated over the entire genome. In addition to characterizing exon regions of genes, probes representing mutated sequences have been utilized to rapidly characterize mutations occurring at known sites, while other probes can be designed to profile micro-RNA or other genetic elements of interest [9,10].

Other profiling techniques can give information about the genome that may be complementary to mRNA expression levels [5,6,11–13]. Comparative genomic hybridization allows a rapid means of determining changes in gene copy number across the genome, relative to that in normal tissues. This technique can be performed with gene arrays similar to those used for profiling mRNA, or can be used without arrays to analyze metaphase chromosomal preparations. For example, specific amplification on chromosome 3q was identified to be associated with squamous cell lung cancer [12]. Profiling of large numbers of single nucleotide polymorphisms (SNPs) allow linkage of phenotype inheritance with specific chromosomal regions in populations as well as uncovering losses of heterozygosity in tumor samples that may be related to malignant transformation and disease phenotype. However, these techniques that measure gene copy number lack the capacity to detect changes in gene expression produced by any of a myriad of other factors regulating gene expression, whereas cDNA microarray experiments assessing mRNA levels can, at least theoretically, detect perturbations reflecting underlying epigenetic mechanisms as well as mutations or chromosomal aberrations. These genomic techniques thus capture less of the complexity responsible for phenotypic variability in lung cancer and, while of demonstrated utility in specific cases such as associating epidermal growth factor receptor (EGFR) amplification with clinical benefit from EGFR tyrosine kinase inhibitors, may be less useful for developing complex predictive models of clinical utility. However, specific genomic alterations may be important in offering insight into the biological relationships discovered by profiling mRNA levels, especially when a single or limited number of genomic alterations drive the biology.

Proteomics

Proteomics encompasses the study of protein expression, including spatial and temporal profiles, posttranslational modifications, and interactions with other molecules. Several important analytical tools and methodologies have been used extensively in proteomic research.

Mass spectrometry (MS) features prominently as the most accurate means of determining the molecular weight of proteins, and is sensitive in detecting proteins in low concentrations. MS can be coupled with a variety of protein separation techniques including gel and column separations, and can also be used directly to assay protein profiles in tissues or blood without a separation step.

A mass spectrometer is an instrument that ionizes molecules from a sample and measures the abundance and the ratio of molecular mass to unit charge (m/z) for all ions produced above a certain sensitivity threshold. A sample is ionized in a vacuum and the m/z ratios of each ionized species are distinguished by different physical properties depending on the type of detector: time-of-flight (TOF), Fourier-transform (FT), quadrupole etc. Two methods of ionization are generally employed: matrix-assisted laser desorption/ionization (MALDI), and electrospray ionization (ESI). The important distinction between MALDI and ESI is that MALDI produces ions by laser irradiation of samples fixed to a solid conductive plate coated with a crystalline layer of organic acid; whereas, ESI produces ions from a sample in solution as it passes through a small-bore highly charge capillary. MALDI, and the closely related technique, surface enhanced laser desorption/ionization (SELDI), can be used to produce protein profiles from frozen tissue sections or whole cell cytological preparations; unfortunately, with limited exceptions, paraffin-embedded tissue cannot be used. Multiple protein mass spectra can be obtained from different positions on a frozen tissue section, allowing analysis of a protein's spatial distribution and production of two-dimensional images of protein location and abundance. Thus, MALDI is useful for discerning field effects or distinguishing protein expression in tumor from proteins found in surrounding stroma or lymphocytic infiltrate. MALDI can also be used to analyze dried droplets of biologic samples such as blood, serum, or plasma, pleural or ascitic fluid, or fractions collected from column separations or extracted proteins from one-dimensional or two-dimensional gel separations. ESI requires samples to be in solution and has been particularly useful for online analysis of proteins and peptides in the eluate of column separations.

MALDI or SELDI experiments have both been used in profiling studies of resected lung tumors and patient serum. Data analysis software is then used to detect and quantitate ions. Various peak detection approaches can be used or alternatively the software can select an *m/z* window surrounding each ion such that the ion abundance data can be put into "bins" across all the samples with the measured ion current in each bin corresponds to the relative expression of a protein. This allows a protein's expression level to be compared between samples and each bin can be used to simplify the data and define molecular variables that are then correlated with clinical parameters in profiling studies. However, these techniques have many drawbacks. Only 10^2–10^3 proteins are typically observed in a MALDI spectrum, falling far short of the number of mRNA species detectable with microarray experiments. Additionally, whereas, oligomer sequences allow the direct identification of the genes expressed in a sample analyzed in a microarray experiment, MALDI spectra identifies a protein only by its *m/z* ratio, which is insufficient for determining its unique identity. Although *m/z* ratios and relative abundance levels may be sufficient for describing a molecular "signature" or "fingerprint" associated with a clinical parameter, the interpretation of such a result in biological context requires knowledge of the identity of proteins responsible for the profile, which requires, at least for profiles derived using MALDI TOF, a laborious separation and purification of each protein of interest followed by sequencing of its amino acids.

More recently the technique of tandem mass spectrometry, also called MS/MS, has enabled direct sequencing of peptides in a mixture. Intact peptide ions are separated in one stage of the mass spectrometer; next a collision gas is introduced into the vacuum, which causes the ions to fragment, producing characteristic fragment ions resulting from cleavage of the carbon–carbon and carbon–nitrogen bonds of the polypeptide backbone. These fragments are then separated and detected in the second stage of the mass spectrometer. This fragmentation does not occur efficiently with full-length proteins, which must first be digested into smaller peptides by proteolytic enzymes such as trypsin. For each peptide undergoing MS/MS analysis, a new mass spectrum is recorded that measures the *m/z* ratios of the fragment ions, and the identity of the parent ion is established by matching to the predicted fragmentation patterns of peptides in a human protein database. These fragmentation patterns can also be used to study posttranslational modifications.

Tandem MS is also a powerful tool for identifying disease-related proteins selected from gel electrophoresis or column-based separations. Two-dimensional gel electrophoresis can be used for proteomic profiling either by directly comparing spot intensity across a set of samples or by using differential in gel electrophoresis (DIGE), in which different samples are labeled with separate fluorescent dyes and are then mixed and separated within the same gel. Tandem MS is then used to determine the primary amino acid sequence and posttranslational modifications of any proteins determined to be of interest.

Tandem MS can also couple with ESI to sequence peptides as they are eluted from a high performance liquid chromatography (HPLC) or reverse phase column separation. Such HPLC/tandem MS analysis has led to a useful form of profiling known as "shotgun" proteomics, in which a biological sample containing proteins is digested and the entire cocktail of proteolytic peptides is separated using HPLC, with MS/MS sequencing providing the identity of these peptides and hence of the original proteins. Although sample analysis is time consuming and analysis of fragmentation spectra is computationally intensive, many more unique proteins are typically observed with shotgun proteomics than with MALDI, and the protein identifications are already established without additional effort. Because of the large number of proteins identified and the additional advantage of investigating posttranslational modifications, shotgun strategies show promise for general proteomic profiling.

Monoclonal antibody-based protein assays are perhaps the oldest and best-established proteomic technologies. They also provide an effective means to detect protein concentrations without the technical complexities of MS analyses, and multiple antibody-based biomarkers are routinely used in clinical lung cancer diagnostic studies. Interestingly, antibodies are often called upon to validate protein signals and relationships determined in MS profiling experiments, for example, by immunohistochemical analysis of tissue microarrays. However, the vast differences between these technologies make this sort of comparison problematic.

Antibody microarrays are another proteomic technique for assaying protein expression. Monoclonal antibodies against a variety of known proteins are fixed to an inert substrate in a two-dimensional array analogous to the DNA oligomers on a gene microarray. Protein lysates with fluorescent labels are applied to individual chips and fluorescence at each antibody position determines the relative expression of the corresponding target protein. These microarrays can be used to look for proteins related to lung cancer phenotypes and underlying similarities between samples in the same way as other proteomic and genomic profiling techniques. Additionally, antibody microarray chips may allow development of practical clinical assays for multifactor predictive markers derived using other technologies.

The development and characterization of new monoclonal antibodies remains laborious, and each antibody may have slightly different optimal binding conditions, so in general, antibodies are not readily applied to high-throughput "comprehensive" discovery efforts.

Data analysis and statistics

Each molecular profiling experiment yields data on the relative abundances of large numbers of mRNA species or proteins in a number of different samples. Statistical algorithms have been developed that allow clustering of different samples with similar expression profiles. When coupled with biologic or clinical data for each sample—response to chemotherapy, metastatic patterns, or survival, for example—statistical correlations between molecular profile clusters and clinical outcome can be made. Although different profiling techniques vary in the type and quantity of molecular analytes measured, the statistical methods used to analyze the data are quite similar. A first step may include removing low quality samples or data values from the analysis and filtering out molecular variables that are either expressed only sporadically, or expressed with low variance across samples. Sophisti-

cated statistical techniques are then required to discover statistically meaningful classifications of samples or relationships between clinical parameters and measured molecular variables. Most studies use a training–testing approach to developing these relationships. A sufficiently large training set is used to define a set of predictive genes or proteins and the accuracy of this model is then assessed in an independent testing set.

Once samples and genes are selected, a number of statistical techniques are applied to discover patterns of gene or protein expression that underlie tumor biology or phenotype. These techniques can be broadly classified as either "supervised" or "unsupervised." Unsupervised techniques use gene expression data without input of nongenetic descriptors to discover subgroups whose members share genetic similarities. Supervised techniques, on the other hand, include one or more clinical covariates such as histologic type, presence of distant metastasis, or clinical outcome data, and use gene expression data to discover relationships that specifically pertain to a clinical question of interest.

Unsupervised clustering is based on the hypothesis that there may exist subgroups that can be discerned solely on the basis of shared gene expression profiles, and that these clusters may exhibit distinct clinical behaviors not previously appreciated without the profiling data. Hierarchical clustering is a common means of defining genetic clusters in which correlations of gene expression between two samples are calculated and a clustering diagram is produced that visually represents underlying similarity of gene expression. Researchers define some number of subgroups based on the clustering results and attempt to discern whether any of these apparent genetic groupings has significance with regard to clinically relevant variables. A common method is to produce Kaplan–Meier survival curves comparing overall or disease-free survival for members of one subgroup against all nonmembers. Any number of subgroups can be defined from the results of a given clustering experiment, depending on the cutoff used to define two tumor samples as similar or dissimilar. A given cutoff may define two patient groups but may fail adequately to capture the genetic complexities of the sample set. A more stringent similarity cutoff can define a larger number of subgroups, each composed of samples that have more uniform gene expression profiles; however, this makes it more difficult for observed differences (e.g., in survival) to reach statistical significance, due to the shrinking number of patients in each group and increase the likelihood of arriving at false conclusions due to multiple subgroup analysis. On the other hand, if newly discovered clinical correlations are statistically robust, the information may be further validated in prospective studies and be applied in individualizing treatment decisions.

Supervised classification schemes start with two or more clinically or biologically defined groups—for instance, node negative versus node positive, responders versus nonresponders, or tumors that express a mutation versus those that do not—and attempt to determine genetic profiles capable of predicting to which group an unknown sample belongs. One can perform a clustering approach similar to that described earlier but with the constraint that the two dominant clusters must differ by the clinical variable of interest. Alternatively, one can use statistical tests to determine individual genes or proteins that may correlate with the clinical variable of interest and then construct a model using weighted linear combinations of these features to make predictions on unknown samples.

Both supervised and unsupervised techniques have the potential to "overtrain" the data, yielding models that perform well on the sample set from which they were derived, but with poor accuracy on independent testing cohorts [14,15]. Validation of results is thus the most important step in a molecular profiling experiment; studies without effective validation deserve little credibility, since even relationships that appear convincing may fail to have significance when applied to an independent set of samples. Some studies have approached this problem by arbitrarily splitting sample sets into separate training and testing groups. However, to be meaningful, the testing set should be used as such only once, without recursive retraining.

It is often underappreciated that high-quality clinical samples are difficult to obtain and costly to collect and store, and maintaining accurate and complete clinical follow-up is labor intensive. Thus,

the limited size of many studies necessitates the most efficient possible use of samples, and setting aside a large number of samples for adequate validation leaves fewer samples for training and less robust predictive models. Furthermore, the genes picked as predictive are very dependent on the patients included in the training set [16]. Cross-validation is an approach that maximizes the size of the training set while still allowing validation of results on a sufficiently large testing set [17–19]. In this method, a single sample or a small number of samples is removed from a set and the remaining samples are used to construct a predictive model. The model is applied to the sample or samples that were left out of the model building process, and its accuracy in predicting the feature of interest is recorded. This is then repeated a large number of times and the combined accuracy over all the left-out samples is reported as an estimate of the classification accuracy rate of the model.

Another method to minimize the necessary number of precious samples required for validating results is to use online databases of previously published gene expression profiles as independent test sets. This is an attractive method made possible by the increasing standardization of some of the technologies [20–26], but there are challenges in integrating data sets from different experiments. There may be substantial differences in the methods used to obtain the expression profiles; for instance, studies use microarray chips from different manufacturers and even arrays produced at in-house microarray facilities. Even data obtained for the same genes from newer versions of chips from a given manufacturer may not be directly comparable to earlier versions. Also, newer microarrays typically have more probes spanning more genetic elements than older versions. Thus, many genes may not be represented in both data sets, and it may be difficult to translate expression data from one set to another. With the advent of exon arrays, it has become clear that the location of the oligo within the putative transcript yields different measurement results. Furthermore, idiosyncratic differences in sample handling and experimental protocol can lead to other systematic differences between gene expression sets. Despite these challenges many studies have shown that relationships observed in one data set can be successfully and convincingly demonstrated to hold true in large independent sets. When efforts are taken to standardize procedures, interlaboratory reproducibility has been shown to be quite good [20–26]. Current microarray-based profiling will likely benefit from such increased standardization across laboratories, as well as the use of a single microarray platform and the ongoing development of bioinformatics tools to permit sharing of large data sets and integrating data optimally despite lab-to-lab differences. These advances will lead not only to more effective validation of models, but will also allow large-scale meta-analyses to look for important molecular–clinical relationships in much larger sample sets, with better statistical power for developing robust molecular classifiers [27–32]. Of course, regardless of its reproducibility in training and validation sets, the real rubric of success for any molecular classification scheme will be its performance in prospective clinical trials that determine whether its clinical use improves patient outcomes.

Clinical applications

Early detection and diagnosis

The peripheral blood is clearly the most readily available and clinically practical biospecimen source for early detection and diagnosis. Pathological states can cause disease-related changes in molecules circulating in the blood, due to altered cellular expression of secreted proteins, proteins being directly released into extracellular fluid after cell death, posttranslational modification by cleavage, glycosylation, or other processes, or as a result of the host's response to the disease. If a change in blood protein composition occurs reproducibly in the presence of a disease, then such a change may be useful for disease detection and diagnosis. For example, the demonstration of proteins leaked from damaged cardiac myocytes has become the gold standard for detection of myocardial infarction, even though they are not themselves causal.

One reason for the abysmal survival rates in lung cancer may be the absence of effective screening for early detection. A variety of screening tests for lung cancer in patients at high risk, including yearly chest X-rays, sputum cytologies, even when coupled with immunofluorescence or PCR, and bronchoscopic screening, have had a discouragingly negligible impact on survival. A recent report of a nonrandomized trial of spiral CT screening of smokers suggests the possibility that very small tumors can be detected with encouraging survival results [33]. However, these results must be validated prospectively, since lead-time bias is a possible explanation for the apparently salutary effect. Moreover, screening detected a number of small, indeterminate nodules, of which a significant minority proved to be benign. The cost of CT screening is not insignificant and a large additional cost—including increased morbidity and potentially mortality—is incurred by the necessity of additional diagnostic testing of suspicious nodules that subsequently prove to be benign. A noninvasive test for cancer detection potentially could be integrated with imaging modalities to help select patients with higher risk nodules for more intensive efforts at diagnosis and follow-up. A very high positive and negative predictive value for the targeted patient population is mandatory, but most important, the screening test or combination of tests must result in improved survival.

MALDI and SELDI have been used to profile blood, serum, and plasma, as have antibody microarrays [34–37]. Other studies have attempted to discover patient antibodies directed against tumor antigens that could have diagnostic utility [37–40]. To date, these studies have been small and incompletely validated and have yielded sensitivities and specificities much lower than what would be required for clinical use. However, as proteomic technology improves, a wider range of low-concentration protein species may be detected, some of which may be useful in detecting early lung cancer.

Other possible avenues for research include proteomic profiling bronchial washings or pleural effusion [41] to determine diagnostic or prognostic indicators. Gene profiles might also be helpful in distinguishing poorly differentiated lung cancers from other malignancies with similar histological appearance [42].

Subclassification and staging

Treatment decisions in lung cancer are based largely on the extent of disease as determined by staging criteria and generalizations on disease behavior associated with histological distinctions. Stage has a strong impact on determining which patients are most likely to benefit from different types of treatment: surgery does not improve survival of stage IV patients since it has no effect on metastatic foci; conversely, patients with stage I lung cancer receive little or no survival advantage as a group from currently available adjuvant chemotherapy because a significant percentage will have no residual disease following surgery and chemotherapy has limited effectiveness for those with micrometastases. Moreover, there is significant variability in the clinical outcome of individual patients within each stage classification; there are differences in metastatic potential, aggressiveness of metastatic disease, and response to chemotherapy. The ability to elucidate factors predicting individual prognosis and response to therapy will be invaluable clinically.

The most important pathologic distinction described so far is that between small cell and nonsmall cell lung cancer (NSCLC). These are readily apparent by histological and immunohistochemical evaluation and have fundamental differences in probable cell of origin, natural history, and response to chemotherapy. Subtype classification of NSCLC has minimal impact on patient care, with a few notable exceptions: e.g., recent studies suggest that EGF-R-targeted therapy may show overall benefit in treating certain patients with adenocarcinoma and especially the subset with receptor mutations. Unfortunately, the behavioral features that most likely affect clinical outcome—aggressiveness, likelihood of metastasis, resistance to apoptosis, and response to therapy, inter alia—are indistinguishable with conventional microscopic evaluation. However, these features clearly have underlying genetic determinants, and uncovering these with molecular profiling may lead to dramatic changes in the management of lung cancer.

Gene profiling experiments in other cancer disciplines have uncovered such determinants [43–55]. Five reproducible genetic clusters within breast cancer have been disclosed by mRNA expression profiling, with corresponding differences in prognosis and response to therapy, including a previously unrecognized subtype, the basal-like, or "triple negative" subtype with a distinctly worse prognosis [48,51–53]. Other expression studies have uncovered independent sets of genes capable of reliably distinguishing good prognosis from poor prognosis patients among women with node-negative, estrogen receptor-positive breast cancer treated with tamoxifen. The Oncotype DX assay (Genomic Health, Redwood City, CA) utilizes a 21-gene marker set, using RT-PCR to profile expression using paraffin-fixed biopsy specimens; from these a 10-year Recurrence Score predicting the rate of distant recurrence among women treated with tamoxifen is generated [49]. Survival benefit with chemotherapy appears to be limited to the poor prognosis group, indicating that this risk stratification may be useful in guiding treatment [50]. These risk predictors, as well as the Affymetrix 70-gene assay [54,55], and the wound response model [44,45], are based on different sets of genes with relatively little overlap, yet they have demonstrated similar ability to distinguish high risk from low risk node-negative, estrogen receptor-positive patients treated with tamoxifen [46]. Further prospective studies are underway to determine whether adding chemotherapy will benefit those patients predicted to have worse prognosis when treated with tamoxifen alone.

Efforts to uncover useful predictive classifiers in lung cancer have also been fruitful. Many studies [6,11,14,15,28–30,56–78] have tried to identify subtypes of lung cancer based on overall similarities in gene and protein expression profiles using similar approaches to those successfully employed in breast and other cancers. The number of patients enrolled in these studies range from approximately 50 to 200, and the number of RNA probes has increased in recent studies as commercial chip technology has advanced. Early studies demonstrated that many clinical or histological groups clustered together by their natural genetic similarity. Normal lung could be distinguished from tumor, NSCLC from SCLC, and adenocarcinomas, squamous cell carcinomas, and large cell carcinomas largely segregated into their respective groups. The ability to differentiate samples with obvious histological differences was not a step forward in itself, but proved the concept that gene profiling experiments could make meaningful classifications. Several studies have demonstrated clustering of samples within one or more histological subtypes [6,14,15,56–58,61–65,71–74,77]. These results suggest that there may be genetic subgroups within the main histologic subtypes, with possible different biologic implications, although the reproducibility of observed subgroups has not been conclusively verified across studies.

Bhattacharjee *et al.* assayed gene profiles of 186 patients and described four distinct clusters of tumors, one of which was said to have worse survival than the others [57]. However, a majority of samples did not fit into distinct clusters, and the prognostic differences have not been validated in subsequent studies. Nevertheless, these were interesting observations about the general appearance of clustering within lung cancer, and the gene data and annotated clinical information has been a valuable resource for deriving and testing new predictive models.

Beer *et al.* studied 86 patients with adenocarcinoma, and described three dominant clusters within this cohort, one cluster differing significantly from the others prognostically [56]. A linear model based on 50 genes that could predict prognostic class in unknown patients was derived using a split sample training–testing approach in "leave-one-out" cross-validation. The conclusions were also tested in the Bhattacharjee *et al.*'s data set and found to be valid. The model was predictive for stage I patients in all testing sets and represents the first well-validated discovery of a prognostic indicator in lung cancer using molecular profiling. Chen *et al.* performed a proteomic analysis of the same patient cohort using two-dimensional PAGE and defined a protein-based risk index predictive of prognosis [6]. The proteins selected did not overlap with the previously developed 50-gene classifier, although the mRNA levels of several proteins were significantly associated with survival. Raponi *et al.* further validated the 50-gene prognostic profile and developed a separate 50-gene classifier through analysis of 129 patients with squamous cell carcinoma [71]. The two classifiers were combined to form a single 100-gene classifier applicable to both histologic types, which was shown to be a significant prognosticator.

Gene expression and annotated clinical data from these early studies and several others, e.g. .[62], were made publicly available, permitting the data to be further investigated through several meta-analyses [27–32]. These studies showed that many underlying genetic relationships were observed in multiple data sets, and that data sets could be combined to make larger training sets or for use as independent testing sets, despite significant differences between sample sets. Furthermore, meta-analyses combining lung cancer microarray studies with studies from other cancer disciplines have discovered profiles of chemotherapy response, metastasis, and oncogenesis that are predictive in multiple types of cancer [27,31,32]. Efforts to standardize microarray platforms and sample handling technique will also likely improve reproducibility across studies and improve the power of future studies.

Potti *et al.* have also recently described a prognostic indicator developed from 89 early-stage lung cancer patients and tested in two independent test sets from cooperative group studies [70]. The results from this work are being used to design a prospective clinical trial to determine whether this classifier can guide recommendations for adjuvant treatment. In one potential design, tumors resected from early-stage patients will be tested to predict good or bad prognostic category. All patients will be randomized to either receive adjuvant chemotherapy or not, in order to test the hypothesis that adjuvant therapy will improve the survival of patients with worse prognosis, regardless of stage, whereas, good prognosis patients will derive little or no benefit from chemotherapy. This would then test whether treatment strategies incorporating molecular predictors to guide treatment are justified.

The above-mentioned and other similar clinical trials may demonstrate that patients have better overall survival when treatment decisions take into account prognostic gene profiles. If this proves to be the case, then molecular profiling may be assimilated into clinical practice as a staging adjunct, particularly to predict which patients may not need chemotherapy. However, it is not at all clear that likelihood of relapse predicts likelihood of benefit from treatment.

Selection of therapy

Although there are numerous chemotherapy single agents and combination regimens with clear clinical activity in the treatment of lung cancer, there is wide variability in their observed effectiveness in individual patients. The ability to select an active regimen de novo in individual patients would be particularly valuable, especially considering the substantial treatment-related morbidity and the tumor morbidity and death associated with ineffective therapy.

In vitro drug sensitivity assays have been touted as a potential means to individualize chemotherapy selection, but so far have had limited clinical utility. If molecular profiling can effectively predict the clinical efficacy of different therapies against a particular tumor, it will profoundly impact patient care, particularly in the age of highly selective targeted therapies [27,69,72,79–87]. It is likely that such selective therapies will be useful only in small subsets of lung cancer patients, and clinical benefit can only be detected if these subsets can be molecularly identified. A number of factors make it more challenging to discover predictors of chemotherapy response using actual patient samples. Surgical resection of NSCLC is typically performed only if it can remove all known disease burden, and this is only possible in about a quarter of NSCLC patients and is rarely an option in SCLC. Thus, while resected primary tumors are well suited for molecular profiling, the requirement for fresh resected tumor tissue poses problems for prediction of chemosensitivity. Chemotherapy is most commonly used in disease diagnosed in advanced stages where fresh tissue is rarely available, in the adjuvant setting, where there is no followable disease, or after local or distant recurrence, in which case the disease may be genetically distinct from the original primary tumor. With effort, tissue specimens can be obtained from metastatic sites to be analyzed for molecular profiling in order to determine correlates with sensitivity; however, this poses new problems. The quality of the specimens may vary, the entirety of the specimen may be required for pathological evaluation, the number of tumor cells observed can be quite small, often too few to perform microarray analysis, highly contaminated with normal tissue elements,

and additionally, a small sample in a heterogeneous tumor may not be representative of the entire tumor. Furthermore, research studies attempting to analyze these samples are often hampered by the frequent opinion that nonclinically indicated biopsies from metastatic lesions are not warranted.

Many groups have applied molecular profiling to panels of cell lines, in which sensitivity to different agents is measured with in vitro techniques, and it is possible that the correlations between drug sensitivity and molecular profile could be translated to patient specimens [79–87]. Studies involving cell lines would allow for greater control of experimental factors affecting microarray assays and a straightforward determination of in vitro drug efficacy. Furthermore, these experiments offer the advantage that large numbers of chemotherapeutics can be economically investigated in parallel, including first-line and second-line agents in lung cancer, drugs used primarily for other types of tumors, and experimental therapies.

However, as for any model, cell lines only partially represent clinical lung cancer and are only hypothesis-generating. Human tumors may differ profoundly from their cell line derivates, and gene expression profiles of cells grown on culture dishes in growth media supplemented with various growth factors are likely quite distinct from those of tumors in vivo. Thus, it may be difficult to translate these molecular assays into a clinically applicable form. If this proves to be the case, it may be possible to develop predictors on other models that better represent human disease, such as implanting cell lines or cells from fresh human tumors into mice.

Molecular profiling may be particularly useful in the selection of targeted therapies. This class of anticancer drugs comprises a growing number of molecular agents that inhibit a particular signaling pathway or other crucial cellular process. Currently available examples of targeted agents include the EGFR inhibitors gefitinib, erlotinib, and cetuximab, the inhibitor of vascular endothelial growth factor (VEGF) receptors, bevacizumab, and the multitargeted agents, sorafenib and sunitinib. These agents can induce dramatic responses in some patients whose tumors are particularly reliant on the targeted pathway, but they often show little benefit in an unselected patient population. Molecular profiles can potentially be correlated with drug response, using methods similar to those described above for conventional agents, or they can be used to determine which tumors have profiles associated with the target gene or protein [80,81,83].

Bild *et al.* observed changes in gene expression after transfection of lung cancer cell lines with different oncogenes, and then used the resulting gene profiles to predict whether patient samples had overexpression or mutations of those genes [80]. Conversely, another approach that has recently been proposed is the compilation of gene expression changes after perturbation of a set of cell lines with a panel of pharmaceutical compounds [83]. These approaches can yield signatures of key molecular pathways and drug effects that can potentially be used to select patients for targeted therapy and may help direct basic research by implicating novel targets for drug design.

Future directions and conclusions

There are many challenges that must be met before profiling techniques can reach their full potential. A major limitation of many studies has been that the number of patient samples investigated has been too small to draw meaningful conclusions. One attractive means of increasing sample sizes is to combine data from multiple laboratories into shared databases. Improved standardization of sample handling, microarray or other analytical platforms, and quality control metrics will be essential for the success of such data sharing [20–26]. Advancements in bioinformatics and computational tools will also be required to efficiently utilize the large quantities of data, to adjust for variability between labs, and to integrate experiments that profile different analytes, e.g., proteomic and genomic studies.

Once a predictive profile has been described and validated, an additional challenge is posed in developing a suitable clinical assay. As already mentioned, this may pose a particular challenge for profiles derived from cell lines or animal models, or from highly technical, limited availability platforms. Once assays are developed, clinical utility will be aided by efforts to accommodate smaller samples and to get accurate results from potentially lower quality real-world clinical samples. MALDI has been shown to be effective in analyzing very small collections of cells, thus allowing analysis of biopsy samples and fine needle aspirates [88]. For microarrays, however, increases in sensitivity are required to expand their clinical utility to these types of specimens. Quantitative real-time PCR can provide such sensitivity and can be clinically used to measure expression levels of each gene used in a profile, and also can be applied to fixed tissue embedded in paraffin, rather than the fresh-frozen samples required for full microarray analysis.

Another challenge is the interpretation of results in a meaningful biological context. Significant clinical predictions and classifications can be made using a gene or protein profile as a "fingerprint" or "signature" without identification of its molecular constituents or knowledge of the biological relationships it represents. The theoretical and statistical framework of molecular profiling does not require that the underlying biology be understood, but such knowledge would undoubtedly aid scientists' ability to form and test hypotheses and identify new targets for therapy. Understanding the biology that underlies clinically significant molecular profiles will require the coordinated efforts of proteomics and genomics researchers, molecular biologists and clinical scientists, as well as statisticians and bioinformatics experts to explore the actions of individual proteins and pathways responsible for various phenotypes and behaviors of lung cancer.

Although many challenges remain, molecular profiling experiments have produced encouraging results in the study of breast, lung, and a variety of other cancers. In breast cancer, gene profiles are already being utilized clinically to predict recurrence risk of certain patients and better inform the decision to include adjuvant chemotherapy. Similar prognostic assays have been developed from microarray analyses of lung cancer, and a prospective clinical trial has been proposed to assess the efficacy of one test in selecting patients for adjuvant treatment of early-stage NSCLC. These early successes attest to the potential of profiling experiments to improve patient outcome through individualized risk assessment and optimal selection of therapy options. As proteomic and genomic technology and methodology continue to mature they will without doubt become more and more integral to research and patient care. The level of information and understanding that can be thus attained will bring about a paradigm shift in the study of cancer biology and the practice of clinical oncology.

Acknowledgments

We gratefully acknowledge Dr Dwight Kaufman, and Dr Angelo Russo, for their invaluable suggestions and insights.

References

1 Martin B, Paesmans M, Berghmans T *et al.* Role of bcl-2 as a prognostic factor for survival in lung cancer: a systematic review of the literature with meta-analysis. *Br J Cancer* 2003; **89**:55–64.

2 Mascaux C, Iannino N, Martin B *et al.* The role of RAS oncogene in survival of patients with lung cancer: a systematic review of the literature with meta-analysis. *Br J Cancer* 2005; **92**:131–9.

3 Mitsudomi T, Hamajima N, Ogawa M, Takahashi T. Prognostic significance of p53 alterations in patients with non-small cell lung cancer: a meta-analysis. *Clin Cancer Res* 2000; **6**:4055–63.

4 Zhu CQ, Shih W, Ling CH, Tsao MS. Immunohistochemical markers of prognosis in non-small cell lung cancer: a review and proposal for a multiphase approach to marker evaluation. *J Clin Pathol* 2006; **59**:790–800.

5 Chen G, Gharib TG, Huang CC *et al.* Discordant protein and mRNA expression in lung adenocarcinomas. *Mol Cell Proteomics* 2002; **1**:304–13.

6 Chen G, Gharib TG, Wang H *et al.* Protein profiles associated with survival in lung adenocarcinoma. *Proc Natl Acad Sci USA* 2003; **100**:13537–42.

7 Nishizuka S, Charboneau L, Young L *et al.* Proteomic profiling of the nci-60 cancer cell lines using new high-density reverse-phase lysate microarrays. *Proc Natl Acad Sci USA* 2003; **100**:14229–34.

8 Quackenbush J. Microarray analysis and tumor classification. *N Engl J Med* 2006; **354**:2463–72.

9 Yanaihara N, Caplen N, Bowman E *et al.* Unique microRNA molecular profiles in lung cancer diagnosis and prognosis. *Cancer Cell* 2006; **9**:189–98.

10 Lu J, Getz G, Miska EA *et al.* Microrna expression profiles classify human cancers. *Nature* 2005; **435**:834–8.

11 Li R, Wang H, Bekele BN *et al.* Identification of putative oncogenes in lung adenocarcinoma by a comprehensive functional genomic approach. *Oncogene* 2006; **25**:2628–35.

12 Massion PP, Kuo WL, Stokoe D *et al.* Genomic copy number analysis of non-small cell lung cancer using array comparative genomic hybridization: implications of the phosphatidylinositol 3-kinase pathway. *Cancer Res* 2002; **62**:3636–40.

13 Shibata T, Uryu S, Kokubu A *et al.* Genetic classification of lung adenocarcinoma based on array-based comparative genomic hybridization analysis: its association with clinicopathologic features. *Clin Cancer Res* 2005; **11**:6177–85.

14 Blackhall FH, Wigle DA, Jurisica I *et al.* Validating the prognostic value of marker genes derived from a non-small cell lung cancer microarray study. *Lung Cancer* 2004; **46**:197–204.

15 Wigle DA, Jurisica I, Radulovich N *et al.* Molecular profiling of non-small cell lung cancer and correlation with disease-free survival. *Cancer Res* 2002; **62**:3005–8.

16 Michiels S, Koscielny S, Hill C. Prediction of cancer outcome with microarrays: a multiple random validation strategy. *Lancet* 2005; **365**:488–92.

17 Braga-Neto UM, Dougherty ER. Is cross-validation valid for small-sample microarray classification? *Bioinformatics* 2004; **30**:374–80.

18 Varma S, Simon R. Bias in error estimation when using cross-validation for model selection. *BMC Bioinformatics* 2005; **7**:91.

19 Simon R, Radmacher MD, Dobbin K, McShane LM. Pitfalls in the use of DNA microarray data for diagnostic and prognostic classification. *J Natl Cancer Inst* 2003; **95**:14–18.

20 Canales RD, Luo Y, Willey JC *et al.* Evaluation of DNA microarray results with quantitative gene expression platforms. *Nat Biotechnol* 2006; **24**:1115–22.

21 Dobbin KK, Beer DG, Meyerson M *et al.* Interlaboratory comparability study of cancer gene expression analysis using oligonucleotide microarrays. *Clin Cancer Res* 2005; **11**:565–72.

22 Guo L, Lobenhofer EK, Wang C *et al.* Rat toxicogenomic study reveals analytical consistency across microarray platforms. *Nat Biotechnol* 2006; **24**:1162–9.

23 Patterson TA, Lobenhofer EK, Fulmer-Smentek SB *et al.* Performance comparison of one-color and

two-color platforms within the microarray quality control (MAQC) project. *Nat Biotechnol* 2006; **24**:1140–50.

24 Shi L, Reid LH, Jones WD *et al*. The microarray quality control (MAQC) project shows inter- and intraplatform reproducibility of gene expression measurements. *Nat Biotechnol* 2006; **24**:1151–61.

25 Shippy R, Fulmer-Smentek S, Jensen RV *et al*. Using RNA sample titrations to assess microarray platform performance and normalization techniques. *Nat Biotechnol* 2006; **24**:1123–31.

26 Tong W, Lucas AB, Shippy R *et al*. Evaluation of external RNA controls for the assessment of microarray performance. *Nat Biotechnol* 2006; **24**:1132–9.

27 Glinsky GV, Berezovska O, Glinskii AB. Microarray analysis identifies a death-from-cancer signature predicting therapy failure in patients with multiple types of cancer. *J Clin Invest* 2005; **115**:1503–21.

28 Guo L, Ma Y, Ward R *et al*. Constructing molecular classifiers for the accurate prognosis of lung adenocarcinoma. *Clin Cancer Res* 2006; **12**:3344–54.

29 Jiang H, Deng Y, Chen HS *et al*. Joint analysis of two microarray gene-expression data sets to select lung adenocarcinoma marker genes. *BMC Bioinformatics* 2004; **5**:81.

30 Parmigiani G, Garrett-Mayer ES, Anbazhagan R, Gabrielson E. A cross-study comparison of gene expression studies for the molecular classification of lung cancer. *Clin Cancer Res* 2004; **10**:2922–7.

31 Ramaswamy S, Ross KN, Lander ES, Golub TR. A molecular signature of metastasis in primary solid tumors. *Nat Genet* 2003; **33**:49–54.

32 Rhodes DR, Yu J, Shanker K *et al*. Large-scale meta-analysis of cancer microarray data identifies common transcriptional profiles of neoplastic transformation and progression. *Proc Natl Acad Sci USA* 2004; **101**:9309–14.

33 Investigators; IELCAP, Henschke CI, Yankelevitz DF *et al*. Survival of patients with stage I lung cancer detected on ct screening. *N Engl J Med* 2006; **355**:1763–71.

34 Gao WM, Kuick R, Orchekowski RP *et al*. Distinctive serum protein profiles involving abundant proteins in lung cancer patients based upon antibody microarray analysis. *BMC Cancer* 2005; **5**:110.

35 Sidransky D, Irizarry R, Califano JA *et al*. Serum protein maldi profiling to distinguish upper aerodigestive tract cancer patients from control subjects. *J Natl Cancer Inst* 2003; **95**:1711–17.

36 Yang SY, Xiao XY, Zhang WG *et al*. Application of serum seldi proteomic patterns in diagnosis of lung cancer. *BMC Cancer* 2005; **5**:83.

37 Zhong L, Hidalgo GE, Stromberg AJ *et al*. Using protein microarray as a diagnostic assay for non-small cell lung cancer. *Am J Respir Crit Care Med* 2005; **172**:1308–14.

38 Matsunaga H, Hangai N, Aso Y *et al*. Application of differential display to identify genes for lung cancer detection in peripheral blood. *Int J Cancer* 2002; **100**:592–9.

39 Zhong L, Coe SP, Stromberg AJ *et al*. Profiling tumor-associated antibodies for early detection of non-small cell lung cancer. *J Thorac Oncol* 2006; **1**:513–19.

40 Zhong L, Peng X, Hidalgo GE *et al*. Identification of circulating antibodies to tumor-associated proteins for combined use as markers of non-small cell lung cancer. *Proteomics* 2004; **4**:1216–25.

41 Tyan YC, Wu HY, Lai WW, Su WC, Liao PC. Proteomic profiling of human pleural effusion using two-dimensional nano liquid chromatography tandem mass spectrometry. *J Proteome Res* 2005; **4**:1274–86.

42 Gordon GJ, Jensen RV, Hsiao LL *et al*. Translation of microarray data into clinically relevant cancer diagnostic tests using gene expression ratios in lung cancer and mesothelioma. *Cancer Res* 2002; **62**:4963–7.

43 Alizadeh AA, Eisen MB, Davis RE *et al*. Distinct types of diffuse large b-cell lymphoma identified by gene expression profiling. *Nature* 2000; **403**:503–11.

44 Chang HY, Nuyten DS, Sneddon JB *et al*. Robustness, scalability, and integration of a wound-response gene expression signature in predicting breast cancer survival. *Proc Natl Acad Sci USA* 2005; **102**:3738–43.

45 Chang HY, Sneddon JB, Alizadeh AA *et al*. Gene expression signature of fibroblast serum response predicts human cancer progression: similarities between tumors and wounds. *PLoS Biol* 2004; **2**:E7.

46 Fan C, Oh DS, Wessels L *et al*. Concordance among gene-expression-based predictors for breast cancer. *N Engl J Med* 2006; **355**:560–9.

47 Golub TR, Slonim DK, Tamayo P *et al*. Molecular classification of cancer: class discovery and class prediction by gene expression monitoring. *Science* 1999; **286**:531–7.

48 Hu Z, Fan C, Oh DS *et al*. The molecular portraits of breast tumors are conserved across microarray platforms. *BMC Genomics* 2006; **7**:96.

49 Paik S, Shak S, Tang G *et al*. A multigene assay to predict recurrence of tamoxifen-treated, node-negative breast cancer. *N Engl J Med* 2004; **351**:2817–26.

50 Paik S, Tang G, Shak S *et al*. Gene expression and benefit of chemotherapy in women with node-negative, estrogen receptor-positive breast cancer. *J Clin Oncol* 2006; **24**:3726–34.

51 Perou CM, Sorlie T, Eisen MB *et al*. Molecular portraits of human breast tumours. *Nature* 2000; **406**:747–52.

52 Sorlie T, Perou CM, Tibshirani R *et al.* Gene expression patterns of breast carcinomas distinguish tumor subclasses with clinical implications. *Proc Natl Acad Sci USA* 2001; **98**:10869–74.

53 Sorlie T, Tibshirani R, Parker J *et al.* Repeated observation of breast tumor subtypes in independent gene expression data sets. *Proc Natl Acad Sci USA* 2003; **100**:8418–23.

54 van't Veer LJ, Dai H, van de Vijver MJ *et al.* Gene expression profiling predicts clinical outcome of breast cancer. *Nature* 2002; **415**:530–6.

55 van de Vijver MJ, He YD, van't Veer LJ *et al.* A gene-expression signature as a predictor of survival in breast cancer. *N Engl J Med* 2002; **347**:1999–2009.

56 Beer DG, Kardia SL, Huang CC *et al.* Gene-expression profiles predict survival of patients with lung adenocarcinoma. *Nat Med* 2002; **8**:816–24.

57 Bhattacharjee A, Richards WG, Staunton J *et al.* Classification of human lung carcinomas by mRNA expression profiling reveals distinct adenocarcinoma subclasses. *Proc Nat Acad Sci USA* 2001; **98**:13790–5.

58 Borczuk AC, Gorenstein L, Walter KL *et al.* Non-small-cell lung cancer molecular signatures recapitulate lung developmental pathways. *Am J Pathol* 2003; **163**:1949–60.

59 Creighton C, Hanash S, Beer DG. Gene expression patterns define pathways correlated with loss of differentiation in lung adenocarcinomas. *FEBS Lett* 2003; **540**:167–70.

60 Cuezva JM, Chen G, Alonso AM *et al.* The bioenergetic signature of lung adenocarcinomas is a molecular marker of cancer diagnosis and prognosis. *Carcinogenesis* 2004; **25**:1157–63.

61 Endoh H, Tomida S, Yatabe Y *et al.* Prognostic model of pulmonary adenocarcinoma by expression profiling of eight genes as determined by quantitative real-time reverse transcriptase polymerase chain reaction. *J Clin Oncol* 2004; **22**:811–19.

62 Garber ME, Troyanskaya OG, Schluens K *et al.* Diversity of gene expression in adenocarcinoma of the lung. *Proc Natl Acad Sci USA* 2001; **98**:13784–9.

63 Hayes DN, Monti S, Parmigiani G *et al.* Gene expression profiling reveals reproducible human lung adenocarcinoma subtypes in multiple independent patient cohorts. *J Clin Oncol* 2006; **24**:5079–90.

64 Inamura K, Fujiwara T, Hoshida Y *et al.* Two subclasses of lung squamous cell carcinoma with different gene expression profiles and prognosis identified by hierarchical clustering and non-negative matrix factorization. *Oncogene* 2005; **24**:7105–13.

65 Larsen JE, Pavey SJ, Passmore LH *et al.* Expression profiling defines a recurrence signature in lung squamous cell carcinoma. *Carcinogenesis* 2007; **28**:760–6.

66 Li C, Chen Z, Xiao Z *et al.* Comparative proteomics analysis of human lung squamous carcinoma. *Biochem Biophys Res Commun* 2003; **309**:253–60.

67 Miura K, Bowman ED, Simon R *et al.* Laser capture microdissection and microarray expression analysis of lung adenocarcinoma reveals tobacco smoking- and prognosis-related molecular profiles. *Cancer Res* 2002; **62**:3244–50.

68 Muller-Tidow C, Diederichs S, Bulk E *et al.* Identification of metastasis-associated receptor tyrosine kinases in non-small cell lung cancer. *Cancer Res* 2005; **65**:1778–82.

69 Petty RD, Kerr KM, Murray GI *et al.* Tumor transcriptome reveals the predictive and prognostic impact of lysosomal protease inhibitors in non-small-cell lung cancer. *J Clin Oncol* 2006; **24**:1729–44.

70 Potti A, Mukherjee S, Petersen R *et al.* A genomic strategy to refine prognosis in early-stage non-small-cell lung cancer. *N Engl J Med* 2006; **355**:570–80.

71 Raponi M, Zhang Y, Yu J *et al.* Gene expression signatures for predicting prognosis of squamous cell and adenocarcinomas of the lung. *Cancer Res* 2006; **66**:7466–72.

72 Takeuchi T, Tomida S, Yatabe Y *et al.* Expression profile-defined classification of lung adenocarcinoma shows close relationship with underlying major genetic changes and clinicopathologic behaviors. *J Clin Oncol* 2006; **24**:1679–88.

73 Talbot SG, Estilo C, Maghami E *et al.* Gene expression profiling allows distinction between primary and metastatic squamous cell carcinomas in the lung. *Cancer Res* 2005; **65**:3063–71.

74 Tomida S, Koshikawa K, Yatabe Y *et al.* Gene expression-based, individualized outcome prediction for surgically treated lung cancer patients. *Oncogene* 2004; **23**:5360–70.

75 Ullmann R, Morbini P, Halbwedl I *et al.* Protein expression profiles in adenocarcinomas and squamous cell carcinomas of the lung generated using tissue microarrays. *J Pathol* 2004; **203**:798–807.

76 Xi L, Lyons-Weiler J, Coello MC *et al.* Prediction of lymph node metastasis by analysis of gene expression profiles in primary lung adenocarcinomas. *Clin Cancer Res* 2005; **11**:4128–35.

77 Yamagata N, Shyr Y, Yanagisawa K *et al.* A training–testing approach to the molecular classification of resected non-small cell lung cancer. *Clin Cancer Res* 2003; **9**:4965–704.

78 Yanagisawa K, Shyr Y, Xu BJ *et al.* Proteomic patterns of tumour subsets in non-small-cell lung cancer. *Lancet* 2003; **362**:433–9.

79 Balko JM, Potti A, Saunders C *et al.* Gene expression patterns that predict sensitivity to epidermal growth factor receptor tyrosine kinase inhibitors in lung cancer cell lines and human lung tumors. *BMC Genomics* 2006; **7**:289.

80 Bild AH, Yao G, Chang JT *et al.* Oncogenic pathway signatures in human cancers as a guide to targeted therapies. *Nature* 2006; **439**:353–7.

81 Coldren CD, Helfrich BA, Witta SE *et al.* Baseline gene expression predicts sensitivity to gefitinib in non-small cell lung cancer cell lines. *Mol Cancer Res* 2006; **4**: 521–8.

82 Gemma A, Li C, Sugiyama Y *et al.* Anticancer drug clustering in lung cancer based on gene expression profiles and sensitivity database. *BMC Cancer* 2006; **6**:174.

83 Lamb J, Crawford ED, Peck D *et al.* The connectivity map: using gene-expression signatures to con-

nect small molecules, genes, and disease. *Science* 2006; **313**:1929–35.

84 Ma Y, Ding Z, Qian Y *et al.* Predicting cancer drug response by proteomic profiling. *Clin Cancer Res* 2006; **12**:4583–9.

85 Potti A, Dressman HK, Bild A *et al.* Genomic signatures to guide the use of chemotherapeutics. *Nat Med* 2006; **12**:1294–300.

86 Rickardson L, Fryknas M, Dhar S *et al.* Identification of molecular mechanisms for cellular drug resistance by combining drug activity and gene expression profiles. *Br J Cancer* 2005; **93**:483–92.

87 Staunton JE, Slonim DK, Coller HA *et al.* Chemosensitivity prediction by transcriptional profiling. *Proc Natl Acad Sci USA* 2001; **98**:10787–92.

88 Amann JM, Chaurand P, Gonzalez A *et al.* Selective profiling of proteins in lung cancer cells from fine-needle aspirates by matrix-assisted laser desorption ionization time-of-flight mass spectrometry. *Clin Cancer Res* 2006; **12**:5142–50.

CHAPTER 11

The Role for Mediastinoscopy in the Staging of Nonsmall Cell Lung Cancer

Carolyn E. Reed

Introduction

The staging of nonsmall cell lung cancer (NSCLC) aids the physician in selecting appropriate treatment, communicating prognosis, and studying treatment results in equivalent patient populations. Once distant metastatic disease has been ruled out, focus shifts to the assessment of lymph node involvement. It is estimated that 26–44% of patients diagnosed with NSCLC will have mediastinal lymph node disease [1,2].

Detection of metastatic disease in contralateral mediastinal or hilar lymph nodes or supraclavicular lymph nodes (stage IIIB) generally renders the patient unresectable. Patients with ipsilateral mediastinal lymph node involvement (stage IIIA) constitute a heterogeneous population with varying treatment options and outcomes. This heterogeneity is emphasized by a study of 702 consecutive patients with N2 disease undergoing surgical resection. Five-year survival varied from 34% when one level was involved with microscopic disease ($n = 244$), 11% when multiple levels were microscopically positive ($n = 78$), 8% when clinical N2 disease in one level was detected ($n = 118$), and only 3% when multiple levels of clinical N2 disease were apparent ($n = 122$) [3]. The need to define the presence and extent of mediastinal lymph node involvement is important

as multimodality therapy has become more common. Therapeutic options will vary for subsets of the N2 patient population, and comparison of study results will require appropriate stratification.

The methods of staging the mediastinum include radiographic modalities, minimally invasive techniques, and invasive procedures as listed in Table 11.1 [4]. This chapter will focus on the role of mediastinoscopy in staging NSCLC, which has been considered the "gold standard." However, discussion of alternate techniques will emphasize that radiographic and endoscopic sophistication in staging has changed the present and probably the future utilization of mediastinoscopy.

Radiographic staging of the mediastinum

The initial staging of the mediastinum usually begins with noninvasive radiographic techniques. These techniques may direct who undergoes invasive staging and/or the most likely location of N2 positivity and therefore modality chosen for staging. There are presently three commonly used methods of radiographic mediastinal assessment: computerized tomography (CT), positron emission tomography (PET), and integrated CT-PET. Table 11.2 illustrates the sensitivity, specificity, positive predictive value (PPV), and negative predictive value (NPV) of each modality [2,5]. CT scanning of the mediastinum has poor accuracy, and denying a patient surgery based on CT-enlarged (>1 cm in

Lung Cancer, 3rd edition. Edited by Jack A. Roth, James D. Cox, and Waun Ki Hong. © 2008 Blackwell Publishing, ISBN: 978-1-4051-5112-2.

Table 11.1 Options for staging the mediastinum.

Noninvasive radiographic imaging
  Chest X-ray
  CT scan
  MRI
  PET scan

Minimally invasive staging
  Transbronchial needle aspiration (TBNA)
  Esophageal endoscopic ultrasonography with
    fine-needle aspiration (EUS-FNA)
  Endobronchial ultrasonography with fine-needle
    aspiration (EBUS-FNA)

Invasive staging
  Mediastinoscopy
  Mediastinotomy
  Extended cervical mediastinoscopy
  Thoracoscopy
  Thoracotomy

Adapted from Pass [4].

diameter) mediastinal lymph nodes should not be accepted without histologic confirmation. Although PET scanning has improved accuracy of mediastinal staging [6], initial hope from early studies that PET would almost eliminate the need for invasive staging has dimmed as more recent reports do not reach the level of accuracy desired [7,8]. PET fails to identify microscopic metastatic disease and certain clinical factors, such as size and location of tumor, need to be considered in the decision to proceed with invasive staging. The integrated CT-PET has the potential to improve accuracy and further refinements are expected [5,9].

Controversy exists over whether invasive mediastinal staging is still needed if radiographic assessment is negative. In a series of 271 clinical stage I CT-negative NSCLC patients undergoing resection after negative mediastinoscopy, N2 disease was found in 9.2% [10]. In a similar study, the negative predictive value of mediastinoscopy was 93.4% [11]. In a small study where both PET and CT scanning did not identify mediastinal lymph node involvement, 8% of patients had pathologically positive nodes [12]. This finding was confirmed in a subsequent report that concluded routine mediastinoscopy is still the most economically reasonable strategy despite negative PET and CT scanning [13]. However, other surgeons have adopted a more selective approach to invasive staging if the mediastinum is negative by radiographic assessment, especially if the tumor is small (<2 cm in diameter) and peripheral. Selective use of mediastinoscopy is further discussed later in the chapter. The additional effectiveness (i.e., percentage of positive lymph nodes) of endoscopic minimally invasive staging in radiographically negative patients awaits further clarification.

Mediastinoscopy

History

Cervical mediastinal exploration using the Jackson laryngoscope was originally described by Harken and associates in 1954 [14]. Carlens, using a specially designed mediastinoscope and a suprasternal notch incision, advanced the technique [15], and Pearson and the Toronto surgical group further developed the indications and popularized the procedure as currently used [16]. Mediastinoscopy subsequently became the "gold standard" by which other methods of evaluating the mediastinum are compared.

Indications for mediastinoscopy

The main indication for mediastinoscopy is enlarged mediastinal lymph nodes detected by CT or PET positivity in any mediastinal lymph node level. There are certain instances where despite a normal CT scan, the incidence of N2 disease is increased and the application of mediastinoscopy is suggested. This includes large lesions and tumors occupying the inner third of the lung field, especially when the histology is adenocarcinoma or large cell carcinoma [17]. As noted previously, the use of mediastinoscopy will vary with surgeon preference and tolerance for an acceptable limit of false negativity. Other techniques are now replacing or being used in a complementary fashion to mediastinoscopy and will be discussed later in this chapter. One of the advantages of mediastinoscopy is the ability to obtain a large fragment of tissue for histopathology or even entire small lymph nodes as

Table 11.2 Radiographic staging of the mediastinum.

Modality	Number of patients	Sensitivity	Specificity	Positive predictive value	Negative predictive value
CT	3438	0.75	0.82	0.56	0.83
PET	1045	0.84	0.89	0.79	0.93
PET-CT	728	0.69	0.94	0.49	0.99

Modified from Toloza *et al.* [2] and Cerfolio *et al.* [5].

compared to clusters of aspirated cells for cytologic examination.

Selective indications for mediastinoscopy in clinical N0 patients include tumor factors (size and location) and histology. In a study of 164 patients with T1 adenocarcinomas or T1 squamous cell carcinomas undergoing mediastinoscopy, true negative (TN) and true positive (TP) rates for tumors 2 cm or less were 96% and 4% compared to large tumors (2–3 cm) with 84% TN and 14% TP rates [18]. In a study of T1N0 patients (N0 defined by CT scan with diameter <1.5 cm) with adenocarcinomas and squamous cell carcinomas undergoing mediastinoscopy, positivity was 9.5% in the adenocarcinoma group. However, none of the T1N0 squamous cell patients had a positive mediastinoscopy [19]. In a meta-analysis of 14 studies involving the size of lymph nodes detected on CT scan, if PET was negative and nodes were 10–15 mm in CT, probability of N2 disease was only 5% [20]. In a cost-effectiveness study of NSCLC patients who were stage I by CT and PET screening, routine mediastinoscopy was found to be of questionable value given the high cost (>$250,000) per life year (0.008) gained [21]. However, the prevalence of N2 disease was low (3%) in this study. As prevalence exceeded 10% in the decision analysis model, the cost-effectiveness increased. In a somewhat similar study comparing PET with selected mediastinoscopy to routine mediastinoscopy, prevalence of mediastinal involvement in potentially resectable NSCLC patients was assumed to be 20% and sensitivities and specificities of modalities were based on literature review [22]. The selective approach of using mediastinoscopy only when PET was positive for N2/N3 disease was shown to offer cost benefit.

Procedure

The technique of cervical mediastinoscopy is described in textbooks of general thoracic surgery. Right and left, high and low paratracheal nodes (levels 2R, 2L, 4R, 4L), pretracheal nodes, and anterior subcarinal nodes (level 7) are accessible via this approach. Correct positioning of the patient is important to facilitate insertion of the mediastinoscope into the pretracheal space. A metal suction catheter can be used to dissect fascial planes. The habit of always aspirating the structure to be biopsied with a spinal needle avoids vascular mishaps.

Ideally, the surgeon should routinely examine and sample five nodal levels (2R, 2L, 4R, 4L, 7). The false-negative rate of mediastinoscopy is undoubtedly affected by the skill and diligence of dissection. A survey of United States cancer practice showed how infrequently mediastinoscopy is done properly and that in over half of cases no tissue is submitted for pathology [23].

Results

In a review of over 5687 patients undergoing cervical mediastinoscopy between 1983 and 1999, the sensitivity was 81% and negative predictive value 91% [1]. In several large series, it has been emphasized that the majority of patients found to have N2 disease at thoracotomy after a negative mediastinoscopy have had abnormal lymph nodes located in levels that are inaccessible by standard mediastinoscopy [24,25].

Complications

The reported mortality rate of cervical mediastinoscopy ranges from 0 to 0.2%, and morbidity rates vary from 0.6 to 3.7% [1]. Ginsberg reported no deaths in 2259 mediastinoscopies [26]. Of the 2.0% of patients having a complication, only 0.3% required surgical treatment (thoracotomy or sternotomy). Significant life-threatening complications include hemorrhage (the most common), tracheobronchial injury, and esophageal injury.

The management of major hemorrhage during mediastinoscopy was reviewed by Park and associates [27]. During a 12-year period at Memorial Sloan Kettering Cancer Center, 3391 mediastinoscopies were performed, and 14 patients (0.4%) experienced major hemorrhage, which was defined as any bleeding that required additional surgical exploration for surgical control. The most common biopsy site resulting in major hemorrhage was the lower right paratracheal region (level 4R), and the most frequently injured vessels were the azygos vein and the pulmonary and innominate arteries. The azygos vein can easily be mistaken for an anthracotic lymph node. Needle aspiration prior to biopsy and avoidance of excessive traction are recommended to avoid bleeding. Possible factors that could increase the risk of hemorrhage include prior radiotherapy, induction therapy, prior surgical procedures in the mediastinum and reoperative mediastinoscopy.

The initial first step to control major hemorrhage is gauze packing. The mediastinoscope should not be removed because direct tamponade is facilitated. Damage to the main pulmonary artery or innominate artery usually requires prompt exploration via median sternotomy and this approach should also be used if packing is unsuccessful and the patient remains unstable. Median sternotomy is the most versatile incision, allows identification and control of most injuries, and facilitates institution of cardiopulmonary bypass if needed. If packing stabilizes the patient but hemorrhage is still ongoing, the surgical approach to repair the injury may include consideration of thoracotomy for possible definitive pulmonary resection.

Injury to the trachea or mainstem bronchi is very rare. It usually responds to packing with absorbable cellulose gauze and closes when the patient is extubated and no longer subjected to positive pressure ventilation [28].

Although unusual, the left recurrent laryngeal nerve can be traumatized if there is excessive dissection, sampling, or cautery at the left tracheobronchial angle occurs. Pneumothorax, wound infections, and arrhythmias are rare minor complications.

Extended cervical mediastinoscopy and anterior mediastinotomy

Standard mediastinoscopy cannot reach lymph nodes in levels 5 and 6, which are major drainage basins for left upper lobe tumors. Extended cervical mediastinoscopy as described by Ginsberg and associates allows exploration of subaortic and anterior mediastinal lymph nodes via the same incision [29]. Blunt dissection with an index finger is used to open the fascia between the innominate and carotid arteries superior to the arch of the aorta. A tunnel is created along the anterolateral surface of the aorta, and the mediastinoscope is inserted into this tunnel and gently advanced over the top of the aorta to the aortopulmonary window [30,31] (Figure 11.1). Electrocautery is not used to avoid injury to the vagus and phrenic nerves. Extended cervical mediastinoscopy when added to standard mediastinoscopy can increase the negative predictive value by 10–20% [1]. However, this technique is not commonly used in the United States.

An alternate approach to the aortopulmonary window is anterior mediastinotomy described by McNeil and Chamberlain in 1966 [32]. Although in the original report a vertical parasternal incision was used with resection of the second and third costal cartilages, more common modifications include a short transverse incision over the second costal cartilage which is excised or a second intercostal incision without cartilage incision. The mediastinal pleura can be bluntly dissected allowing access to the aortopulmonary window without entering the pleural space. A mediastinoscope can be inserted through the incision and regional lymph nodes identified and biopsied (Figure 11.2). When performed alone as directed by CT scan, the sensitivity of anterior mediastinotomy is 63–86% and

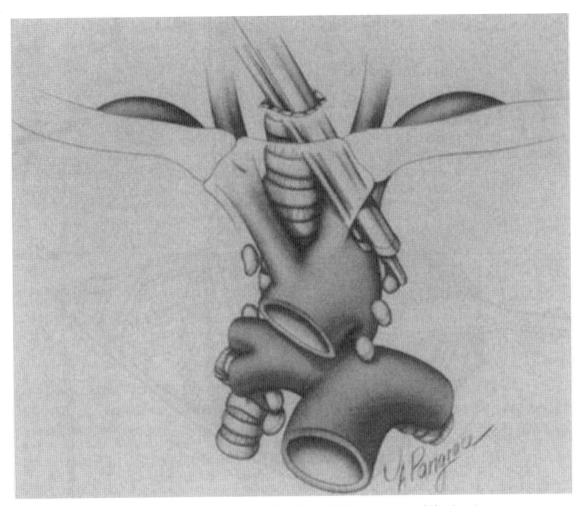

Figure 11.1 Extended cervical mediastinoscopy. Reproduced from [31] by permission of Elsevier.

the NPV 89–100% [1]. Today, anterior mediastinotomy is most commonly used to obtain large biopsies of anterior mediastinal masses as other techniques have become available to assess aortopulmonary lymphadenopathy.

Video-assisted mediastinoscopy

Video-assisted mediastinoscopy was introduced in 1994 by Sortini and associates [33]. The use of the video mediastinoscope allows wide and magnified operative exposure, ability to perform bimanual surgery, excisional biopsy of entire lymph nodes, and is an excellent teaching tool. It does increase the cost when compare to standard mediastinoscopy. In a study of 240 consecutive patients undergoing video-assisted mediastinoscopy, the mean number of biopsies was 6, mean number of lymph node levels sampled was 2.3, and mean operating room time was 36.6 minutes [34]. The sensitivity, specificity, and accuracy for the 154 patients with NSCLC were 97.3, 100, and 98.0%, respectively. There were no deaths, and there were two complications (0.83%), a pneumothorax and injury to the innominate artery requiring manubrial split and direct repair.

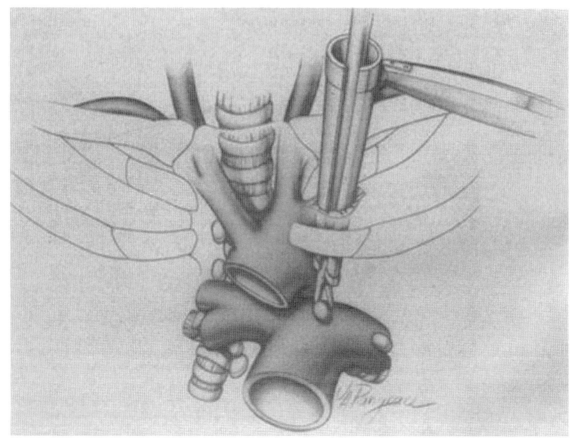

Figure 11.2 Anterior mediastinotomy. Reproduced from [31] by permission of Elsevier.

Redo mediastinoscopy

Multiple studies utilizing induction chemotherapy or chemoradiotherapy have documented increased survival in the subset of N2 patients found to have N0 or N1 disease at the time of surgery [35–37]. Although the use of PET scanning to assess response to induction therapy is being investigated, histopathologic confirmation of residual N2 disease is required if alternate therapies to surgery are being considered. Most surgeons are fearful of redo mediastinoscopy secondary to expected fibrosis and difficulty reaching the original biopsy site and the danger of increased complications.

In a small study of patients undergoing neoadjuvant chemotherapy for N2 disease, 24 patients underwent redo mediastinoscopy to assess response

[38]. It was possible to obtain a biopsy at the same level that was positive at the initial mediastinoscopy. There were no complications other than a wound infection. Of the 12 patients found to be N2 negative, 5 had residual N2 disease after thoracotomy and lymphadenectomy. The sensitivity for redo mediastinoscopy was 0.70 and accuracy 0.80. It was admitted that the technique was more complex secondary to peritracheal adhesions. The authors emphasized digital dissection and gradual access created by using the electrocautery. It was noted that the mediastinoscope was more easily inserted via the left side of the trachea. Dissection to create a left paratracheal tunnel until the posterior arch of the aorta is reached is also emphasized in a series reported by Van Schil and associates [39]. Dissection using the suction tip is then carried back to the

mid line and right side of the trachea. Bleeding controlled by tamponade was encountered in two of 27 patients. The accuracy of redo mediastinoscopy in this series was 85%. It was noted that subcarinal nodes were the most difficult to reach.

Video-assisted mediastinoscopy has also been successfully used in the postinduction setting [40]. The anticipated increased difficulty when radiotherapy is added requires further evaluation.

Although redo mediastinoscopy is feasible, the use of alternate minimally invasive techniques to evaluate the mediastinum offers a simpler and less risky method to reassess the postinduction mediastinum. Although limited by fine-needle aspirations, the level of initial positivity can always easily be rebiopsied and multiple procedures are possible.

Alternative methods to mediastinoscopy

Both endobronchial ultrasonography (EBUS) and esophageal endoscopic ultrasonography (EUS) allow excellent visualization of the mediastinum. By adding real-time fine-needle aspiration (FNA) to both techniques, histologic confirmation of mediastinal disease can be obtained in an outpatient setting with conscious sedation, and even minor complications are rare (i.e., these methods are minimally invasive). As shown in Figure 11.3, the diagnostic reach of EBUS-FNA and EUS-FNA is complementary [41]. EUS-FNA allows access to the retrotracheal space (level 3), the lower paratracheal region on the left (4L), the radiographic subaortic space (5), and the posterior mediastinum (levels 7, 8, and 9). EBUS-FNA provides access to the superior mediastinum (levels 2R, 2L, 4R, 4L), the subcarinal space (7), as well as hilar (10), interlobar (11) and lobar (12) lymph node levels.

EUS-FNA

In a large series of 242 consecutive patients with suspected or proven NSCLC and enlarged (>1 cm short-axis diameter) lymph nodes by CT, the sensitivity, specificity, and accuracy for EUS in mediastinal analysis were 91, 100, and 93%, respectively [42]. In patients with suspicious nodes by CT and/or

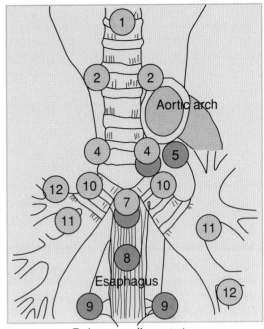

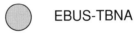 EBUS-TBNA

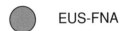 EUS-FNA

Figure 11.3 The diagnostic reach of EUS-FNA and EBUS-FNA (TBNA).(Reproduced with permission from Elsevier.)

PET in the posterior mediastinum, the sensitivity ranged from 92.5 to 96% and accuracy has been 97–98% [43,44].

EUS-FNA can prevent up to 70% of invasive staging in patients with radiographic evidence of N2/N3 disease [45,46] and therefore can clearly impact on patient management [47]. The utility of EUS-FNA in the setting of a radiographic negative mediastinum has yet to be clarified. In a study by Wallace and associates [48], a small cohort of patients (n = 24) without enlarged mediastinal lymph nodes underwent EUS-FNA and a surprising 42% had stage III or IV disease detected by EUS. In a study specifically assessing EUS-FNA in the CT-negative mediastinum, surgery was precluded by the finding of stage IIIA or IIIB disease in 12% of patients with NSCLC [49]. Malignant mediastinal adenopathy was detected significantly more frequently in lower lobe and hilar cancers combined compared with upper lobe cancers.

EUS also has the ability to detect T4 disease and allows biopsy of suspicious left adrenal lesions. The use of EUS-FNA is not meant to supplant mediastinoscopy as the methods are complementary. When used as a first approach to accessible enlarged mediastinal lymph nodes, EUS-FNA has been found by decision analysis to be cost-effective [50,51].

EBUS-FNA

Transbronchial needle aspiration has not been widely used in the staging of NSCLC as the reported yield has been variable, success is related to the size and location of the lesion, and the technique is essentially "blind" and highly operator dependent. Using EBUS as a guide, the diagnostic yield was increased (71%) and lymph node size and location did not influence success [52]. In a randomized trial of conventional versus ultrasound-guided transbronchial needle aspiration to assess 200 patients, EBUS guidance significantly increased the yield in all stations except in the subcarinal region [53].

As technology evolved, linear array EBUS has been coupled with fine-needle aspiration capability via the biopsy channel. In an initial report, the sensitivity, specificity, and accuracy of EBUS-FNA in distinguishing benign from malignant lymph nodes were 95.7, 100, and 97.1%, respectively [54]. EBUS-FNA was recently evaluated in NSCLC patients with no evidence of enlarged lymph nodes in CT scan [55]. Of 100 patients evaluated, 119 lymph nodes with a mean size of 8.1 mm were biopsied. Unnecessary surgical exploration was avoided in 19 patients, and malignancy was missed in two patients. Sensitivity was therefore 92.3%, specificity was 100%, and the negative predictive value was 96.3%.

The accuracy of the combination of EBUS-FNA and EUS-FNA has been reported to be 100% [56]. In a study of patients with enlarged lymph nodes in one of eight lymph node stations with a crossover design, EBUS-FNA was successful in 85% and EUS-FNA was successful in 78%[57]. Combining both approaches produced successful biopsies in 97% and diagnoses in 94%.

The learning curve for thoracic surgeons is probably least with EBUS. If both EBUS and EUS are available, it is recommended that EBUS be performed first unless lower mediastinal lymph nodes other than level 7 are the only enlarged nodes. In view of the minimal invasiveness of these techniques, the yield and cost-effectiveness of assessing a CT and PET-negative mediastinum should be further defined.

Video-assisted thoracoscopy

Video-assisted thoracoscopy can be utilized to assess all lymph node levels if performed on both right and left sides. It has been most frequently used to assess level 5 and 6 lymph nodes or when tumor invasion or pleural tumor seeding is suspected. It may be useful after induction therapy when both assessment of the N2 positive site and/or tumor status could alter attempt at surgical resection.

Future recommendations

The staging of the mediastinum will continue to be critical for optimal management of NSCLC. The combined use of EBUS-FNA and EUS-FNA offers the potential of more comprehensive access to mediastinal and hilar lymph nodes than is usual by standard mediastinoscopy. These minimally invasive approaches avoid anesthesia, do not necessitate clinical admission, and reduce risk. The same lymph node level can be repeatedly biopsied and this ability becomes increasingly important if downstaging is essential to surgical intervention, chemotherapeutic regimens could be added or changed, and correlation with PET findings need to be corroborated. There will continue to be instances when despite negative evaluation of CT-enlarged or PET-positive mediastinal nodes by EBUS and/or EUS, mediastinoscopy is still warranted by tumor characteristics, surgeon judgment, or patient risk profile.

References

1 Toloza EM, Harpole L, Detterbeck F, McCrory DC. Invasive staging of non-small cell lung cancer: a review of the current evidence. *Chest* 2003; **123**:157S–66S.

2 Toloza EM, Harpole L, McCrory DC. Noninvasive staging of non-small cell lung cancer: a review of the current evidence. *Chest* 2003; **123**:137S–46S.

3 Andre F, Grunenwald D, Pignon J-P *et al.* Survival of patients with resected N2 non-small cell lung cancer: evidence for a subclassification and implications. *J Clin Oncol* 2000; **18**:2981–9.

4 Pass HI. Mediastinal staging 2005: pictures, scopes, and scalpels. *Semin Oncol* 2005; **32**:269–78.

5 Cerfolio RJ, Ojha B, Bryant AS, Raghuveer V, Mountz JM, Bartolucci AA. The accuracy of integrated PET-CT compared with dedicated PET alone for the staging of patients with non small cell lung cancer. *Ann Thorac Surg* 2004; **78**:1017–23.

6 Birim O, Kappetein AP, Stijnen T, Bogers AJJC. Meta-analysis of positron emission tomographic and computed tomographic imaging in detecting mediastinal lymph node metastases in nonsmall cell lung cancer. *Ann Thorac Surg* 2005; **79**:375–81.

7 Reed CE, Harpole DH, Posther KE *et al.* Results of the American College of Surgeons Oncology Group Z0050 trial: the utility of positron emission tomography in staging potentially operable non-small cell lung cancer. *J Thorac Cardiovasc Surg* 2003; **126**:1943–51.

8 Gonzalez-Stawinski GV, Lemaire A, Merchant F *et al.* A comparative analysis of positron emission tomography and mediastinoscopy in staging non-small cell lung cancer. *J Thorac Cardiovasc Surg* 2003; **126**:1900–5.

9 Lardinois D, Weder W, Hany TF *et al.* Staging of non-small cell lung cancer with integrated positron-emission tomography and computed tomography. *N Engl J Med* 2003; **348**:2500–7.

10 Choi YS, Shim YM, Kim J, Kim K. Mediastinoscopy in patients with clinical stage I non-small cell lung cancer. *Ann Thorac Surg* 2003; **75**:364–6.

11 Gürses A, Turna A, Bedirhan MA *et al.* The value of mediastinoscopy in preoperative evaluation of mediastinal involvement in non-small cell lung cancer patients with clinical N0 disease. *Thorac Cardiovasc Surg* 2002; **50**:174–7.

12 Kempstine KH, Stanford W, Mullan BF *et al.* PET, CT, and MRI with Combidex for mediastinal staging in non-small cell lung carcinoma. *Ann Thorac Surg* 1999; **68**:1022–8.

13 Kelly RF, Tran T, Holmstrom A, Murar J, Segurola RJ. Accuracy and cost-effectiveness of [18F]-2-Fluoro-Deoxy-D-Glucose-positron emission tomography scan in potentially resectable non-small cell lung cancer. *Chest* 2004; **125**:1413–23.

14 Harken DE, Black H, Clauss R, Farrand RE. A simple cervicomediastinal exploration for tissue diagnosis of intrathoracic disease. *N Engl J Med* 1954; **251**: 1041–4.

15 Carlens E. Mediastinoscopy: a method for inspection and tissue biopsy of the superior mediastinum. *Dis Chest* 1959; **36**:343–52.

16 Pearson FG. An evaluation of mediastinoscopy in the management of presumably operable bronchial carcinoma. *J Thorac Cardiovasc Surg* 1968; **55**:617–25.

17 Daly BD, Mueller JD, Faling LJ *et al.* N2 lung cancer: outcome in patients with false-negative computed tomographic scans of the chest. *J Thorac Cardiovasc Surg* 1993; **105**:904–10.

18 Funatsu T, Matsubara Y, Ikeda S, Hatakenaka R, Hanawa T, Ishida H. Preoperative mediastinoscopic assessment of N factors and the need for mediastinal lymph node dissection in T1 lung cancer. *J Thorac Cardiovasc Surg* 1994; **108**:321–8.

19 De Leyn P, Vansteenkiste J, Cuypers P *et al.* Role of cervical mediastinoscopy in staging of non-small cell lung cancer without enlarged mediastinal lymph nodes on CT scan. *Eur J Cardiothorac Surg* 1997; **12**:706–12.

20 de Langen AJ, Raijmakers P, Riphagen I, Paul MA, Hoekstra OS. The size of mediastinal lymph nodes and its relation with metastatic involvement: a meta-analysis. *Eur J Cardiothorac Surg* 2006; **29**:26–9.

21 Meyers BF, Haddad F, Siegel BA *et al.* Cost-effectiveness of routine mediastinoscopy in computed tomography—and positron emission tomography—screened patients with stage I lung cancer. *J Thorac Cardiovasc Surg* 2006; **131**:822–9.

22 Yap KK, Yap KS, Byrne AJ *et al.* Positron emission tomography with selected mediastinoscopy compared to routine mediastinoscopy offers cost and clinical outcome benefits for pre-operative staging of non-small cell lung cancer. *Eur J Nucl Med Mol Imaging* 2005; **32**:1033–40.

23 Little AG, Rusch VW, Bonner JA *et al.* Patterns of surgical care of lung cancer patients. *Ann Thorac Surg* 2005; **80**:2051–6.

24 Luke WP, Pearson FG, Todd TR, Patterson GA, Cooper JD. Prospective evaluation of mediastinoscopy for assessment of carcinoma of the lung. *J Thorac Cardiovasc Surg* 1986; **91**:53–6.

25 Hammoud ZT, Anderson RC, Meyers BF *et al*. The current role of mediastinoscopy in the evaluation of thoracic disease. *J Thorac Cardiovasc Surg* 1999; **118**:894–9.

26 Ginsberg RJ. Evaluation of the mediastinum by invasive techniques. *Surg Clin North Am* 1987; **67**:1025–35.

27 Park BJ, Flores R, Downey RJ, Bains MS, Rusch VW. Management of major hemorrhage during mediastinoscopy. *J Thorac Cardiovasc Surg* 2003; **126**:726–31.

28 Pubakka HJ. Complications of mediastinoscopy. *J Laryngol Otol* 1989; **103**:312–5.

29 Ginsberg RJ, Rice TW, Goldberg M, Waters PF, Schmocker BJ. Extended cervical mediastinoscopy: a single staging procedure for bronchogenic carcinoma of the left upper lobe. *J Thorac Cardiovasc Surg* 1987; **94**:673–8.

30 Ginsberg RJ. Extended cervical mediastinoscopy. *Chest Surg Clin North Am* 1996; **6**:21–30.

31 Kirby TJ, Fell SC. Mediastinoscopy. In: Pearson FG, Cooper JD, Delauriers J *et al*. (eds). *Thoracic Surgery*. Philadelphia, PA: Churchill Livingstone, 2002:98–103.

32 McNeill TM, Chamberlain JM. Diagnostic anterior mediastinotomy. *Ann Thorac Surg* 1966; **2**:532–9.

33 Sortini A, Navarra G, Santini M *et al*. Video-assisted mediastinoscopy: a new application of television technology in surgery. *Minerva Chir* 1994; **49**:803–5.

34 Venissac N, Alifano M, Mouroux J. Video-assisted mediastinoscopy: experience from 240 consecutive cases. *Ann Thorac Surg* 2003; **76**:208–12.

35 Albain K, Rusch VW, Crowley JJ *et al*. Concurrent cisplatin/etoposide plus chest radiotherapy followed by surgery for stages IIIA (N2) and IIIB non-small cell lung cancer: mature results of Southwest Oncology Group phase II study 8805. *J Clin Oncol* 1995; **13**:1880–92.

36 Bueno R, Richards WG, Swanson SJ *et al*. Nodal stage after induction therapy for stage IIIA lung cancer determines patient survival. *Ann Thorac Surg* 2000; **70**:1826–31.

37 Betticher DC, Hsu Schmitz SF, Tötsch M *et al*. Mediastinal lymph node clearance after docetaxel-cisplatin neoadjuvant chemotherapy is prognostic of survival in patients with stage IIIA pN2 non-small cell lung cancer. A multicenter phase II trial. *J Clin Oncol* 2003; **21**:1752–9.

38 Mateu-Navarro M, Rami-Porta R, Bastus-Piulats R, Cirera-Nogueras L, González-Pont G. Remediastinoscopy after induction chemotherapy in non-small cell lung cancer. *Ann Thorac Surg* 2000; **70**:391–5.

39 Van Schil P, van der Schoot J, Poniewierski J *et al*. Remediastinoscopy after neoadjuvant therapy for non-small cell lung cancer. *Lung Cancer* 2002; **37**:281–5.

40 Lardinois D, Schallberger A, Betticher D, Ris HB. Postinduction video-mediastinoscopy is as accurate and safe as video-mediastinoscopy in patients without pretreatment for potentially operable non-small cell lung cancer. *Ann Thorac Surg* 2003; **75**:1102–6.

41 Yasufuku K, Chiyo M, Koh E *et al*. Endobronchial ultrasound guided transbronchial needle aspiration for staging of lung cancer. *Lung Cancer* 2005; **50**:347–54.

42 Annema JT, Versteegh MI, Veselic M, Voigt P, Rabe KF. Endoscopic ultrasound-guided fine-needle aspiration in the diagnosis and staging of lung cancer and its impact on surgical staging. *J Clin Oncol* 2005; **23**:8357–61.

43 Eloubeidi MA, Cerfolio RJ, Chen VK, Desmond R, Syed S, Ojha B. Endoscopic ultrasound-guided fine needle aspiration of mediastinal lymph node in patients with suspected lung cancer after positron emission tomography and computed tomography scans. *Ann Thorac Surg* 2005; **79**:263–8.

44 Savides TJ, Perricone A. Impact of EUS-guided FNA of enlarged mediastinal lymph nodes on subsequent thoracic surgery rates. *Gastrointest Endosc* 2004; **60**:340–6.

45 Annema JT, Hoekstra OS, Smit EF, Veselic M, Versteegh MIM, Rabe KF. Towards a minimally invasive staging strategy in NSCLC: analysis of PET positive mediastinal lesions by EUS-FNA. *Lung Cancer* 2004; **44**:53–60.

46 Kramer H, van Putten JWG, Post WJ *et al*. Oesophageal endoscopic ultrasound with fine needle aspiration improves and simplifies the staging of lung cancer. *Thorax* 2004; **59**:596–601.

47 Larsen SS, Krasnik M, Vilmann P *et al*. Endoscopic ultrasound guided biopsy of mediastinal lesions has a major impact on patient management. *Thorax* 2002; **57**:98–103.

48 Wallace MB, Silvestri GA, Sahai AV *et al*. Endoscopic ultrasound-guided fine needle aspiration for staging patients with carcinoma of the lung. *Ann Thorac Surg* 2001; **72**:1861–7.

49 LeBlanc JK, Devereaux BM, Imperiale TF *et al*. Endoscopic ultrasound in non-small cell lung cancer and negative mediastinum on computed tomography. *Am J Respir Crit Care Med* 2005; **171**:177–82.

50 Aabakken L, Silvestri GA, Hawes R, Reed CE, Marsi V, Hoffman B. Cost-efficacy of endoscopic ultrasonography with fine-needle aspiration vs. mediastinotomy in patients with lung cancer and suspected mediastinal adenopathy. *Endoscopy* 1999; **31**:707–11.

51 Harewood GC, Wiersema MJ, Edell ES, Liebow M. Cost-minimization analysis of alternative diagnostic approaches in a modeled patient with non-small cell

lung cancer and subcarinal lymphadenopathy. *Mayo Clin Proc* 2002; **77**:155–64.

52 Herth FJ, Becker HD, Ernst A. Ultrasound-guided transbronchial needle aspiration: an experience in 242 patients. *Chest* 2003; **123**:604–7.

53 Herth F, Becker HD, Ernst A. Conventional vs endobronchial ultrasound-guided transbronchial needle aspiration: a randomized trial. *Chest* 2004; **125**:322–5.

54 Yasufuku K, Chiyo M, Sekine Y *et al*. Real-time endobronchial ultrasound-guided needle aspiration of mediastinal and hilar lymph nodes. *Chest* 2004; **126**:122–8.

55 Herth FJF, Ernst A, Eberhardt R, Vilmann P, Dienemann H, Krasnik M. Endobronchial ultrasound-guided transbronchial needle aspiration of lymph nodes in the radiologically normal mediastinum. *Eur Resp J* 2006; **28**: 910–14.

56 Vilmann P, Krasnik M, Larsen SS, Jacobsen GK, Clementsen P. Transesophageal endoscopic ultrasound-guided fine-needle aspiration (EUS-FNA) and endobronchial ultrasound-guided transbronchial needle aspiration (EBUS-TBNA) biopsy: a combined approach in the evaluation of mediastinal lesions. *Endoscopy* 2005; **37**:833–9.

57 Herth FJ, Lunn W, Eberhardt R, Becker HD, Ernst A. Transbronchial versus transesophageal ultrasound-guided aspiration of enlarged mediastinal lymph nodes. *Am J Respir Crit Care Med* 2005; **171**:1164–7.

CHAPTER 12

Minimally Invasive Surgery for Lung Cancer

Michael Kent, Miguel Alvelo-Rivera, and James Luketich

Introduction

Minimally invasive surgery has revolutionized the management of many benign diseases. As an example, laparoscopy has largely supplanted open techniques for the treatment of morbid obesity and gastroesophageal reflux disease. However, this has not been the case for patients with malignant disease. For lung cancer in specific, only a few centers have developed significant experience with thoracoscopic lobectomy. Proponents of this operation note the decreased morbidity and equivalent long-term survival that can be achieved with the minimally invasive approach. Despite these claims, the procedure has not found widespread acceptance. In fact, among the 40,000 lobectomies performed annually in the United States, only 5% are performed thoracoscopically [1].

There are several reasons for this. The most important is that nearly all the data supporting thoracoscopic lobectomy are retrospective. Although some centers have extensive experience with the operation and have reported outstanding results [1,2], no large, multi-institutional trials have been conducted. Furthermore, the few randomized trials comparing thoracoscopic lobectomy to open resection are either small [3] or were performed when the procedure was still in its infancy [4]. Thus, critics of the operation emphasize that strong evidence

demonstrating decreased morbidity and equivalent long-term survival is lacking.

The other issue that has limited widespread adoption of the procedure is the potential for uncontrolled bleeding. Injury to the pulmonary artery or vein may occur during lobectomy, particularly for more central tumors or those with nodal involvement. Injury to these vessels is not more common during thoracoscopic lobectomy, but the concern is that valuable time will be spent while the procedure is converted to an open thoracotomy. Large series of thoracoscopic lobectomy have shown that this complication is extremely rare. However, this will remain an issue until the procedure becomes commonplace at training programs for thoracic surgery, regardless of the level of evidence that supports thoracoscopic lobectomy.

In this chapter the technique of thoracoscopic lobectomy, and the evidence that it leads to lower morbidity and equivalent long-term survival will be critically evaluated. In addition, the controversy surrounding the role of thoracoscopic wedge resection for early-stage lung cancer will be briefly discussed.

Technique of thoracoscopic lobectomy

Unfortunately there is no universally accepted definition for what distinguishes a thoracoscopic from an open lobectomy. In either procedure a thoracotomy is required for removal of the

Lung Cancer, 3rd edition. Edited by Jack A. Roth, James D. Cox, and Waun Ki Hong. © 2008 Blackwell Publishing, ISBN: 978-1-4051-5112-2.

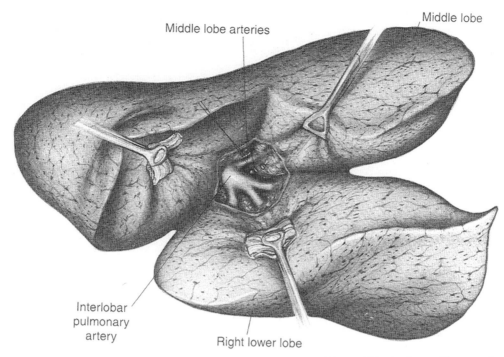

Figure 12.1 During an open lobectomy, the pulmonary artery is visualized from within the fissure. The parenchymal division that is required may lead to postoperative air leaks. (Reproduced with permission from *General Thoracic Surgery*, 6th edn, Lipincott Williams and Wilkins, 2005.)

specimen. For a thoracoscopic lobectomy this small (or "access") thoracotomy is usually limited to 5 cm in length, and a rib-spreading retractor is not used. The surgeon may use standard instruments for dissection, but visualization of the operative field is provided by a thoracoscope. In contrast, during a "VATS-*assisted* lobectomy" the surgeon uses a rib-spreading retractor and operates directly through the thoracotomy (usually 8–10 cm in length). In these cases the camera is only used for illumination. These two procedures are probably not equivalent in terms of postoperative pain and length of stay. Confusion over this terminology has made it more difficult to document the benefits of the minimally invasive approach. In this chapter we therefore define a thoracoscopic lobectomy by the avoidance of rib-spreading and use of the thoracoscope for visualization. The total number of ports is not relevant in this definition, but is typically between 2 and 4.

The technique of thoracoscopic lobectomy is similar to an open lobectomy in many respects. In both cases the hilar structures are individually dissected and divided. Similarly, the extent of lymph node dissection should not differ between the two techniques. However, one important difference is that in an open lobectomy the pulmonary artery is usually identified from *within* the fissures of the lung (see Figure 12.1). Unless the fissure is absent, this approach entails some division of parenchyma that overlies the pulmonary artery. The parenchyma is usually divided with either scissors or electrocautery, neither of which provides an airtight closure. This may lead to a postoperative air leak that could potentially increase length of stay. In the thoracoscopic approach, dissection within the fissure is usually avoided (see Figure 12.2). Identification and division of the pulmonary artery is instead performed from the hilum. The fissures are then completed with staplers. This technical difference is important, as it is claimed that the thoracoscopic approach leads to a lower incidence of prolonged air leaks, allowing earlier removal of chest tubes and

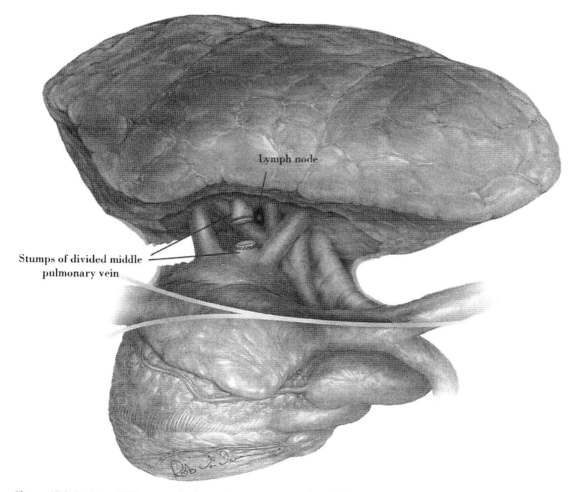

Figure 12.2 During a VATS approach, the pulmonary artery is identified from the hilum. In this figure the artery is visualized once the middle lobe vein has been divided. The fissures are divided with a stapler once the hilar dissection is complete. (Reproduced with permission from *Operative Techniques in Thoracic and Cardiovascular Surgery* 2004; **9**:98–114.)

discharge from the hospital. It should be noted that this distinction in technique is not absolute. On occasion the pulmonary artery is dissected from within the fissure during thoracoscopy, although this is less common than during open lobectomy.

Contraindications to thoracoscopic lobectomy

There are few absolute contraindications to thoracoscopic lobectomy. A prior thoracotomy is certainly not a contraindication. In fact, adhesions from prior surgery may be easier to visualize during thoracoscopy than through a thoracotomy incision. Complete pleural symphysis is a contraindication for any thoracoscopic procedure, as is the inability to tolerate single lung ventilation. However, complete pleural symphysis is rare in the absence of prior chemical pleurodesis, high-dose radiation therapy or a history of empyema. Moreover, most minimally invasive surgeons would at least attempt thoracoscopy to determine if the operation is feasible before converting to a thoracotomy.

Another contraindication is involvement of the chest wall by tumor. Although the pulmonary resection may be performed thoracoscopically, the requirement for a chest wall resection would obviate any benefit gained from the thoracoscopic approach. Thoracoscopy is certainly useful to determine if the chest wall is involved, but if so the procedure should be converted to a thoracotomy.

There are also relative contraindications to thoracoscopic lobectomy, although these are being challenged in experienced centers. The first is the presence of a central tumor, in which involvement of the hilar structures is suspected. Most surgeons would consider these cases inappropriate for VATS for the following reasons: (1) injury to a hilar vessel is more likely in this setting, with the possibility of significant blood loss, and (2) some patients may be spared a pneumonectomy if a sleeve resection can be performed, and this is difficult to perform thoracoscopically.

However, minimally invasive pneumonectomies for central tumors have been performed [5]. Experience with this operation is very limited, in fact the largest series has only reported seven patients [6]. In this report, a total of 25 pneumonectomies were performed over the study period. Only seven were attempted thoracoscopically, and one was converted to a thoracotomy. As such one can only conclude that the operation is technically feasible in a highly selected group of patients. However for most surgeons, even those with significant experience in thoracoscopy, a central tumor or bulky adenopathy would mandate a thoracotomy.

In most centers induction therapy is also considered a contraindication to VATS lobectomy. Reasons for this are twofold: (1) preoperative therapy may fuse the normal anatomic planes, rendering hilar dissection more hazardous, and (2) many patients will have residual nodal disease within the mediastinum, and this may be difficult to completely resect during thoracoscopy. However, one report has documented that thoracoscopic lobectomy can be safely performed in the setting of induction therapy [7]. In this series 97 consecutive patients were reviewed, 12 of whom had a thoracoscopic lobectomy. There were no significant complications in the thoracoscopic group, and median survival between the open and minimally invasive groups was equivalent. It should be noted that these results come from a highly experienced center, and represent a carefully selected group of patients. For most surgeons thoracoscopic lobectomy is reserved for peripheral, early-stage tumors, although this may change as experience with the technique increases.

Benefits of thoracoscopic lobectomy

Proponents of thoracoscopic lobectomy claim that there are several advantages to the minimally invasive approach. Specifically, these are:
– equivalent nodal clearance
– decreased pain
– lower perioperative morbidity
– earlier discharge and return to work
– equivalent long-term survival
A detailed review of the literature that supports or challenges these claims follows.

Adequacy of nodal clearance
The benefit of a complete lymphadenectomy versus nodal sampling for nonsmall cell lung cancer has not been resolved. Hopefully, a multi-institutional trial sponsored by the American College of Surgeons Oncology Group (ACOSOG protocol Z0030) will provide definitive data on this issue. What is clear at the present time is that mediastinal lymph nodes should be adequately sampled during pulmonary resection. This is important for two reasons: (1) it is critical for prognosis, and (2) decisions regarding adjuvant therapy are driven by accurate staging. The issue of adequate sampling is so important that some have suggested it be used to measure quality of care in thoracic surgery [8].

Three prospective trials, all from Japan, have investigated the adequacy of nodal sampling during thoracoscopic lobectomy. The first is a small trial of 29 patients who underwent thoracoscopic lobectomy with mediastinal nodal dissection [9]. What is remarkable about this study is that following thoracoscopic dissection, a thoracotomy was carried out *by another surgeon* and any remaining mediastinal lymph nodes were removed. For right-sided tumors,

40 nodes on average were removed during thoracoscopy. During open thoracotomy, only one additional lymph node was removed on average. Similar results were found for left-sided tumors. Based on weight and number of nodes, the authors concluded that only 2–3% of nodal tissue was "missed" with thoracoscopic techniques. Unfortunately, despite the excellent design of this study the results are not clearly interpretable. This is because it does not appear that a true "VATS lobectomy" was performed. The authors describe using an 8-cm thoracotomy with a "retractor." Furthermore, approximately 50% of the operation was performed under direct vision, the remainder using the thoracoscope. This does not meet the currently accepted definition of a VATS lobectomy, and it is not clear if the same degree of nodal clearance could be achieved using a true minimally invasive approach.

Two randomized studies have also documented the degree of lymph node clearance that can be achieved during thoracoscopic lobectomy. In the first study, 100 patients with clinical stage IA lung cancer were randomized to either a conventional or VATS lobectomy [3]. The mean number of hilar and mediastinal nodes removed during open lobectomy were 8 and 13 respectively, exactly the same as in the thoracoscopy group. Furthermore, an equal number of patients were upstaged to N1 or N2 disease in each group. Unfortunately, this study has been criticized for not describing the thoracoscopic technique in sufficient detail. The thoracotomy incision was 8 cm in size, and the authors do not state if a rib-spreading retractor was used.

In the second trial, 39 patients were randomized to undergo either a "complete VATS lobectomy" (in which the access incision was 4 cm in length and rib-spreading was not used) or an "assisted VATS lobectomy" (in which the thoracotomy was 10 cm in length and rib-spreading was used) [10]. Given the length of the thoracotomy and the use of a rib-spreading retractor in the "assisted" group, we would argue that this trial really compares the true VATS procedure to an open lobectomy technique. In the complete VATS group 32 nodes were submitted for pathologic review, compared to 29 in the control group ($p = 0.12$).

Decreased pain

Pain after thoracotomy can be considerable. For several reasons, minimizing this pain may have a significant impact on both morbidity and long-term quality of life. First, pain related to thoracic incisions has a significant impact on chest wall mechanics [11]. Patients with significant pain have a reduced functional residual volume, and are more prone to develop atelectasis, sputum retention, and pneumonia. Secondly, regimens to treat postoperative pain are themselves associated with morbidity. Opiates, for example, are associated with decreased ventilatory drive, hypotension, nausea, and urinary retention. These side effects persist even when pain control is supplemented with an epidural catheter [12]. Perhaps most important, pain in the perioperative period is a significant risk-factor for the development of chronic postthoracotomy pain syndrome [13]. This syndrome is characterized by a burning pain in the distribution of the thoracotomy incision that responds poorly to medication and may have a significant impact on quality of life.

Postthoracotomy pain is primarily related to two issues. The first is trauma to the intercostal nerve that occurs during rib-spreading [14]. The second is shoulder dysfunction caused by division of the latissimus dorsi muscle. Thoracoscopy is likely to lead to less pain, as the ribs are not spread and the latissimus muscle is largely preserved.

However, the evidence to support these claims is largely retrospective. Only three randomized studies have reported pain control as an outcome measure. The first study randomized patients to either a thoracoscopic lobectomy without rib-spreading or a "VATS-assisted lobectomy" with rib-spreading and a large access incision. The design of this trial was discussed previously [10]. In this trial analgesic requirements were less in the completely thoracoscopic group, although this did not reach statistical significance ($p = 0.07$). Unfortunately, this was the only measure of pain control that was reported. Neither pain measured by a visual analogue scale (VAS) nor the duration of narcotic use after discharge was reported. In an earlier trail from the United States, 55 patients were randomized to either a conventional muscle-sparing thoracotomy or a thoracoscopic lobectomy [15]. Acute pain was not reported in this study, although the authors did note that there was no difference in disabling postthoracotomy pain between the two groups. The final study randomized 47 patients with an undiagnosed pulmonary nodule to undergo either thoracoscopic or open surgery [16]. The majority of patients had a wedge resection; only seven had a lobectomy. However, we believe that this study is relevant given that rib-spreading was not used in the VATS group and the incisions were similar in size to those used during VATS lobectomy. Pain as measured by a VAS was significantly lower in the thoracoscopic group up to 72 hours after surgery. Similarly, narcotic requirements were less in the VATS group at all time points.

Several retrospective studies have also shown that the VATS approach is associated with less pain in the immediate postoperative period [17–19]. While this is important, evidence that VATS could lessen the incidence of *chronic* postoperative pain would be more significant. Chronic postthoracotomy pain is surprisingly common and can be quite disabling. For example, in a prospective study from Finland 61% of patients had pain 1 year after thoracotomy [20]. Pain was considered severe in only 5% of patients, however more than half of the patients said that pain interfered with their daily activities.

Unfortunately, there is no large study that documents the prevalence of chronic pain following thoracoscopic lobectomy. One small study compared 22 patients who underwent a thoracoscopic lobectomy versus an equal number who underwent open lobectomy [21]. Patients were surveyed by questionnaire at a mean of 13 months in the VATS group and 34 months in the open group. Although the follow-up was longer in the open group, four of these patients (18%) still required narcotics for pain control, compared to none in the VATS group. A similar study from our center concluded that thoracoscopy patients had less pain and narcotic requirements than those who underwent a thoracotomy [22]. However, these differences did not persist beyond the first postoperative year. Other studies without a control group have drawn similar conclusions. In a large series of 173 VATS patients (16 had a lobectomy), 75% had no complaints at 6 months after surgery, and no patient had severe

pain [23]. By 2 years, only 4% of patients had any residual discomfort.

Shoulder dysfunction is another potential complication of thoracotomy. Preservation of shoulder function is necessary for many activities of daily living. The restriction of shoulder function after thoracotomy may delay resumption of full activity, and could lead to significant long-term disability. To date two retrospective and one prospective study have documented that shoulder dysfunction is less after VATS lobectomy. In the first retrospective study, shoulder dysfunction was the same in both the VATS and muscle-sparing thoracotomy groups in the first 3 days after surgery. However, shoulder function returned to normal within 3 weeks in the VATS group, whereas it remained significantly impaired in the thoracotomy group [24]. A follow-up study compared shoulder function in 178 patients who had a VATS resection (wedge or lobectomy) to 165 patients who had a thoracotomy [22]. Within the first year following surgery 25% of patients in the open group had shoulder dysfunction versus 10% in the VATS group ($p < 0.001$).

One prospective study has validated these earlier reports. In this report, 29 consecutive patients who underwent lobectomy through a thoracotomy ($n = 11$) or VATS ($n = 18$) were followed [25]. Shoulder function was measured preoperatively and at 1 week, 1 month, and 3 months following surgery. Strength and function were determined by a physiotherapist using the American Shoulder and Elbow Surgeons Standardized Assessment forms. Shoulder strength and range of motion were found to be significantly improved in the VATS group throughout the study period. Importantly, the analgesic requirement was also lower in the VATS group, and this persisted for up to 1 month after surgery.

Lower morbidity

The prevalence of complications following open lobectomy has been prospectively measured by the Z0030 trial, a randomized study sponsored by the American College of Surgeons [26]. In this study, 1111 patients undergoing thoracotomy and anatomic resection for lung cancer were randomized to either lymph node sampling or a complete nodal dissection. Overall, 38% of patients had

Table 12.1 Morbidity following open and thoracoscopic lobotomy.

Author	Procedure	Evidence	Number	Mortality	Air leak	Arrhythmia	MI	Pneumonia	Length of stay
Allen (Z0030 trial)	Open	Prospective, randomized	1111	1.4%	11.5%	14%	1%	2.5%	Not Stated
McKenna	VATS	Retrospective	1100	0.8%	5%	3%	1%	1%	3 days
Onaitis	VATS	Retrospective	500	1.2%	4%	10%	0.4%	5%	3 days

one or more complications following surgery. However, the majority of these complications were minor: atrial arrhythmias (14%) and prolonged air leak (11.5%) were the most common. More significant complications such as pneumonia (2.5%) and myocardial infarction (1%) were rare. The operative mortality was 1.4%. This multi-institutional series represents a benchmark against which series of thoracoscopic lobectomy can be compared (Table 12.1).

The largest VATS lobectomy series was reported by McKenna [27]. Among 1100 cases, the operative mortality was 0.8%. There were no intraoperative deaths and only six patients required conversion to a thoracotomy for bleeding. Overall 85% of patients had no complications. Prolonged air leak (5%) and atrial fibrillation (3%) were the most common complications. Pneumonia and myocardial infarction occurred in 1% of patients.

Similar results were reported from Duke University [28]. Among 500 consecutive patients, the mortality was 1.2%, and conversion to a thoracotomy was required in 1.6% of cases. Atrial fibrillation and pneumonia were the most common complications, occurring in 10% and 5% of cases, respectively. Prolonged air leak occurred in 4% of patients.

What is clear from these series is that outstanding results with very low mortality can be achieved in dedicated centers. Massive intraoperative bleeding is extremely rare, and the conversion rate to thoracotomy is low. The incidence of minor complications such as atrial fibrillation and prolonged air leak seem to be lower after thoracoscopic lobectomy when compared to the Z0030 trial. Although

these complications are not life-threatening, they may have a significant impact on length of stay. Serious complications such as pneumonia and myocardial infarction are rare after thoracoscopic lobectomy, although comparable to open series.

However, outstanding results from dedicated centers need to be interpreted with caution. The most important issue is whether such a low complication rate could be achieved in smaller centers without the same degree of experience. The second issue is whether results from a single center with a few dedicated surgeons can be fairly compared to outcomes from a large randomized trial that enrolled patients from 63 institutions.

There is no question that there is a learning curve associated with thoracoscopic lobectomy. The approach to the hilar structures is different, and the thoracoscopic view can be disorienting for those used to open surgery. In our opinion, at least 30 cases are required before a surgeon experienced in open pulmonary resection will be comfortable performing a VATS lobectomy. Experience with other minimally invasive procedures, such as thoracoscopic wedge resection or laparoscopic surgery will shorten this learning curve.

The issue of whether outstanding results can be replicated in smaller centers will only be answered by a multi-institutional trial. Although the results have not yet been published, such a trial has been concluded by the Cancer and Leukemia Group B (CALGB protocol 93802). This prospective trial was designed to determine the perioperative morbidity and mortality of patients undergoing thoracoscopic lobectomy, without an open control group. A follow-up registry study is planned, in which surgeons can prospectively enter patients who have undergone either an open or thoracoscopic lobectomy. This study was designed in lieu of a randomized trial comparing the two procedures. Unfortunately, it has been estimated that an adequately powered randomized study would require approximately 800 patients. Accrual to such a study would be limited by an unwillingness of centers with experience in thoracoscopic lobectomy to randomize patients to an open procedure. A registry study may provide some data to support claims of decreased morbidity following thoracoscopic lobectomy, although issues regarding outcomes in smaller centers may remain unanswered.

Earlier discharge and return to work

Outside of a randomized trial it is difficult to substantiate claims that length of stay is shorter after thoracoscopic lobectomy. This is because length of stay is not only related to pain control and the incidence of complications, but also to the practices of the institution and country where the procedure is performed. It is therefore difficult to compare length of stay from different institutions or from separate time periods within a single institution. However, a trend toward earlier discharge has been demonstrated by several retrospective series.

For example, a comparative study from the University of Missouri evaluated 19 patients who had undergone VATS lobectomy [29]. These patients were matched to a cohort of open lobectomy patients on the basis of age, gender, and pulmonary function. In this study length of stay was markedly reduced in the VATS group (5.2 versus 12.2 days). The median time required to return to full activity was 2.2 months in the VATS group compared to 3.6 months in the open group ($p < 0.01$).

Similar results have been reported from Japan. In the largest study, the outcomes of 90 patients who underwent VATS lobectomy in three institutions were compared with 55 patients treated with an open lobectomy [10]. The thoracoscopic lobectomy group was subdivided into those who had a completely thoracoscopic procedure (no rib-spreading) and an "assisted" VATS procedure (a small thoracotomy with rib-spreading). There was a clear relationship between the invasiveness of the procedure

and length of stay: 11.8 days in the completely thoracoscopic group, 15.3 days in the assisted group, and 17.9 days in the open group.

Within the United States the largest series to report length of stay is from McKenna [1]. Among 1100 patients who underwent VATS anatomic resection, the median length of stay was 3 days (mean 4.8 days). Median length of stay was also 3 days in the series from Duke University [28]. Although there is no comparison group, these series clearly demonstrate that patients can anticipate a short hospital stay when thoracoscopic lobectomy is performed in a dedicated center. It may be argued that these short stays reflect efficient postoperative care and discharge planning as much as the operative approach. However, we would note that a *median* length of stay of 3 days would be most unusual in series of open lobectomies.

Equivalent long-term survival

Critics of thoracoscopic lobectomy suggest that inadequate nodal sampling and the potential for port site contamination by tumor will lead to inferior survival compared to open lobectomy. However, several retrospective series and a single randomized trial have minimized the significance of these concerns (Table 12.2).

The single randomized trial to report survival data was published in 2000 from Japan [3]. In this trial 100 consecutive patients with clinical stage IA lung cancer were randomized to either a thoracoscopic or open lobectomy. The median follow-up was 4.9 years. Within this period, 6% of patients in both the thoracoscopic and open group developed a local recurrence. The 5-year survival was 85% in the open group and 90% in the thoracoscopic group ($p = 0.91$). Although this study stands as the only randomized study on the topic, it is unfortunately underpowered to document equivalency between the two procedures. For comparison, the Clinical Outcomes of Surgery Study Group (COST) trial was an adequately powered study to evaluate laparoscopic colectomy for colon cancer [31]. The primary endpoint was time to recurrence. To document equivalency between the open and laparoscopic groups, a sample size of 1200 patients was deemed necessary.

Table 12.2 Survival following thoracoscopic lobectomy for lung cancer.

Author	Year	Evidence	Number	Mean follow-up	Stage	5-yr survival
Shiraishi [36]	2006	Retrospective	81 VATS, 79 open	46 mo	IA	89% VATS, 78% open
Shigemura [10]	2006	Retrospective	145 VATS	39 mo	IA	96%
McKenna [1]	2006	Retrospective	1015 VATS	NR	IA-IIIB	Stage IA: 80%
Onaitis [2]	2006	Retrospective	416 VATS	NR	IA-IIIB	Stage I: 85% at 2 yr
Iwasaki [35]	2004	Retrospective	140 VATS	NR	I/II	Stage I: 81%, stage II: 70%
Walker [30]	2002	Prospective	158 VATS	38 mo	I/II	Stage I: 78%, stage II: 51%
Sugi [3]	2000	Prospective, randomized	48 VATS, 52 open	NR	IA	90% VATS, 85% open

NR, not reported.

However, two large single-institution series have shown that stage-specific survival is comparable to historical series of open lobectomy. In the McKenna series, 1015 patients underwent thoracoscopic lobectomy for nonsmall cell lung cancer. For those with pathologic stage IA disease, the 5-year survival was 78%. Similar data was reported in the Duke series (2-year survival for stage I cancer was 85%). By comparison, Mountain reported survival data of 1524 patients treated by open lobectomy in 1997; this data was used to validate the current TNM staging system [32]. In that series, the 5-year survival of stage IA patients was only 67%.

The local recurrence rate was not reported in either the McKenna or Duke series. However, this data was provided in some smaller reports. For example, in an earlier paper from McKenna of 298 patients, recurrence in the incision occurred in one patient (0.3%) [33]. Comparable results were reported in a large series from France [34]. In that report, outcomes of 110 patients with stage I lung cancer treated thoracoscopically were compared with 405 patients resected through a thoracotomy. The recurrence rates (distant and local) were 25% for the VATS group and 23% for the open group. No patients in either group developed a recurrence at a port site or the thoracotomy incision. Several other retrospective series have documented similar findings—that overall and recurrence-free survival are equivalent among patients treated by open and VATS lobectomy [9,35,36].

VATS lobectomy summary

No appropriately powered study has documented decreased morbidity and equivalent survival with VATS lobectomy compared to the open approach. However, smaller studies have documented that nodal clearance is equivalent and that perioperative morbidity may be less with the minimally invasive approach. Certainly, large single-institution series have shown that the risk of uncontrolled bleeding during the procedure is extremely rare. It is likely that a well-designed randomized study to substantiate these findings will never be performed, given the reluctance of surgeons skilled in thoracoscopic lobectomy to randomize patients to a thoracotomy. A prospective study evaluating VATS lobectomy in a multi-institutional setting has been completed, and a comparative registry study is being planned. Currently, only a small percentage of lobectomies are performed thoracoscopically in the United States. Positive findings from these studies may increase this percentage, despite the lack of a randomized trial.

Limited resection for lung cancer

Lobectomy with mediastinal node dissection is considered the standard of care for patients with early-stage nonsmall cell lung cancer. Resection of the primary tumor by less than a lobectomy (i.e., anatomic segmentectomy or a wedge resection) is considered a "limited resection." Whether such an operation is appropriate for any subset of patients has been intensely debated for 25 years [37]. The clear benefit of a limited resection is that more pulmonary parenchyma is conserved. Consequently, it has been argued that a limited resection should be offered to those patients with pulmonary disease severe enough that a lobectomy is contraindicated. However, two additional issues have made this debate more relevant for a larger population of patients. The first is that screening for lung cancer in high-risk patients has become more common [38]. As such an increasing number of patients with subcentimeter tumors are presenting for resection. It has been argued that removing the entire lobe may not offer any survival benefit in these patients. The other issue is that a thoracoscopic wedge resection is technically straightforward. Most thoracic surgeons are very comfortable with this procedure, although this is not the case for thoracoscopic lobectomy. Therefore, in many centers the distinction between a wedge resection and a lobectomy is that the former can be performed thoracoscopically whereas the latter will mandate a thoracotomy.

The single randomized trial designed to resolve this debate was conducted by the Lung Cancer Study Group, and reported in 1995 [39]. In this study, 276 patients with clinical stage I lung cancer were randomized to receive either a lobectomy or a limited resection (both wedge resection and segmentectomy were allowed). Although the trial predated the era of high-resolution CT and PET scanning, the study required hilar and mediastinal nodes to be sampled before resection to confirm stage I disease. The authors found no difference in perioperative morbidity or mortality between the two groups. Also, there was no difference in pulmonary function at 6 months. Most importantly, the local recurrence rate was three times higher in the limited resection group, and this was associated with a 50% increase in disease-specific mortality.

Although the conclusions of this trial would appear definitive, the methodology of the study has been questioned. First, the survival advantage seen with lobectomy was calculated on the basis of a one-sided statistical test. If a more rigorous two-sided test was used, the reported survival advantage would not be significant at a p-value of 0.05. Second, only 60% of patients were able to undergo pulmonary function testing at 6 months. It is stressed by critics that the poor follow-up in this study should preclude any conclusions regarding pulmonary function from being made.

Since the Lung Cancer Study Group report, several retrospective series have confirmed a higher local recurrence after limited resections [40–42]. In some of these series overall survival was also decreased in patients who underwent limited resection [40,41]. Some studies have suggested that limited resection may be appropriate for smaller tumors. For instance, Warren [40] demonstrated that the survival advantage for lobectomy was only evident if the tumor was greater than 3 cm in size. However, in another study [42] that only included tumors smaller than 1 cm, 5-year survival was still higher after lobectomy than limited resection (71% versus 33%).

It should be noted that excellent survival following limited resection have been reported from Japan [43–45]. These studies have consistently shown that 5-year survival rates above 80% can be achieved with limited resection. A uniform conclusion of these studies is that limited resection is an acceptable alternative to lobectomy for "selected patients."

Therefore, the critical issue is to determine the criteria by which patients should be selected for limited resection. Unfortunately, retrospective series contain significant biases that make it difficult to establish these criteria. For example, wedge resection is often reserved for marginal surgical candidates with multiple comorbidities. Survival in the limited resection group will be lower because of comorbid disease, regardless of the effectiveness of the operation. Another issue is the potential understaging of patients who undergo limited resection. The rate of lymph node metastases in tumors less than 2 cm in size is approximately 20% [46,47]. It is certainly possible that a significant number of patients who undergo wedge resection with limited nodal sampling will be erroneously staged as N0, whereas they may harbor occult nodal micrometastases. Thus reports that claim to be restricted to stage IA patients likely include some with stage II or III disease. A recent paper from our institution supported this concern [48]. Over a 13-year period 784 patients with stage I lung cancer were reviewed: 577 underwent a lobectomy and 207 a sublobar resection. Those who underwent limited resection were much more likely to have limited nodal sampling: 43% of patients in the limited group had no nodes sampled compared to 3% in the lobectomy group. Furthermore, a 2% decrease in mortality was observed for every additional node resected, an observation that likely reflects more accurate staging with increased nodal sampling.

Another issue that may impact on mortality after limited resection is age. Although limited resection may have a survival disadvantage, this may not be relevant for older patients who have a limited life expectancy. This hypothesis was examined in a review of 14,555 patients with lung cancer registered in the Surveillance, Epidemiology and End Results Database [49]. In this study age itself was a significant predictor of both overall and disease-specific mortality. For younger patients (less than 65 yr), lobectomy conferred a significant survival advantage over wedge resection. However, for older patients (75 yr or above) the choice of surgical procedure had no impact on survival (Figure 12.3). This paper suggests that age is a confounding factor in series that compare limited resection to lobectomy. It also supports the practice of offering wedge resection to elderly patients, although this should be individualized. For example, an otherwise healthy elderly patient would likely benefit from lobectomy. On the other hand, an older patient with multiple comorbidities and a limited life expectancy may be appropriately managed with a wedge resection.

Adjuvant radiation therapy has been suggested as a means to reduce the high local recurrence rate following limited resection. The largest study to investigate this was a prospective, multi-institutional trial sponsored by the Cancer and Leukemia Group B (CALGB) [50]. This trial only included patients with clinical T1 lesions considered to be "high-risk" for lobectomy on the basis of pulmonary function testing. Surgeons were required to show proficiency

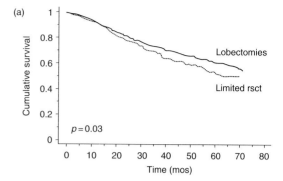

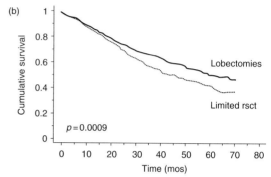

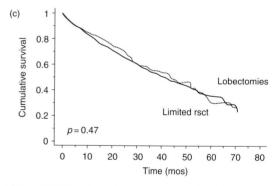

Figure 12.3 Survival of patients undergoing lobectomy or limited resection based on SEER data. Panel (a): Patients < 65 years of age; Panel (b): 65–74 years old; Panel (c): > 75 years. As illustrated, lobectomy offers no survival benefit for patients older than 75 years of age. (Reproduced with permission from *Chest* 2005; **128**:237–45.)

in thoracoscopy to participate in the trial, although the manner by which this was established was not specified. However, the results of surgical resection of these small tumors were poor: conversion to thoracotomy occurred in 17% of cases, and resection margins were positive in 9% of patients. Furthermore, a resection margin of more that 1 cm was present in only 44% of pathologically staged T1 lesions and 33% of those with T2 lesions. Fortunately, complications after surgery and radiotherapy were low in this high-risk population: the rates of perioperative mortality, postoperative respiratory failure, and radiation pneumonitis were each 4%. The median survival after combined therapy was 27 months. The authors of this study concluded that thoracoscopic wedge resection had a high technical failure rate, although radiation therapy could be administered safely.

Another technique to decrease the risk of local failure is to combine wedge resection with placement of brachytherapy mesh [51–53]. In contrast to external beam radiation, brachytherapy allows radiation to be precisely delivered to the staple line, with 100% patient compliance. At the moment the data to support the use of brachytherapy is retrospective. In one series from our center [52] the addition of brachytherapy to sublobar resection was demonstrated to lower the local recurrence rate from 17% to 3%.

One issue with limited resections is whether functional lung tissue is being preserved. In fact, patients with severe emphysema have been shown to improve their pulmonary function after lobectomy [54,55]. In these patients lobectomy is thought to improve pulmonary mechanics in much the same way as long-volume reduction surgery—by improving diaphragmatic excursion and restoring the elastic recoil of the remaining lung. Although it may be difficult to predict which patients will benefit from lobectomy, what is clear is that not all patients with COPD should be consigned to limited resection or nonoperative therapy.

Future directions

Radiofrequency ablation and stereotactic radiosurgery have both been explored as alternatives to conventional radiation therapy for high-risk patients with early-stage lung cancer. These patients have such severe cardiopulmonary dysfunction that they are unlikely to tolerate even a thoracoscopic wedge resection. At the present, data on these modalities is from small, single-institution series [56]. However, a nonrandomized clinical trial has begun accruing patients treated with RFA. This prospective trial, sponsored by the American College of Surgeons, will document technical complications associated with the procedure and the rates of local recurrence and overall survival.

In addition, two upcoming randomized trials will provide more data on the role of limited resection and brachytherapy. The first is a trial sponsored by the CALGB which will randomize patients with early-stage lung cancer to either lobectomy or sublobar resection. This study will essentially revisit the issues raised earlier by the Lung Cancer Study Group trial. The second is a trial sponsored by the American College of Surgeons Oncology Group (protocol Z4032). The study seeks to enroll patients with compromised pulmonary function and early-stage lung cancer (less than 3 cm). Patients are randomized to receive sublobar resection with or without brachytherapy. The primary endpoint of the trial is local recurrence. Hopefully, the results of these trials will allow the treatment of early-stage lung cancer to be guided by the highest levels of clinical evidence.

References

1 McKenna R, Houck W, Fuller C. Video-assisted thoracic surgery lobectomy: experience with 1,100 cases. *Ann Thorac Surg* 2006; **81**:421–6.

2 Onaitis M, Peterson R, Balderson S. Thoracoscopic lobectomy is a safe and versatile procedure: experience with 500 consecutive patients. *Ann Thorac Surg* 2006; **244**:420–5.

3 Sugi K, Kaneda Y, Esato K. Video-assisted thoracoscopic lobectomy achieves a satisfactory long-term prognosis in patients with clinical stage IA lung cancer. *World J Surg* 2000; **24(1)**:27–31.

4 Kirby T, Mack M, Landreneau R, Rice T. Initial experience with video-assisted thoracoscopic lobectomy. *Ann Thorac Surg* 1993; **56**:1248–52.

5 Conlan A, Sandor A. Total thoracoscopic pneumonectomy: indications and technical considerations. *J Thorac Cardiovasc Surg* 2003; **126**:2083.

6 Nwogu C, Glinanski M, Demmy T. Minimally invasive pneumonectomy. *Ann Thorac Surg* 2006; **82**:e3–4.

7 Peterson R, DuyKhanh P, Toloza E *et al*. Thoracoscopic lobectomy: a safe and effective strategy for patients receiving induction therapy for non-small cell lung cancer. *Ann Thorac Surg* 2006; **82**:214–9.

8 Little A. No nodes is good nodes. *Ann Thorac Surg* 2006; **82**:4–5.

9 Sagawa M, Sato M, Sakurada A *et al*. A prospective trial of systematic nodal dissection for lung cancer by video-assisted thoracic surgery: can it be perfect? *Ann Thorac Surg* 2002; **73**: 900–904.

10 Shigemura N, Akashi A, Nakagiri T, Ohta M, Matsuda H. Complete versus assisted thoracoscopic approach: a prospective trial comparing a variety of video-assisted thoracoscopic lobectomy techniques. *Surg Endosc* 2004; **18**:1492–7.

11 Ochroch A, Gottschalk A. Impact of acute pain and its management for thoracic surgical patients. *Thorac Surg Clin* 2005; **15**:105–21.

12 Richardson J, Sabanathan S, Jones J *et al*. A prospective, randomized comparison of preoperative and continuous balanced epidural or paravertebral bupivacaine on post-thoracotomy pain, pulmonary function and stress responses. *Br J Anaesth* 1999; **83**:387–92.

13 Gotoda Y, Kambara N, Sakai T *et al*. The morbidity, time course and predictive factors for persistent post-thoracotomy pain. *Eur J Pain* 2001; **5**:89–96.

14 Benedetti F, Amanzio M, Casadio C *et al*. Postoperative pain and superficial abdominal reflexes after posterolateral thoracotomy. *Ann Thorac Surg* 1997; **64**:207–10.

15 Kirby T, Mack M, Landreneau R, Rice T. Lobectomy-video-assisted thoracic surgery versus muscle-sparing thoracotomy. *J Thorac Cardiovasc Surg* 1995; **109**:997–1001.

16 Tschernko EM, Hofer S, Bieglmeyer C *et al*. Early postoperative stress: video-assisted wedge resection/lobectomy vs conventional axillary thoracotomy. *Chest* 1996; **109(6)**:1636–42.

17 Walker WS, Pugh GC, Craig SR *et al*. Continued experience with thoracoscopic major pulmonary resection. *Int Surg* 1996; **81(3)**:235–6.

18 Ohbuchi T, Morikawa T, Takeuchi E *et al*. Lobectomy: video-assisted thoracic surgery versus posterolateral thoracotomy. *Jpn J Thorac Cardiovasc Surg* 1998; **46(6)**:519–22.

19 Nomori H, Horio H, Naruke T, Suemasu K. What is the advantage of a thoracoscopic lobectomy over a limited thoracotomy procedure for lung cancer surgery? *Ann Thorac Surg* 2001; **72**:879–84.

20 Pertunnen K, Tasmuth T, Kalso E. Chronic pain after thoracic surgery: a follow-up study. *Acta Anaesthesiol Scand* 1999; **43**:563–7.

21 Sugiura H, Morikawa T, Kaji M *et al*. Long-term benefits for the quality of life after video-assisted thoracoscopic lobectomy in patients with lung cancer. *Surg Lap Percut Tech* 1999; **9**:403–8.

22 Landreneau RJ, Mack MJ, Hazelrigg SR *et al*. Prevalence of chronic pain after pulmonary resection by thoracotomy or video-assisted thoracic surgery. *J Thorac Cardiovasc Surg* 1994; **107**:1079–86.

23 Stammberger U, Steinacher C, Hillinger S *et al*. Early and long-term complaints following video-assisted thoracoscopic surgery: evaluation in 173 patients. *Eur J Cardiothorac Surg* 2000; **18(1)**:7–11.

24 Landreneau RJ, Hazelrigg SR, Mack MJ *et al*. Postoperative pain-related morbidity: video-assisted thoracic surgery versus thoracotomy. *Ann Thorac Surg* 1993: **56(6)**:1285–9.

25 Li W, Lee R, Lee, T *et al*. The impact of thoracic surgical access on early shoulder function: video-assisted thoracic surgery versus posterolateral thoracotomy. *Eur J Cardiothorac Surg* 2003; **23**:390–6.

26 Allen M, Darling G, Pechet T *et al*. Morbidity and mortality of major pulmonary resections in patients with early-stage lung cancer: initial results of the randomized, prospective ACOSOG Z0030 trial. *Ann Thorac Surg* 2006; **81**:1013–20.

27 McKenna R, Houck W, Fuller C. Video-assisted thoracic surgery lobectomy: experience with 1,100 cases. *Ann Thorac Surg* 2006; **81**:421–6.

28 Onaitis M, Peterson R, Balderson S *et al*. Thoracoscopic lobectomy is a safe and versatile procedure: experience with 500 consecutive patients. *Ann Surg* 2006; **244**:420–5.

29 Demmy T, Curtis J. Minimally invasive lobectomy directed toward frail and high-risk patients: a case–control study. *Ann Thorac Surg* 1999; **68**:194–200.

30 Walker WS, Codispoti M, Soon SY *et al*. Long-term outcomes following VATS lobectomy for non-small cell bronchogenic carcinoma. *Eur J Cardiothorac Surg* 2003; **23**:397–402.

31 Clinical Outcomes of Surgery Study Group. A comparison of laparoscopically assisted and open colectomy for colon cancer. *N Engl J Med* 2004; **350**:2050–9.

32 Mountain CF. Revisions in the international system for staging lung cancer. *Chest* 1997; **111**: 1710–7.

33 McKenna R, Wolf R, Brenner M, Fischel R, Wurning P. Is lobectomy by video-assisted thoracic surgery an adequate cancer operation? *Ann Thorac Surg* 1998; **66**:1903–8.

34 Thomas P, Doddoli C, Yena S *et al*. VATS is an adequate oncological operation for stage I non-small cell lung cancer. *Eur J Cardiothorac Surg* 2002; **21**:1094–9.

35 Iwasaki A, Shirakusa T, Shiraishi T, Yamamoto S. Results of video-assisted thoracic surgery for stage I/II non-small cell lung cancer. *Eur J Cardiothorac Surg* 2004; **26**:158–64.

36 Shiraishi T, Shirakusa T, Hiratsuka M *et al*. Video-assisted thoracoscopic surgery lobectomy for c-T1N0M0 primary lung cancer: its impact on locoregional control. *Ann Thorac Surg* 2006; **82**:1021–6.

37 Peters RM. The role of limited resection in carcinoma of the lung. *Am J Surg* 1982; **143**:706–10.

38 Henschke C, Yankelevitz D, Libby D *et al*. Survival of stage I lung cancer detected on CT screening. *N Engl J Med* 2006; **335**:1763–71.

39 Lung Cancer Study Group. Randomized trial of lobectomy versus limited resection for T1 N0 non-small cell lung cancer. *Ann Thorac Surg* 1995; **60**:615–23.

40 Warren W, Faber P. Segmentectomy versus lobectomy in patients with stage I pulmonary carcinoma. *J Thorac Cardiovasc Surg* 1994; **107**:187–94.

41 Landreneau R, Sugarbaker D, Mack M *et al*. Wedge resection versus lobectomy for stage I (T1N0M0) non-small cell lung cancer. *J Thorac Cardiovasc Surg* 1997; **113**:691–700.

42 Miller D, Rowlang C, Deschamps C *et al*. Surgical treatment of non-small cell lung cancer 1 cm or less in diameter. *Ann Thorac Surg* 2002; **73**:1545–51.

43 Kodama K, Doi O, Higashiyama M *et al*. Intentional limited resection for selected patients with T1N0M0 non-small cell lung cancer: a single institution study. *J Thorac Cardiovasc Surg* 1997; **114**:347–53.

44 Sagawa M, Koike T, Sato M *et al*. Segmentectomy for roentgenographically occult bronchogenic carcinoma. *Ann Thorac Surg* 2001; **71**:1100–4.

45 Yoshikawa K, Tsubot N, Kodama K *et al*. Prospective study of extended segmentectomy for small lung tumors: final report. *Ann Thorac Surg* 2002; **73**:1055–9.

46 Asamura H, Nakayama H, Kondo H *et al*. Lymph node involvement, recurrence and prognosis in resected, small, peripheral non-small cell lung carcinomas: are these carcinomas candidates for video-assisted lobectomy? *J Thorac Cardiovasc Surg* 1996; **111**:1125–34.

47 Takizawa T, Terishima M, Koike T *et al*. Lymph node metastases in small, peripheral adenocarcinoma of the lung. *J Thorac Cardiovasc Surg* 1998; **116**:276–80.

48 El-Sherif A, Gooding W, Santos R *et al*. Outcomes of sublobar resection versus lobectomy for stage I non-small cell lung cancer: a 13 year analysis. *Ann Thorac Surg* 2006; **82**:408–16.

49 Mery C, Pappas A, Bueno R *et al*. Similar long-term survival of elderly patients with non-small cell lung cancer treated with lobectomy or wedge resection within the surveillance, epidemiology and end results database. *Chest* 2005; **128**:237–45.

50 Shennib H, Bogart J, Herndon J *et al*. Video-assisted wedge resection and local radiotherapy for peripheral lung cancer in high-risk patients: The Cancer and Leukemia Group B (CALGB) 9335, a phase II multi-institutional cooperative group study. *J Thorac Cardiovasc Surg* 2005; **129(4)**:813–8.

51 Santos R, Colonias A, Parda D *et al*. Comparison between sublobar resection and 125 Iodine brachytherapy after sublobar resection in high-risk patients with stage I non-small cell lung cancer. *Surgery* Oct 2003; **134(4)**:691–7.

52 Fernando HC, Santos RS, Benfield JR *et al*. Lobar and sublobar resection with and without brachytherapy for small stage IA non-small cell lung cancer. *J Thorac Cardiovasc Surg* Feb 2005; **129(2)**:261–7.

53 Birdas TJ, Koehler RP, Colonias A *et al*. Sublobar resection with brachytherapy versus lobectomy for stage IB nonsmall cell lung cancer. *Ann Thorac Surg* Feb 2006; **81(2)**:434–8.

54 Korst R, Ginsberg R, Ailawadi *et al*. Lobectomy improves ventilatory function in selected patients with severe COPD. *Ann Thorac Surg* 1998; **66**:898–902.

55 Sekine Y, Iwata T, Chiyo M *et al*. Minimal alteration of pulmonary function after lobectomy in lung cancer patients with chronic obstructive pulmonary disease. *Ann Thorac Surg* 2003; **76**:356–61.

56 Fernando H, de Hoyos A, Landreneau R. Radiofrequency ablation for the treatment of non-small cell lung cancer in marginal surgical candidates. *J Thorac Cardiovasc Surg* 2005; **129**:639–44.

CHAPTER 13

Extended Resections for Lung Cancer

Philippe G. Dartevelle, Bedrettin Yildizeli, and Sacha Mussot

Introduction

Lung cancer remains the most fatal cancer worldwide with over 1,300,000 deaths estimated for the year 2000 [1,2]. Only 10% of patients with lung cancers diagnosed in the European population are alive at 5 years, a figure that compares quite poorly with the 50 and 70% 5-year survival rates for colon and breast cancer, respectively [3]. Using the tumor node metastasis (TNM) classification to direct treatment can eliminate some patients from potentially curative surgery. For example, Stage IIIb includes T1N3 which is not curable by surgery as well as T4N0 which is sometimes amenable to surgical resection and possible long-term survival.

Locally advanced lung cancer encompasses T3 tumors with direct extension into the chest wall, diaphragm, mediastinal pleura, or within 2 cm of the carina and nearly all T4 tumors invading the mediastinum, heart, great vessels, trachea, esophagus, vertebral body, or carina.

Extended resections for tumors that are locally advanced according to T status imply that surgical resection is being performed under circumstances that are technically challenging and beyond the usual scope of an operation for lung cancer (Table 13.1).

Likewise, the development of preoperative chemotherapy or chemoradiotherapy is said to make curative treatment possible for tumors that are locally advanced according to N status. However,

Lung Cancer, 3rd edition. Edited by Jack A. Roth, James D. Cox, and Waun Ki Hong. © 2008 Blackwell Publishing, ISBN: 978-1-4051-5112-2.

surgery after induction therapy poses special perioperative risks and technical challenges because the difference it is often difficult to distinguish between sclerotic tissue and tumor margins; moreover the "down staging" phenomenon does not occur with a high frequency.

Patients with T4 tumors with N0 or N1 disease should benefit most from surgery because these tumors are often more local-regionally than systemically aggressive.

This chapter will try to define the subsets of patients with locally advanced nonsmall cell lung cancer (NSCLC) who are most likely to benefit from surgery.

Chest wall invasion

Five to eight percent of patients undergoing resection for NSCLC have involvement of the chest wall [4]. Patients' complaints are the most reliable indications of chest wall involvement, as infiltration between the ribs may result in false-negative bone or computed tomography (CT) scans. It was claimed that CT scan could be inaccurate in assessing direct parietal pleura invasion of lung cancer [5]. However, Ratto *et al.* [6] and Rendina *et al.* [7] reported that thickening of the pleura is not useful and obliteration of the extrapleural fat pad is the most sensitive and specific finding in CT scan. Furthermore, visible rib destruction from direct invasion is a very specific sign (and a bad prognosis) for chest wall invasion. Although magnetic resonance imaging (MRI) is not routinely used, it has the theoretic advantage of being able to determine if the muscle

Table 13.1 New technical advances in T4 tumors surgery.

Vascular resection/reconstruction
Tracheal/carinal resection
Anterior approach to thoracic inlet tumors
Vertebrectomy
Safety of surgery after induction chemoradiation therapy

---

layers are involved. Positron emission tomography (PET) is useful for detecting distant metastases but is not useful for determining local invasion because the resolution is not adequate to determine chest wall invasion. McCaughan *et al.* [8] reported an elevated serum alkaline phosphatase level in 34% of the patients; however, this abnormality is not a specific finding. Pulmonary function tests and quantitative perfusion lung scan are necessary to assess the patient's ability to withstand operation and whether the paradox motion of the residual wall requires stabilization.

The goals of surgery are to completely resect the primary tumors with clear surgical margins and maintain a normal respiratory physiology by restoring the rigidity of the chest wall and resected soft tissue. Knowledge of chest wall invasion preoperatively is important because entering the chest at a site remote from the chest wall invasion lessens the risk of tumor spillage, allows the surgeon to assess the extent of involvement, and avoids placement of the prosthetic material directly beneath the incision. As a general rule, all tumors except those invading the thoracic inlet or the anterior thoracic cage are approached through a standard posterolateral thoracotomy. Resection should include at least one segment of rib (with the related intercostal muscle) above and below the involved rib(s) and 3–5 cm laterally and medially. To prevent tumor spillage, the entire tumor-bearing area should be resected en bloc, and it is frequently easier to do the chest wall resection initially (small involvements) and then proceed with the pulmonary resection. For large involvements, it is easier to do a wedge excision of the tumor-bearing area with a mechanical stapler and to resect the remainder of the collapsed lobe later. Frozen sections on the soft-tissue margins

are mandatory to confirm completeness of the resection.

Majority of the chest wall resections do not require prosthetic reconstruction. Resection of a portion of three or fewer ribs posteriorly rarely requires prosthetic replacement, as the scapula lessens the cosmetic and functional impact of the chest wall resection. Resection of larger defect, especially when located anterolateral aspects of the lower ribs, may require prosthetic replacement, yet the risks of infection should be balanced against the cosmetic and functional benefit of prosthetic replacement.

Reconstruction can be accomplished using non-reinforced materials like Marlex mesh or Gore-tex patch. The advantage of Marlex mesh (Bard Inc.), over Gore-tex patch (W. L. Gore and Assoc., Flagstaff), is that it allows the ingrowth of the surrounding tissue and remains rigid over time [9]. For small defects, the Marlex mesh is doubled crosswise at a 90° angle for added strength, and tailored and sutured to the edges of the defect with nonabsorbable sutures. With larger and unsupported defects, the chest wall rigidity can be obtained by utilizing methylmethacrylate between two layers of Marlex mesh as described by Eschapasse *et al.* [9] and McCormack *et al.* [10].

In recent years, we adapted a more anatomical reconstruction, which is less prone to infection [11]. Following the chest wall resection, the Marlex mesh is anchored to the surrounding tissues so that it remains beneath the ribs; 28-Fr silicone chest wall tubes are then tailored so that they can be interposed between the healthy portion of the previously resected rib to cover the Marlex mesh. The methylmethacrylate is then spread into chest tubes, and while it becomes settled, the tubes are shaped according to the course of the resected ribs. Once hard and cool enough, the tube edges are telescoped and fixed with nonabsorbable sutures to the edges of the corresponding ribs. Presently, chest wall reconstruction rarely requires the interposition of a myocutaneous flap. As with all other prosthetic substitutes, absolute sterility is required, and the amount of air leaks should be minimal.

All T3 tumors are resectable, but the prognosis varies according to the involved site. A T3 tumor involving the chest wall provides the most favorable

Table 13.2 Results after complete resection of NSCLC invading the chest wall.

Author [ref.]	Year	Number of patients	Operative mortality (%)	Survival rates, 5 yr (%)			
				Overall	N0	N1	N2
Piehler et al. [12]	1982	66	15.2	32.9	54.0	7.4*	7.4*
Patterson et al. [13]	1982	35	8.5	38.0	NS	NS	0.0
McCaughan et al. [8]	1985	125	4.0	40.0	56.0	21.0*	21.0*
Ratto et al. [6]	1991	112	1.7	NS	50.0	25.0	0.0
Allen et al. [14]	1991	52	3.8	26.3	29.0	11.0	NS
Shah and Goldstraw [15]	1995	58	3.4	37.2	45.0	38.0	0.0
Downey et al. [16]	1999	175	6.0	36.0	56.0	13.0	29.0
Facciolo et al. [17]	2001	104	0.0	61.4	67.0	100.0	17.0
Magdeleinat et al. [18]	2001	201	7.0	21.0	25.0	21.0	20.0
Burkhart et al. [19]	2002	94	6.3	38.7	44.0	26*	26.0*
Chapelier et al. [20]	2000	100	1.8	18	22	9	0
Riquet et al. [21]	2002	125	7	22.5	30.7	0	11.5
Roviaro et al. [22]	2003	146	0.7	NS	78.5	7.2*	7.2*
Matsuoka et al. [23]	2004	97	NS	34.2[†]	44.2	40.0	6.2

*N1 and N2 patients combined.
[†]Complete resection.
NS, not stated.

prognosis among the resected T3 lesions. If completely excised, T3 (chest wall) N0 lung cancers provide a 5-year survival in excess of 50% (Table 13.2). The strongest determinants of 5-year survival, by far, are completeness of resection, depth of chest wall invasion, and nodal status. Patients with incomplete resection may survive less than 2.5 years [6,8,12–23]. Likewise, the depth of chest wall invasion affects prognosis, as extension to the parietal pleura only is associated with twofold increase of 5-year survival (62% versus 35%) when compared to deeper involvements [8]. Different opinions exist as to whether tumors confined to the parietal pleura can be resected by simple extrapleural mobilization, without resecting en bloc the adjacent soft and bony tissues, as long as the resection margins are negative. While McCaughan et al. [8] showed that extrapleural mobilization was sufficient for a significant number of patients whose tumors invaded the parietal pleura only, Piehler et al. [12] reported a high incidence of local recurrence after extrapleural dissection for tumors invading the parietal pleura. Chapelier et al. [20] also found that patients with a tumor infiltration confined to the parietal pleura had a significantly better 5-year survival than those

with chest wall infiltration. Current trend for this decision depends on the extent of the tumor. When only flimsy adhesions are found, these can be safely divided without a problem. When there is a question of whether the tumor invades into the chest wall, however, an extrapleural resection is not adequate and only an en bloc chest wall resection should be performed. We believe that when a lung cancer invades at least the parietal pleura, a wide resection of the chest wall with attached lung should be performed [20].

Most if not all series report no 5-year survivors with positive N2, compared to 5-year survival exceeding 50% for N0 patients. In this sense, both PET scan and mediastinoscopy is advocated for patients with chest wall involvement and enlarged lymph nodes. If patients are found to have N2 disease before thoracotomy, they should receive either preoperative chemotherapy or chemoradiotherapy, either as induction or definitive treatment.

The final area of controversy is whether radiation therapy, administered either pre- or postoperatively, is indicated in patients who have lung cancer that invade the chest wall. Potential benefits of preoperative therapy include the following: downstaging the tumor, allowing potentially unresectable tumors to be resected, decreasing the rate of close margins, and decreasing the risk of tumor spillage at the time of resection [24]. However, recent reports showed decreased survival rates in those patients who received radiation therapy [14,18]. Currently, radiotherapy is proposed to reduce the incidence of local recurrence, and should be reserved for patients with close surgical margins, or those with hilar or mediastinal nodal involvement. Adjuvant chemotherapy had no apparent effect on survival, but the number of patients was too small to obtain statistically meaningful data.

Superior sulcus tumors

Superior sulcus lesions include a constellation of benign or malignant tumors extending to the superior thoracic inlet. They cause steady, severe, and unrelenting shoulder and arm pain along the distribution of the eighth cervical nerve trunk and first and second thoracic nerve trunks. They also cause Horner's syndrome and weakness and atrophy of the intrinsic muscles of the hand, a clinical entity known as Pancoast–Tobias syndrome. Bronchial carcinoma represents the most frequent cause of superior sulcus lesions. Superior sulcus lesions of nonsmall cell histology account for less than 5% of all bronchial carcinomas. These tumors may arise from either upper lobe and tend to invade the parietal pleura, endothoracic fascia, subclavian vessels, brachial plexus, vertebral bodies, and first ribs. However, their clinical features are influenced by their location. Tumors located anterior to the anterior scalene muscle may invade the platysma and sternocleidomastoid muscles, external and anterior jugular veins, inferior belly of the omohyoid muscle, subclavian and internal jugular veins and their major branches, and the scalene fat pad. They invade the first intercostal nerve and first rib more frequently than the phrenic nerve or superior vena cava (SVC), and patients usually complain of pain distributed to the upper anterior chest wall.

Tumors located between the anterior and middle scalene muscles may invade the anterior scalene muscle with the phrenic nerve lying on its anterior aspect; the subclavian artery with its primary branches, except the posterior scapular artery; and the trunks of the brachial plexus and middle scalene muscle (Figure 13.1). As the tumor involves the brachial plexus, symptoms develop in the distribution of T1 (ulnar distribution of the arm and elbow) and C8 nerve roots (ulnar surface of the forearm and small and ring fingers).

Tumors lying posterior to the middle scalene muscles are usually located in the costovertebral groove and invade the nerve roots of T1, the posterior aspect of the subclavian and vertebral arteries, paravertebral sympathetic chain, inferior cervical (stellate) ganglion, and prevertebral muscles. Some of these posterior tumors can invade transverse process indeed the vertebral bodies (only abutting the costovertebral angle or extending into the intraspinal foramen without intraspinal extension may yet be resected). Because of the peripheral location of these lesions, pulmonary symptoms, such as cough, hemoptysis, and dyspnea, are uncommon in the initial stages of the disease. Abnormal sensation and pain in the axilla and medial aspect of the upper arm in the distribution of the intercostobrachial (T2) nerve are more frequently observed in the early stage of the disease process. With further tumor growth, patients may present with full-blown Pancoast's syndrome.

Superior sulcus tumors are extremely difficult to diagnose at initial presentation. The time elapsed between the onset of the Pancoast–Tobias syndrome and diagnosis is still around 6 months. These patients usually present with small apical tumors that are hidden behind the clavicle and the first rib on routine chest radiographs. The diagnosis is established by history and physical examination, biochemical profile, chest radiographs, bronchoscopy and sputum cytology, fine-needle transthoracic or transcutaneous biopsy and aspiration, and CT of the chest. If there is evidence of mediastinal adenopathy on chest radiographs, computed tomographic scanning or PET scan, histological proof is mandatory because patients with clinical N2 disease are not suitable for operation. Neurologic examination, MRI, and electromyography delineate the tumor's extension to the brachial plexus, phrenic nerve, and epidural space. Vascular invasion is evaluated

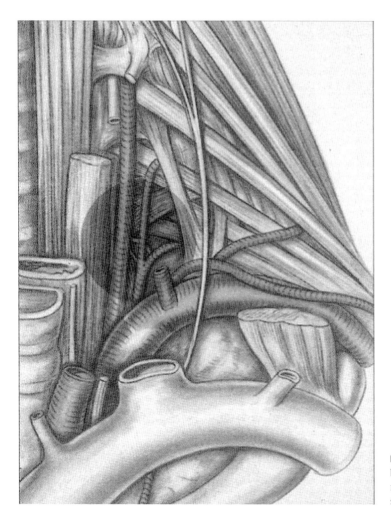

Figure 13.1 A left superior sulcus bronchial carcinoma invading the middle thoracic inlet, including the subclavian artery.

by venous angiography, subclavian arteriography, Doppler ultrasonography (cerebrovascular disorders may contraindicate sacrifice of the vertebral artery), and MRI. Magnetic resonance imaging has to be performed routinely when tumors approach the intervertebral foramina to rule out invasion of the extradural space.

The initial evaluation also includes all preoperative cardiopulmonary functional tests routinely performed before any major lung resection and investigative procedures to identify the presence of any metastatic disease.

Although it is now established that radical surgery represents the only hope for long-term survival and cure, optimal management for superior sulcus tumors continues to be a major challenge. The traditional approach to superior sulcus tumors has been preoperative radiotherapy followed by resection, although this standard was established 45 years ago solely on the basis of encouraging short-term survival as compared with historical controls [25]. Then, high-dose curative primary radiotherapy [26], "sandwich" preoperative and postoperative radiotherapy [27], postoperative radiotherapy alone [28], or intraoperative brachytherapy combined with preoperative radiation therapy and operation [29] have been reported as the treatment modalities of superior sulcus tumors. In 2001,

SWOG 9416 (Intergroup 0160) [30], evaluated the role of induction chemoradiotherapy and surgery for patients with superior sulcus tumors in multi-institutional setting and updated their results in 2003 [31] for the treatment of these tumors. And then, preoperative concurrent chemotherapy and radiotherapy has been explored by several other groups [32,33]. The rate of complete resection was 92% as opposed to an average of 66% among historical series of conventional treatment [30,34]. The consistency of the data regarding preoperative chemoradiotherapy and regarding preoperative radiotherapy alone is convincing that preoperative chemoradiotherapy represents a new standard of care for patients with Pancoast tumors. Although no randomized data are available comparing these approaches [35]. As to whether surgery should proceed or follow radiation therapy in newly diagnosed superior sulcus tumors, our strong opinion is to first resect, because dissecting on a previously (chemo)irradiated thoracic inlet unquestionably increases the technical difficulties and postoperative morbidity. Radiation therapy is to be discussed in the postoperative course.

Absolute surgical contraindications in the management of superior sulcus tumors are the presence of extra-thoracic sites of metastasis, histologically confirmed N2 disease, extensive invasion of the cervical trachea, esophagus and the brachial plexus above the T1 nerve root; this because it indicates that the tumor is locally too extensive to achieve a complete resection or that limb amputation is necessary. Invasion of the subclavian vessels should no longer be considered a surgical contraindication. Massive vertebral invasion, diagnosed preoperatively, is synonymous with unresectability. Invasions limited to the intervertebral foramen without extension into the spinal canal are resectable.

As a general rule, superior sulcus tumors not invading the thoracic inlet are completely resectable through the classic posterior approach of Shaw and associates [25] alone. Because the posterior approach does not allow direct and safe visualization, manipulation, and complete oncologic clearance of all anatomic structures that compose the thoracic inlet, superior sulcus lesions extending to the thoracic inlet should be resected by the ante-

rior transcervical approach as described by Dartevelle and colleagues [28]. This operative procedure is increasingly accepted as a standard approach for all benign and malignant lesions of the thoracic inlet structures, including nonbronchial cancers (e.g., osteosarcomas of the first rib and tumors of the brachial plexus), and for exposing the anterolateral aspects of the upper thoracic vertebrae. Contraindications to this approach include extrathoracic metastasis, invasion of the brachial plexus above the T1 nerve root, invasion of the vertebral canal and sheath of the medulla, massive invasion of the scalene muscles and extrathoracic muscles, mediastinal lymph node metastasis, and significant cardiopulmonary disease.

Our technique of anterior transcervical approach has been reviewed in detail elsewhere [36]. Only some specific points are presented herein. Following double-lumen endotracheal intubation, the patient is in the supine position with the neck hyperextended and the head turned away from the involved side. An L-shaped cervicotomy incision is made, including a vertical presternocleidomastoid incision carried horizontally below the clavicle up to the deltopectoral groove (Figure 13.2).

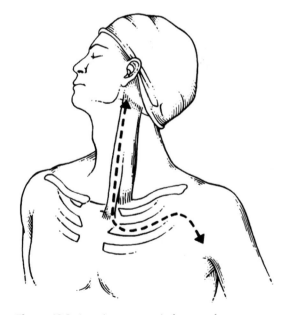

Figure 13.2 Anterior transcervical approach.

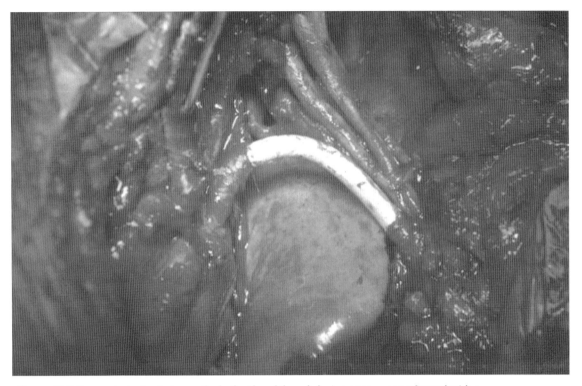

Figure 13.3 Revascularization between the both sides of the subclavian artery was performed with a polytetrafluoroethylene graft.

A myocutaneous flap is then folded back, providing full exposure of the neck and cervicothoracic junction. The scalene fat pad is dissected and pathologically examined to exclude scalene lymph node metastasis. Inspection of the ipsilateral superior mediastinum after division of the sternothyroid and sternohyoid muscles is then made by the operator's finger along the tracheoesophageal groove. The tumor's extension to the thoracic inlet is then carefully assessed. We recommend resection of the medial half of the clavicle only if the tumor is deemed respectable. Before dealing with the anterior scalene muscle, the status of the phrenic nerve is carefully assessed because its unnecessary division has a deleterious influence on the postoperative course. The vertebral artery is resected only if invaded and if no significant extracranial occlusive disease was detected on preoperative Doppler ultrasound. If there is invasion of the arterial wall, resection and reconstruction of the artery to obtain tumor-free margins

is necessary. Revascularization is performed at the end of the procedure either with a polytetrafluoroethylene graft (6 or 8 mm) (Figure 13.3) or, more often, with an end-to-end anastomosis after freeing the carotid and subclavian arteries (Figure 13.4). During these maneuvers, the pleural space is usually opened by dividing Sibson's fascia. The middle scalene muscle is divided above its insertion on the first rib or higher, as indicated by the extension of the tumor. The nerve roots of C8 and T1 are then easily identified and dissected free from outside to inside up to where they join to form the lower trunk of the brachial plexus. The T1 nerve root is usually divided proximally beyond visible tumor, just lateral to the T1 intervertebral foramen. Although the tumor's spread to the brachial plexus may be high, neurolysis is usually achieved without division of the nerve roots above T1. Injury of the lateral and long thoracic nerves should be avoided because it may result in a winged scapula. Before the upper

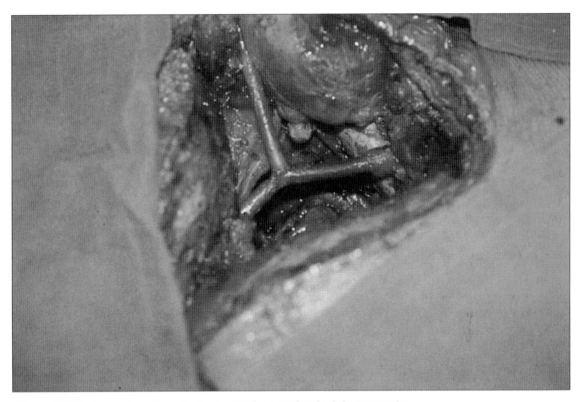

Figure 13.4 End-to-end anastomosis after freeing the carotid and subclavian arteries.

lobectomy, the chest wall resection is completed. It is through this cavity that an upper lobectomy can be performed to complete the operation, although it is technically demanding. Unlike our original description [28], it has become evident that an additional posterior thoracotomy is usually not required.

There is increasing concern about the functional and esthetic benefit of preserving the clavicle. We believe that the indications for preserving and reconstructing the clavicle are limited to the combined resection of the serratus anterior muscle and the long thoracic nerve because this causes the scapula to rotate and draw forward. This entity (*scapula alata*), combined with the resection of the internal half of the clavicle, pushes the shoulder anteriorly and medially and leads to severe cosmetic and functional discomfort. If this circumstance is anticipated, we recommend an oblique section of the manubrium that fully preserves the sternoclavicular articulation, its intra-articular disc, and the

costoclavicular ligaments rather than the simple sternoclavicular disarticulation. Clavicular osteosynthesis can then be accomplished by placing metallic wires across the lateral clavicular edges and across the divided manubrium.

We also developed a technique for resecting posteriorly located superior sulcus tumors extending into the intervertebral foramen without intraspinal extension in collaboration with a spinal surgeon [37]. The underlying principle is that one can perform a radical procedure by resecting the intervertebral foramen and dividing the nerve roots inside the spinal canal by a combined anterior transcervical and posterior midline approach. After division of the ipsilateral hemivertebral bodies, the specimen is resected en bloc with the lung, ribs, and vessels through the posterior incision (Figure 13.5). On the side of the tumor, spinal fixation is performed from the pedicle above to the pedicle below the resected hemivertebrae; on the contralateral side, a

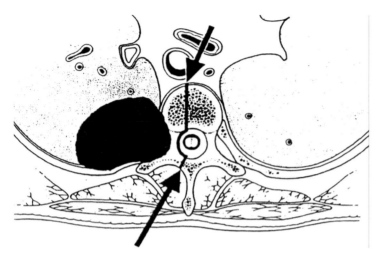

Figure 13.5 Right-sided apical tumor involving the costo-transverse space and intervertebral foramen and part of the ipsilateral vertebral body; this tumor is first approached anteriorly and then the operation is completed through a hemivertebrectomy performed through the posterior midline approach. (Adapted from Dartevelle *et al.* [28].)

screw is placed in each pedicle. However, the presence of an anterior spinal artery penetrating the spinal canal through an invaded intervertebral foramen may contraindicates surgery. Tumors involving transverse processes should be resected with the anterior approach. The maneuver is similar to what is used with the posterior approach but from the front to the back, with a finger placed behind the transverse process of T1 and T2 to give the correct direction of the chisel.

The reported surgical morbidity ranges from 7 to 38% with surgical mortality generally around 5–10% [38]. Surgical complications include spinal fluid leakage, Horner's syndrome and nerve deficits, hematothorax, chylothorax, and prolonged ventilatory support due to atelectasis because of the concomitant extended chest wall resection and phrenic nerve resection.

The overall 5-year survival rates after combined radiosurgical (posterior approach) treatment of superior sulcus tumors due to bronchial carcinoma range from 18 to 56% (Table 13.3). The best prognosis is found in patients without nodal involvement who have had a complete resection. We reported a complete resection rate of 100% with no postoperative mortality or major complications. The 5-year and median survival rates were approximately 35% and 18 months, respectively. The local recurrence rate was less than 1.8% using our approach. Fadel *et al.* [37] reported 17 en bloc resections of NSCLCs invading the thoracic inlet and intervertebral foram-

ina with a 5-year and median survival rates of 20% and 27 months, respectively. Among the adverse prognostic factors, the nodal status is the only predictor of disease-free survival.

Carinal resections

Refinement in techniques of tracheal surgery and bronchial sleeve lobectomy has made carinal resection and reconstruction possible. However, the potential for complications remains high and few centers only have cumulated sufficient expertise to safely perform the operation. Surgery is still infrequently proposed because of its complexity and the paucity of data demonstrating benefit in the long term. However, results from recent series demonstrate that carinal resection is safe in experienced centers with an operative mortality of less than 10% and can be associated with good to excellent long-term survival in selected patients. The current results are considerably better than those from earlier reported series and likely accounts for the improvement in surgical and anesthetic techniques.

Careful patient selection and detailed evaluation of the lesion is a key component to good surgical results in carinal resection. All patients should be evaluated to ascertain that they can tolerate the operation and withstand the necessary removal of pulmonary parenchyma. The preoperative workup

Table 13.3 Results of patients treated surgically for superior sulcus tumors.

Author (year)	Number of cases	5-yr survival (%)	Mortality (%)
Paulson [39] (1985)	79	35	3
Anderson *et al.* [40] (1986)	28	34	7
Devine *et al.* [41] (1986)	40	10	8
Miller *et al.* [42] (1979)	36	31	NS
Wright *et al.* [43] (1987)	21	27	—
Shahian *et al.* [27] (1987)	18	56	—
McKneally [44] (1987)	25	51	NS
Komaki *et al.* [26] (1990)	25	40	NS
Sartori *et al.* [45] (1992)	42	25	2.3
Maggi *et al.* [46] (1994)	60	17.4	5
Ginsberg *et al.* [47] (1994)	100	26	4
Okubo *et al.* [48] (1995)	18	38.5	5.6
Dartevelle [49] (1997)	70	34	—
Martinod *et al.* [50] (2002)	139	35	7.2
Alifano *et al.* [51] (2003)	67	36.2	8.9
Goldberg *et al.* [52] (2005)	39	47.9	5%
Total	807	34.5 ± 11.7	5.6 ± 2.2

Values are number ± standard deviation.
NS, not stated.

consists of chest radiography, chest CT scan, pulmonary function tests, arterial blood gas, ventilation/perfusion scan, electrocardiography, and echocardiography. Stress thallium studies, maximum oxygen uptake, and exercise testing are used when indicated. The operation is an elective procedure and efforts should be made to prepare the patients for surgery with chest physiotherapy, deep breathing, and cessation of smoking. Airway obstruction, bronchospasm, and intercurrent pulmonary infection should be reversed. Steroids should be discontinued before surgery.

Flexible or rigid bronchoscopy is crucial to evaluate the overall length of the tumor, the adequacy of the remaining airway, and the feasibility of a tension-free anastomosis. Besides routine investigation to rule out extrathoracic metastasis for patients with bronchogenic carcinoma, we also routinely perform a mediastinoscopy at the time of surgery in patients presenting with bronchogenic carcinoma to exclude N2 or N3 disease.

Pulmonary angiography is performed for carinal tumors arising from the anterior segment of the right upper lobe, because invasion of right upper lobe (mediastinal) artery usually indirectly reveals invasion of the posterior aspect of the SVC. Superior cavography is performed if the SVC is potentially involved. Transesophageal echography is occasionally performed to evaluate tumor extension to the posterior mediastinum, especially the esophagus or the left atrium.

Indications and contraindications

The safe limit of resection between the lower trachea and the contralateral main bronchus is usually considered to be 4 cm. This is particularly important if a right carinal pneumonectomy is performed and the left mainstem bronchus is to be reanastomosed end-to-end to the distal trachea. Upward mobilization of the left mainstem bronchus is limited because of the aortic arch and can easily result in excessive anastomotic tension.

In patients with bronchogenic carcinoma, carinal resection should be considered for tumors invading the first centimeter of the ipsilateral main bronchus, the lateral aspect of the lower trachea, the carina, or the contralateral main bronchus. This applies usually for right-sided tumor, since left-sided tumor rarely extend up to the carina without massively invading structures situated in the subaortic space. The long-term results of carinal resection for patients with bronchogenic carcinoma and N2 or N3 disease is poor, and therefore the findings of positive mediastinal nodes at the time of mediastinoscopy is usually considered a contraindication to surgery. Induction therapy may be offered for these patients, but we have found that this increases the technical difficulty of the operation and is associated with greater operative mortality, particularly if carinal pneumonectomy is required.

Surgical technique

Our technique of carinal resection has been reviewed in detail elsewhere [53,54]. Only some specific points are presented herein. Ventilation during carinal resection has always been a major concern. Our technique is similar to Grillo *et al.* [55]. The patient is initially intubated with an extra-long armored oral endotracheal tube that can be advanced into the opposite bronchus if one-lung ventilation is desired. Once the carina has been resected, the opposite main bronchus is intubated with a cross-field sterile endotracheal tube connected to a sterile tubing system. The tube can be safely removed intermittently to place the sutures precisely. Any blood spillage into the contralateral lung should be carefully suctioned to preserve the lung. Once the trachea and the bronchus are ready to be approximated, the cross-field tube is withdrawn, and ventilation resumed with the original oral tube once the anastomosis is completed. If a secondary end-to-side anastomosis is required between the other bronchus and the lateral trachea, the oral tube is advanced across the first anastomosis and ventilation can proceed uninterrupted until the secondary anastomosis is completed.

Approaches

The incision varies according to the type of carinal resection. Carinal resection without sacrifice of pulmonary parenchyma is approached through a median sternotomy. The pericardium is opened anteriorly and the tracheobronchial bifurcation is exposed between the SVC and the ascending aorta. The exposure is facilitated by completely mobilizing the ascending aorta and both main pulmonary arteries. The ligamentum arteriosum is systematically sectioned. As previously reported by Pearson *et al.* [56], we find that this approach offers several advantages over a right posterolateral thoracotomy. It allows any type of pulmonary resection, includ-

ing a left pneumonectomy, can provide access to a cervical collar incision for laryngeal or suprahyoid release procedure, and affords access to both a right and a left pulmonary hilar release if it is found to be necessary intraoperatively.

For carinal resection with sacrifice of pulmonary parenchyma approach depends on the lung concerned by resection. On the right side, a right posterolateral thoracotomy in the fifth intercostal space gives perfect exposure of the lower trachea and the origin of both main bronchi. On the left side, exposure of the lower trachea and right main bronchus is hindered by the aortic arch that is why the median sternotomy is our preferred approach for left carinal pneumonectomy. It provides superb exposure to the tracheobronchial bifurcation, causes less incisional discomfort and results in less ventilatory restriction than a thoracotomy. The main disadvantages are that freeing pleuroparietal adhesions can be difficult and mobilization of the left hilum requires cardiac retraction that may cause some hemodynamic instability.

Type of carinal resection

Carinal resection without pulmonary resection

Carinal resection without pulmonary resection is limited to the tumors located at the carina or at the origin of the right or left main bronchus. Depending on the extent of invasion, different modes of reconstruction exist. For very small tumors implanted on the carina only, the medial wall of both main bronchi can be approximate together to fashion a new carina that is then anastomosed to the trachea (Figure 13.6). The main problem with this reconstruction is that the "neocarina" has very limited mobility because of the aortic arch and therefore the trachea needs to be pulled down to the newly created carina.

When the tumor is more extensive, requiring a larger portion of the trachea to be resected, end-to-end plus end-to-side anastomosis is the method of choice. Various methods of reconstruction have been described according to the length of resection of the trachea, right and left main bronchi. The technique described by Barclay *et al.* [57] involves end-to-end anastomosis between the trachea and right

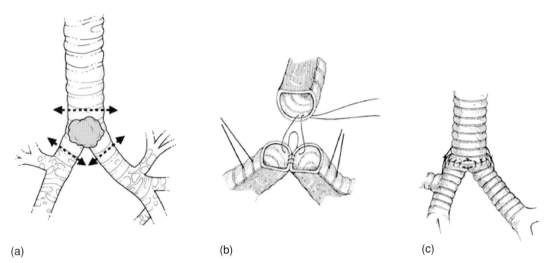

(a)   (b)   (c)

Figure 13.6 Carinal resection with "neo-carina" reconstruction. (a) Carinal lesion involving little of the trachea. Resection lines are indicated. (b) The medial walls of the right and left main bronchi are approximated with interrupted 4–0 PDS sutures to form a new carina. Note the midlateral traction sutures in the lateral walls, one ring distant from the cut edges. After the neocarina is completed, sutures for anastomosis between the trachea and the bronchial circumference are placed. The joined main bronchi are treated as a single unit. The anterior mattress suture at the confluence of the trachea and both bronchi is shown. (c) After all anastomotic sutures are placed, the paired lateral traction sutures are tied on each side simultaneously. Note the mattress suture in the anterior midpoint.

main bronchus with end-to-side anastomosis of the left main bronchus across the mediastinum into the bronchus intermedius (Figure 13.7). This reconstruction is possible only if the right main bronchus is left sufficiently long, but presents difficult access for the end-to-side anastomosis, often requiring hypoventilation of the right lung. Grillo *et al.* [55] described anastomosing the left main bronchus into the lateral wall of the trachea after an end-to-end anastomosis between the trachea and the right main bronchus. This technique has rare indication and is technically very demanding. In our experience, the right main bronchus can usually be anastomosed to the lateral wall of the trachea after adequate release maneuvers, regardless of the residual length of the right main bronchus (Figure 13.8).

Right carinal pneumonectomy

Right carinal pneumonectomy is the most frequent type of carinal resection for bronchogenic carcinoma. No irrevocable step should be taken until resection is certain. After division of the azygos vein, the tracheobronchial bifurcation is gently mobilized and dissected. Dissection should be limited to the anterior surface of the lower trachea while preserving the lateral blood supply as much as possible. Umbilical tapes are passed around the distal trachea and contralateral main bronchus. The hilum and esophagus are then dissected and the esophagus is retracted posteriorly. If there is no SVC involvement, the pulmonary artery and veins are stapled at their extrapericardial origin in order to have the lung attached by the main bronchus only. Subsequently, the cross-field intubation system is installed. The trachea and contralateral main bronchus are divided by sharp, straight transection lines. The trachea is always sectioned first to provide better exposure to section the left main bronchus. In order to accomplish a tension-free anastomosis, it is crucial to limit the length of resection between the distal trachea and left main bronchus to less than 4 cm. Frozen section are obtained on the tracheal and bronchial margins. The decision to resect further trachea or bronchus or leave residual tumor at the bronchial margin in case of positive margins is balanced by the necessity to perform a tension-free anastomosis. Enlarged subcarinal nodes can be resected, but otherwise the soft tissue

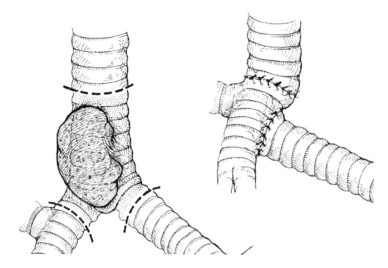

Figure 13.7 Barclay technique; resection of the carina and a significant length of the trachea. *Right*: The length of trachea resected (dotted lines) exceeds 4 cm. The trachea and left main bronchus will not approximate safely. *Left*: The elevated right main bronchus is anastomosed to the trachea after intrapericardial hilar mobilization. The left main bronchus is then anastomosed to the medial wall of the bronchus intermedius.

around the carina should be preserved as much as possible to ensure adequate vascularization of the anastomosis and good lymphatic drainage for the contralateral lung. After completing the anastomosis, the endotracheal tube is pulled back a sufficient distance from the suture line to avoid any damage from the tip of the tube and the anastomosis is checked for airtightness. The anastomosis is then covered by the surrounding tissue.

If segmental resection of the SVC is planed, the vascular procedure is usually performed before division of the airway. The SVC is clamped proximally at the confluence of the brachiocephalic veins and distally at the cavoatrial junction, and divided on each side of the tumor. Section of the SVC facilitates exposure and stapling of the right pulmonary artery in the interaorto-caval groove. The SVC is reconstructed with a ring-less straight 18- or 20-sized polytetrafluoroethylene (PTFE) graft. The PTFE graft is protected with gauze soaked in beta-dine during reconstruction of the airway to prevent graft contamination.

Carinal resection with lobar resection

Occasionally, the bronchogenic tumor can extend from the right upper lobe to the carina and lower trachea. The fissure is completed and the vessels for the right upper lobe are ligated and sectioned before dividing the lower trachea and left main bronchus as for a right carinal pneumonectomy. The bronchus intermedius is then transected below the take off of the right upper lobe bronchus. After completing the anastomosis between the trachea and the left main bronchus, the bronchus intermedius is anastomosed 1 cm below the initial anastomosis to the left main bronchus (Figure 13.9). We do not suggest to perform an anastomosis of the bronchus intermedius above the initial anastomosis of the trachea and left main bronchus (Figure 13.9b). Mobilization of the pulmonary ligament and a right hilar release is always required to limit the tension on the anastomosis. Occasionally, the bronchus intermedius can be anastomosed to the lateral wall of the trachea if the tension on this anastomosis is not excessive.

Left carinal pneumonectomy

The aortic arch greatly hinders performance of the anastomosis in left carinal pneumonectomy and renders the procedure technically challenging through a left thoracotomy. A one-step procedure with mobilization of the aortic arch should, however, be preferred to a two-stage approach in which a left proximal pneumonectomy with positive bronchial margin is followed 2–3 weeks later by the resection of the carina through a right thoracotomy or a sternotomy. In our experience, we have favored a median sternotomy over a left thoracotomy in the past few years if a left carinal pneumonectomy is anticipated [58].

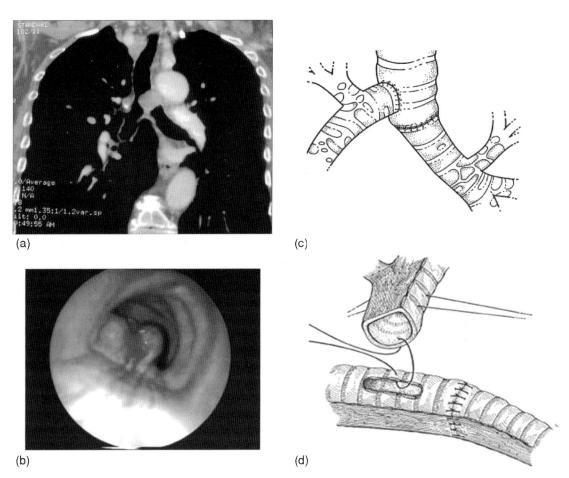

(a)

(b)

(c)

(d)

Figure 13.8 Extended resection of the carina and the trachea. (a) Computed tomographic scan of a 74-year-old female patient with adenocarcinoma of the trachea obstructing distal lumen of the trachea. (b) Fiberoptic bronchoscopy showing the lesion. (c) Anastomosis is first completed between the trachea and left main bronchus. The long proximal endotracheal tube is then advanced into the left main bronchus. The right main bronchus, which has been freed by intrapericardial hilar mobilization, is anastomosed to an orifice in the lateral wall of the trachea. On rare occasions, it may be preferable to implant the right main bronchus into the medial wall of the left main bronchus. The decision is based on evaluation of relative tensions intraoperatively. (d) Anastomosis of the right main bronchus to the trachea. The oval orifice in the trachea is located entirely within the cartilaginous wall. The lung is retracted anteriorly. The opening is as long as the bronchus is wide, but the width of the aperture is somewhat less than the anteroposterior diameter of the bronchus. Note the location of the orifice about two rings above the prior anastomosis. The initial anastomotic suture is shown.

Exposure of the carina and main bronchi through a median sternotomy requires a transpericardial approach. The anterior pericardium is divided vertically to permit circumferential mobilization of the ascending aorta and aortic arch, which is then encircled and retracted laterally to the left of the patient. The key to an adequate exposure of the left main bronchus through a median sternotomy is to perform a large mobilization of the ascending aorta and aortic arch, and to section the ligamentum arteriosum. Then, excellent exposure of the mediastinal trachea and carina can be displayed

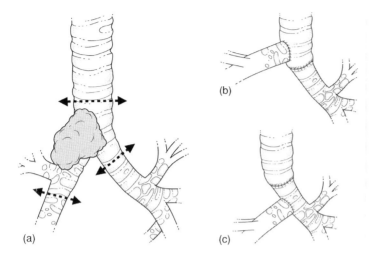

(a)

(b)

(c)

Figure 13.9 Carinal resection with lobar resection. (a) A right upper lobe tumor extending to the carina and lower trachea. (b) An anastomosis of the bronchus intermedius above the initial anastomosis of the trachea and left main bronchus is not suggested. (c) Following the anastomosis between the trachea and the left main bronchus, the bronchus intermedius is anastomosed 1 cm below the initial anastomosis.

by encircling and retracting the SVC to the right and the right main pulmonary artery inferiorly. The posterior pericardium can then be divided vertically to improve accessibility to both the right and left main bronchi (Figure 13.10).

The left mediastinal pleura is opened anteriorly below the sternal edge to access the left pleural space and perform the left pneumonectomy. The hilum is dissected to expose the left pulmonary artery and both pulmonary veins. The pericardium can be opened anteriorly and posteriorly around the hilum to improve exposure and facilitate stapling of both pulmonary veins and the pulmonary artery. The pericardial opening should be limited around the hilum and closed at the end of the procedure to avoid luxation of the heart into the left chest. The left lung can then be removed after transecting the distal trachea and right main bronchus. An end-to-end anastomosis between the trachea and right main bronchus is performed. The left pleura should then be closed in order to contain fluid accumulation into the pleural space. The anastomosis can be covered with surrounding tissue and the anterior pericardium closed. The left pleural space and the pericardium should be drained separately.

Anastomotic technique

The tracheobronchial anastomosis is usually performed in an end-to-end fashion first. Our technique consists in applying a running 4/0 poly-diaxone (PDS) suture on the deepest aspect of the airway with respect to the surgeon. For instance, in right carinal pneumonectomy, this represents the left aspect of the cartilage wall of the trachea and left main bronchus. The running suture is then tied at each end with two independent PDS sutures whose knots are made outside the lumen. Thereafter, several interrupted stitches of 3/0 PDS or 3/0 vicryl are placed in the remaining part of the anastomosis. They are tied after all of them have been placed to correct for size discrepancies. The stitches applied on the membranous portion are tied at the end to avoid any traction and potential tears. If an end-to-side anastomosis is required, the lateral side of the trachea is opened in an ovoid fashion corresponding to the size of the bronchus to be implanted. The opening is performed at least 1 cm away from the first anastomosis and is placed on the cartilaginous part of the trachea or bronchus to avoid any devascularization of the initial anastomosis and to provide additional rigidity to the end-to-side anastomosis. Again, a running suture of 4/0 PDS is used for the posterior part and interrupted stitches of 3/0 PDS or 3/0 vicryl are used for the anterior part of the anastomosis.

The development of anastomotic complications is likely due to technical factors at the time of airway resection and reconstruction. Careful dissection and

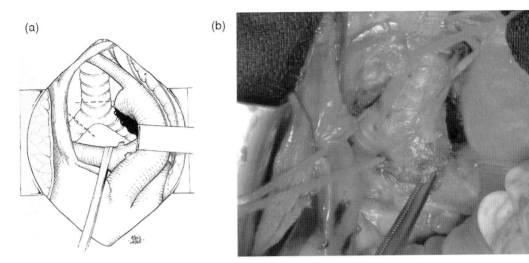

(a)　　　　　　　　(b)

Figure 13.10 (a) Mediastinal approach to the entire trachea. The sternum is fully divided, the anterior pericardium is opened vertically between the superior vena cava (SVC) and the aorta. The posterior pericardium is similarly opened retraction of the vena cava and aorta exposes a quadrilateral space in which the lower trachea and carina are seen. The right pulmonary artery lies just below the carina. A tape around the right pulmonary artery helps exposure. (b) Intraoperative photograph showing the exposure of the carina for a patient who underwent a left carinal pneumonectomy. The aorta is retracted to the left and the SVC is to the right. The tapes are around the right main bronchus and the trachea.

precise placement of anastomotic sutures should limit tissue trauma and avoid devascularization of the anastomotic site. In addition, airway resection should be limited to a maximum of 4 cm at the carinal level, in particular if a right carinal pneumonectomy is performed and the left mainstem bronchus is to be reanastomosed end-to-end to the distal trachea. Upward mobilization of the left mainstem bronchus is limited because of the aortic arch and can easily result in excessive anastomotic tension.

Release maneuvers

Dissection of the pretracheal plane is always performed (usually at the time of the mediastinoscopy) to reduce the tension at the anastomotic site. Hilar release with a U-shaped incision of the pericardium starting on the anterior pericardium behind the phrenic nerve at the level of the upper pulmonary vein, coming down below the inferior pulmonary vein, and rising up behind the pulmonary veins along the posterior pericardium up the pulmonary artery can allow the hilar structures to advance by about 2 cm upward and reduce the anastomotic tension. Additional length may be gained by completely incising the pericardium around the hilar vessels. We do not find that laryngeal or supralaryngeal release is useful to reduce the anastomotic tension at the level of the carina and we do not routinely use a chin stitch in these patients.

Postoperative care

The anastomosis is always controlled by bronchoscopy at the end of the procedure and secretions are cleaned up from the airways. All patients are extubated in the operating room or shortly after arrival in the recovery room. Pain relief is achieved with epidural analgesia or patient-controlled analgesia.

Inadequate epithelial ciliary motility of the residual lung usually occur after resection of the carina, but this can be controlled by adequate chest physiotherapy and occasionally repeated aspiration by flexible bronchoscopies in the first few days postoperatively. A temporary tracheostomy can be performed to reduce the physiological respiratory

Author (year)	Number of patients	Operative mortality (%)	5-yr survival (%)
Jensik et al. [59] 1982	34	29	15
Deslauriers et al. [60] 1989	38	29	13
Tsuchiya et al. [61] 1990	20	40	59 (2 yr)
Mathisen and Grillo [62] 1991	37	18.9	19
Roviaro et al. [63] 1994	28	4	20
Dartevelle et al. [64] 1995	60	6.6	43.3
Mitchell et al. [65] 1999	143	12.7	42
Roviaro et al. [66] 2001	49	8.2	24.5
Porhanov et al. [67] 2002	231	16	24.7
Regnard et al. [68] 2005	65	7.7	26.5
de Perrot et al. [58] 2006	119	7.6	44
Macchiarini et al. [69] 2006	50	4	51
Total	874	10.4 ± 11.6	25.6 ± 15.2

Table 13.4 Mortality and 5-year survival rates after carinal pneumonectomy.

dead space and facilitate direct aspiration whenever the predicted residual ventilatory functional reserve is borderline or the patient's collaboration reduced. The tracheostomy should be performed early in the postoperative period to prevent possible complications.

The results of carinal resection for bronchogenic carcinoma have improved over time. Recent series have shown that carinal resection is relatively safe in experienced centers and can be associated with good long-term survival in selected patients [58–69]. The median operative mortality is less than 7% and the median 5-year survival is 43.3% in our experience (Table 13.4).

Patients with positive mediastinal lymph node metastasis have a dismal prognosis; therefore, carinal resection should be considered a potential contraindication. This also underscores the importance of performing routine preoperative mediastinoscopy in these patients. We recommend performing the mediastinoscopy at the time of the planed carinal resection in order to avoid the development of scaring tissue along the trachea and to take advantage of the tracheal mobilization to reduce tension at the anastomotic site.

Further studies should determine the role of induction therapy in patients presenting with bronchogenic carcinoma and N2 disease. Induction therapy seems to improve survival if the mediastinal nodes can be sterilized prior to the lung resection. However, induction therapy could potentially be associated with increased operative morbidity and mortality in patients requiring right carinal pneumonectomy. Recently, we reported that operative mortality increased from 6.7 to 13% after induction therapy in patients undergoing right carinal pneumonectomy [58]. Martin et al. [70] also reported an operative mortality as high as 24% after right pneumonectomy following induction therapy.

SVC invasion

SVC syndrome is a distressing manifestation of benign and malignant disease obstructing venous return through the SVC. Invasion of the SVC by the right-sided bronchogenic carcinomas occurs in less than 1% of operable patients [71] and is usually regarded as an absolute surgical contraindication because of the dismal prognosis, absence of suitable graft material for reconstruction, and technical fear concerning the effects of SVC clampage, graft thrombosis, and infection. However, recent experimental and clinical advances increased the popularity of SVC replacement and expanded its therapeutic role in the management of patients with thoracic neoplasm [70–82]. Although, SVC resection and revascularization is a technically demanding procedure, a favorable outcome is possible for selected patients with advanced lung cancer.

The clinical picture of a patient with SVC syndrome is routinely simple because the symptoms and signs are typical and unmistakable. The most common symptoms in descending order are dyspnea, suffusion, cough, and arm or facial swelling. Less common symptoms include chest pain, dysphagia, syncope, obtundation, hemoptysis, and headache. The most common signs are facial and extremity edema, engorged neck, and chest veins, cyanosis, and plethora. In most patients, the syndrome is insidious, with slow development of symptoms. A short interval to presentation is highly correlated with either an underlying malignancy or catheter-induced thrombotic occlusion, whereas nonmalignant etiologies other than catheters are associated with long-standing symptoms. In this group of patients, the median time from onset of first symptom to actual presentation ranged from 3.2 to 6.5 weeks for patient with malignant disease.

These patients usually present with a mediastinal mass as noted by a widened superior mediastinum on routine chest radiographs. CT of the chest provides a detailed radiographic analysis of SVC, its tributaries and critical anatomic structures. MRI provides multiplanar anatomic detail that allows for easy visualization of the extrinsic mass in transverse, sagittal, and coronal planes. Superior vena cavography (simultaneous injection through both upper limbs) is an essential procedure when surgical intervention is contemplated. Echocardiography eliminates thrombosis extension into the right atrium and detects the patency of the jugular and axillary veins. Brain CT scan should always be performed to eliminate brain diseases that may increase brain edema during SVC clamping. Histologic diagnosis can be established by sputum histology, bronchoscopy, supraclavicular lymph node biopsy, thoracentesis, mediastinoscopy, bone marrow biopsy, and thoracotomy.

To perform an adequate and safe SVC resection and reconstruction, the greatest emphasis should be directed to adequately: evaluate the tumoral and vascular indications; keep in mind the hemodynamic effects of venous clamping; and select the material for SVC revascularization.

Vascular indications

Graft thrombosis may develop in the postoperative period and has deleterious consequences because of the risk of pulmonary embolism. In this sense, the status of the cephalic venous collateral pathway plays a major role. Since the proximal anastomosis needs to be performed either at the origin of the SVC or at the level of one or both brachiocephalic veins, SVC revascularization can be done only if there is an excellent patency at the level of the cephalic venous bed. Moreover, the proximal veins should have normal venous walls.

Hemodynamic effects of SVC clampage

The effects of SVC clampage are different according to the degree of obstruction of the SVC. For patients whose SVC is completely obstructed or tightly stenosed, intraoperative venous clamping results in a negligible hemodynamic compromise since a functioning collateral venous network already exists and supplements the flow obstruction to SVC. By contrast, when the intrathoracic or mediastinal disease does not obstruct the SVC, an even, sharp venous clamping might induce a hemodynamic cascade of events, including decreases cardiac inflow and outflow, increased venous pressure of the cephalic territory, and alterations of the cerebral arterial–venous gradient, leading to brain damage and intracranial bleeding. In fact, we have found that it is not difficult to reverse the hemodynamic effects of SVC clamping by using fluid supplementation and pharmacologic agents, reducing the venous clamping time, and giving adequate anticoagulation therapy [73].

A standard right posterolateral thoracotomy in the fifth intercostal space is the routine approach as opposed to the median sternotomy usually performed for replacing the SVC invaded by malignant mediastinal tumors. When the circumference of the involved caval wall is less than 30%, a partial resection of the vein is possible. Its reconstruction can be made either directly with a running suture or indirectly with the interposition of a prosthetic patch. Closure of up to 50% of the caval circumference can be made without hemodynamic imbalance.

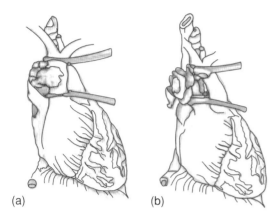

(a)   (b)

Figure 13.11 (a) Clamping and division of the superior vena cava beyond each side of the tumor. (b) This maneuver facilitates the exposure and stapling of the retrocaval pulmonary artery.

However, when there is a greater circumferential involvement, one should not hesitate to perform a total replacement of the SVC for both oncologic and hemodynamic reasons. Truncular replacement requires a tumor-free confluence of both brachiocephalic veins.

After the resectability of the lung is assessed, the SVC is clamped proximally at the confluence of the brachiocephalic veins and distally at the cavoatrial junction. Before that, the azygos vein is ligated, the tumor is dissected, the patient is loaded with fluid, and heparin (0.5 mg/kg) is given. The SVC is clamped and divided on each side of the tumor (Figure 13.11a), facilitating the exposure and stapling of the retrocaval pulmonary artery (Figure 13.11b). The reconstruction of the SVC follows. Although a heterologous bovine custom-made pericardium was used [83], we prefer a ringless, straight, size 18 or 20 PTFE graft. The proximal anastomosis is performed first, and the graft is flushed and deaired before completing the distal anastomosis. Because of the risk of infection while opening the airways, the PTFE is protected with an absorbed gauze of polyvinyl pyrolidone. After the vascular step, the pneumonectomy procedure is completed with or without carinal reconstruction. At the end of the procedure the PTFE graft is wrapped with a pleural flap. To avoid prosthesis kinking, the length of the graft should be adapted so that the distal anastomosis rests under mild tension.

Several complications might be associated with SVC revascularization and include anastomotic stenosis, graft thrombosis, and infection.

Spaggiari *et al.* [84] reported an analysis of the literature review regarding 109 patients who underwent SVC resection to identify the prognostic factors for patients with SVC invasion. This study has shown that SVC resection for lung cancer results in 30% major postoperative morbidity and 12% mortality rates. Five-year survival is 21%, with median survival at 11 months. Patients who had an induction treatment presented with an increased risk of major complications. The type of pulmonary resection (i.e., pneumonectomy) and the type of SVC resection (i.e., complete resection with prosthetic replacement) are the prognostic factors with the greatest adverse effect on survival.

Recently, Suzuki *et al.* [81] and Shargall *et al.* [82] reported a total of 55 patients with 12% of mortality rate. For their 40 patients, Suzuki *et al.* [81] found 24% of a 5-year survival and concluded that patients with direct tumor invasion to the SVC have a 30% of a 5-year survival whereas those with SVC invasion by metastatic nodes have a 6.6%.

We have performed SVC resection with a right carinal pneumonectomy in 25 patients with bronchogenic carcinoma. The SVC was completely resected en bloc with the tumor in 13 patients and was reconstructed with PTFE. The SVC cross-clamped time ranged between 15 and 45 minutes (median 23 min). The remaining 12 patients had only partial resection of the SVC and did not require graft interposition. One patient had complete agenesia of the inferior vena cava (IVC) and developed large collaterals draining into the azygos vein. The azygos vein was anastomosed to the right atrium after being sectioned from the SVC to maintain adequate venous return from the lower part of the body. Part of the left atrium was resected in 10 patients, the muscular wall of the esophagus in 4 patients, and the chest wall (2 ribs) or the diaphragm in 1 patient each.

Morbidity and mortality is linked with the association of a carinal pneumonectomy, excision of the SVC alone does not change anything.

Invasion of the left atrium, aorta, and main pulmonary trunk

Complete resections in patients with tumors invading the left atrium, aorta, and main pulmonary trunk are often not possible and are associated with a high mortality. There are no consistent data regarding these resections of T4 lung cancers. Systemic arterial invasion of T4 lung cancer carry the poorest long-term outcome. Limited local invasion of the intrapericardial pulmonary artery or left atrium can be resected completely with expected 5-year survival rates of 20–30% [85]. In general, if there is less than 1–1.5 cm of intrapericardial involvement of these structures, they can usually be resected with negative margins and a safe vascular closure. Although most authorities have viewed the need for more complex reconstructions that require cardiopulmonary bypass (CPB) as a contraindication to resection, recent reports encourage the application of CPB in extended pulmonary resection to achieve complete resection [74,86–94]. It had been estimated that less than 0.1% of all thoracic resections were done with CPB.

The indication for the surgical radical therapy is based on the individual situation of the patients after interdisciplinary evaluation and discussion of treatment options. Distant metastatic disease or extrathoracic sites of disease have to be excluded. All elective procedures are to be done in curative intention; no palliative indication is considered acceptable in these advanced tumors.

In most patients, locally advanced bronchogenic carcinoma can be resected without the need of CPB. Cardiopulmonary bypass is used to resect carcinoma invading the aortic arch, the descending aorta, the pulmonary artery bifurcation, the left atrium, and the carina. The potential side effects of CPB on lung function and other organ function is well described in the literature, but the oncologic side effect is less known. The observation that some patients with carcinomas, sarcoma and other tumors are disease-free survivors over many years, despite the resection which occurs on CPB, indicates that the use of CB does not necessarily increase the risk of tumor dissemination although it has been observed occasionally [86]. The key issue for a favorable outcome justifying extended resection of advanced thoracic malignancies on CPB is patient selection.

Preoperative evaluation

For preoperative work-up chest CT is the primary mode of evaluation for all patients. A full biologic and radiographic work-up is to be performed to exclude brain, abdominal, and bone metastasis. An angiography of the aortic arch and supraaortic trunks as well as a transesophageal ultrasound should be performed to demonstrate presence of any invasion of the left subclavian artery and the esophageal wall. Duplex scan of both carotid and vertebral arteries have to be performed to assure good patency of all four vessels. MRI is necessary to exclude an invasion of the intervertebral foramen.

The invasion of the left atrium by NSCLC is typically discovered at thoracotomy in less than 4% of patients undergoing curative resection for NSCLC. The left atrium is usually invaded more frequently by direct extension rather than by tumor emboli protruding from the pulmonary veins. In most cases, resection of the left atrium can be achieved by apposing a vascular clamp on the left atrium to remove the tumor along with both pulmonary veins and by directly suturing the defect. If a larger portion of the left atrium is invaded, the tumor is often not completely resectable because of prolonged microscopic infiltration of the myocardium. Thus, CPB has rarely been used for left atrial resection in our experience. Some authors have found that CPB could be useful if the tumor extends into the lumen of the left atrium with a risk of systemic tumor embolization. Cardiopulmonary bypass allowed opening the left atrium after aortic cross-clamping and instillation of cardioplegia or after the induction of hypothermic ventricular fibrillation to avoid air embolism. After opening the pericardium, the cannulas are placed in the superior and IVC or in the right atrium, and in the ascending aorta. The pulmonary artery is then stapled at its bifurcation without compromising the lumen of the main pulmonary artery. Then bronchus and left atrium is stapled at distance from their origin to obtain complete resection of the tumor.

Complete resection of tumors with partial invasion of the left atrial wall should not be denied because this procedure represents the only hope for cure [11,74,90–93].

The results of invasion of the aorta by NSCLC are limited to scattered reports, mainly because tumors are so locally extensive that resection is often impossible. Aortic invasion by NSCLC is usually limited to the adventitia. However, in rare instances, the media of the aorta is also invaded and resection requires cross-clamping of the aorta proximally and distally to remove the infiltrated wall. A shunt prosthesis between the ascending and descending aorta in order to resect and reconstruct the infiltrated portion of the aorta has been suggested. However, we believe that CPB was the easiest way to achieve perfusion of the upper and lower part of the body during aortic cross-clamping.

Surgical access is achieved by posterolateral thoracotomy or median sternotomy and sometimes by an initial anterior transcervical approach that allows dissection of the thoracic inlet at distance from the tumor confirming resectability of the tumor. In case where the subclavian artery is invaded by the tumor, the artery is sectioned distally from the tumor and anastomosed in a terminolateral fashion to the carotid artery (Figure 13.12). To perform lobectomy, patient is then turned in a right lateral decubitus position. The cannulas for CPB are inserted in the main pulmonary artery and the descending aorta. Perfusion of the upper part of the body is thus achieved by the beating heart and the lower part of the body was perfused by normothermic partial bypass. Adequate perfusion of the upper part of the body is controlled with an arterial line in the right radial artery. The aorta can then be cross-clamped between the innominate artery and the left carotid artery to resect the distal part of the aortic arch and the origin of the subclavian artery. Cannulation of the main pulmonary artery and descending aorta through a left posterolateral thoracotomy can also be useful when the aortic wall of the descending aorta is unexpectedly invaded by the tumor and the femoral vessels are not kept in the operating field. Using this technique, the venous cannula should be placed proximally in the left pulmonary artery after having cut the arterial ligament, and the tip of the

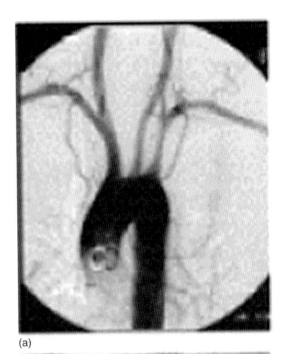

(a)

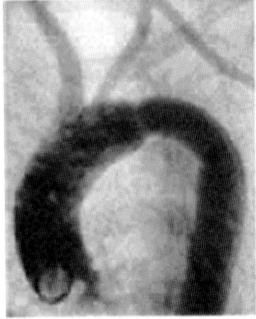

(b)

Figure 13.12 Angiography of a patient before (a) and after (b) surgery showing that the left subclavian artery was sectioned and anastomosed in a terminolateral fashion to the left carotid artery and the distal aortic arch was replaced with a Dacron graft.

venous cannula should be placed in the main pulmonary artery or in the right ventricle. Care should be taken to avoid placing the tip of the cannula in the right pulmonary artery, since it may prevent adequate ejection from the right ventricle. When the tumor invades the aortic arch more proximally than the left carotid artery, or if the lesser curvature of the aortic arch is invaded, CPB with selective cerebral perfusion or with circulatory arrest can be required. The aorta is then reconstructed with a Dacron patch. Patients with large tumors occluding the left main pulmonary artery at its origin, precluding any resection of the pulmonary artery without having to reconstruct the main pulmonary artery, also need resection with CPB. In this case, a median sternotomy is preferred.

Complications

There is considerable evidence that CPB is associated with deterioration of pulmonary function as assessed by measuring the alveolar–arterial oxygenation gradient, intrapulmonary shunt, degree of pulmonary edema, pulmonary compliance, and pulmonary vascular resistance. More frequent and more severe complications with extended periods of mechanical ventilation are expected, if CPB is applied. In our experience [86] pulmonary edema, acute respiratory distress syndrome, and atelectasis associated with recurrent nerve palsy were the most common complications observed following T4 lung cancer resection with CPB. Bleeding is another frequent complication following CPB-assisted procedures. In a series of lung resection during cardiac operations with CPB, bleeding complications were reported to affect 21% of patients.

Surgical reports dealing with tumors invading the pulmonary artery trunk are limited. Ricci *et al.* [94] reported pulmonary angioplasty under CPB in three patients whose NSCLC invaded the main pulmonary trunk; however, all patients died within 25 months following operation. Tsuchiya *et al.* [74] replaced the bifurcation of the pulmonary artery on CPB in six patients. Because all patients died within 30 months from operation, invasion of the pulmonary artery trunk was considered technically resectable but incurable biologically.

Vascular resection and reconstruction of the aorta, and left atrium have been safely described with 5-year survival rates of 20%. Combined pulmonary and aorta resection is described by Fukuse *et al.* [89] with 5-year survival rates of 31% ($n = 15$). Combined pulmonary and left atrial resection has been described most recently by Bobbio *et al.* [90] with 5-year survival rates of 10% ($n = 23$). Recently, Ohta and colleagues [95] reported 16 patients underwent thoracic aorta resection along with a lung resection with the mortality rate 12.5% and 5-year survival rates were 70% for patients with N0 disease and 16.7% for patients with N2 or N3 disease.

We have recently reported our CPB experience in resecting NSCLC [86]. We operated on seven patients with 0% mortality and 28% ($n = 2$) morbidity. Among the seven patients, one died of pulmonary emboli 6 months after surgery, three patients are alive without recurrences, and remaining three patients are alive with recurrences.

The use of CPB does not appear to increase the risk of cancer dissemination. Several series have reported combining lung resection for bronchogenic carcinoma with aortocoronary bypass surgery during the same operative procedure with good early and long-term results despite the use of CPB.

Long-term outcome of patients with locally advanced lung cancer depends primarily of completeness of resection. Martini *et al.* [92] have reported a series of lung cancer invading the mediastinum, and observed that the 5-year survival rate was 30% if the tumor was completely resected, whereas it was only 14% if it was incompletely resected. Similar observations were reported in a series of lung cancer invading the heart or great vessels with 5-year survival ranging between 23 and 40% if the tumor was completely resected, whereas no patients survived greater than 3 years if the tumor was incompletely resected.

Further studies will be necessary to confirm these findings in patients undergoing resection of locally advanced NSCLC under CPB. Patients with locally advanced NSCLC should be treated with aggressive multidisciplinary therapy in a manner that maximizes the chance for long-term cure while minimizing the overall risks of treatment.

Invasion of the vertebral body

Direct invasion of the vertebral body or the costovertebral angle by an NSCLC other than a superior sulcus tumor is rarely observed. Treatment options vary among the radiation therapy alone, resection by shaving off the bone, and tangential or hemivertebrectomy. DeMeester and colleagues [96] provide evidence that for tumors limited invasion of periosteum below the third vertebral body, long-term survival (5-year survival, 42%) and cure for selected patients can be anticipated by combining a preoperative radiation therapy (30 Gy) and en bloc resection of the primary tumor and involved vertebral body. Resectability was based on the preoperative radiological absence of bony erosion and intraoperative absence of invasion into costotransverse foramen. For tumors with more extensive invasion, McCormack [71] reported a 10% survival at 5 years by performing a total vertebrectomy and spinal stabilization; however, no conclusions were drawn as to its value.

Conclusion

Improved surgical techniques have increased the feasibility and radicality of extended operations for patients with potentially resectable but locally invasive NSCLC. Advances in the perioperative management and postoperative care, along with a careful patient selection, will likely make the operative mortality and morbidity less prohibitive and a more favorable prognosis.

It has been well demonstrated that the prognosis after operations for T3/T4 tumors mainly depends on the N stage. Patients with N0 or minimal N1 disease do significantly better after radical resection, a finding that clearly justifies operative therapy in these patients. On the other hand, both the technical complexity of the operation and its rare occurrence therefore suggest centralization of the procedure to departments that express profound and continuous interest in such problems and that at the same time have a high degree of experience with both general thoracic and vascular procedures.

Our policy regarding locally advanced lung cancer patients is to perform surgery on first intention, whenever a complete resection is thought to be technically possible. Complete resection resulting in good mean 5-year survival is possible, especially for tumors invading the trachea or carina (5-year survival is 40%). In our opinion, any attempt to downstage the disease in these particular patients introduced a new dilemma for the surgeon concerning the type of resection to be performed: the one that was required initially to remove all the disease, or the one dictated by the residual disease?

The thoracic medical and surgical community should promote all efforts to extend the surgical indications for locally advanced NSCLC, making these operations available whenever possible to patients in whom a cure can be achieved.

References

1 Murray CJL, Lopez AD (eds). *The Global Burden of Disease: A Comprehensive Assessment of Mortality and Disability from Disease Injuries and Risk Factors in 1990 and Projected to 2020.* Cambridge: Harvard University Press, 1996.

2 Parker SL, Long T, Bolden S *et al.* Cancer statistics, 1997. *CA Cancer J Clin* 1997; **47**:5–27.

3 Berrino F, Capocaccia R, Esteve J (eds). Survival of cancer patients in Europe. In: *The EUROCARE 2 Study*, Vol. 151. Lyon, France: IARC Scientific Publications, 1999:1–572.

4 Grillo HC. Pleural and chest wall involvement. *Int Trends Gen Thorac Surg* 1985; **1**:134–8.

5 Akay H, Cangir AK, Kutlay H *et al.* Surgical treatment of peripheral lung cancer adherent to the parietal pleura. *Eur J Cardiothorac Surg* Oct 2002; **22(4)**:615–20.

6 Ratto GB, Piacenza G, Frola C *et al.* Chest wall involvement by lung cancer: computed tomographic detection and results and prognostic factors. *Ann Thorac Surg* 1991; **51**:182–8.

7 Rendina EA, Bognolo DA, Mineo TC *et al.* Computed tomography for the evaluation of intrathoracic invasion by lung cancer. *J Thorac Cardiovasc Surg* 1987; **94**:57–63.

8 McCaughan BC, Martini N, Bains MS *et al.* Chest wall invasion in carcinoma of the lung. *J Thorac Cardiovasc Surg* 1985; **89**:836–41.

9 Eschapasse H, Gaillard J, Henry F *et al.* Repair of large chest wall defects. *Ann Thorac Surg* 1981; **31**:45–51.

10 McCormack PM, Bains M, Beattie EJ, Jr, Martini N. New trends in skeletal reconstruction after resection of chest wall tumors. *Ann Thorac Surg* 1981; **31**:45–52.

11 Macchiarini P, Dartevelle P. Extended resections for lung cancer. In: Roth JA, Cox J, Hong WK (eds). *Lung Cancer*, 2nd edn. London: Blackwell Science, 1998:135–61.

12 Piehler JM, Pairolero PC, Weiland LH *et al.* Bronchogenic carcinoma with chest wall invasion: factors affecting survival following en bloc resection. *Ann Thorac Surg* 1982; **34**:684–91.

13 Patterson GA, Ilves R, Ginsberg RJ *et al.* The value of adjuvant radiotherapy in pulmonary and chest wall resection for bronchogenic carcinoma. *Ann Thorac Surg* 1982; **34**:692–7.

14 Allen MS, Mathisen DJ, Grillo HC. Bronchogenic carcinoma with chest wall invasion. *Ann Thorac Surg* 1991; **51**:948–51.

15 Shah SS, Goldstraw P. Combined pulmonary and thoracic wall for resection for stage III lung cancer. *Thorax* 1995; **50**:782–4.

16 Downey RJ, Martini N, Rusch VW *et al.* Extent of chest wall invasion and survival in patients with lung cancer. *Ann Thorac Surg* 1999; **68**:188–93.

17 Facciolo F, Cardillo G, Lopergolo M *et al.* Chest wall invasion in non-small cell lung carcinoma: a rationale for en bloc resection. *J Thorac Cardiovasc Surg* Apr 2001; **121**:649–56.

18 Magdeleinat P, Alifona M, Benbrahem C *et al.* Surgical treatment of lung cancer invading the chest wall: results and prognostic factors. *Ann Thorac Surg* 2001; **71**:1094–9.

19 Burkhart HM, Allen MS, Nichols FC, III *et al.* Results of en bloc resection for bronchogenic carcinoma with chest wall invasion. *J Thorac Cardiovasc Surg* Apr 2002; **123(4)**:670–5.

20 Chapelier A, Fadel E, Macchiarini P *et al.* Factors affecting long-term survival after en-bloc resection of lung cancer invading the chest wall. *Eur J Cardiothorac Surg* 2000; **18**:513–8.

21 Riquet M, Lang-Lazdunski L, Le PB *et al.* Characteristics and prognosis of resected T3 non-small cell lung cancer. *Ann Thorac Surg* Jan 2002; **73(1)**:253–8.

22 Roviaro G, Varoli F, Grignani F *et al.* Non-small cell lung cancer with chest wall invasion: evolution of surgical treatment and prognosis in the last 3 decades. *Chest* May 2003; **123(5)**:1341–7.

23 Matsuoka H, Nishio W, Okada M *et al.* Resection of chest wall invasion in patients with non-small cell lung cancer. *Eur J Cardiothorac Surg* Dec 2004; **26(6)**:1200–4.

24 Allen MS. Chest wall resection and reconstruction for lung cancer. *Thorac Surg Clin* 2004; **14**:211–6.

25 Shaw RR, Paulson DL, Kee JL, Jr. Treatment of superior sulcus tumors by irradiation followed by resection. *Ann Surg* 1961; **154**:29–40.

26 Komaki R, Mountain CF, Holbert JM *et al.* Superior sulcus tumors: treatment selection and results for 85 patients without metastasis (M0) at presentation. *Int J Radiat Oncol Biol Phys* 1990; **19**:31.

27 Shahian DM, Neptune WB, Ellis FH, Jr. Pancoast tumors: improved survival with preoperative and postoperative radiotherapy. *Ann Thorac Surg* 1987; **43**:32.

28 Dartevelle P, Chapelier A, Macchiarini P *et al.* Anterior transcervical–thoracic approach for radical resection of lung tumors invading the thoracic inlet. *J Thorac Cardiovasc Surg* 1993; **105**:1025.

29 Hilaris BS, Martini N, Wong GY *et al.* Treatment of superior sulcus tumors (Pancoast tumor). *Surg Clin North Am* 1987; **67**:965–77.

30 Rusch VW, Giroux DJ, Kraut MJ *et al.* Induction chemoradiation and surgical resection for non-small cell lung carcinomas of the superior sulcus: Initial results of Southwest Oncology Group Trial 9416 (Intergroup Trial 0160). *J Thorac Cardiovasc Surg* 2001; **121**:472–83.

31 Rusch VW, Giroux D, Kraut MJ *et al.* Induction chemoradiotherapy and surgical resection for non-small cell lung carcinomas of the superior sulcus (Pancoast tumors): mature results of Southwest Oncology Group trial 9416 (Intergroup 0160). *Proc Am Soc Clin Oncol* 2003; **22**:2548.

32 Wright CD, Menard MT, Wain JC *et al.* Induction chemoradiation compared with induction radiation for lung cancer involving the superior sulcus. *Ann Thorac Surg* 2002; **73**:1541–4.

33 Kunitoh H, Kato H, Tsuboi M *et al.* A phase II trial of pre-operative chemoradiotherapy followed by surgical resection in Pancoast tumors: initial report of Japan Clinical Oncology Group trial (JCOG 9806). *Proc Am Soc Clin Oncol* 2003; **22**:2549.

34 Detterbeck FC, Jones DR, Rosenman JG. Pancoast tumors. In: Detterbeck FC, Rivera MP, Socinski MA, Rosenman JG (eds). *Diagnosis and Treatment of Lung Cancer: An Evidence-Based Guide for the Practicing Clinician.* Philadelphia: WB Saunders, 2001:233–43.

35 Detterbeck FC. Changes in the treatment of Pancoast tumors. *Ann Thorac Surg* Jun 2003; **75(6)**:1990–7.

36 Dartevelle PG, Mussot S. Anterior approach to superior sulcus lesions. In: Shields TW, Locicero J, III,

Ponn RB, Rusch VW (eds). *General Thoracic Surgery*, 6th edn. Philadelphia: Lippincott Williams and Wilkins, 2005:545–53.

37 Fadel E, Missenard G, Chapelier A *et al*. En bloc resection of non-small cell lung cancer invading the thoracic inlet and intervertebral foramina. *J Thorac Cardiovasc Surg* Apr 2002; **123(4)**:676–85.

38 Pitz CC, de la Riviere AB, van Swieten HA *et al*. Surgical treatment of Pancoast tumours. *Eur J Cardiothorac Surg* Jul 2004; **26(1)**:202–8.

39 Paulson DL. Technical considerations in stage T3 disease: the superior sulcus lesion. In: Delarue NC, Eschapasse H (eds). *International Trends in Thoracic Surgery*, Vol. 1. Philadelphia: WB Saunders, 1985:121.

40 Anderson TM, Moy PM, Holmes EC. Factors affecting survival in superior sulcus tumors. *J Clin Oncol* 1986; **4**:1598.

41 Devine JW, Mendenhall WM, Million RR *et al*. Carcinoma of the superior pulmonary sulcus treated with surgery and/or radiation therapy. *Cancer* 1986; **57**:941.

42 Miller JI, Mansour KA, Hatcher CR, Jr. Carcinoma of the superior pulmonary sulcus. *Ann Thorac Surg* 1979; **28**:44.

43 Wright CD, Moncure AC, Shepard JA *et al*. Superior sulcus lung tumors. Results of combined treatment (irradiation and radical resection). *J Thorac Cardiovasc Surg* 1987; **94**:69.

44 McKneally M. Discussion of Shahian DM, Neptune WB, Ellis FH Jr: Pancoast tumors: improved survival with preoperative and postoperative radiotherapy. *Ann Thorac Surg* **43**:32, 1987.

45 Sartori F, Rea F, Calabro F *et al*. Carcinoma of the superior pulmonary sulcus. Results of irradiation and radical resection. *J Thorac Cardiovasc Surg* 1992; **104**:679.

46 Maggi G, Casadio C, Pischedda F *et al*. Combined radiosurgical treatment of Pancoast tumor. *Ann Thorac Surg* 1994; **57**:198.

47 Ginsberg RJ, Martini N, Zaman M *et al*. Influence of surgical resection and brachytherapy in the management of superior sulcus tumors. *Ann Thorac Surg* 1994; **57**:1440.

48 Okubo K, Wada H, Fukuse T *et al*. Treatment of Pancoast tumors. Combined irradiation and radical resection. *Thorac Cardiovasc Surg* 1995; **43**:84.

49 Dartevelle P. Extended operations for lung cancer. *Ann Thorac Surg* 1997; **63**:12.

50 Martinod E, D'Audiffret A, Thomas P *et al*. Management of superior sulcus tumors: experience with 139 cases treated by surgical resection. *Ann Thorac Surg* 2002; **73**:1534–9.

51 Alifano M, D'Aiuto M, Magdeleinat P *et al*. Surgical treatment of superior sulcus tumors: results and prognostic factors. *Chest* Sep 2003; **124(3)**:996–1003.

52 Goldberg M, Gupta D, Sasson AR *et al*. The surgical management of superior sulcus tumors: a retrospective review with long-term follow-up. *Ann Thorac Surg* 2005; **79(4)**:1174–9.

53 Dartevelle P, Macchiarini P. Carinal resection for bronchogenic cancer. *Semin Thorac Cardiovasc Surg* 1996:414–25.

54 Dartevelle P, Macchiarini P. Techniques of pneumonectomy. Sleeve pneumonectomy. *Chest Surg Clin N Am* 1999:407–17.

55 Grillo HC, Bendixen HH, Gephart T. Resection of the carina and lower trachea. *Ann Surg* 1963; **158**:889–93.

56 Pearson FG, Todd TRJ, Cooper JD. Experience with primary neoplasms of the trachea and carina. *J Thorac Cardiovasc Surg* 1984; **88**:511–8.

57 Barclay RS, McSwann N, Welsh TM. Tracheal reconstruction without the use of grafts. *Thorax* 1957; **12**:177–80.

58 de Perrot M, Fadel E, Mercier O *et al*. Long-term results after carinal resection for carcinoma: does the benefit warrant the risk? *J Thorac Cardiovasc Surg* Jan 2006; **131(1)**:81–9.

59 Jensik RJ, Faber LP, Kittle CF, Miley RW, Thatcher WC, El-Baz N. Survival in patients undergoing tracheal sleeve pneumonectomy for bronchogenic carcinoma. *J Thorac Cardiovasc Surg* 1982; **84**:489–96.

60 Deslauriers J, Beaulieu M, McClish A. Tracheal-sleeve pneumonectomy. In: Shields TW (ed). *General Thoracic Surgery*, 3rd edn. Philadelphia: Lea & Febiger, 1989:383–7.

61 Tsuchiya R, Goya T, Naruke T, Suemasu K. Resection of tracheal carina for lung cancer. Procedure, complications, and mortality. *J Thorac Cardiovasc Surg* May 1990; **99(5)**:779–87.

62 Mathisen DJ, Grillo HC. Carinal resection for bronchogenic carcinoma. *J Thorac Cardiovasc Surg* 1991; **102**:16–23.

63 Roviaro GC, Varoli F, Rebuffat C *et al*. Tracheal sleeve pneumonectomy for bronchogenic carcinoma. *J Thorac Cardiovasc Surg* 1994; **107**:13–8.

64 Dartevelle P, Macchiarini P, Chapelier A. Superior vena cava resection and reconstruction. In: Faber LP (ed). *Techniques of Pulmonary Resection*. Philadelphia: WB Saunders, 1995.

65 Mitchell JD, Mathisen DJ, Wright CD *et al*. Clinical experience with carinal resection. *J Thorac Cardiovasc* 1999; **117**:39–53.

66 Roviaro G, Varoli C, Romanelli A *et al.* Complications of tracheal sleeve pneumonectomy: personal experience and overview of the literature. *J Thorac Cardiovasc* 2001; **121**:234–40.

67 Porhanov V, Poliakov IS, Selvaschuk AP *et al.* Indications and results of sleeve carinal resection. *Eur J Cardiothorac Surg* 2002; **22**:685–94.

68 Regnard JF, Perrotin C, Giovannetti R *et al.* Resection for tumors with carinal involvement: technical aspects, results, and prognostic factors. *Ann Thorac Surg* Nov 2005; **80(5)**:1841–6.

69 Macchiarini P, Altmayer M, Go T *et al.* Technical innovations of carinal resection for nonsmall-cell lung cancer. *Ann Thorac Surg* Dec 2006; **82(6)**:1989–97.

70 Martin J, Ginsberg RJ, Abolhoda A *et al.* Morbidity and mortality after neoadjuvant therapy for lung cancer: the risks of right pneumonectomy. *Ann Thorac Surg* 2001; **72**:1149–54.

71 McCormack PM. Extended pulmonary resections. In: Pearson FG, Deslauriers J, Ginsberg RJ *et al.* (eds). *Thoracic Surgery.* New York: Churchill Livingstone, 1995:897–908.

72 Spaggiari L, Regnard JF, Magdeleinat P *et al.* Extended resections for bronchogenic carcinoma invading the superior vena cava system. *Ann Thorac Surg* 2000; **69**:233–6.

73 Dartevelle P, Macchiarini P, Chapelier A. Technique of superior vena cava resection and reconstruction. *Chest Surg Clin N Am* May 1995; **5(2)**:345–58.

74 Tsuchiya R, Asamura H, Kondo H, Goya T, Naruke T. Extended resection of the left atrium, great vessels, or both for lung cancer. *Ann Thorac Surg* 1994; **57**:960–5.

75 Thomas P, Magnan PE, Moulin G, Giudicelli R, Fuentes P. Extended operation for lung cancer invading the superior vena cava. *Eur J Cardiothorac Surg* 1994; **8**:177–82.

76 Nakahara K, Ohno K, Mastumura A *et al.* Extended operation for lung cancer invading the aortic arch and superior vena cava. *J Thorac Cardiovasc Surg* 1989; **97**:428–33.

77 Dartevelle P, Chapelier A, Navajas M *et al.* Replacement of the superior vena cava with polytetrafluoroethylene grafts combined with resection of mediastinal-pulmonary malignant tumors. Report of thirteen cases. *J Thorac Cardiovasc Surg* 1987; **94**:361–6.

78 Dartevelle PG, Chapelier AR, Pastorino U *et al.* Long-term follow-up after prosthetic replacement of the superior vena cava combined with resection of mediastinal-pulmonary malignant tumors. *J Thorac Cardiovasc Surg* 1991; **102**:259–65.

79 Grunenwald DH, Andre F, Le Pechoux C *et al.* Benefit of surgery after chemoradiotherapy in stage IIIB (T4 and/or N3) non-small cell lung cancer. *J Thorac Cardiovasc Surg* 2001; **122**:796–802.

80 Spaggiari L, Thomas P, Magdeleinat P *et al.* Superior vena cava resection with prosthetic replacement for non-small cell lung cancer: long-term results of a multicentric study. *Eur J Cardiothorac Surg* 2002; **21**:1080–6.

81 Suzuki K, Asamura H, Watanabe S *et al.* Combined resection of superior vena cava for lung carcinoma: prognostic significance of patterns of superior vena cava invasion. *Ann Thorac Surg* Oct 2004; **78(4)**:1184–9.

82 Shargall Y, de Perrot M, Keshavjee S *et al.* 15 years single center experience with surgical resection of the superior vena cava for non-small cell lung cancer. *Lung Cancer* 2004; **45**:357–63.

83 Spaggiari L, Veronesi G, D'Aiuto M *et al.* Superior vena cava reconstruction using heterologous pericardial tube after extended resection for lung cancer. *Eur J Cardiothorac Surg* Sep 2004; **26(3)**:649–51.

84 Spaggiari L, Magdeleinat P, Kondo H *et al.* Results of superior vena cava resection for lung cancer. Analysis of prognostic factors. *Lung Cancer* Jun 2004; **44(3)**:339–46.

85 DiPerna CA, Wood DE. Surgical management of T3 and T4 lung cancer. *Clin Cancer Res* Jul 1, 2005; **11(13, Pt 2)**:5038s–44s.

86 de Perrot M, Fadel E, Mussot S, de Palma A, Chapelier A, Dartevelle P. Resection of locally advanced (T4) non-small cell lung cancer with cardiopulmonary bypass. *Ann Thorac Surg* May 2005; **79(5)**:1691–6.

87 Vaporciyan AA, Rice D, Correa AM *et al.* Resection of advanced thoracic malignancies requiring cardiopulmonary bypass. *Eur J Cardiothorac Surg* 2002; **22**:47–52.

88 Wiebe K, Baraki H, Macchiarini P *et al.* Extended pulmonary resections of advanced thoracic malignancies with support of cardiopulmonary bypass. *Eur J Cardiothorac Surg* Apr 2006; **29(4)**:571–7.

89 Fukuse T, Wada H, Hitomi S. Extended operations for non-small cell lung cancers invading great vessels and left atrium. *Eur J Cardiothorac Surg* 1997; **11**:664–9.

90 Bobbio A, Carbognani P, Grapeggia M *et al.* Surgical outcome of combined pulmonary and atrial resection for lung cancer. *Thorac Cardiovasc Surg* Jun 2004; **52**:180–2.

91 Shirakusa T, Kimura M. Partial atrial resection in advanced lung carcinoma with and without cardiopulmonary bypass. *Thorax* 1991; **46**:484–7.

92 Martini N, Yellin A, Ginsberg RJ *et al.* Management of non-small cell lung cancer with direct mediastinal involvement. *Ann Thorac Surg* 1994; **58**:1447–51.

93 Ratto GB, Costa R, Vassallo G *et al.* Twelve-year experience with left atrial resection in the treatment of non-small cell lung cancer. *Ann Thorac Surg* Jul 2004; **78(1)**:234–7.

94 Ricci C, Rendina E, Venuta F *et al.* Reconstruction of the pulmonary artery in patients with lung cancer. *Ann Thorac* 1994; **57**:627–33.

95 Ohta M, Hirabayasi H, Shiono H *et al.* Surgical resection for lung cancer with infiltration of the thoracic aorta. *J Thorac Cardiovasc Surg* 2005; **129**:804–8.

96 DeMeester TR, Albertucci M, Dawson PJ *et al.* Management of tumors adherent to the vertebral column. *J Thorac Cardiovasc Surg* 1989; **97**:373–8.

CHAPTER 14

Adjuvant Chemotherapy Following Surgery for Lung Cancer

Benjamin Besse and Thierry Le Chevalier

Introduction

For many years, surgery has been the standard treatment for patients with early-stage nonsmall cell lung cancer (NSCLC). Despite complete resection, 5-year survival rates have been disappointing, ranging from 67% for stage I patients to 23% in patients with ipsilateral mediastinal lymph node involvement [1]. Following surgery, 10–15% of patients will experience a local relapse, while a distant recurrence will occur in 15–60% of the cases, generally leading to death. Efforts at improving local control and survival for patients with operable NSCLC have examined the addition of chemotherapy and/or radiation in the postoperative (adjuvant) setting.

Mediastinal postoperative radiation therapy (PORT) has been shown to decrease local recurrence but this local control advantage did not translate to a survival benefit [2]. The PORT Meta-Analysis Trialists Group analyzed individual patient data from prospective trials of patients with resected early-stage NSCLC [3]. Nine trials (involving >2000 patients) were included in the analysis, some of them initiated as early as 1965. The results strongly suggested that PORT had a detrimental effect on survival, presumably through the increased incidence of intercurrent death. The detriment of PORT was inversely related to nodal

status, with significantly reduced survival noted for N0 and N1 disease while results for stage III and N2 patients slightly favored PORT. Radiation oncologists were critical of the study for several reasons, including patient selection, the use of outdated treatment modalities and inappropriately high radiation doses. However, these data do not support the routine use of adjuvant radiation therapy in completely resected stage I or II patients. It may be recommended for patients at high risk of local relapse, i.e., with extensive nodal involvement or positive surgical margins. It should be evaluated in totally resected N2 patients in a prospective randomized trial.

As the majority of deaths occur as a result of recurrent disease, unrecognized micrometastases present at the time of surgery may be a crucial prognostic factor. It is of concern that sensitive immunohistochemical techniques (using antibody to cytokeratin 18) have demonstrated the presence of micrometastatic disease in the bone marrow of as many as 28–60% of patients undergoing surgical resection thought not to show evidence of extrathoracic disease after conventional staging [4,5]. Circulating cells related to NSCLC primary tumor can also be characterized by quantitative PCR in patients, even before surgery [6,7]. Postoperative chemotherapy may eliminate micrometastatic disease and prevent the subsequent emergence of incurable clinical disease. In experimental models, potential curability of tumors by drugs has been inversely correlated to the tumor burden, thus supporting this concept. Adjuvant chemotherapy has

Lung Cancer, 3rd edition. Edited by Jack A. Roth, James D. Cox, and Waun Ki Hong. © 2008 Blackwell Publishing, ISBN: 978-1-4051-5112-2.

Table 14.1 Overview of recent randomized platin-based adjuvant trial and pooled analysis.

	n	IA	IB	II	IIIA
			Randomized trials		
ALPI [16]	1209			0.96 [0.81–1.13]	
CALGB [21]	344		0.8 [0.6–1.07]		
BLT [18]	381			1.02 [0.77–1.35]	
IALT [17]	1867			0.86 [0.76–0.98]	
ANITA [20]	840				0.8 [0.66–0.96]
BR10 [19]	482			0.69 [0.52–0.91]	
			Pooled analysis		
LACE [22]	4584			0.89 [0.82–0.96]	

been validated in breast cancer and colorectal cancer, especially in node-positive patients, with an absolute 5-year benefit ranging from 5 to 10% [8,9]. A growing list of other tumor types, including early-stage ovarian cancer and soft tissue sarcomas of the extremities, appears to contain good candidates for adjuvant chemotherapy.

In NSCLC, early trials of postoperative adjuvant chemotherapy revealed a detrimental effect of alkylating agents and older chemotherapy regimens on survival. Subsequent randomized trials of postoperative cisplatin-based chemotherapy failed to demonstrate individually relevant benefit. These studies were pooled in an individual patient data-based meta-analysis reported in 1995 [10]. Eight

trials used cisplatin in a range of doses (50–240 mg/m^2 total dose) and in various combinations with doxorubicine, cyclophosphamide, and vindesine. The overall hazard ratio (HR) was 0.87 ($p = 0.08$) in favor of chemotherapy and corresponded to a 13% reduction in the risk of death. This study suggested an absolute benefit for chemotherapy of 3% at 2 years (95% CI, 0.5% detriment to 7% benefit) and 5% at 5 years (95% CI, 1% detriment to 10% benefit). Although these results were not significant, they prompted many groups to launch adjuvant platin-based chemotherapy trials in completely resected NSCLC (Tables 14.1–14.3).

A platin-free chemotherapy alternative was developed in Japan in the adjuvant setting.

Summary of recent randomized adjuvant platin-based chemotherapy trials

The North American Intergroup Trial INT0115

The North American Intergroup Trial INT0115 evaluated the efficacy of a combination of four courses of cisplatin and etoposide plus concomitant thoracic radiotherapy compared with radiotherapy alone given at the same dose for resected stage II and stage IIIA NSCLC patients [11]. Thoracic radiotherapy was given at a dose of 50 Gy. A total of 463 patients were included in the trial between

Table 14.2 Recent randomized platin-based adjuvant trials and pooled analysis.

Trial	Number of patients	Stage	Chemotherapy	5-yr benefit (%)	Hazard ratio [95% CI]	p
ALPI [16]	1209	I-IIIA	MVdP*	3	0.96 [0.81–1.13]	0.589
IALT [17]	1867	I-IIIA	VincaP or EP*	4	0.86 [0.76–0.98]	0.03
BLT [18]	381	I-IIIA	Platin-based*	−2 (2yr)	1.02 [0.77–1.35]	0.90
BR10 [19]	482	IB-II	VnrP	15	0.69 [0.52–0.91]	0.04
CALGB [21]	344	IB	PacCb	2	0.8 [0.6–1.07]	0.1
ANITA [20]	840	IB-IIIA	VnrP*	9	0.8 [0.66–0.96]	0.017
LACE [22]	4584	I-IIIA	Cisplatin-based*	5	0.89 [0.82–96]	0.004

*Optional adjuvant radiotherapy.
EP, etoposide/cisplatin; ALPI, Adjuvant Lung Project Italy; MVdP, mitomycin/vindesine/cisplatin; IALT, International Adjuvant Lung Trial; VincaP, vinorelbine, vindesine, or vinblastine/cisplatin; BLT, Big Lung Trial; BR10: from NCIC-CTG, National Institute of Canada Clinical Trials Group; VnrP, vinorelbine/cisplatin; CALGB, Cancer and Leukemia Group B; PacCb, paclitaxel/carboplatin; ANITA, Adjuvant Navelbine International Trialist Association; LACE, Lung Adjuvant Ciplatin Evaluation.

Table 14.3 Regimens, compliance, and toxicity of recent randomized platin-based adjuvant trial.

| Trial | Regimen | | Nb of cycles | Compliance | RT | % death |
	Cisplatin	Other				
IALT [17]	80–120 mg/m^2 q3w or q4w	Vindesine 3 mg/m^2/w* Vinblastine 4 mg/m^2/w* Vinorelbine 30 mg/m^2/w Etoposide 100 mg/m^2 d1, d2, d3	3–4	73% received >240 mg/m^2 cisplatin	31%	0.8%
ALPI [16]	100 mg/m^2 q3w	Mitomycin C (8 mg/m^2), Vindesine (3 mg/m^2 d1, d8)	3	69% received 3 cycles, 31% received full dose	70%	0.5%
BR10 [19]	100 mg/m^2 q4w	Vinorelbine 25 mg/m^2/w	4	58% received ≥3 cycles, 77% had a dose reduction	0	0.8%
CALGB [21]		Carboplatin AUC 6 Paclitaxel 200 mg/m^2 q3w	4	NR	0	0%
ANITA [20]	100 mg/m^2 q4w	Vinorelbine 30 mg/m^2/w	4	63% received >260 mg/m^2 cisplatin	28%	2%

*Weekly then modified.
EP, etoposide/cisplatin; ALPI, Adjuvant Lung Project Italy; IALT, International Adjuvant Lung Trial; BR10: from NCIC-CTG, National Institute of Canada Clinical Trials Group; CALGB, Cancer and Leukemia Group B; ANITA, Adjuvant Navelbine International Trialist Association; RT, radiotherapy.

1991 and 1997. The two groups were well balanced in terms of patterns and there was no significant difference in terms of failure rates, nor in the median time to recurrence. In addition, p53 mutation or protein expression and K-ras mutations had no impact on the outcome in a subset of 197 patients [12]. The possible enhancement of the toxic effects of radiation by cytotoxic agents may explain this lack of efficacy, particularly for those patients with stage II disease (as reported in the PORT meta-analysis).

Italian stage IB study

Between January 1988 and December 1994, investigators in Italy conducted a randomized trial enrolling patients with completely resected IB (pT2N0) NSCLC, comparing six cycles of adjuvant chemotherapy to observation alone [13]. Chemotherapy consisted of cisplatin (100 mg/m^2 on day 1) and etoposide (120 mg/m^2 on days 1–3). Eligible patients were <75 years old, had a Karnofsky over 90%, and had to be able to begin CT within 30 days after surgery. Postoperative

radiotherapy was not administered. The study was reported initially with 66 patients and subsequently published with a larger cohort and a 10-year follow-up [14]. A hundred and forty patients were included, seventy in each group; groups were homogenous for conventional risk factors. There were no treatment-related deaths. Sixty-three percent of the chemotherapy patients received the six planned courses of chemotherapy. Median survival was 84.8 months for the chemotherapy group and 41.6 months in the control arm ($p = 0.02$). Five-year and 10-year survival rates were 62% and 44% in the adjuvant group and 42% and 20% in the control group, respectively. Median disease-free survival was 78.4 months in the chemotherapy arm and 25.6 months in the control group ($p = 0.0001$).

Japanese Clinical Oncology Group Trial 9304

The Japan Clinical Oncology Group Trial 9304 aimed to determine whether three courses of cisplatin and vindesine was superior to observation only in patients with completely resected NSCLC patients with ipsilateral mediastinal lymph node involvement [15]. Three courses of chemotherapy (cisplatin 80 mg/m² day 1, vindesine 3 mg/m² days 1 and 8) were administered in the experimental arm. Chemotherapy started within 6 weeks after surgery, and was repeated every 4 weeks. Postoperative radiotherapy was not delivered. Eligible patients were under 75 years of age, had a WHO PS of 0 or 1, and could not have been previously treated with chemotherapy or radiotherapy. The two groups were well balanced, even though patients were stratified only by treatment center. Accrual was discontinued prior to accumulation of the planned number of registrations because of the slow accrual rate. From January 1994 to July 1998, a total of 119 patients were randomized (59 in the chemotherapy arm and 60 in the surgery alone arm). The intended dose of chemotherapy was administered to 58% of patients. Median survival was 36 months in both groups and 5-year survival was 28% in the chemotherapy arm and 36% in the control arm ($p = 0.89$). Median disease-free survival was 18 months in the chemotherapy arm and 16 months in the control arm ($p = 0.66$).

Adjuvant Lung Project Italy

Investigators from the Adjuvant Lung Project Italy (ALPI) and the European Organisation for Research and Treatment of Cancer randomly assigned patients with completely resected stage I, II, or IIIA NSCLC to either MVP (mitomycin [8 mg/m² on day 1], vindesine [3 mg/m² on days 1 and 8], and cisplatin [100 mg/m² on day 1]) every 3 weeks for three cycles or observation, within 42 days after radical surgery [16]. Patients were stratified by center, tumor size, lymph node involvement, and the intention to perform radiotherapy. Patients received radiotherapy according to the policy of the individual participating center. For the patients in the MVP arm, radiotherapy was initiated 3–5 weeks after the last chemotherapy, and for patients in the control arm, radiotherapy was initiated 4–6 weeks after surgery. In both groups, the total radiotherapy dose was 50–54 Gy (2 Gy/day, 5 days per week) over 5–6 weeks. The primary endpoint was overall survival.

Secondary endpoints were progression-free survival and toxicity associated with adjuvant treatment. The trial was designed to have 80% power to detect a 20% relative reduction in mortality (increasing 5-yr survival from 50 to 57%) corresponding to a hazard rate of 0.8, with a two-sided alpha of 0.05. The authors anticipated that 1300 patients would have to be recruited over 5 years. However, the trial closed after having enrolled 93% of the planned sample size since the accrual rate slowed down during the last 6 months. From January 1994 to January 1999, 1209 patients were enrolled, 606 to the MVP arm, and 603 to the control arm. Thirteen patients were excluded from the analysis because of eligibility violations. One hundred eight patients from one center were excluded from the final analysis because of serious concerns about data integrity. Thus, the final report was based on 548 patients in the MVP arm, and 540 patients in the control arm. Patients were well balanced between the two arms of the study: 39% had stage I disease, 33% had stage II disease, and 28% had stage IIIA disease. Median age was 61 years. Sixty-nine percent of the MVP patients completed the three planned cycles of chemotherapy. Sixty-five percent of patients received radiotherapy in the MVP arm, and 82% in the control arm. The MVP chemotherapy was associated with grade 3 or 4 neutropenia in 16 and 12% of patients, respectively. There were 10 treatment-related deaths in the study; three in the chemotherapy arm and seven in the control arm. After a median follow-up of 64.5 months, no significant difference in overall survival was seen with an HR of 0.96 (95% CI, 0.81–1.13; $p = 0.589$), nor in progression-free survival (HR = 0.89, 95% CI, 0.76–1.03; $p = 0.128$). Median overall survival was 55 months in the MVP arm and 48 months in the control arm. Disease stage and sex were associated with survival in the multivariable analysis. Several molecular and biologic features of NSCLC (including Ki 67, p53, K-ras mutation status) were investigated for their prognostic value. No statistically significant association between disease stage or tumor histology and tumor expression of p53 or Ki67 was found. Mutations of K-ras were found in 22% of the 117 tumor specimens identified as adenocarcinoma or large-cell carcinoma. No association between any of these 3 tumor tissue markers and overall survival or progression-free survival was found.

International Adjuvant Lung Cancer Trial

The International Adjuvant Lung Cancer Trial (IALT) Collaborative Group evaluated the effect of cisplatin-based adjuvant chemotherapy on survival in completely resected NSCLC [17]. They randomly assigned 1867 patients to either 3 or 4 cycles of cisplatin-based chemotherapy or to observation. Chemotherapy was one of four different regimens combining cisplatin (80–120 mg/m^2, every 3–4 weeks) with vindesine (3 mg/m^2 weekly, then every 2 weeks), vinblastine (4 mg/m^2 weekly then every 2 weeks), vinorelbine (30 mg/m^2 weekly), or etoposide (100 mg/m^2 days 1–3 per cycle). Each participating center could determine the pathologic stage of disease to include, the dose of cisplatin given per cycle, the drug that was combined with cisplatin, and the postoperative radiotherapy policy. This open-choice design was chosen to facilitate accrual, allow broad generalization of the results, and take into account the uncertainty regarding the best available chemotherapy regimen. Eligible patients had completely resected stage I, II, or III NSCLC, and were between 18 and 75 years of age. Patients were randomly assigned within 60 days of surgery and were stratified by treatment center, type of surgery, and pathological stage. Chemotherapy was to begin within 60 days of surgery and within 14 days of randomization. Postoperative radiotherapy consisted of 60 Gy or less, delivered to the mediastinal lymph nodes. The primary endpoint was overall survival. Secondary endpoints were disease-free survival, second primary cancers, and adverse effects. The trial was designed to demonstrate an absolute improvement in overall survival of 5%, from 50 to 55% at 5 years. A total of 3300 patients were required to have a 90% power with a type I one-sided error rate. The data-monitoring committee recommended reformulation of the trial with a two-sided test to provide 83% power to detect a 5% difference and 90% power to detect a 5.6% difference. Enrollment began in February 1995, but slowed down significantly in 1999, and the steering committee decided to discontinue recruitment on December 31,

2000. A total of 1867 patients had been randomly assigned, recruited by 148 centers in 33 countries (932 were enrolled into the chemotherapy arm and 935 into the control group). Patients were well balanced between the two arms of the study, with 10% having stage IA disease, 27% stage IB, 24% stage II, and 39% stage III. Median age was 59 years, 7% had a WHO PS of 2. Twenty percent were women, 40% had adenocarcinoma, and 35% of the patients underwent pneumonectomy. A regimen combining 100 mg/m^2 cisplatin for three or four cycles with etoposide was selected for 49.3% of the patients. Of the patients assigned to the chemotherapy arm, 74% received at least 240 mg/m^2 of cisplatin. Twenty-seven percent of patients received postoperative radiotherapy. In the chemotherapy arm, 23% of patients experienced grade 3 or 4 toxicity, and 7 patients (0.8%) died of chemotherapy-related toxicity. In the chemotherapy group, 7.8% did not receive chemotherapy. The median duration of follow-up was 56 months. Patients assigned to chemotherapy had a significantly higher overall survival rate than patients assigned to observation (44.5% versus 40.4% at 5 yr, respectively; HR = 0.86 [0.76–0.98], $p < 0.03$). Disease-free survival was also significantly improved with chemotherapy (HR = 0.83 [0.74–0.94], $p < 0.003$). Median survival was 50.8 months in the chemotherapy arm and 44.4 months in the control arm, while median disease-free survival was 40.2 months and 30.5 months, respectively. Five-year disease-free survival rates were 39.4% and 34.3% in the chemotherapy group and in the control group, respectively.

Big Lung Trial

Investigators in Great Britain reported a randomized trial (Big Lung Trial) examining the role of cisplatin-based chemotherapy in a variety of treatment settings in patients with completely resected stage I–III NSCLC [18]. A total of 381 patients were randomly assigned to surgery alone (189 patients) or to three cycles of pre- (4%) or postoperative (96%) cisplatin-based chemotherapy (192 patients). This trial was not designed to specifically answer a question about postoperative chemotherapy and was underpowered to detect a clinically significant survival difference. Chemotherapy consisted of three

3-weekly cycles of cisplatin (50–80 mg/m^2 day 1), given with either vindesine (3 mg/mg^2 days 1 and 8), or mitomycin (6 mg/m^2) and ifosfamide (3 gm/m^2), or mitomycin (6 mg/m^2) and vinblastine (6 mg/m^2), or vinorelbine (30 mg/m^2, days 1 and 8). Median age was 61 years, 69% of patients were male, 48% had squamous cell carcinoma and 37% had adenocarcinoma. Twenty-seven percent of patients were stage I, 38% were stage II, and 34% stage III. A macroscopic complete resection was achieved in approximately 95% of patients, and an incomplete microscopic resection was reported in 15% of cases. Sixty-four patients in the chemotherapy group received all three cycles, 40% of whom required a dose adjustment, and 30% had grade 3 or 4 toxicity (mainly hematological or nausea/vomiting); 14% of patients received postoperative radiation. With a median follow-up of only 2.9 years, there was no evidence of a benefit in overall survival to the chemotherapy group (HR: 1.02; $p = 0.90$).

National Cancer Institute of Canada Clinical Trials Group JBR.10

The National Cancer Institute of Canada Clinical Trials Group (NCIC CTG) randomly assigned completely resected stage IB and II (excluding T3N0) NSCLC patients to postoperative chemotherapy or to surgery alone [19]. Chemotherapy consisted of vinorelbine 25 mg/m^2 weekly (originally 30 mg/m^2, but reduced shortly after study initiation because of hematologic toxicity) and cisplatin 50 mg/m^2 on days 1 and 8, every 4 weeks for four cycles, to start within 6 weeks of surgery. Patients did not receive postoperative thoracic radiotherapy. Patients were stratified by nodal status (N0 versus N1) and Ras mutation (present versus absent versus unknown). The primary study endpoint was overall survival; principal secondary endpoints were recurrence-free survival, quality of life, and toxicity. Between 1994 and 2001, 482 patients underwent randomization to chemotherapy (242 patients) or observation alone (240 patients). The two groups were well balanced: the median age was 61 years (eldest patient was 82 yr), all had PS 0 or 1, and 35% were women. Forty-five percent of the patients had T2N0 disease, 40% had T2N1, and 15%

had T1N1 disease extent. Fifty-three percent had adenocarcinoma and Ras mutations were present in 24% of the samples. Grade 3 or 4 neutropenia occurred in 76% of patients. However, febrile neutropenia occurred in only 7%. Common nonhematologic toxicities included fatigue (81%), nausea (80%), anorexia (55%), vomiting (48%), sensory neuropathy and constipation (48 and 47%, respectively), but severe (grade 3 or greater) toxic effects were rare (<10%). There were two chemotherapy-related deaths (febrile neutropenia and pulmonary fibrosis). The most common cause of death was NSCLC (including one patient with second primary NSCLC), while three patients died from toxicity related to later anticancer therapy, nine patients died of other primary malignancies, and 21 from other causes. Overall survival was significantly increased in the chemotherapy group (94 mo versus 73 mo; HR = 0.69; $p = 0.011$), as was recurrence-free survival (not reached versus 47 mo; HR = 0.6; $p = 0.0003$). The 5-year survival rates were 69 and 54% in the chemotherapy and control group, respectively ($p = 0.03$).

ANITA 01

Investigators in France reported a randomized trial comparing the effect of adjuvant vinorelbine plus cisplatin to observation alone on survival in patients with completely resected NSCLC [20]. Patients with stage IB–IIIA NSCLC from 101 centers in 14 countries were randomly assigned to observation, or to vinorelbine (30 mg/m^2 on days 1, 8, 15, and 22 for a maximum of 16 doses) plus cisplatin (100 mg/m^2 on days 1, 29, 57, 85). Postoperative radiotherapy was undertaken according to each center's policy and was recommended for patients with node-positive disease. Patients were stratified by center, stage, and histology (squamous versus other). The primary endpoint was overall survival. Secondary endpoints were disease-free survival and safety. By assuming a 2-year survival of 30% in the control group, the trial was designed to have a 90% power to detect an absolute improvement of 10% indicating a benefit for adjuvant chemotherapy, with a two-sided alpha of 0.05. The planned sample size for the study was 400 patients per treatment group. An interim analysis of safety was planned at 6 months, 12 months, and when 600 patients had been enrolled, to allow study discontinuation if treatment tolerability was unacceptable. From December 1994 to December 2000, 840 patients were enrolled: 407 to the chemotherapy arm and 433 to the observation group. Patients were well balanced between the two arms of the study, with 36% having stage IB disease, 24% stage II disease, and 39% stage IIIA disease. In the chemotherapy group, 368 received vinorelbine and 367 concurrently received cisplatin. Thirty-eight percent of them received more than 66% of the total planned dose of vinorelbine, and 63% received more than 66% of the total planned dose of cisplatin. Fifty percent of patients completed the planned four cycles. Chemotherapy was associated with grade 3 or 4 neutropenia in 92% of patients, and febrile neutropenia in 9% of patients. At the time of analysis, median follow-up was 76 months in the chemotherapy group and 77 months in the observation group. Median survival was 65.7 months (95% CI, 47.9–88.5) and 43.7 months (95% CI, 37.7–52.3) for the chemotherapy group and the control group, respectively (HR = 0.80 [0.66–0.96], $p = 0.017$). Overall survival at 5 years improved by 8.6% with chemotherapy, and was maintained at 7 years (8.4%). A subgroup analysis indicated that the benefit was restricted to patients with stage II and IIIA disease.

Cancer and Leukemia Group B

The Cancer and Leukemia Group B (CALGB) trial 9633 randomly assigned completely resected stage IB (T2N0) patients to four postoperative cycles of paclitaxel (200 mg/m^2) and carboplatin (AUC = 6) chemotherapy versus surgery alone [21]. This trial was initially presented at ASCO 2004 as positive after a follow-up of 34 months, then updated as a negative trial at ASCO 2006. Chemotherapy was started within 4–8 weeks of surgery and there was no planned thoracic radiotherapy. The trial started in September 1996 and was initially planned to accrue 500 patients over 3.5 years. Because of slow accrual, accumulation of events over time and the results of IALT, the data monitoring committee recommended early closure on November 2003 following accrual of 344 patients. The design was changed from a two-sided to a one-sided hypothesis analysis. The trial

had a power of 40% to demonstrate a significant difference with 155 deaths and HR of 0.8. Median age was 61 years (eldest patient treated was 81 yr), all had PS 0 or 1. The two arms of the study were well balanced with regard to age, sex, race, weight loss, ethnicity, histology, tumor differentiation, and resection type. Adjuvant chemotherapy was well tolerated, and there were no chemotherapy-related deaths. Grade 3 or 4 neutropenia occurred in 35% of patients. At a median follow-up of 54 months, there were 64 deaths from any cause among 173 patients in the chemotherapy group compared with 73 deaths among 171 patients in the observation group (HR = 0.80 [0.60–1.07], $p = 0.10$). Overall survival at 5 years was 59% (95% CI, 63–75%) and 57% (95% CI, 50–64%) in the chemotherapy group and observation group, respectively. There was a significant advantage in failure-free survival favoring the chemotherapy group (HR = 0.74; 95% CI, 0.57–0.96; $p = 0.03$). In an unplanned subgroup analysis, the CALGB investigators found a benefit restricted to patients with tumors larger than 4 cm.

Pooled analysis of recent randomized adjuvant cisplatin-based chemotherapy trials

The LACE pooled analysis, presented at ASCO 2006, pooled individual data of 4584 patients from the 5 recent randomized adjuvant cisplatin-based chemotherapy trials [22]. The ALPI, IALT, ANITA, BLT, and JBR10 trials were selected because they were conducted after the IGR-MRC 1995 meta-analysis and their cohorts were superior to 300 patients [16–18,20,23]. In the five selected trials, 80% of the patients were male and the median age was 59 years (9% of patients were over 70 yr). Patients were roughly equally divided between the pathological stages (IA: 8%, IB: 30%, II: 35%, III: 27%). A pneumonectomy was performed in 31% of cases. Approximately half the tumors (49%) were squamous cell carcinomas, 39% were adenocarcinomas, and 12% were of other histologies. With a median follow-up of 5.1 years (3.1–5.9), 5-year survival was significantly better in the chemotherapy group

(HR for death = 0.89 [0.82–0.96], *p* = 0.004) corresponding to an absolute benefit of 5.3% with chemotherapy. There was no heterogeneity of chemotherapy effect among trials. The benefit varied with stage (test for trend, *p* = 0.046) with an HR of 1.41 [0.96–2.09] for stage IA, 0.93 [0.78–1.10] for stage IB, 0.83 [0.73–0.95] for stage II, and 0.83 [0.73–0.95] for stage III. The effect of chemotherapy did not vary significantly (test for interaction, *p* = 0.10) with the associated drugs: vinorelbine (HR = 0.80 [0.70–0.91]) etoposide/vinca-alcaloide (0.93 [0.80–1.07]) or other (0.98 [0.84–1.14]). There was no interaction between chemotherapy and sex, age, planned radiotherapy or planned total dose of cisplatin. The authors concluded that cisplatin adjuvant-based chemotherapy should be considered for stage II and IIIA disease while it is not recommended for stage IA disease. Benefit for stage IB disease was not statistically significant but the study may have lacked sufficient power to demonstrate this.

The known and the unknown

Which stages should be treated?

In the largest randomized trial, IALT, the 4.3% benefit of cisplatin-based chemotherapy was independent of the stage [17]. Other studies suggested that stage IA or all stage I patients did not benefit from adjuvant chemotherapy. If adjuvant chemotherapy is consistently active for stage II and III resected NSCLC, as has been confirmed in the LACE pooled analysis, its role remains controversial for the earliest stages.

Stage IA

BLT, ALPI, and IALT were the only cisplatin-based chemotherapy trials to include stage IA disease. This group accounted for 347 patients in total [17,18,20]. Individual data have been analyzed in the LACE pooled analysis [22]. The latter suggested a detrimental effect in that subgroup, taking into account that some of the patients were treated by the toxic mitomycin C/vindesin/cisplatin regimen. Nevertheless, adjuvant cisplatin-based chemotherapy is not a standard of care in stage IA disease.

Stage IB

The statistically negative CALGB study is the only large platin-based adjuvant trial focusing on patients with stage IB disease [21]. Many hypotheses have been advanced to explain the negative results of this study, including the lower activity of the paclitaxel/carboplatin doublet in comparison with cisplatin-based doublets and the lack of power due to the early discontinuation of accrual. In a subgroup analysis of JBR10 and ANITA trials, no benefit was observed for patients with stage IB disease [20,23]. In the LACE pooled analysis, a trend toward a benefit for adjuvant chemotherapy was reported but it is insufficient to recommend it as a standard [22]. Identification of other prognostic factors and the large meta-analysis including ongoing and/or unreported trials may help to clarify this issue in the near future.

Which conventional cytotoxic regimen to use?

Doublets versus triplets

Cisplatin-based doublets are the only validated chemotherapy regimens in advanced disease as in the adjuvant setting [24]. Old triplets are known to be equally effective as modern doublets (platinum compound with vinorelbine, gemcitabine, or taxanes), and may be partly responsible for negative trials such as ALPI [16,25]. In the JBR10 trial, which reported the highest benefit (up to 15% absolute 5-yr benefit), the conventional cisplatin-vinorelbine regimen was used. This doublet seems to be more active than older doublets or triplets, according to the LACE pooled analysis. However, the protocol dose of cisplatin was higher with vinorelbine than with other drugs and the interaction with the associated drug(s) may be confounded by the cisplatin dose [22]. Although taxanes and gemcitabine may be often used in daily practice, no randomized data has proven a benefit for this drugs combined with platinum compounds.

Carboplatin versus cisplatin

The CALGB study is the only reported trial evaluating the paclitaxel/carboplatin combination [21]. Its negativity raised concern about the efficacy of the doublet in the adjuvant setting, taking in account that it has not been demonstrated whether or not cisplatin and carboplatin are likely to be equivalent. A recent study questions the equivalence of the two platinum compounds [26]. In this study, 618 patients were randomized to receive paclitaxel 200 mg/m^2 in combination with either carboplatin at an area under the curve (AUC) of 6 or cisplatin at 80 mg/m^2 every 3 weeks. A survival update after 22 months of additional follow-up yielded a median survival of 8.2 months in the paclitaxel/carboplatin arm and 9.8 months in the paclitaxel/cisplatin arm (HR = 1.22, 90% CI, 1.06–1.40; p = 0.019); the 2-year survival rates were 9 and 15%, respectively. Excluding neutropenia and thrombocytopenia, which were more frequent in the paclitaxel/carboplatin arm, and nausea/vomiting and nephrotoxicity, which were more frequent in the paclitaxel/cisplatin arm, the rate of severe toxicities was generally low and equivalent between the two arms. The CISCA (cisplatin versus carboplatin) meta-analysis based on individual data of 2968 patients and presented at ASCO 2006 concludes along the same lines [27] showing a better response rate with cisplatin than with carboplatin-based chemotherapy: 33% versus 26%, which correlated to an HR of 1.37 (p < 0.001). Thus, in the absence of contraindications, cisplatin should be the platinum compound of choice in the adjuvant setting.

Neoadjuvant or adjuvant setting?

The role of induction chemotherapy in NSCLC is still under debate while it has been established that adjuvant cisplatin-based chemotherapy improves overall survival in completely resected patients. The theoretical advantages of neoadjuvant chemotherapy over adjuvant chemotherapy are numerous, including improved patient compliance, a reduction in size of the primary tumor and a pathological evaluation of treatment efficacy. In the neoadjuvant setting, a 32–60% response rate is expected and a near to 10% pathological complete response rate. Nevertheless, the only large randomized phase III trial has not demonstrated that induction chemotherapy prolongs overall patient survival [28]. Suboptimal cytotoxic combinations and increased surgical mortality might explain this result. Exploratory studies have suggested that patient subgroups (such as downstaged N2 disease) could benefit from induction treatment. Recent randomized trials evaluating neoadjuvant chemotherapy versus surgery alone were prematurely discontinued after publication of the first positive adjuvant trials in 2004 and were unable to demonstrate any benefit favoring neoadjuvant chemotherapy [29,30]. Ongoing phase III trials comparing a single chemotherapy regimen in the adjuvant and neoadjuvant setting (NATCH, IFCT0002) will be of particular assistance in clarifying the place of neoadjuvant chemotherapy in the NSCLC armatorium. However, adjuvant chemotherapy remains the best-validated perioperative treatment currently available.

Customized chemotherapy

There is at present no validated prognostic factor to identify subgroups of patients who will derive particular benefit from adjuvant treatment. A treatment decision-making process based on the analysis of biomarkers of response and resistance to cytotoxic drugs is likely to be a major issue in the near future. Biomarkers such as p53 mutation, p53 protein expression, or K-ras mutations have not proved to have either a prognostic or a predictive value in published adjuvant trials [12,16,31]. Resistance mechanisms to chemotherapy have been actively investigated in recent years. Overexpression of DNA repair mechanisms may be crucial for the tumor cell to overcome apoptosis caused by chemotherapy-induced DNA damage. Recent studies have focused on various players involved in nucleotide excision repair, which is known to have a central role in DNA repair and to be associated with resistance to platinum compounds. In particular, the excision repair cross-complementation group 1 (ERCC1) enzyme plays a rate-limiting role in the nucleotide excision repair pathway that recognizes and removes cisplatin-induced DNA adducts. ERCC1 protein expression has been evaluated by immunohistochemistry in 761 tumors of the IALT, assuming the hypothesis that a high expression rate would correlate to a relative chemoresistance [32]. Cisplatin-based chemotherapy significantly prolonged survival among patients with

ERCC1-negative tumors (56% of the cases, HR = 0.65 [0.50–0.86], $p = 0.002$) while in patients with ERCC1-positive tumor, adjuvant chemotherapy had no effect (HR = 1.14 [0.84–1.55], $p = 0.40$). The interest of customized chemotherapy based on ERCC1 level (assessed by quantitative RT PCR) has been prospectively evaluated in advanced NSCLC [33]. Early results suggest that nonplatinum doublets could be of interest in patients with ERCC1-positive tumors. Other biomarkers may predict the benefit of selected drugs. For example, gemcitabine efficacy may be related to RRM1 expression (encoding the regulatory subunit of ribonucleotide reductase, a molecular target of gemcitabine), and the benefit of taxanes linked to beta-tubulin mutations [34,35]. The value of these biomarkers needs to be validated before any translation to the neoadjuvant setting. The improvement of patient selection is a highly interesting area for further studies.

Better understanding of the biology of lung cancer has led to the development of novel therapies directed at tumor-specific targets. Most of these targets are tumor growth factor signal pathways. However, tumor proliferation, angiogenesis, and apoptosis may also be targeted, particularly by targeting the epidermal growth factor receptor (EGFR) pathway since overexpression of EGFR is found in NSCLC. Erlotinib and gefitinib inhibit the tyrosine kinase activity of EGFR and have been extensively evaluated in NSCLC [36,37]. A randomized phase III trial proved a survival benefit for erlotinib compared with placebo in patients with previously treated NSCLC (overall survival: 6.7 and 4.7 mo, respectively, HR: 0.70; $p < 0.001$) [37]. Nevertheless, the combination of cytotoxic doublets combined with EGFR inhibitors has failed to demonstrate any substantial benefit in phase III trials [38–40]. Various clinical and biological predictive factors of response to erlotinib have been identified: adenocarcinomas, females, nonsmokers, Asian ethnicity, EGFR mutation, EGFR gene or protein expression [41]. These predictive factors should be used to select a population which might experience a survival benefit when given EGFR TKI as an adjuvant treatment although this has not yet been demonstrated. More recently, the Eastern Cooperative Oncology Group (ECOG) reported the results of a randomized trial in 878 patients with chemo-naïve inoperable NSCLC, which evaluated the effectiveness of the addition of bevacizumab, an antiangiogenic agent, to the standard paclitaxel–carboplatin combination [42]. Median survival was significantly increased in the bevacizumab arm (12.5 mo versus 10.2 mo; $p = 0.0075$). This trial is the first to show that the addition of a targeted agent to a standard cytotoxic doublet could prolong survival. A large randomized trial will investigate the benefit of adding bevacizumab to different cytotoxic regimens.

Brief guidelines

–Cisplatin-based chemotherapy is standard in totally resected stage II and IIA patients.

–Cisplatin-based chemotherapy is optional for stage IB patients; prognostic factors need to be clarified to better select patients.

–Cisplatin-based chemotherapy is not recommended for stage IA patients.

–Three to four cycles of cisplatin-based chemotherapy are recommended (total dose of cisplatin from 300 to 400 mg/m^2)

–Vinorelbine–cisplatin is the most validated regimen in randomized trials.

–Carboplatin should not be used in the absence of contraindications to cisplatin.

–Adjuvant chemotherapy has been validated in patients under 75 years, PS 0 or 1 without surgical complications.

–Adjuvant chemotherapy should begin within 2 months after surgery. Its value after 2 months is not clear.

References

1 Mountain CF. Revisions in the International system for staging lung cancer. *Chest* 1997; **111(6)**:1710–7.
2 The Lung Cancer Study Group. Effects of postoperative mediastinal radiation on completely-resected stage II and stage III epidermoid cancer of the lung. *N Engl J Med* 1986; **315(22)**:1377–81.
3 PORT Meta-analysis Trialists Group. Postoperative radiotherapy in non-small-cell lung cancer: systematic review and meta-analysis of individual patient data

from nine randomised controlled trials. *Lancet* 1998; **352(9124)**:257–63.

4 Pantel K, Izbicki J, Passlick B *et al*. Frequency and prognostic significance of isolated tumour cells in bone marrow of patients with non-small-cell lung cancer without overt metastases. *Lancet* 1996; **347(9002)**:649–53.

5 Osaki T, Oyama T, Gu CD *et al*. Prognostic impact of micrometastatic tumor cells in the lymph nodes and bone marrow of patients with completely-resected stage I non-small-cell lung cancer. *J Clin Oncol* 2002; **20(13)**:2930–6.

6 Sher YP, Shih JY, Yang PC *et al*. Prognosis of non-small-cell lung cancer patients by detecting circulating cancer cells in the peripheral blood with multiple marker genes. *Clin Cancer Res* 2005; **11(1)**:173–9.

7 Yamashita J, Matsuo A, Kurusu Y, Saishoji T, Hayashi N, Ogawa M. Preoperative evidence of circulating tumor cells by means of reverse transcriptase-polymerase chain reaction for carcinoembryonic antigen messenger RNA is an independent predictor of survival in non-small cell lung cancer: a prospective study. *J Thorac Cardiovasc Surg* 2002; **124(2)**:299–305.

8 Andre T, Boni C, Mounedji-Boudiaf L *et al*. Oxaliplatin, fluorouracil, and leucovorin as adjuvant treatment for colon cancer. *N Engl J Med* 2004; **350(23)**:2343–51.

9 Early Breast Cancer Trialists' Collaborative Group (EBCTCG). Effects of chemotherapy and hormonal therapy for early breast cancer on recurrence and 15-year survival: an overview of the randomised trials. *Lancet* 2005; **365(9472)**:1687–717.

10 Non-small Cell Lung Cancer Collaborative Group. Chemotherapy in non-small cell lung cancer: a meta-analysis using updated data on individual patients from 52 randomised clinical trials. *BMJ* 1995; **311(7010)**:899–909.

11 Keller SM, Adak S, Wagner H *et al*., for Eastern Cooperative Oncology Group. A randomized trial of postoperative adjuvant therapy in patients with completely-resected stage II or IIIA non-small-cell lung cancer. *N Engl J Med* 2000; **343(17)**:1217–22.

12 Schiller JH, Adak S, Feins RH *et al*. Lack of prognostic significance of p53 and K-ras mutations in primary resected non-small-cell lung cancer on E4592: a Laboratory Ancillary Study on an Eastern Cooperative Oncology Group Prospective Randomized Trial of Postoperative Adjuvant Therapy. *J Clin Oncol* 2001; **19(2)**:448–57.

13 Mineo TC, Ambrogi V, Corsaro V, Roselli M. Postoperative adjuvant therapy for stage IB non-small-cell lung cancer. *Eur J Cardiothorac Surg* 2001; **20(2)**:378–84.

14 Roselli M, Mariotti S, Ferroni P *et al*. Postsurgical chemotherapy in stage IB non-small-cell lung cancer: long-term survival in a randomized study. *Int J Cancer* 2006; **119(4)**:955–60.

15 Tada H, Tsuchiya R, Ichinose Y *et al*. A randomized trial comparing adjuvant chemotherapy versus surgery alone for completely-resected pN2 non-small-cell lung cancer (JCOG9304). *Lung Cancer* 2004; **43(2)**:167–73.

16 Scagliotti GV, Fossati R, Torri V *et al*. Randomized study of adjuvant chemotherapy for completely-resected stage I, II, or IIIA non-small-cell lung cancer. *J Natl Cancer Inst* 2003; **95(19)**:1453–61.

17 Arriagada R, Bergman B, Dunant A *et al*., for International Adjuvant Lung Cancer Trial Collaborative Group. Cisplatin-based adjuvant chemotherapy in patients with completely-resected non-small-cell lung cancer. *N Engl J Med* 2004; **350(4)**:351–60.

18 Waller D, Peake MD, Stephens RJ *et al*. Chemotherapy for patients with non-small-cell lung cancer: the surgical setting of the Big Lung Trial. *Eur J Cardiothorac Surg* 2004; **26(1)**:173–82.

19 Winton T, Livingston R, Johnson D *et al*. Vinorelbine plus cisplatin vs. observation in resected non-small-cell lung cancer. *N Engl J Med* 2005; **352(25)**:2589–97.

20 Douillard JY, Rosell R, De Lena M *et al*. Adjuvant vinorelbine plus cisplatin versus observation in patients with completely-resected stage IB-IIIA non-small-cell lung cancer (Adjuvant Navelbine International Trialist Association [ANITA]): a randomised controlled trial. *Lancet Oncol* 2006; **7(9)**:719–27.

21 Strauss GM, Herndon JE, II, Maddaus MA *et al*. Adjuvant chemotherapy in stage IB non-small-cell lung cancer (NSCLC): update of Cancer and Leukemia Group B (CALGB) protocol 9633 [Meeting Abstracts]. *J Clin Oncol* 2006; **24(Suppl 18)**:7007.

22 Pignon JP, Tribodet H, Scagliotti GV *et al*. Lung adjuvant cisplatin evaluation (LACE): a pooled analysis of five randomized clinical trials including 4,584 patients [Meeting Abstracts]. *J Clin Oncol* 2006; **24(Suppl 18)**:7008.

23 Winton TL, Livingston R, Johnson D *et al*., National Cancer Institute of Canada CKOC, National Cancer Institute of Canada CTG KOC. A prospective randomised trial of adjuvant vinorelbine (VIN) and cisplatin (CIS) in completely-resected stage 1B and II non-small-cell lung cancer (NSCLC) Intergroup JBR.10 [Abstract]. *Proc Am Soc Clin Oncol* 2004; **22**:7018.

24 Schiller JH, Harrington D, Belani CP *et al*. Comparison of four chemotherapy regimens for advanced non-small-cell lung cancer. *N Engl J Med* 2002; **346(2)**:92–8.

25 Delbaldo C, Michiels S, Syz N, Soria JC, Le Chevalier T, Pignon JP. Benefits of adding a drug to a single-agent or a 2-agent chemotherapy regimen in advanced non-small-cell lung cancer: a meta-analysis. *JAMA* 2004; **292(4)**:470–84.

26 Rosell R, Gatzemeier U, Betticher DC *et al*. Phase III randomised trial comparing paclitaxel/carboplatin with paclitaxel/cisplatin in patients with advanced non-small-cell lung cancer: a cooperative multinational trial. *Ann Oncol* 2002; **13(10)**:1539–49.

27 Ardizzoni A, Tiseo M, Boni L *et al*. CISCA (cisplatin vs. carboplatin) meta-analysis: an individual patient data meta-analysis comparing cisplatin versus carboplatin-based chemotherapy in first-line treatment of advanced non-small-cell lung cancer (NSCLC) [Meeting Abstracts]. *J Clin Oncol* 2006; **24(Suppl 18)**:7011.

28 Depierre A, Milleron B, Moro-Sibilot D *et al*. Preoperative chemotherapy followed by surgery compared with primary surgery in resectable stage I (except T1N0), II, and IIIa non-small-cell lung cancer. *J Clin Oncol* 2002; **20(1)**:247–53.

29 Pisters K, Vallieres E, Bunn P *et al*. S9900: a phase III trial of surgery alone or surgery plus preoperative (preop) paclitaxel/carboplatin (PC) chemotherapy in early stage non-small-cell lung cancer (NSCLC): preliminary results [Meeting Abstracts]. *J Clin Oncol* 2005; **23(Suppl 16)**:LBA7012.

30 Scagliotti GV, On Behalf of Ch. Preliminary results of Ch. E.S.T.: A phase III study of surgery alone or surgery plus preoperative gemcitabine-cisplatin in clinical early stages non-small-cell lung cancer (NSCLC) [Meeting Abstracts]. *J Clin Oncol* 2005; **23(Suppl 16)**:LBA7023.

31 Shepherd FA, Dancey J, Ramlau R *et al*. Prospective randomized trial of docetaxel versus best supportive care in patients with non-small-cell lung cancer previously treated with platinum-based chemotherapy. *J Clin Oncol* 2000; **18(10)**:2095–103.

32 Olaussen KA, Dunant A, Fouret P *et al*. DNA repair by ERCC1 in non-small-cell lung cancer and cisplatin-based adjuvant chemotherapy. *N Engl J Med* 2006; **355(10)**:983–91.

33 Rosell R, Gandara DR, Cobo M *et al*. Customizing cisplatin (CIS) based on quantitative excision repair cross-complementing 1 (ERCC1) mRNA expression: a phase III randomized trial in non-small-cell lung cancer (NSCLC). *Ann Oncol* 2006; **17(Suppl 9)**.

34 Bepler G, Kusmartseva I, Sharma S *et al*. RRM1 modulated in vitro and in vivo efficacy of gemcitabine and platinum in non-small-cell lung cancer. *J Clin Oncol* 2006; **24(29)**:4731–7.

35 Monzo M, Rosell R, Sanchez JJ *et al*. Paclitaxel resistance in non-small-cell lung cancer associated with beta-tubulin gene mutations. *J Clin Oncol* 1999; **17(6)**:1786.

36 Thatcher N, Chang A, Parikh P, Pemberton K, Archer V. Results of a phase III placebo controlled study (ISEL) of gefitinib (IRESSA) plus best supportive care (BSC) in patients with advanced non-small-cell lung cancer (NSCLC) who had received 1 or 2 prior chemotherapy regimens [AACR Meeting Abstracts]. 2005; **LB-6**.

37 Shepherd FA, Rodrigues Pereira J, Ciuleanu T *et al*. Erlotinib in previously treated non-small-cell lung cancer. *N Engl J Med* 2005; **353(2)**:123–32.

38 Herbst RS, Prager D, Hermann R *et al*. TRIBUTE: a phase III trial of erlotinib hydrochloride (OSI-774) combined with carboplatin and paclitaxel chemotherapy in advanced non-small-cell lung cancer. *J Clin Oncol* 2005; **23(25)**:5892–9.

39 Giaccone G, Herbst RS, Manegold C *et al*. Gefitinib in combination with gemcitabine and cisplatin in advanced non-small-cell lung cancer: a phase III trial–INTACT 1. *J Clin Oncol* 2004; **22(5)**:777–84.

40 Herbst RS, Giaccone G, Schiller JH *et al*. Gefitinib in combination with paclitaxel and carboplatin in advanced non-small-cell lung cancer: a phase III trial–INTACT 2. *J Clin Oncol* 2004; **22(5)**:785–94.

41 Tsao MS, Sakurada A, Cutz JC *et al*. Erlotinib in lung cancer–molecular and clinical predictors of outcome. *N Engl J Med* 2005; **353(2)**:133–44.

42 Sandler A, Gray R, Brahmer J *et al*. Randomized phase II/III Trial of paclitaxel (P) plus carboplatin (C) with or without bevacizumab (NSC # 704865) in patients with advanced non-squamous non-small-cell lung cancer (NSCLC): an Eastern Cooperative Oncology Group (ECOG) Trial - E4599 [Meeting Abstracts]. *J Clin Oncol* 2005; **4**.

CHAPTER 15

Induction Chemotherapy for Resectable Lung Cancer

Katherine M.W. Pisters

Introduction

In 2007, 213,380 new cases of lung cancer will be diagnosed in the United States; 160,390 patients are expected to die [1]. Lung cancer is the leading cause of cancer-related death in both men and women [1]. Nonsmall cell lung cancer (NSCLC) accounts for roughly 80–85% of these cases. At present, there is no standardized screening procedure for early detection of NSCLC; lung cancer is most often asymptomatic in its early stages. Consequently, the majority of patients are diagnosed with advanced, incurable disease.

For patients with early stage NSCLC, surgery offers the best hope for cure. However, despite complete resection, survival rates are disappointing. Five-year survival rates range from 67% for T1N0 disease to 23% for patients with T1-3N2 extent [2]. Clinical or preoperative staging often underestimates the extent of disease (particularly if positron-emission tomography and mediastinoscopy are not used) and the estimated survival rates for a given clinical stage are much worse than the corresponding surgical/pathological stage (see Table 15.1) [3]. Given the poor survival rates seen with surgery alone, investigators have studied adjuvant therapies such as chemotherapy and thoracic irradiation in an attempt to improve survival.

Lung Cancer, 3rd edition. Edited by Jack A. Roth, James D. Cox, and Waun Ki Hong. © 2008 Blackwell Publishing, ISBN: 978-1-4051-5112-2.

For many years, postoperative adjuvant chemotherapy was studied, and the majority of trials did not find a survival benefit [4]. A meta-analysis examining the role of chemotherapy in the treatment of NSCLC was published in 1995 [5]. Part of this meta-analysis examined the role of postoperative chemotherapy compared to surgery alone. For regimens containing cisplatin, the pattern of results was consistent with most trials favoring chemotherapy. However, despite an overall hazard ratio (HR) of 0.87 corresponding to a 13% reduction in the risk of death and an absolute benefit from cisplatin-based chemotherapy of 5% at 5 years, the results did not achieve statistical significance ($p = 0.08$). More recently, randomized trials have found postoperative chemotherapy beneficial in completely resected stage II and IIIA NSCLC [6–8]. Postoperative adjuvant chemotherapy is reviewed in greater detail elsewhere in this textbook.

Preoperative or induction chemotherapy trials were designed based on the poor survival following surgical resection and, at that time, a lack of evidence in support of postoperative chemotherapy. Further support to pursuing this concept came from positive data in locally advanced, unresectable patients where chemotherapy administered prior to definitive chest radiation therapy had led to a survival improvement over radiation alone [9,10]. Moreover, induction therapy has several theoretical advantages. Administration of chemotherapy prior to surgery allows assessment of radiographic and pathologic tumor response to

Table 15.1 Expected outcome based on clinical and surgical staging for early-stage NSCLC.

Stage	TNM	Estimated 5-yr survival (%) Pathological staging	Clinical staging
IA	T1N0M0	67	61
IB	T2N0M0	57	38
IIA	T1N1M0	55	34
IIB	T2N1M0	39	24
	T3N0M0	38	22
IIIA	T3N1M0	25	9
	T1-3N2M0	23	13

Adapted from Mountain [2].

chemotherapy, earliest treatment of clinically undetectable micrometastatic disease, and improved compliance compared to adjuvant therapy [3,11]. The focus of this chapter will be the use of preoperative or induction chemotherapy in resectable NSCLC.

Phase II trials

Stage III disease

Second-generation regimens
Initial phase II trials evaluating preoperative chemotherapy in stage IIIA NSCLC occurred following reports from MSKCC of the poor outcome of surgery alone in this patient subset [12]. Martini *et al.* demonstrated that patients with ipsilateral mediastinal lymph node involvement could have 5-year survival rates as high as 24% following complete resection, but that a subgroup of patients with bulky ipsilateral nodal involvement (mediastinal lymphadenopathy so large as to be apparent on chest X-ray or causing splaying of the carina at bronchoscopy) had only an 8% survival at 3 years [12]. Based on these observations, a preoperative regimen of mitomycin, vinca alkaloid (vindesine or vinblastine) and high dose cisplatin (MVP) was administered to this poor risk, bulky N2 patient population [13]. In their large phase II trial of 136 patients, the investigators at MSKCC found

a radiographic major response rate of 77%, with 65% of patients undergoing complete surgical resection. Pathologically, 14% achieved a complete response with no evidence of viable tumor in the resected surgical specimen. Median survival for the 136 patients was 19 months. Three-year survival was 41% in patients who were completely resected; an improvement over the historical experience of 8% for surgery alone. A confirmatory phase II trial was conducted by investigators in Canada [14]. The Toronto group enrolled 65 mediastinoscopy-proven stage IIIA NSCLC patients and treated them with two cycles of preoperative mitomycin, vindesine and cisplatin, followed by thoracotomy and two further cycles of postoperative chemotherapy. The radiographic response rate to induction chemotherapy was 68%, and 54% had complete surgical resection. The median survival of the entire patient group was 18.6 months, with a 5-year survival of 29%, and 10-year survival of 22%.

A number of other phase II trials have been completed assessing the role of induction chemotherapy with or without radiation therapy followed by surgery for stage III disease [15–21]. These trials have demonstrated that radiographic response rates range from 39 to 76%, surgical resection is feasible following induction therapy, and pathologic complete responses are seen [14]. In trials utilizing induction chemotherapy alone, the pathologic complete response rate has been reported as high as 18%, while those using chemotherapy and radiation have been as high as 26% [14,21]. Patients who have been found to have pathologic complete responses have been noteworthy for significantly prolonged survival [22]. Another important finding of these trials was that radiographic response did not always correlate with pathological response, with both more and less extensive disease found at surgery than would have been predicted radiographically [11,14]. Finally, survival does not appear to be substantially different in studies using combined radiation and chemotherapy as compared with those using induction chemotherapy alone [23]. A current intergroup study comparing induction chemoradiation to induction chemotherapy alone in stage IIIA/N2 NSCLC will help to clarify this issue.

Table 15.2 Phase II induction trials with newer agents in stage III NSCLC.

Study	Stage	Regimen	Number of patients	Radiographic response rate (%)	Complete resection rate (%)	Median survival (mo)	1-yr survival (%)	Pathologic complete response (%)
Betticher et al. [24,25]	IIIA- N2	DP	90	66	48	NR	NR	NR
Van Zandwijk et al. [26]	IIIA- N2	GP	47	70	NR	19	69	NR
Migliorino et al. [27]	IIIA-N2/IIIB	GP	70	57	41	15	67	3
Choi et al. [28]	IIIA- N2	PacP	34	65	74	24	70	6
Garrido et al. [29]	IIIA/B	DGP	136	72	50	16	NR	NR
Esteban et al. [30]	IIIA/B	GPVn	62	65	NR	NR	NR	NR
		GP	66	66	NR	NR	NR	NR
Lorent et al. [31]	IIIA-N2	VdIP	131	54	47	24	21 (5 yr)	5
Cappuzzo et al. [32]	IIIA-N2/IIIB	GPacP	42	71	38	22	92	7
De Marinis et al. [33]	IIIA-N2	GPacP	49	74	55	23	85	16
Brechot et al. [34]	IIIA	MIP vs. GP	30	NR	NR	NR	NR	NR

DP, docetaxel, cisplatin; GP, gemcitabine, cisplatin; PacP, paclitaxel, cisplatin; DGP, docetaxel, gemcitabine, cisplatin; GPVn, gemcitabine, cisplatin, vinorelbine; VdIP, vindesine, ifosfamide, cisplatin; GPacP, gemcitabine, paclitaxel, cisplatin; MIP, mitomycin, ifosfamide, cisplatin.
NR, not reported.

Third-generation regimens

More recent phase II investigations have examined third-generation chemotherapy agents such as the taxanes and gemcitabine in the induction setting. Some of these trials have employed a two-drug regimen, while others have examined a three-drug combination. Some trials have focused only on stage IIIA/N2 patients, while others have allowed selected entry of stage IIIB patients. Although comparison of these phase II trials is hampered by differences in patient selection and subsequent use of either surgery or thoracic radiation, there are no striking differences between the two- and three-drug regimens, and second- versus third-generation agents. Randomized trials would be required to detect real differences, but are unlikely to occur. A summary of these trials is presented in Table 15.2.

Betticher and colleagues from Switzerland have studied docetaxel and cisplatin in stage IIIA/N2 NSCLC [24]. In this trial, 90 patients with potentially operable IIIA/N2 NSCLC were treated with three cycles of docetaxel/cisplatin. Chemotherapy was well tolerated with 96% of patients completing all three cycles. The radiographic response rate was 66%, and 48% underwent complete resection [25]. With mature follow-up, those patients who

were completely resected had a median survival of 5.2 years (range 0.3–6.3 yr). Multivariate analysis found that mediastinal lymph node downstaging and complete resection were independent predictors for long-term survival.

Van Zandwijk and colleagues have evaluated gemcitabine and cisplatin as an induction therapy in stage IIIA/N2 NSCLC (EORTC 08955). Radiographic responses were seen in 70% of the 47 eligible patients. Patients in this study were randomized to surgery or thoracic radiation therapy as part of the ongoing EORTC 08941 trial. Those patients who were randomized to surgery had encouraging resection and survival rates and the investigators concluded that gemcitabine/cisplatin was highly active and should be investigated further in early stage NSCLC [26].

Gemcitabine/cisplatin induction in stage IIIAN2 and selected IIIB NSCLC has also been evaluated by investigators from Italy [27]. In this phase II trial of 70 patients, radiographic response was seen in 57% of patients. Twenty-eight patients were able to undergo complete resection (41%), with pathologic complete response seen in two patients. With a median follow-up of only 16 months, the median survival was 15 months. The investigators felt the activity seen with this regimen warranted further study.

Paclitaxel and cisplatin have been administered as induction therapy to 34 patients with stage IIIA, clinical N2 NSCLC [28]. Clinical N2 disease was defined as lymphadenopathy greater than 1.5 cm, or multiple nodes measuring 1.0 cm on CT imaging. A radiographic response was seen in 65% of patients and 74% were completely resected. The median overall survival was 24 months. Although the resection rate appears encouraging in this study, the definition of "clinical N2" disease utilized by these investigators would have included less extensive disease than defined in other studies.

A three-drug regimen of docetaxel, cisplatin, and gemcitabine has been evaluated by investigators in Spain [29]. One hundred thirty-six patients with pathologically proven IIIA/N2 or IIIB/T4N0-1 were included. The radiographic response rate was 72% and complete surgical resection was achieved in 50% of evaluable patients. Median survival for the entire group was 16 months and had not been reached for the patients who underwent complete surgical resection. No differences in survival between stage IIIA/N2 and IIIB/T4N0-1 were seen. The investigators concluded that the three-drug regimen was feasible in the neoadjuvant setting and that surgery may play a role in selected stage IIIB patients.

Another group in Spain has studied gemcitabine/cisplatin with or without vinorelbine as induction therapy in stage III NSCLC. In this study of 128 patients, there was no difference in radiographic response between the two- and three-drug regimens (66% versus 65%, respectively). Predictably, hematologic toxicity and fatigue were more frequent with the three-drug regimen. Preliminary results found no difference between the two regimens for resection rates and survival, although specific data were not given in the preliminary report [30].

Three cycles of preoperative vindesine, ifosfamide, and cisplatin were given to 131 patients with stage IIIA/N2 NSCLC by investigators in Belgium [31]. Radiographic response occurred in 54% and the median and 5-year survival rates for the entire patient group were 24 months and 21%, respectively. Seventy-five patients underwent surgery, with complete resection in 47%. Although survival in the entire cohort appeared to correlate with response following chemotherapy, this effect was not seen in patients who underwent complete resection. Resection rates were lower in the subgroup of patients with stable disease; however, the authors emphasized that long-term survival following complete resection was seen in some patients who did not have major radiographic response [31].

Gemcitabine, paclitaxel, and cisplatin have also been studied as an induction regimen. In one study, this three-drug regimen was given to 42 patients with stage IIIA/N2 and IIIB NSCLC. Major radiographic response was seen in 71%, and 21 patients underwent thoracotomy with 16 complete resections (38%). Pathologic complete responses were seen in 7%. With short median follow-up (14 mo), the median survival was 22 months [32]. This same regimen was studied as an induction treatment in 49 patients with stage IIIA/N2 disease [33]. In this cohort of 49 patients, 74% achieved radiographic response, and 55% were completely resected. In this small study, 8/49 (16%) had pathologic complete response at surgery. With a median follow-up of 15.6 months, the median overall survival was 23 months.

The regimen of mitomycin, ifosfamide, and cisplatin has also been compared to gemcitabine and cisplatin in a randomized phase II trial in clinically operable stage IIIA NSCLC [34]. Thirty patients have been studied and response, resection, and survival rates were similar between the two arms of this small study. Increased postoperative pulmonary toxicity led to the premature closure of the MIP arm of the trial [34].

Earlier stage disease

After the use of induction chemotherapy appeared promising in stage III NSCLC, clinical trials were designed and conducted which examined this approach in earlier stages of NSCLC. These trials are summarized in Table 15.3. The first such study was the Bimodality Lung Oncology Team Trial (BLOT) [11]. This phase II trial enrolled two sequential cohorts of patients with clinical stage IB, II, and IIIA patients. Clinical staging was defined by CT imaging

Table 15.3 Phase II induction trials with early-stage NSCLC.

Study	Stage	Regimen	Number of patients	Radiographic response rate (%)	Complete resection rate (%)	Overall survival (%) yr	Pathologic complete response (%)
Pisters et al. [11,35]	IB-IIIA	PacCb	134	51	86	(42) 5	5
Marks et al. [36]	T1-3N0-1	PacCb	51	59	71	(73) 2	NA
Tsuboi et al. [37]	IB-IIIA	PacCb	62	61	87	(52) 3	6
Kunitoh et al. [38]	IB-II	DP	40	45	95	NR	5
		D	39	15	85	NR	0
Lothaire et al. [39]	I-IIIA	MIP vs.	18	67	83	NR NR	17
		GVbP	18	67	72	NR	0
Abratt et al. [40]	IB-IIIA	PacGCb	44	75	82	NR	11
Socinski et al. [41]	I-II	GCb	82	NR	73*	(74)* 1	1
		GPac		NR			
		GCb		NR			
		GP		NR			
Sommers et al. [42]	IB-III	GVn	62	34	77	(68) 2	3

*Data given as combined figure for all 82 patients in the trial.
PacCb, paclitaxel, carboplatin; DP, docetaxel, cisplatin; D, docetaxel; MIP, mitomycin, ifosfamide, cisplatin; PacGCb, paclitaxel, gemcitabine, carboplatin; GCb, gemcitabine, carboplatin; GPac, gemcitabine, paclitaxel; GCb, gemcitabine, carboplatin; GP, gemcitabine, cisplatin; GVn, gemcitabine, vinorelbine.
NR, not reported.

and all patients were required to undergo mediastinoscopy. PET imaging was not routinely performed in this study. Patients with mediastinoscopy proven N2 disease or superior sulcus tumors were excluded from this trial. Patients were treated with paclitaxel and carboplatin before and after surgery (number of cycles in cohort I: 2 pre and 3 post; cohort II: 3 pre and 4 post). For the two cohorts combined, the radiographic response rate was 51%, complete resection rate was 86%, and pathologic complete response rate was 5%. Three- and five-year survival rates were 61 and 42%, respectively [35]. There were no significant differences in patient characteristics or outcome between the two cohorts. Based on this encouraging data, a randomized phase III trial was initiated and is discussed below.

The North Central Cancer Treatment Group (NCCTG) also evaluated paclitaxel and carboplatin given for three cycles preoperatively to early-stage NSCLC (clinical stage T1-3N0-1M0) [36]. Fifty-one evaluable patients were treated. The radiographic response rate was 59%, 71% had complete resection. The 2-year survival rate was 73%. No further follow-up has been presented on this study.

Japanese investigators have administered weekly paclitaxel with carboplatin given monthly for two cycles prior to surgery in clinical stage IB, II, and IIIA NSCLC [37]. In 62 patients, they found a radiographic response rate of 61%, with 87% of patients undergoing complete resection and 6% having pathologic complete response. The 3-year survival was 52%.

Induction docetaxel and cisplatin has been compared to docetaxel alone in a randomized phase II trial from the Japan Clinical Oncology Group. This study of 79 clinical stage IB and II NSCLC patients found improved results with the doublet. With docetaxel/cisplatin, 45% of patients had radiographic response, 95% were completely resected and 5% had pathologic complete response. Disease-free survival at 1 year was 77%, but no overall survival data were given [38].

A three-drug regimen of mitomycin, ifosfamide, and cisplatin is being compared to another triplet of gemcitabine, vinorelbine, and cisplatin in a randomized phase II trial conducted in Europe by Lothaire and colleagues. When last reported, this trial had randomized 36 clinical stage I-IIIA NSCLC patients.

Response rates were 67% in both arms, and complete resection rates were 83% and 72%, respectively [39].

Gemcitabine, carboplatin and paclitaxel have been used as induction therapy in a phase II trial of 44 clinical stage IB, II, and IIIA NSCLC. Radiographic response in 75% and complete resection occurred in 82% and pathologic complete response in 11%. No survival data has been reported to date [40].

The GINEST Project consisting of two similar randomized phase II trials is testing platin and nonplatin regimens preoperatively in clinical stage I or II NSCLC. At last report, 82 patients had been randomized onto these trials comparing gemcitabine/carboplatin to gemcitabine/paclitaxel and gemcitabine/carboplatin to gemcitabine/cisplatin. Complete resection has occurred in 73% of all patients and 1-year survival for all patients is 74%. The authors concluded that induction chemotherapy with gemcitabine as part of a platin or nonplatin doublet is feasible, well tolerated, and results in rates of resection, response, and survival similar to other regimens in this setting [41].

A nonplatin regimen of gemcitabine and vinorelbine for two preoperative cycles was given to clinical stage IB-III NSCLC [42]. This study enrolled 62 patients. Although the radiographic response rate was low at 34%, 77% underwent complete resection, and 3% had pathologic complete response. A 2-year survival of 68% was seen with a median of 38 months. The authors concluded that although the response to chemotherapy was lower than platin-doublets, the preliminary survival results appeared similar.

Randomized phase II and phase III trials

Following the initial encouraging phase II reports of induction chemotherapy, randomized trials were undertaken comparing induction chemotherapy and surgery to surgery alone. These trials are summarized in Table 15.4. These induction chemotherapy trials were designed and conducted before the publication of the positive results for chemotherapy in the adjuvant setting [6–8].

Stage III trials

The first randomized phase II trial of induction chemotherapy for resectable NSCLC came from France [43]. This study stopped accrual after only 26 patients had been entered. Of the 13 patients randomized to receive induction cisplatin, cyclophosphamide and vindesine chemotherapy, 11 agreed to receive treatment. Five had radiographic response (45%) and four patients had disease progression causing cancellation of surgical resection in two. Given the rate of disease progression observed, the investigators terminated the study.

Roth and colleagues conducted a phase III randomized trial of perioperative chemotherapy with cyclophosphamide, etoposide, and cisplatin followed by surgery compared to a control arm of surgery alone in potentially resectable clinical stage IIIA NSCLC [44,45]. Patients randomized to chemotherapy were to receive three cycles of chemotherapy before surgery; an additional three cycles were given after surgery to patients with preoperative radiographic response. Following an interim analysis, the trial was closed after 60 patients had been accrued because of a clinically meaningful survival benefit in favor of the induction chemotherapy arm [44]. Long-term follow-up of this trial after a median time from randomization of 82 months confirmed the beneficial effect of induction chemotherapy. Median and 5-year survival rates were 21 months and 36% versus 14 months and 15% for surgery alone [45].

A similar phase III trial conducted by Rosell and colleagues from Barcelona was reported at the same time [46]. In this study, clinical stage IIIA NSCLC patients were randomized to immediate surgery or surgery preceded by three cycles of mitomycin, ifosfamide, and cisplatin chemotherapy. Both treatment groups received postoperative mediastinal radiation therapy to 50 Gy. Interim analysis after 24 months follow-up with 60 eligible patients showed a significant difference in survival favoring induction chemotherapy and enrollment was stopped. Reassessment with 7-year follow-up found median and 5-year survival rates of 22 months and 17% in the chemotherapy arm compared to 10 months and 0% in the surgery alone arm [47].

Table 15.4 Randomized trials of induction therapy in operable NSCLC.

Study	Stage	Regimen	Number of patients	Radiographic response rate (%)	Complete resection rate (%)	Median survival (mo)	1-yr survival (%)	Pathologic complete response (%)
Dautzenberg et al. [43]	III	PCV	13	45	NR	NR	NR	NR
		Control	13	—	NR	NR	NR	—
Roth et al. [44,45]	IIIA	CEP	28	35	39	21	36	0
		Control	32	—	31	14	15	—
Rosell et al. [46,47]	IIIA	MIP	30	60	77	22	17	3
		Control	30	—	90	10	0	—
Pass et al. [48]	IIIAN2	EP	13	62	85	29	46 (2 yr)	8
		Control	14	—	86	16	21 (2 yr)	—
Wu et al. [49]	IIIA	DP	26	73	65	NR	NR	NR
		Control	22	—	NR	NR	NR	—
Zhou et al. [50]	III	Varied	414	73	94	NR	34	15
		Control	310	—	92	NR	24	—
Nagai et al. [51]	IIIAN2	VdP	31	28	65	17	10	NR
		Surgery	31	—	77	16	22	—
Yang et al. [52]	IIIA	GCborP	19	58	90	NR	NR	NR
		Surgery	21	—	91	NR	NR	—
DePierre et al. [54,55]	IB, II, IIIA (+N2)	MIP	179	64	92	37	41	11
		Surgery	176	—	86	26	32	—
Sorensen et al. [56]	IB, II, IIIA	PacCb	44	46	79	34	36	NR
		Surgery	46	—	70	23	24	—
Pisters et al. [57]	IB, II, IIIA	PacCb	168	41	94	47	69 (2 yr)	NR
		Surgery	167	—	89	40	63 (2 yr)	—

PCV, cisplatin, cyclophosphamide, vindesine; CEP, cyclophosphamide, etoposide, cisplatin; MIP, mitomycin, ifosfamide, cisplatin; EP, etoposide, cisplatin; DP, docetaxel, cisplatin; VdP, vindesine, cisplatin; GcborP, gemcitabine and carboplatin or cisplatin; PacCb, paclitaxel, carboplatin.
NR, not reported.

Another phase III randomized study of induction chemotherapy was conducted at the National Cancer Institute. This trial randomized stage IIIA/N2 patients to receive two cycles of cisplatin/etoposide chemotherapy prior to surgery (and four postoperative cycles if evidence of radiographic response) or surgery followed by 54–60 Gy of mediastinal radiation. After 4 years of accrual only 27 patients had agreed to participate. An interim analysis published in 1992 found a trend toward improved survival in the chemotherapy arm of the study—median survival of 29 versus 16 months, $p = 0.095$ [48].

Investigators in China have conducted a phase II randomized trial of surgery alone versus two cycles of induction docetaxel and carboplatin chemotherapy in resectable stage IIIA NSCLC. At the time of last report, 48 patients had been entered with 26 randomized to chemotherapy. Radiographic response was seen in 73% and complete resection achieved in 65% of the chemotherapy treated patients. Slightly more patients had died on the surgery alone control arm (8/22 versus 5/26), but no information on median or overall survival rates were reported [49].

A large randomized trial of neoadjuvant chemotherapy in stage III NSCLC from China has been reported in abstract form only [50]. This study randomized 724 patients over a 12-year period to preoperative chemotherapy or a control group of surgery alone. Of the 414 patients assigned to two cycles of chemotherapy, 21 had bronchial artery interventional chemotherapy (details not listed). The other 393 patients were given intravenous chemotherapy (130 pts-gemcitabine/cisplatin, 68-mitomycin/vinca/cisplatin, 67-etoposide/cisplatin, 36-cyclophosphamide/doxorubicin/cisplatin, 32-vindesine/cisplatin, 30-paclitaxel/vinorelbine, and 30-paclitaxel/cisplatin). Response to induction chemotherapy was reported for 73% of patients with pathologic complete responses seen in 15%. Complete resection rates were 94% in the chemotherapy arm and 92% in the surgery group. No significant differences in operative complications or mortality were reported. Five- and ten-year survival rates were 34% and 29% versus 24% and 22%, $p < 0.01$. It is disappointing that the results of this trial have not been published in manuscript form. The response, resection, survival, and pathologic complete response rates are higher than what has been reported in other trials. Also of concern is the marked variation in induction regimen.

Nagai and colleagues from the Lung Cancer Surgical Study Group of the Japan Clinical Oncology Group have published their experience of a phase III randomized trial in stage IIIA/N2 NSCLC [51]. The trial was designed to accrue 200 patients over a 3-year period. However, the trial was closed secondary to slow accrual after only 62 patients had entered in 5 years. The authors cited lack of rewarding compensation to the patients, prolonged hospitalization in the induction chemotherapy group, and wide reports in the domestic media of the ineffectiveness of chemotherapy for NSCLC as the major reasons for poor accrual. With a median follow-up of 6.2 years, there was no difference in survival between the two arms in terms of median or 5-year survival rates (17 mo and 10% versus 16 mo and 22% in the surgery alone arm) [51].

A randomized phase III trial comparing neoadjuvant gemcitabine plus carboplatin or cisplatin to surgery alone in potentially resectable clinical stage IIIA NSCLC was attempted in China [52]. Unfortu-nately, after 5 years, only 40 patients could be enrolled and the study was closed. Of the patients randomized to chemotherapy, 56% had radiographic response and 90% were completely resected. A similar proportion of the surgery alone patients had complete resection (91%). After a median follow-up of 28 months, 8 of 19 patients had died on the chemotherapy arm versus 12 of 21 in the surgery control group [52].

Earlier stage disease

The first report of a randomized induction chemotherapy trial in early stage NSCLC (patients without mediastinal lymph node involvement) came from the Royal Brompton Hospital in London, England. This feasibility study was performed in 22 patients with early stage (IB, II, and IIIA) resectable NSCLC. Patients were randomized to either three cycles of mitomycin, vinblastine, and cisplatin chemotherapy followed by surgery ($n = 11$) or to surgery alone ($n = 11$). Of 40 patients who were potentially eligible for the study, 22 agreed to participate. Patients assigned to chemotherapy tolerated treatment well and did not have increased operative morbidity or mortality [53]. Based on this limited experience, the authors recommended a large, multicenter phase III trial in all patients with operable NSCLC and supported accrual to the Medical Research Council Lung Group trial—the UK Big Lung Trial.

In 2001, the results of a phase III randomized trial of induction mitomycin, ifosfamide, and cisplatin chemotherapy in resectable stage IB, II, and IIIA were reported [54]. Three hundred fifty-five eligible patients were randomized to surgery alone or combined modality therapy with two cycles of chemotherapy followed by surgery. Responding patients (radiographically or pathologically) received two additional cycles of chemotherapy postoperatively. The arms were well balanced for patient characteristics with the exception that less clinical N2 patients were assigned to the surgery-only arm (28% versus 40%, $p = 0.65$). A non-significant excess of postoperative morbidity in the chemotherapy arm was seen (24/167 versus 22/171). Postoperative mortality was 6.7% in the chemotherapy arm and 4.5% in the surgery arm ($p = 0.38$). Median survival was improved by

11 months (37 versus 26 mo) and at 4 years, there was an 8.6% increase in survival in the chemotherapy arm, but this did not achieve statistical significance. In a subset analysis, the benefit of chemotherapy was confined to patients with N0 to N1 disease with a relative risk of death of 0.68, $p = 0.027$. After a nonsignificant excess of deaths in the combined modality arm during the treatment period, the effect of induction chemotherapy was favorable on survival. No difference was seen in local recurrence rates. A significant decrease in distant metastases was observed favoring the chemotherapy arm with a relative risk of 0.54, $p = 0.01$. Follow-up data on this trial was presented in 2003, when minimal follow-up exceeded 60 months [55]. The 3- to 5-year survival differences were stable around 10% ($p = 0.04$ at 3 yr and $p = 0.06$ at 5 yr). Statistically significant benefits in the N0-1 subgroup were confirmed with 5-year survival rates of 49% compared to 34% ($p = 0.02$) [55].

The Scandinavians have recently reported their randomized trial of neoadjuvant paclitaxel/carboplatin chemotherapy in clinical stage IB, II, and IIIA (excluding N2 patients) NSCLC [56]. The study was closed prematurely secondary to slow accrual (90 patients in 6 yr). Of the 44 patients randomized to chemotherapy, major radiographic responses were seen in 46% and 79% had complete resection. In the 46 patients treated with surgery alone, complete resection was achieved in 70%. Median and 5-year survival rates were 34 months and 36% compared to 23 months and 24% in the control arm. Although the results were not statistically significant, a beneficial effect was suggested by these results [56].

The Southwest Oncology Group trial, S9900, was a phase III randomized study comparing induction paclitaxel/carboplatin chemotherapy for three cycles followed by surgery to surgery alone in clinical stage IB, II, and IIIA NSCLC (excluding superior sulcus and N2 disease). The study called for 600 patients to detect a 33% increase in median survival or 10% increase in 5-year survival. Unfortunately, accrual to this trial was suspended after data from randomized adjuvant chemotherapy trials in completely resected NSCLC revealed a survival benefit. Total accrual reached 354 patients, and preliminary results were presented at ASCO 2005 [57]. Patient

characteristics were well balanced between the two groups. Of the patients randomized to chemotherapy, 41% had radiographic response and 94% had complete resection. Eighty-nine percent of patients on the control arm had complete resection. With a median follow-up of 31 months, median and 2-year survival rates were 47 months versus 40 months, and 69% versus 63% for the chemotherapy/surgery and surgery alone arms, respectively. Although the use of chemotherapy was associated with a 16% reduction in the risk of death (HR, 0.84; $p = 0.32$), this difference did not achieve statistical significance.

Preliminary results from the CH.E.S.T. (Chemotherapy in Early Stages in NSCLC Trial) trial were also presented at ASCO 2005 [58]. This phase III randomized trial compared three cycles of induction gemcitabine/cisplatin chemotherapy administered before resection to surgery alone. The primary endpoint of this study was progression-free survival and the original study design required 700 randomized patients. Similar to the S9900 study, the CH.E.S.T. trial was closed to patient accrual at 267 patients following the results of the positive adjuvant trials. At a median follow-up time of 10 months, 6-month progression-free survival was 89% versus 80%, favoring the combined approach [58].

Finally, there is an ongoing three-arm randomized trial in Spain comparing induction chemotherapy followed by surgery, surgery followed by adjuvant chemotherapy and surgery alone. The trial is designed with disease-free survival as the primary endpoint and at the time of last report, has accrued 492 of a planned 628 patients [59].

Meta-analyses

To date, there have been two meta-analyses examining the efficacy of induction chemotherapy in resectable NSCLC [60,61]. Both these meta-analyses were not IDP (individual patient data) meta-analyses, but were based on data extracted from abstracts and manuscripts. An IPD meta-analysis is considered vastly superior to one based on abstracted or pooled data, as it allows verification of randomization and patient data, updates the

Table 15.5 Meta-analyses of randomized trials in operable NSCLC.

	Berghmans et al. [60]	Burdett et al. [61]
Number of trials	6	7
Number of patients	590	988
Hazard ratio	0.66 (0.48–0.93)	0.82 (0.69–0.97)
Trials included	Katzenberg	Dautzenberg
	Rosell	Rosell
	Roth	Roth
	Depierre	Depierre
	Nagai	Nagai
	Pass	Sorensen
		Pisters

data, and is highly reliable. Drawbacks to the IPD meta-analysis are increased cost and length of time required [62]. Meta-analyses based on abstracted data are based only on published trial results or abstracts and thus do not allow updated patient outcomes, which are crucial in interpreting combined modality data. Although less time-consuming and costly, meta-analyses based on abstracted data are much less reliable [62]. As such, these meta-analyses should be interpreted with caution. Summary data from these two meta-analyses are presented in Table 15.5.

The first meta-analysis by Berghmans et al., looked at both induction and adjuvant randomized studies reported between 1965 and June 2004 [60]. They found an HR of 0.66 (95% CI, 0.48–0.93) for the addition of induction chemotherapy and an HR of 0.84 (95% CI, 0.78–0.89) for the addition of adjuvant (postoperative chemotherapy). The randomized neoadjuvant trials included in this meta-analysis are a subset of those reviewed above [43,45,47,48,51,55], and included six trials enrolling 590 patients. When examining the effect of induction chemotherapy in the subgroup of patients with clinical stage III NSCLC, the HR became 0.65 (95% CI, 0.41–1.04) and although strongly trended in favor of the use of chemotherapy in stage III disease, did not achieve statistical significance. In a subsequent letter to the editor, the statistical methodology used to compare the effects of induction chemotherapy in stages I/II versus stage

III NSCLC was questioned and it was suggested that the nonsignificant result may have been related to numbers of patients included or because of the use of the random effects model [63].

The second meta-analysis by Burdett et al. was also based on data extracted from abstracts and manuscripts from randomized trials [61]. Literature searches identified 12 eligible randomized controlled trials. Five of these trials were excluded as insufficient data could be extracted from the published results [49,53,58,64,65]. The remaining seven trials on which the meta-analysis is based included 988 patients [43,45,47,51,55–57]. The authors found that preoperative chemotherapy improved survival with an HR of 0.82 (0.69–0.97, $p = 0.02$). This is equivalent to an absolute benefit of 6% at 5 years. An analysis grouping trials according to the type of chemotherapy administered was also performed. All patients received a platinum-based chemotherapy—either cisplatin or carboplatin—that was combined with other agents. These other agents were split into the three groups: vinca alkaloid/etoposide, taxane, or other. There was no clear evidence of a difference of treatment effect shown by chemotherapy group. The authors concluded that the meta-analysis suggests a significant survival benefit for patients with NSCLC who receive preoperative chemotherapy compared to those who do not. The value of this treatment will be further assessed through an ongoing IPD meta-analysis [61].

Surgical morbidity and mortality after induction therapy

The use of chemotherapy prior to surgery has raised concern that surgical complications may be increased. Data from large series address this issue. Siegenthaler et al. from MDACC have reported on a series of 380 consecutive patients undergoing lobectomy or greater resection for NSCLC [66]. Following exclusion of 45 patients (history of prior lung cancer, prior radiation or chemoradiation to the chest, prior malignancy etc.), a population of 335 patients (259 surgery alone, 76 chemotherapy followed by surgery) was studied from the MDACC

Thoracic Surgery database. The use of preoperative chemotherapy did not significantly affect morbidity or mortality overall, based on clinical stage, postoperative stage, or extent of resection. No significant differences in overall or subset mortality or morbidity including pneumonia, acute respiratory distress syndrome, reintubation, tracheostomy, wound complication, or length of hospitalization were seen [66].

All patients undergoing thoracotomy after induction chemotherapy from 1993 through 1999 at MSKCC were the subject of a review [67]. Four hundred seventy patients treated with induction chemotherapy and surgery were reviewed. Univariate and multivariate methods for logistic regression model were used to identify predictors of adverse events. Overall, the MSKCC group found a surgical mortality rate of 3.8%, which compared favorably to other primary surgery studies. Total morbidity and major complication rates were 38.1% and 26.6%; similar to previous primary surgery studies. The authors concluded that overall morbidity rates were not significantly affected by the use of induction therapy. They did find an operative mortality rate of 23.9% for patients undergoing right pneumonectomy following induction therapy. This number was higher than previous mortality rates seen in trials where patients did not have induction therapy. The authors recommended that right pneumonectomy after induction therapy be performed very selectively and only when no alternative resection is possible [67].

A third series from investigators in France reviewed 114 patients who underwent thoracotomy following induction chemotherapy [68]. In this series, there was only 1 death following pneumonectomy in 55 patients. Overall morbidity rate was 28.9%, similar to other surgical series. The authors concluded that preoperative chemotherapy did not increase postoperative morbidity and mortality.

Conclusions

Induction chemotherapy has been extensively evaluated and appears promising based on phase II and phase III trials. The number of patients studied in individual phase III trials has been inadequate to clearly determine the efficacy of this approach. Two meta-analyses that extracted data from published trials and abstracts have both shown statistically significant benefits in favor of induction chemotherapy. A meta-analysis employing individual patient data is underway and should yield more reliable results. Randomized trials comparing preoperative to postoperative chemotherapy are warranted.

References

1 Jemal A, Siegel R, Ward E et al. Cancer Statistics, 2007. *CA Cancer J Clin* 2007; **57**:43–66.
2 Mountain CF. Revisions in the international system f staging lung cancer. *Chest* 1997; **111**:1710–7.
3 Patel J, Blum M, Argiris A. Induction chemotherapy for resectable non-small cell lung cancer. *Oncology* 2004; **18**:1591–602.
4 Pisters KMW, Le Chevalier T. Adjuvant chemotherapy in completely resected non-small cell lung cancer. *J Clin Oncol* 2005; **23**:3270–8.
5 Non-Small Cell Lung Cancer Collaborative Group. Chemotherapy in non-small cell lung cancer: a meta-analysis using updated data on individual patients from 52 randomized clinical trials. *BMJ* 1995; **311**:899–909.
6 The International Adjuvant Lung Cancer Trial Collaborative Group. Cisplatin-based adjuvant chemotherapy in patients with completely resected non-small cell lung cancer. *N Engl M Med* 2004; **350**:351–60.
7 Winton T, Livingston R, Johnson D et al. Vinorelbine plus cisplatin vs. observation in resected non-small cell lung cancer. *N Engl J Med* 2005; **353**:2589–97.
8 Douillard J, Rosell R, De Lena M et al. Adjuvant vinorelbine plus cisplatin versus observation in patients with completely resected stage IB-IIIA non-small cell lung cancer (Adjuvant Navelbine International Trialist Association [ANITA]): a randomized controlled trial. *Lancet Oncol* 2006; **7**:719–27.
9 Dillman R, Seagren S, Herndon J et al. Improved survival in stage III non-small cell lung cancer: seven-year followup of CALGB 8433. *J Natl Cancer Inst* 1996; **88**:1210–5.
10 Sause WT, Scott C, Taylor S et al. Radiation Therapy Oncology Group 88-08 and Eastern Cooperative Oncology Group 4588: preliminary results of a phase III trial of regionally advanced, unresectable non-small cell lung cancer. *J Natl Cancer Inst* 1995; **87**:198–205.

11 Pisters K, Ginsberg R, Giroux D *et al*. Induction chemotherapy before surgery for early-stage lung cancer: a novel approach. *J Thorac Cardiovasc Surg* 2000; **119**:429–39.

12 Martini N, Flehinger B, Zaman M *et al*. Prospective study of 445 lung carcinomas with mediastinal lymph node metastases. *J Thorac Cardiovasc Surg* 1980; **80**:390–7.

13 Martini N, Kris M, Flehinger B *et al*. Preoperative chemotherapy for stage IIIa(N2) lung cancer: the Memorial Sloan-Kettering experience with 136 patients. *Ann Thorac Surg* 1993; **55**:1365–74.

14 Burkes R, Shepherd R, Blackstein M *et al*. Induction chemotherapy with mitomycin, vindesine, and cisplatin for stage IIIA (T1-3N2) unresectable non-small cell lung cancer: final results of the Toronto phase II trial. *Lung Cancer* 2005; **47**:103–9.

15 Darwish S, Minotti V, Crino L *et al*. Neoadjuvant cisplatin and etoposide for stage IIIA (clinical N2) non-small cell lung cancer. *Am J Clin Oncol* 1994; **17**:64–7.

16 Vokes E, Bitran J, Hoffman P *et al*. Neoadjuvant vindesine, etoposide and cisplatin for locally advanced non-small cell lung cancer. *Chest* 1989; **96**:110–3.

17 Elias A, Skarin A, Leong T *et al*. Neoadjuvant therapy for surgically staged IIIA N2 non-small cell lung cancer (NSCLC). *Lung Cancer* 1997; **17**:147–61.

18 Albain K, Rusch V, Crowley J *et al*. Concurrent cisplatin/etoposide plus chest radiotherapy followed by surgery for stage IIIA (N2) and IIIB NSCLC: mature results of Southwest Oncology Group phase II study 8805. *J Clin Oncol* 1995; **13**:1880–92.

19 Faber LP, Kettle F, Warren WH *et al*. Preoperative chemotherapy and irradiation for stage III non-small cell lung cancer. *Ann Thorac Surg* 1989; **47**:266–72.

20 Strauss G, Herndon J, Sherman D *et al*. Neoadjuvant chemotherapy and radiotherapy followed by surgery in stage IIIA non-small cell lung carcinoma of the lung: report of a Cancer and Leukemia Group B phase II study. *J Clin Oncol* 1992; **10**:1237–44.

21 Eberhardt W, Wilke H, Stamatis G *et al*. Preoperative chemotherapy followed by concurrent chemoradiation therapy based on hyperfractionated accelerated radiotherapy and definitive surgery in locally advanced non-small cell lung cancer: mature results of a phase II trial. *J Clin Oncol* 1998; **16**:622–34.

22 Pisters K, Kris M, Gralla R *et al*. Pathologic complete response in advanced non-small cell lung cancer following preoperative chemotherapy: implications for the design of future non-small cell lung cancer combined modality trials. *J Clin Oncol* 1993; **11**:1757–62.

23 Martin J, Ginsberg R, Venkatraman E *et al*. Long-term results of combined-modality therapy in resectable non-small cell lung cancer. *J Clin Oncol* 2002; **20**:1989–95.

24 Betticher D, Hsu Schmitz S, Roth A *et al*. Neoadjuvant therapy with docetaxel and cisplatin in patients with non-small cell lung cancer, stage IIIA, pN2: a large phase II study with 59 months of follow-up. *Lung Cancer* 2005; **49**:S14.

25 Betticher D, Hsu Schmitz S, Totsch M *et al*. Mediastinal lymph node clearance after docetaxel–cisplatin neoadjuvant chemotherapy is prognostic of survival in patients with stage IIIA pN2 non-small cell lung cancer: a multicenter phase II trial. *J Clin Oncol* 2003; **21**:1752–9.

26 Van Zandwijk N, Smit E, Kramer G *et al*. Gemcitabine and cisplatin as induction regimen for patients with biopsy-proven stage IIIA N2 non-small cell lung cancer: a phase II study of the European Organization for Research and Treatment of Cancer Lung Cancer Cooperative Group (EORTC 08955). *J Clin Oncol* 2000; **18**:2658–64.

27 Migliorino M, De Marinis F, Nelli F *et al*. A 3-week schedule of gemcitabine plus cisplatin as induction chemotherapy for stage III non-small cell lung cancer. *Lung Cancer* 2002; **35**:319–27.

28 Choi I, Oh D, Kwon J *et al*. Paclitaxel/platinum-based perioperative chemotherapy and surgery in stage IIIA non-small cell lung cancer. *Jpn J Clin Oncol* 2005; **35**:6–12.

29 Garrido P, Rosell R, Torres A *et al*. Docetaxel, cisplatin and gemcitabine as neoadjuvant treatment in stage IIIAN2 and T4N0-1 non-small cell lung cancer patients. Final results of SLCG phase II trial 9901. *Lung Cancer* 2005; **49**:S14.

30 Esteban E, Fernancez y, Vieitez J *et al*. Cisplatin plus gemcitabine with or without vinorelbine as neoadjuvant therapy for radically treatable stage III non-small cell lung cancer. Preliminary results of a randomized study of the GON. *Lung Cancer* 2005; **49**:S40.

31 Lorent N, De Leyn P, Lievens Y *et al*. Long term survival of surgically staged IIIA-N2 non-small cell lung cancer treated with surgical combined modality approach: analysis of a 7-year prospective experience. *Ann Oncol* 2004; **15**:1645–53.

32 Cappuzzo F, De Marinis F, Nelli F *et al*. Phase II study of gemcitabine-cisplatin-paclitaxel triplet as induction chemotherapy in inoperable, locally advanced non-small cell lung cancer. *Lung Cancer* 2003; **42**:355–61.

33 De Marinis F, Nelli F, Migliorino M *et al*. Gemcitabine, paclitaxel, and cisplatin as induction chemotherapy for

patients with biopsy-proven stage IIIA(N2) non-small cell carcinoma. *Cancer* 2003; **98**:1707–15.

34 Brechot J, Saintigny P, Azorin J *et al.* A phase II randomized study of gemcitabine-cisplatin versus mitomycin-ifosfamide-cisplatin as neoadjuvant chemotherapy in resectable stage IIIA non-small cell lung cancer. *Lung Cancer* 2005; **49**:S175.

35 Pisters K, Ginsberg R, Giroux D *et al.* Bimodality lung oncology team trial of induction paclitaxel/carboplatin in early stage non-small cell lung cancer: long term followup of a phase II trial [Abstract]. *Proc Am Soc Clin Oncol* 2003; **22**:2544.

36 Marks R, Streitz J, Deschamps C *et al.* Response rate and toxicity of preoperative paclitaxel and carboplatin in patients with resectable non-small cell lung cancer: a North Central Cancer Treatment Group study [Abstract]. *Proc Am Soc Clin Oncol* 2001; **20**:1355.

37 Tsuboi M, Ohira T, Hayashi A *et al.* Preoperative induction chemotherapy with weekly paclitaxel and carboplatin for clinical-stage IB-IIIA non-small cell lung cancer. *Lung Cancer* 2005; **49**:S175.

38 Kunitoh H, Hato H, Tsuboi M *et al.* A randomized phase II trial of preoperative docetaxel and cisplatin or docetaxel alone in clinical stage IB/II non-small cell lung cancer: initial resort of Japan Clinical Oncology Group Trial. *J Clin Oncol, 2005 ASCO Ann Mtg Proc* 2005; **23(16S)**:7119.

39 Lothaire P, Berghmans Th, Lafitte J *et al.* Resectability after two different chemotherapy regimens: results of the first step of a phase II randomized trial in initially resectable stage I-IIIA non-small cell lung cancer conducted by the European Lung Cancer Working Party. *Lung Cancer* 2003; **41(Suppl 2)**:S63.

40 Abratt R, Lee J, Han J *et al.* Phase II trial of gemcitabine-carboplatin-paclitaxel as neoadjuvant chemotherapy for operable non-small cell lung cancer. *Lung Cancer* 2005; **49**:S92.

41 Socinski M, Detterbeck F, Gralla R *et al.* Induction chemotherapy with gemcitabine-containing regimens in stage I-II non-small cell lung cancer: initial results of the GINEST Project. *Lung Cancer* 2005; **49**: S40.

42 Sommers E, Ramnath N, Robinson L *et al.* Neoadjuvant chemotherapy with gemcitabine and vinorelbine in resectable non-small cell lung cancer. *Lung Cancer* 2005; **49**:S96–7.

43 Dautzenberg B, Benichou J, Allard P *et al.* Failure of the perioperative PCV neoadjuvant polychemotherapy in resectable bronchogenic non-small cell carcinoma. Results from a randomized phase II trial. *Cancer* 1990; **65(11)**:2435–41.

44 Roth J, Fossella F, Komaki R *et al.* A randomized trial comparing perioperative chemotherapy and surgery with surgery alone in resectable stage IIIA non-small cell lung cancer. *J Natl Cancer Inst* 1994; **86**:673–80.

45 Roth J, Atkinson E, Fossella F *et al.* Long-term followup of patients enrolled in a randomized trial comparing perioperative chemotherapy and surgery with surgery alone in resectable stage IIIA non-small cell lung cancer. *Lung Cancer* 1998; **21**:1–6.

46 Rosell R, Gomez-Codina J, Camps C *et al.* A randomized trial comparing preoperative chemotherapy plus surgery with surgery alone in patients with non-small cell lung cancer. *N Engl J Med* 1994; **330**:153–8.

47 Rosell R, Gomez-Codina J, Camps C *et al.* Preresectional chemotherapy in stage IIIA non-small cell lung cancer: a 7-year assessment of a randomized controlled trial. *Lung Cancer* 1999; **47**:7–14.

48 Pass H, Pogrebniak H, Steinberg S *et al.* Randomized trial of neoadjuvant therapy for lung cancer: interim analysis. *Ann Thorac Surg* 1992; **53**:992–8.

49 Wu Y, Gu L, Weng Y *et al.* Neoadjuvant chemotherapy with docetaxel plus carboplatin for non-small cell lung cancer [Abstract]. *Ann Oncol* 2002; **13(Suppl 5)**:140.

50 Zhou Q, Liu L, Li L *et al.* A randomized clinical trial of preoperative neoadjuvant chemotherapy followed by surgery in the treatment of stage III non-small cell lung cancer. *Lung Cancer* 2003; **41(Suppl 2)**:S45–46.

51 Nagai K, Tsuchiya R, Mori T *et al.* A randomized trial comparing induction chemotherapy followed by surgery with surgery alone for patients with stage IIIA N2 non-small cell lung cancer (JCOG 9209). *J Thorac Cardiovasc Surg* 2003; **125**:254–60.

52 Yang X, Wu Y, Chen G *et al.* A randomized trial comparing neoadjuvant gemcitabine plus carboplatin or cisplatin followed by surgery with surgery alone in clinical stage IIIA non-small cell lung cancer. *Lung Cancer* 2005; **49**:S288.

53 de Boer R, Smith I, Pastorino U *et al.* Preoperative chemotherapy in early stage resectable non-small cell lung cancer: a randomized feasibility study justifying a multicenter phase III trial. *Br J Cancer* 1999; **79**:1514–8.

54 Depierre A, Milleron B, Moro-Sibilot D *et al.* Preoperative chemotherapy followed by surgery compared with primary surgery in resectable stage I (except T1N0), II, and IIIA non-small cell lung cancer. *J Clin Oncol* 2001; **20**:247–53.

55 Depierre A, Westeel V, Milleron B *et al.* 5 year results of the French Randomized study comparing preoperative chemotherapy followed by surgery and primary surgery in resectable stage I (except T1N0), II and

IIIA non-small cell lung cancer. *Lung Cancer* 2003; **41(Suppl 2)**:S62.

56 Sorensen J, Riska H, Ravn J *et al.* Scandinavian phase III trial of neoadjuvant chemotherapy in NSCLC stages IB-IIIA/T3. *J Clin Oncol, 2005 ASCO Ann Mtg Proc* 2005; **23(16S)**:7146.

57 Pisters K, Vallieres E, Bunn P *et al.* S9900: a phase III trial of surgery alone or surgery plus preoperative paclitaxel/carboplatin chemotherapy in early stage non-small cell lung cancer: preliminary results. *J Clin Oncol, 2005 ASCO Ann Mtg Proc* 2005; **23(16S)**:7012.

58 Scagliotti G on behalf of the CH.E.S.T. Investigators. Preliminary results of CH.E.S.T.: a phase III study of surgery alone or surgery plus preoperative gemcitabine-cisplatin in clinical early stages non-small cell lung cancer. *J Clin Oncol, 2005 ASCO Ann Mtg Proc* 2005; **23(16S)**:7023.

59 Canela M, Maestre J, Rodriguez-Paniagua M *et al.* NATCH Trial update. *Lung Cancer* 2005; **49**:S93.

60 Berghmans T, Paesmans M, Meert A *et al.* Survival improvement in resectable non-small cell lung cancer with (neo)adjuvant chemotherapy: results of a meta-analysis of the literature. *Lung Cancer* 2005; **49**:13–23.

61 Burdett S, Stewart L, Rydzewska L. A systematic review and meta-analysis of the literature: chemotherapy and surgery versus surgery alone in non-small cell lung cancer. *J Thorac Oncol* 2006; **1**:611–21.

62 Piedbois P, Buyse M. Editorial: meta-analyses based on abstracted data: a step in the right direction, but only a first step. *J Clin Oncol* 2004; **22**:3839–40.

63 Pignon JP, Burdett S. Letter to the Editor. *Lung Cancer* 2005; **51**:261–2.

64 Waller D, Peake MD, Stephens RJ *et al.* Chemotherapy for patients with non-small cell lung cancer: the surgical setting of the Big Lung Trial. *Eur J Cardiothorac Surg* 2004; **26**:173–82.

65 Yi X, Zhang R, Ding J *et al.* A clinicopathologic study on neoadjuvant chemotherapy in the treatment of non-small cell lung cancer. *Chin J Lung Cancer* 2003; **6**:124–8.

66 Siegenthaler M, Pisters K, Merriman K *et al.* Preoperative chemotherapy for lung cancer does not increase surgical morbidity. *Ann Thorac Surg* 2001; **71**:1105–12.

67 Martin J, Ginsberg R, Abolhoda A *et al.* Morbidity and mortality after neoadjuvant therapy for lung cancer: the risks of right pneumonectomy. *Ann Thorac Surg* 2001; **72**:1149–54.

68 Perrot E, Guibert B, Mulsant P *et al.* Preoperative chemotherapy does not increase complications after non-small cell lung cancer resection. *Ann Thorac Surg* 2005; **80**:423–7.

CHAPTER 16
Image-Guided Radiation Therapy

Kenneth E. Rosenzweig and Sonal Sura

Introduction

Local control continues to be a major challenge when treating nonsmall cell lung cancer (NSCLC) with radiation therapy. Even with newer techniques such as three-dimensional conformal radiation therapy (3D-CRT) and intensity modulated radiation therapy (IMRT) [1–7], 2-year local failure rates have been reported between 22 and 50% [3,6]. Traditional imaging used for identifying tumor size, location, geometry and patient anatomy has been through fluoroscopy, or more recently, static computed tomography (CT) scans done prior to treatment planning.

However, conventional imaging modalities such as CT may be inadequate for visualization of disease. One strategy to improve tumor delineation has been the incorporation of FDG-PET scanning into the treatment planning process. This provides both anatomic and biologic imaging of the tumor.

Another challenge in treating tumors in the thorax is organ and tumor motion during respiration. This motion may change the exact location of the tumor during treatment and from the time of the planning scan and the time of actual treatment.

Image-guided radiation therapy (IGRT) involves the production of images in the radiation therapy treatment room prior to the initiation of treatment. The images are either three-dimensional images similar to CT or two-dimensional images, such as

X-rays that are aided by fiducial markers in, or near, the tumor [8]. There are a number of techniques that are able to provide these images.

PET and PET-CT in radiation treatment planning

A crucial component of lung cancer radiation treatment planning is accurate tumor delineation. Often patients present with locally advanced disease that is not detected by CT alone or have abnormalities on PET that do not represent areas of cancer. PET scans have been compared to thoracotomy and mediastinoscopy for detecting mediastinal lymphadenopathy and determining stage. In two meta-analyses the sensitivity and specificity of PET for nodal staging in NSCLC ranged from 84 to 88% and 89 to 92%, respectively [9,10]. PET scans have been shown to have a good negative predictive value ranging from 87 to 100% [11–13] and less notable positive predictive values reported as <80% in several studies [11,13,14].

The effect of FDG-PET imaging on radiation treatment planning has been investigated. To assess the adequacy of coverage of RT fields planned with CT or X-ray data, Kiffer *et al.* retrospectively performed a graphical coregistration of PET and AP simulator images using coordinates measured from the carina. In 4/15 patients, they found inadequate coverage by the AP portals due to abnormal mediastinal nodes detected on PET but not CT [15]. Munley *et al.* found that PET data increased target volumes (expressed in terms of beam apertures) by up to 15 mm in 34% of patients in their series, using the union of

Lung Cancer, 3rd edition. Edited by Jack A. Roth, James D. Cox, and Waun Ki Hong. © 2008 Blackwell Publishing, ISBN: 978-1-4051-5112-2.

PET- and CT-defined volumes [16]. Nestle *et al.* performed a retrospective evaluation of AP/PA portal sizes as altered by PET data. Thirty-five percent of cases had a change in the size or shape of the original CT portals, mostly a reduction in size, and mostly in patients with atelectasis [17]. Schmucking *et al.* report decreases in the planning target volume (PTV) of up to 21% due to distinction of atelectasis from tumor after integrating PET data, with subsequent decreases in the volume of normal lung irradiated (V20) [18].

The use of software registered PET/CT images in radiation treatment planning has also been studied. Caldwell *et al.* evaluated 30 patients who were to be treated with definitive RT for NSCLC who had features of atelectasis on CT scan. The majority of the patients had smaller PTVs when contoured using fused PET and CT images as compared with volumes generated from CT alone, resulting in decreases of dose to normal lung and spinal cord [19]. In a study of 11 patients with NSCLC, Erdi *et al.* found that registered PET/CT altered the PTV that had previously been contoured on CT images in all cases. Increases in volume were due to inclusion of positive lymph nodes not detected on CT and decreases were due to exclusion of atelectatic lung [20]. Bradley *et al.* studied differences in gross target volumes (GTVs) contoured with CT data alone versus PET/CT fusion images. The addition of PET information altered the inclusion of tumor and/or nodal regions in 14 of 24 patients receiving 3D-CRT. Two of these were decreases due to atelectasis distinguished from tumor by PET. In such cases, parameters calculated to predict for normal tissue toxicity such as mean lung dose (MLD), mean esophageal dose (MED), and the volume of lung receiving >20 Gy (V20) were decreased as well, theoretically decreasing the risk of radiation pneumonitis or esophagitis [21]. Giraud *et al.* reported results consistent with these studies using PET images from dual-head coincidence (CDET) gamma cameras fused with simulation CT images by use of external fiducial markers [22]. The above findings suggest that the use of PET data can potentially improve patient outcomes, both by identifying areas of disease that would not have been contoured on CT alone, and by decreasing the amount of normal lung tissue included in the target volume and thus the volume at risk for pulmonary toxicity.

Tumor motion

Managing respiratory motion during radiation treatments is an important aspect of treating thoracic malignancies. For patients who are medically unfit for surgery or whose tumors are inoperable based on stage and/or location, radiotherapy is the primary treatment option often in conjunction with chemotherapy [23]. Organ motion during respiration can limit the accuracy with which radiation can be delivered to the tumor volume. Some investigators have shown underdosing as high as 30% with conventional radiation therapy techniques [24]. Stevens *et al.* have reported that lung tumors move during free breathing from 5 to 10 mm and in some cases as much as 4.5 cm [25]. To account for these inaccuracies larger margins are added to the GTV to create a PTV. The increase in volume may limit dose escalation to tumoricidal doses based on predictors of normal tissue toxicity, such as the V20 [26]. Limiting the effects of organ and tumor motion during treatment planning and delivery may help in increasing accuracy and allow for further dose escalation and more favorable survival outcomes while maintaining an acceptable toxicity profile.

Two distinct techniques have been used to reduce the effects of respiratory motion. The first involves confining radiation delivery to a specified phase in the breathing cycle by gating the linear accelerator while the patient breathes freely. Breathing is monitored with devices that trigger radiation delivery during specific phases of the patient's respiratory cycle [27]. In the second approach, breathing is controlled either voluntarily by the patient or by using an occlusion valve, such as the active breathing control (ABC) developed by Wong *et al.* [28,29] or the deep inspiration breath hold (DIBH) technique [30].

Another approach uses images obtained during inspiration and expiration to create an internal target volume (ITV). This ITV would therefore theoretically account for the full extent of organ motion during the entire treatment [31].

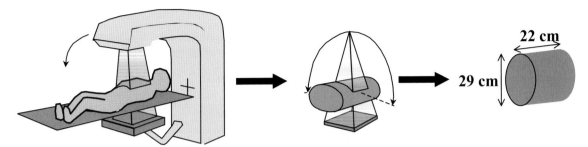

Figure 16.1 Megavoltage cone beam CT. The linear accelerator rotates around the patient megavoltage beams are used to acquire three-dimensional imaging of a volume of normal tissue. Unlike a conventional CT scanner where the images are "slices" of the volume, the cone beam image acquires information from the entire volume at the same time.

Image-guided radiation therapy

Day-to-day changes in organ motion, tumor shape, and patient position can lead to variability in tumor location while patients are being treated. IGRT attempts to account for this variability which can lead to more accurate treatment. In addition, due to the increased precision of the radiation therapy treatment plan, regions that have not been typically considered for treatment, such as the liver, and radiation fraction sizes not conventionally delivered, such as 2000 cGy can now be safely delivered (Plate 16.1). There are numerous commercially available technical solutions for IGRT in the treatment room. They include cone beam CT (CBCT), tomotherapy, orthogonal kilovoltage (kV) X-rays, and CT scanning in the treatment room.

Cone beam CT

Newer therapies, such as IMRT, have high-dose gradients which make it particularly important to verify accurate treatment. Currently, most patient treatments are verified using two-dimensional portal imaging using anatomic structures such as bones or air cavities. CBCT is a method to assess tumor position for patients on the treatment table. There are two technologies available for producing cone beam images. The first uses the linear accelerator's megavoltage (MV) beam to produce the image. This is called megavoltage cone beam CT (MVCBCT, Figure 16.1). The other uses a separate imaging source with kV energy to produce the images (KVCBCT, Figure 16.2). Although there are several CBCT technologies available [32–40], the basic concept behind the CBCT system is that the ability to obtain information about anatomy and tumor location immediately before each treatment that may lead to more accurate delivery of radiation. By monitoring these daily changes, treatment plans can be tailored for each fraction [41].

The value of CBCT for lung cancer has not yet been thoroughly studied. As the implementation of stereotactic body radiotherapy (SBRT) hypofractionated treatments increases, the use of CBCT may become more important in the treatment of lung carcinomas. Even with standard margins of 5–10 mm that are added to the GTV to account for setup error and target motion, it has shown that significant deviations occur between the planned and actual target position at the time of treatment and bony landmarks are not always reliable for target localization [42,43]. With CBCT, a 3D image can be acquired in the treatment position immediately prior to each treatment without having to reposition the patient on a different imaging machine, which further minimizes the variation in the planned versus actual target position. Increased precision in target localization with image guidance in the form of CBCT can also allow for reduction in the safety margin added to the GTV [44]. Megavoltage and kilovoltage CBCT may facilitate the use of high-dose radiotherapy for the treatment of NSCLC by accounting for both inter- and intrafractional tumor motion and improving treatment accuracy [45].

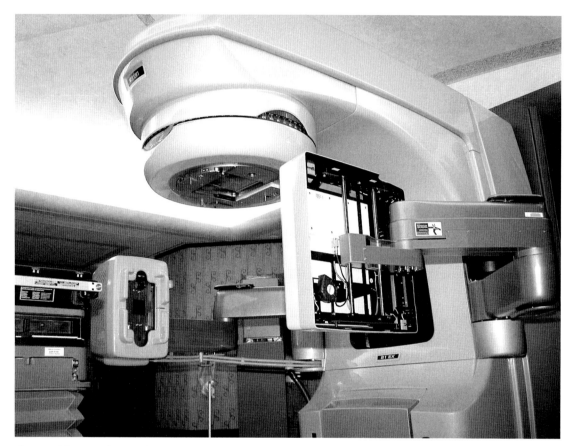

Figure 16.2 Varian kV Imaging system (OBI). The kV source, kV detector, and MV detector are all mounted on robotic arms.

Tomotherapy

The helical tomotherapy unit is an innovative device used for radiation delivery that combines a linear accelerator and a helical CT scanner allowing for the targeted region to be imaged before, during, and after each treatment. This allows for improved tumor localization and can help account for target motion during and between treatments. CT scans provide improved soft tissue resolution over the standard port films, thereby providing increased anatomical detail. With tomotherapy the concept of "adaptive radiotherapy" can be implemented allowing for daily adjustments in radiation delivery based on changes in tumor position and size [46,47]. By using information obtained during previous fractions to modify an ongoing treatment, errors in dose and tumor location can be better accounted [48,49]. Another concept that is equally important in radiotherapy for lung cancer is "conformal avoidance" which emphasizes the importance of protecting normal structures from radiation damage. With the use of tomotherapy both conformal radiotherapy and "conformal avoidance" can be achieved by daily imaging of target motion and changes in size and position [46,50,51].

The unit is designed to deliver IMRT treatments using a binary multileaf collimator but has the ability to deliver radiation along every possible gantry angle. This translates into higher degrees of freedom when compared to linac-based IMRT. The clinical relevance for lung cancer treatment, however, has not been fully studied [52].

Markers and respiratory gating

Fiducial markers provide another way to localize lung tumors. These markers are placed within the lung tumor or external to the tumor and monitored during all aspects of radiotherapy. The markers are radio-opaque and can be a simple gold seed or more complex, such as a coil. The role of the marker is to act as a surrogate for the tumor's location.

BrainLab (Munich, Germany) has developed a system that allows for image guidance and respiratory gating using the Exactrac Adaptive Gating system (Version 4.5, Gating Version 1). The system itself consists of an infrared camera, 2 amorphous silicon plates, and 2 kV X-ray tubes and uses a combination of X-ray and optical tracking to monitor internal target motion. Signals are sent to the linear accelerator to turn on the beam when the target is located at the machine's isocenter. For thoracic tumors, this system can be used to track tumor motion by X-ray localization of internal fiducials along with optical tracking of external landmarks [53–55]. The system works by allowing the placement of internal fiducials as surrogate for tumor location. X-rays are then used to determine the location of the internal target to the linac isocenter and displacement of the internal target is corrected by optical tracking. These X-rays are registered to digitally reconstructed images from the treatment-planning CT. This gating system has been shown to have an accuracy of 1.7 mm for tumor localization with motion up to 2 cm in the anteroposterior and superoinferior directions [56].

The Cyberknife system (Accuray, Sunnyvale, CA) is another system that allows for imaging of tumor motion and variation by monitoring gold seeds placed near the tumor. The system consists of a linear accelerator radiation source that is mounted on a robotic arm and through the use of image-guided cameras can precisely track tumor motion during the treatment. Also with the addition of the Synchrony™ option, dynamic radiosurgery during respiration is possible. By recording the breathing movements of a patient's chest the Synchrony option combines that information with sequential X-ray pictures of the fiducials to facilitate delivery of radiation during any point in the respiratory cycle. This allows further precision during radiation delivery and reduces normal tissue exposure [57,58].

Orthogonal kV X-rays

The use of orthogonal kV X-rays provides another method of onboard imaging allowing for daily target localization while exposing the patient to lower doses of radiation as compared to MV radiographs [59]. Similar to the MV CBCT system, the kV X-ray source and two fluoroscopic imaging systems (one for the kV X-ray beam and the other for the MV beam) are installed on a linear accelerator. The kV X-ray beam is mounted orthogonally to the MV treatment beam and the two fluoroscopic systems are placed perpendicular to the corresponding beam axis. Three-dimensional target localization is then assessed by measurements of 2D shifts in four orthogonal images (anteroposterior, posteroanterior, and right and left lateral images). Each image provides a way of measuring shifts of the tumor relative to the treatment machine isocenter and simulation films. The benefit of using a kV imaging X-ray system may be that it exposes the patient to less radiation because of its lower imaging dose thereby allowing for more routine use of 2D imaging for daily tumor localization when compared to MV radiographs [60].

In-room CT

Many systems have been developed that incorporate use in-room CT scanners but the basic steps and concepts are the same. First, the patient is positioned by aligning the initial setup marks with the treatment positioning lasers. Then the table is rotated 180° to obtain a CT scan of the patient that is limited to the treatment area. Finally, the planning CT scan is compared with the CT just obtained to determine if a shift in patient position is necessary and adjustments can be made accordingly.

An example of a system that incorporates the in-room CT with a linear accelerator is a CT-on-Rails. The system consists of a CT scanner that slides on rails in the floor so the patient does not have to move between the time of the scan and treatment. It slides over the patient's treatment table and then is pushed out of the way during treatment. The system allows for corrections to be made based on changes in the patient's daily positioning between treatments to assure the accurate delivery of radiation [52].

The role of image guidance in stereotactic body radiotherapy

Based on the experience and effectiveness stereotactic radiotherapy for the treatment of small intracranial tumors [61,62], the use of extracranial SBRT for treating small-volume lung tumors has increases. The use of hypofractionated regimens requires highly accurate daily patient setup. As demonstrated by Bortfeld et al., respiratory motion may have no significant effect (<1%) on the planned versus the delivered dose when treatment is delivered in 30 or more fractions [63]. However, with the use of small-volume hypofractionated IGRT, daily variation in organ and target motion becomes more of a concern and can lead to inadequate dosing. Uematsu et al. developed frameless unit (focal unit) that consisted of a linac, CT scanner, simulator, and couch which they used for treatment delivery allowing them to make intra- and interfractional adjustments based on changes in tumor and patient motion [64].

Standard techniques used in SBRT to reduce respiration-related organ motion include frames, belts, and ABC which requires patients to hold their breath at different points during the treatment [64,65]. However, often times these patients are unable to tolerate frames or have poor baseline pulmonary function and are unable to hold their breath long enough. Another method of image guidance in hypofractionated radiotherapy involves fusing the clinical target volumes (CTVs) derived from CT scans from different phases of respiration to represent the ITV which would then account for the effects of respiratory motion. Onimaru et al. implemented this method of analyzing tumor motion through CT scans at inspiration, expiration, and while the patient was breathing normally. CTV was defined for each respiratory cycle and then fused together when determining the PTV. This method was thought to account for the effects of respiratory motion [66]. A similar technique for PTV definition through fusion of CTVs derived from CT scans taken at different phases of respiration was applied by Fukumoto et al. when treating patients with NSCLC with SBRT [67].

Conclusions

The definitive role of IGRT for lung cancer treatment has yet to be established. With local control as the main goal of radiotherapy, precision and accuracy through all parts of the treatment process, including initial staging, treatment planning, and treatment delivery, remains a challenge. Image guidance, whether through PET-CT fusion for staging or MV CBCT, orthogonal kV X-rays and CT-based SBRT for treatment, may change how patients with thoracic malignancies are treated in the future.

References

1 Armstrong JG, Burman C, Leibel SA et al. Three-dimensional conformal radiation therapy may improve the therapeutic ratio of high dose radiation therapy for lung cancer. Int J Radiat Oncol Biol Phys 1993; **26**:685–9.

2 Hayman JA, Martel MK, Ten Haken RK et al. Dose escalation in non-small cell lung cancer using three-dimensional conformal radiation therapy: update of a phase I trial. J Clin Oncol 2001; **19**:127–36.

3 Narayan S, Henning GT, Randall TK et al. Results following treatment to doses of 92.4 or 102.9 Gy on a phase I dose escalation study for non-small cell lung cancer. Lung Cancer 2004; **44**:79–88.

4 Rosenzweig KE, Mychalzhak B, Fuks Z et al. Final report of the 70.2-Gy and 75.6-Gy dose levels of a phase I dose escalation study using three-dimensional conformal radiotherapy in the treatment of inoperable non-small cell lung cancer. Cancer 2000; **6**:82–7.

5 Rosenzweig KE, Fox JL, Leibel SA *et al*. Results of a phase I dose-escalation study using three-dimensional conformal radiotherapy in the treatment of inoperable nonsmall cell lung carcinoma. *Cancer* 2005; **103**:2118–27.

6 Bradley J, Graham MV, Winter K *et al*. Toxicity and outcome results of RTOG 9311: a phase I-II dose-escalation study using three-dimensional conformal radiotherapy in patients with inoperable non-small-cell lung carcinoma. *Int J Radiat Oncol Biol Phys* 2005; **61**:318–28.

7 Schwarz M, Alber M, Lebesque LV *et al*. Dose heterogeneity in the target volume and intensity-modulated radiotherapy to escalate the dose in the treatment of non–small-cell lung cancer. *Int J Radiat Oncol Biol Phys* 2005; **62(2)**:561–70.

8 Grau C, Hoyer M, Lindegaard J, Overgaard J. The emerging evidence for stereotactic body radiotherapy. *Acta Oncologia* 2006; **45**:771–4.

9 Toloza E, Harpole L, McCrory DC. Noninvasive staging of non-small cell lung cancer, a review of the current evidence. *Chest* 2003; **123**:137S–46S.

10 Reske SN, Kotzerke J. FDG-PET for clinical use: Results of the 3rd German Interdisciplinary Consensus Conference. *Eur J Nucl Med* 2001; **28**:1707–23.

11 Vansteenkiste JF, Stroobants SG, Dupont PJ *et al* The Leuven Lung Cancer Group, FDG-PET scan in potentially operable non-small cell lung cancer. Do anatometabolic PET-CT fusion images improve the localization of regional lymph node metastases? *Eur J Nucl Med* 1998; **25**:1495–501.

12 Steinert HC, Hauser M, Allemann F *et al*. Non-small cell lung cancer Nodal staging with FDG PET versus CT with correlative lymph node mapping and sampling. *Radiology* 1997; **202**:441–6.

13 Pieterman RM, van Putten JW, Meuzelaar JJ *et al*. Preoperative staging of non-small-cell lung cancer with positron-emission tomography. *N Engl J Med* 2000; **203**:254–61.

14 Poncelet AJ, Lonneux M, Coche E *et al*. PET-FDG scan enhances but does not replace preoperative surgical staging in non-small cell lung carcinoma. *Eur J Cardiothorac Surg* 2001; **20**:468–75.

15 Kiffer JD, Berlangieri SU, Scott AM *et al*. The contribution of 18F-fluoro-2-deoxy-glucose positron emission tomographic imaging to radiotherapy planning in lung cancer. *Lung Cancer* 1998; **19**:167–77.

16 Munley MT, Marks LB, Scarfone C *et al*. Multimodality nuclear medicine imaging in three-dimensional radiation treatment planning for lung cancer: challenges and prospects. *Lung Cancer* 1999; **23**:105–14.

17 Nestle U, Hellwig D, Schmidt S *et al*. 2-Deoxy-2-[18F]fluoro-D-glucose positron emission tomography in target volume definition for radiotherapy of patients with non-small-cell lung cancer. *Mol Imaging Biol* 2002; **4**:257–63.

18 Schmucking M, Baum RP, Bonnet R *et al*. Correlation of histologic results with PET findings for tumor regression and survival in locally advanced non-small cell lung cancer after neoadjuvant treatment. *Pathologe* May 2005; **26**:178–89.

19 Caldwell CB, Mah K, Ung YC *et al*. Observer variation in contouring gross tumor volume in patients with poorly defined non-small-cell lung tumors on CT: the impact of 18FDG-hybrid PET fusion. *Int J Radiat Oncol Biol Phys* 2001; **51(4)**:923–31.

20 Erdi YE, Rosenzweig K, Erdi AK *et al*. Radiotherapy treatment planning for patients with non-small cell lung cancer using positron emission tomography (PET). *Radiother Oncol* 2002; **62**:51–60.

21 Bradley J, Thorstad WL, Mutic S *et al*. Impact of FDG-PET on radiation therapy volume delineation in non-small-cell lung cancer. *Int J Radiat Oncol Biol Phys* 2004; **59**:78–86.

22 Giraud P, Grahek D, Montravers F *et al*. CT and (18)F-deoxyglucose (FDG) image fusion for optimization of conformal radiotherapy of lung cancers. *Int J Radiat Oncol Biol Phys* 2001; **49**:1249–57.

23 Vora SA, Daly B, Blaszkowsky L *et al*. High dose radiation therapy and chemotherapy as induction treatment for Stage III non-small cell lung carcinoma RTOG 7311. *Cancer* 2000; **89(9)**:1946–52.

24 Ross CS, Hussey DH, Pennington EC, Stanford W, Doornbos JF. Analysis of movement of intrathoracic neoplasms using ultrafast computerized tomography. *Int J Radiat Oncol Biol Phys* 1990; **18**:671–7.

25 Stevens CW, Munden RF, Forster KM *et al*. Respiratory-driven lung tumor motion is independent of time size, tumor location, and pulmonary function. *Int J Radiat Oncol Biol Phys* 2001; **51**:62.

26 Bradely J, Graham MV, Winter K *et al*. Toxicity and outcome results of RTOG 9311: a phase I-II dose-escalation study using three-dimensional conformal radiotherapy in patients with inoperable non-small cell lung carcinoma. *Int J Radiat Oncol Biol Phys* 2005; **61**:318–28.

27 Kubo HD, Hill BC. Respiration gated radiotherapy treatment: a technical study. *Phys Med Biol* 1996; **41**:83.

28 Wong JW, Sharpe MB, Jaffray DA *et al*. The use of active breathing control (ABC) to minimize breathing motion during radiation therapy [Abstract]. *Int J Radiat Oncol Biol Phys* 1997; **39(Suppl 2)**:164.

29 Stromberg JS, Sharpe MB, Kini VR *et al*. Active breathing control (ABC) for Hodgkin's disease: reduction in normal tissue irradiation with deep inspiration and implication for treatment [Abstract]. *Int J Radiat Oncol Biol Phys* 1998; **42(1S)**:140.

30 Rosenzweig KE, Hanley J, Mah D *et al*. The deep inspiration breath-hold technique in the treatment of inoperable non-small cell lung cancer [Abstract]. *Int J Radiat Oncol Biol Phys* 2000; **48**:81.

31 Liu H, Koch N, Starkschall G *et al*. Evaluation of internal lung motion for respiratory-gated radiotherapy using MRI: Part II—margin reduction of internal target volume. *Int J Radiat Oncol Biol Phys* 2004; **60(5)**:1473–83.

32 Ma CM, Paskalev K. In-room CT techniques for image-guided radiation therapy. *Med Dosim* 2006; **31**:30–9.

33 Wong JR, Cheng CW, Grimm L *et al*. Clinical implementation of the world's first Primatom, a combination of CT scanner and linear accelerator, for precise tumor targeting and treatment. *Med Phys* 2001; **17**: 271–6.

34 Jaffray DA, Siewerdsen JH, Wong JW *et al*. Flat-panel cone-beam computed tomography for image-guided radiation therapy. *Int J Radiat Oncol Biol Phys* 2002; **53**:1337–49.

35 Oelfke U, Tucking T, Nill S *et al*. Linac-integrated KV cone-beam CT Technical features and first applications. *Med Dosim* 2006; **31**:62–70.

36 Sorensen SP, Chow E, Kriminski S *et al*. Image guided radiotherapy using a mobile kilovoltage x-ray device. *Med Dosim* 2006; **31**:40–50.

37 Sillanpaa J, Chang J, Mageras G *et al*. Developments in megavoltage cone beam CT with an amorphous silicon EPID Reduction of exposure and synchronization with respiratory gating. *Med Phys* 2005; **32**:819–29.

38 Pouliot J, Bani-Hashemi A, Chen J *et al*. Low-dose megavoltage cone-beam CT for radiation therapy. *Int J Radiat Oncol Biol Phys* 2005; **61**:552–60.

39 Gildersleve J, Dearnaley DP, Evans PM *et al*. A randomised trial of patient repositioning during radiotherapy using a megavoltage imaging system. *Radiother Oncol* 1994; **31**:161–8.

40 Evans PM, Gildersleve JQ, Rawlings C *et al*. Technical note: the implementation of patient position correction using a megavoltage imaging device on a linear accelerator. *Br J Radiol* 1993; **66**:833–8.

41 Morin O, Gillis A, Chen J *et al*. Megavoltage cone-beam CT: system description and clinical applications. *Med Dosim* 2006; **31(1)**:51–61.

42 Herfarth KK, Debus J, Lohr F *et al*. Extracranial stereotactic radiation: set-up accuracy of patients treated for liver metastasis.*Int J Radiat Oncol Biol Phys* 2000; **46**:329–35.

43 Wulf J, Hardinger U, Oppitz U *et al*. Stereotactic radiotherapy of extracranial targets: CT-simulation and accuracy of treatment in the stereotactic body frame. *Radiother Oncol* 2000; **57**:225–36.

44 Guckenberger M, Meyer J, Wilbert J *et al*. Cone-beam CT based image-guidance for extracranial stereotactic radiotherapy of intrapulmonary tumors. *Acta Oncol* 2006; **45**:897–906.

45 Sidhu K, Ford EC, Spirou S *et al*. Optimization of conformal thoracic radiotherapy using cone-beam CT imaging for treatment verification.*Int J Radiat Oncol Biol Phys* 2003; **55(3)**:757–67.

46 Welsh JS, Patel R, Ritter MA *et al*. Helical tomotherapy: an innovative technology and approach to radiation therapy. *Technol Cancer Res Treat* 2002; **1(4)**:311–16.

47 Ruchala KJ, Olivera GH, Kapatoes JM *et al*. Megavoltage CT image reconstruction during tomotherapy treatments. *Phys Med Biol* 2000; **45**:3545–62.

48 Olivera GH, Shepard DM, Ruchala KJ *et al*. Tomotherapy. In: Van Dyk J (ed). *Modern Technology of Radiation Oncology*. Madison, WI: Medical Physics Publishing, 1999:521–87.

49 Mackie TR. Tomotherapy: rethinking the process of radiotherapy. In: Leavitt DD, Starkshall G (eds). *XII International Conference on the Use of Computers in Radiation Therapy*. Salt Lake City, UT: Medical Physics Publishing, 1997.

50 Kapatoes JM, Olivera GH, Ruchala KJ *et al*. On the verification of the incident energy fluence in tomotherapy IMRT. *Phys Med Biol* 2001; **46**:2953–65.

51 Yan D, Ziaga E, Jaffray D *et al*. The use of adaptive radiation therapy to reduce set-up error: a prospective clinical study. *Int J Radiat Oncol Biol Phys* 1998; **41**:715–20.

52 Mah D. IGRT: in-room technologies. *Med Imaging* October 2006; **21**:26–9.

53 Meeks SL, Tome WA, Willoughby TR *et al*. Optically guided patient positioning techniques. *Semin Radiat Oncol* 2005; **15**:192–201.

54 Medin PM, Solberg TD, De Salles AA *et al*. Investigations of a minimally invasive method for treatment of spinal malignancies with LINAC stereotactic radiation therapy: accuracy and animal studies. *Int J Radiat Oncol Biol Phys* 2002; **52**:1111–22.

55 Krupelian PA, Willoughby TR, Meeks SL *et al*. Intraprostatic fiducials for localization of the prostate gland: monitoring intermarker distances during radiation therapy to for the marker stability. *Int J Radiat Oncol Biol Phys* 2005; **62**:1291–6.

56 Willoughby TR, Forbes AR, Buchholz D *et al.* Evaluation of an infrared camera and X-ray system using implanted fiducials in patients with lung tumors for gated radiation therapy. *Int J Radiat Oncol Biol Phys* 2006; **66(2)**:568–75.

57 Whyte RI, Crownover R, Murphy MJ *et al.* Stereotactic radiosurgery for lung tumors: preliminary report of a phase I trial. *Ann Thorac Surg* 2003; **75**:1097–101.

58 El-Sherif A, Luketich JD, Landreneau RJ *et al.* New therapeutic approached for early stage non-small cell lung cancer. *Surgical Oncol* 2005; **14(1)**:27–32.

59 Jaffray DA, Chawla K, Yu C *et al.* Dual-beam imaging for online verification of radiotherapy field placement. *Int J Radiat Oncol Biol Phys* 1995; **33**:1273–80.

60 Pisani L, Lockman D, Jaffray D *et al.* Set-up error in radiotherapy: on-line correction using electronic kilovoltage and megavoltage radiographs. *Int J Radiat Oncol Biol Phys* 2000; **47(3)**:825–39.

61 Kihlstrom L, Karlsson B, Lindqvist C. Gamma knife surgery for cerebral metastases. Implications for survival based on 16 years' experience. *Stereotact Funct Neurosurg* 1993; **61**:45–50.

62 Flickinger JC, Kondoziolka D, Lunsford LD *et al.* A multi-institutional experience with stereotactic radiosurgery for solitary brain metastasis. *Int J Radiat Oncol Biol Phys* 1994; **28**:797–802.

63 Bortfeld T, Jokivarsi K, Goitein M *et al.* Effects of intrafraction motion on IMRT dose delivery: statistical analysis and simulation. *Phys Med Biol* 2002; **47(13)**:2209–20.

64 Uematsu M, Shioda A, Tahara K *et al.* Focal, high dose, and fractionated modified stereotactic radiation therapy for lung carcinoma patients. *Cancer* 1998; **82**:1062–70.

65 Blomgren H, Lax I, Naslund I, Svanstrom R. Stereotactic high dose fraction radiation therapy of extracranial tumors using an accelerator. *Acta Oncol* 1995; **34**:861–70.

66 Onimaru R, Shirato H, Shimizu S *et al.* Tolerance of organs at risk in small-volume, hypofractionated, image-guided radiotherapy for primary and metastatic lung cancers. *Int J Radiat Oncol Biol Phys* 2003; **56(1)**:126–35.

67 Fukumoto S, Shirato H, Shimzu S *et al.* Small-volume image-guided radiotherapy using hypofractionated, coplanar, and noncoplanar multiple fields for patients with inoperable stage I non-small cell lung carcinomas. *Cancer* 2002; **95(7)**:1546–53.

CHAPTER 17

Stereotactic Body Radiation Therapy for Lung Cancer

Robert D. Timmerman and Brian D. Kavanagh

Introduction

Stereotactic body radiation therapy (SBRT) has rather quickly emerged as an important cancer treatment strategy that challenges dogmas associated with conventional fractionated radiation therapy (CFRT) [1]. Whereas CFRT is typically administered in daily doses, or fractions, in the range of 1.8–2.0 Gy to total doses of 60–70 Gy or so, with SBRT much higher doses per fraction are applied, generally in the range of 10–20 Gy per fraction, in an abbreviated, hypofractionated regimen of 5 or fewer fractions. Such high doses per treatment were unthinkable in the past because of limitations in treatment delivery technology that raised concerns about potential toxicity if large volumes of normal tissues were exposed to so much radiation each treatment.

SBRT has definitely been facilitated by recent refinements in technology including image-guided techniques, motion assessment and control techniques, and advanced treatment planning dosimetry. This technology has allowed what was previously unattainable, namely, the delivery of very large or ablative dose treatments without necessarily resulting in unacceptable late toxicity. Careful, disciplined analyses of the results of well-designed clinical trials of SBRT have led to new understandings of the nuances of normal

Lung Cancer, 3rd edition. Edited by Jack A. Roth, James D. Cox, and Waun Ki Hong. © 2008 Blackwell Publishing. ISBN: 978-1-4051-5112-2.

tissue responses to high-dose ionizing radiation. As clinician-researchers at more institutions become familiar with the principles and adept in the application of SBRT, this new treatment paradigm will likely become an established alternative in numerous clinical indications.

Interestingly, SBRT has been most commonly applied in either early stage cancer or in metastatic cancer with few indications for intermediate stage cancer [2]. As a primary therapy for early stage lung cancer, for example, SBRT offers an elegantly noninvasive and highly efficient treatment option. And for patients with metastatic disease, SBRT can serve as a physically targeted systemic cytoreductive agent, envisioned as complementary to novel biologically targeted agents that retard cancer growth generally but provide low response rates in sites of gross disease. In the latter indication, the conceptual approach is aligned with the Norton-Simon hypothesis of cancer growth within a host, whereby it is proposed that reductions in systemic disease burden will render cancers more susceptible to systemic therapy by increasing the proportion of cells within more sensitive phases of the cell cycle.

While mostly used in frail medically inoperable patients with lung cancer, SBRT should still be viewed as a most potent treatment against gross tumor deposits. Local control with SBRT has been shown to be dramatically superior to historical controls using CFRT for early stage lung cancer. Indeed, local control with SBRT rivals surgical resection for most indications. Limitations definitely exist as will be discussed in this review. With careful clinical

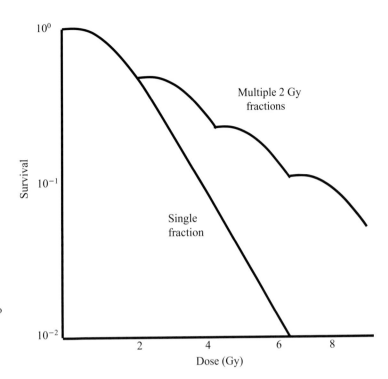

Figure 17.1 Total dose versus log of survival probability (retained ability to form colonies, clonogenicity) for idealized treatments given in a single fraction and for similar doses given in multiple fractions.

testing, SBRT is finding a prominent place within the cancer treatment arsenal.

History of SBRT

The negative effects suffered by normal tissue related to very large dose per fraction treatment are well known. Soon after the discovery of radiation at the turn of the last century, large dose per treatment irradiations were performed against accessible tumors. Responses were impressive and hopes were high for a true cancer cure. Unfortunately, late toxic effects appeared months and even years after therapy that were severe. This late toxicity associated with large dose per fraction treatment appeared mostly to affect the normal tissue stroma such as soft tissues, connective tissues, and bone. The toxicity was sclerosing and tissues had definite signs of reduced vasculature. The experience led to an abandonment of using limited numbers of large dose treatments in favor of what became CFRT.

CFRT exploited inherent differences between normal and neoplastic tissues. In particular, neoplastic tissues were noted to allocate much of the cellular machinery to proliferation (via a characteristic called clonogenicity). On the other hand, normal tissues have potential for proliferation, but relatively more capability to repair life's day to day injuries. CFRT gives small multiple small daily doses of radiation resulting in injury to both normal tissues and tumors. On a given day, the normal tissues with greater repair capability will fix relatively more of this modest damage than tumor tissues as shown in Figure 17.1. Over the course of very many days (e.g., 30 or more treatments), the cumulative damage to the tumor is greater than the cumulative damage to the normal tissues. Hence, there is a therapeutic benefit as was first explained decades ago by Coutard and Baclesse. This is very different than SBRT where all tissues exposed to the high prescription doses, whether normal tissue or tumor, are equally and irreversibly destroyed.

The problem with CFRT as demonstrated throughout the modern era of oncology is that even after many days and large cumulative doses of radiation, some populations of tumor clonogens still survive. This puts the patient at substantial risk of local, regional, and distance tumor recurrence with associated morbidity in addition to shortened survival. Oncologists have tried to overcome this inherent radioresistance to CFRT by adding "sensitizers" like chemotherapy or by using CFRT as an adjunct to surgery. While gains have been made, considerable room for improvement remains for many cancer presentations.

The success of brain radiosurgery pioneered by Swedish neurosurgeon Lars Leksell forms the basis of SBRT [3]. Leksell broke from the perceived wisdom of CFRT by using large dose single sessions of radiation delivery in, of all places, the radio-intolerant CNS. Although a single large dose radiation treatment was historically intolerable, Leksell's approach defied conventional wisdom by its technology and conduct. Unlike CFRT which often irradiates much larger volumes of normal tissue to the prescription dose than the tumor itself, Leksell's stereotactic radiosurgery (SRS) went to great lengths to avoid delivering high dose to nontargeted tissues. Whatever normal tissue was included, either by being adjacent to the target or by inferior dosimetry, was likely damaged. However, if this damaged tissue was small in volume or noneloquent, the patient did not suffer clinically apparent toxicity, even as a late event. On the other hand, it is undeniable that the large dose per fraction treatments are biologically extremely potent by overwhelming repair mechanisms. The net result was a convenient and effective treatment.

The earliest examples of treatments mimicking the SRS treatments outside of the brain were reported for treating spine tumors by Hamilton and colleagues [4]. These treatments employed the same rigid immobilization principles of SRS by screwing a frame to the spinous processes. While reports were encouraging, the conduct of the treatment was not as gratifying as natural and inherent motion confounded accuracy. The brain can be practically immobilized by immobilizing the skull. Once the skull is immobilized, targets within the brain have very little additional movement. Such is not the case outside of the skull. Tumors in the body may be displaced as a function of time by forces exerted by muscle contraction, breathing, gastrointestinal peristalsis, cardiac activity, and many other important physiological processes. We cannot eliminate or account for all of these forces. As such, SBRT is inherently less accurate than SRS.

Not to be dissuaded, researchers again from Sweden, Ingmar Lax and Henric Blomgren, constructed a body frame that would both comfortably immobilize the patient's torso as well as dampen the internal motion relating to respiration [5]. Subsequently, they treated patients with localized tumors using dosimetry plans that mimicked SRS. The dosimetry was constructed using multiple noncoplanar beams with aperture dimensions on the order of the target dimensions. Each of the many beams carried relatively lower weight than with CFRT such that the target dose at the convergence could be dramatically escalated. The team treated patients with mostly metastases initially. Local tumor control was better than expected leading them to treat more limited stage cancer patients. Blomgren and Lax shared their results via publications and eventually trained others in this new technique [6].

Nearly simultaneously with the work carried out by Blomgren and Lax, investigators from Japan were exploring radiosurgery-like treatments in the chest. Shirato and colleagues pioneered investigation into characterization and accounting of respiratory motion [7]. While initially they did not use dose schedules similar to current SBRT regimens, the understanding of target motion control was very important for the ultimate feasibility of SBRT as it currently exists. Uematsu and colleagues again from Japan worked in the early 1990s on developing technologies for delivering multiple focused beams of radiation for extracranial targets [8]. In addition, Uematsu's group started treating patients with lung tumors and following their outcomes.

With acquisition of more sophisticated technology, the groups at University of Heidelberg, University of Wuerzburg, Kyoto University, and Indiana University refined and broadened their approach for extracranial treatments and began formalized prospective testing [9–12]. Initially, dose escalation toxicity studies were carried out in the liver and lung trying to find the most potent dose schedules for typically radioresistant primary and metastatic tumors. These prospective trials are maturing and will add a wealth of understanding for the use of SBRT. It already appears that local tumor control will be higher with SBRT than has been observed with CFRT. However, true rates of tumor control will require years of follow-up on all treated patients and such data is still maturing. Furthermore, toxicity from large dose per fraction radiation schedules often appears quite "late" from time of treatment. Therefore, it is unlikely that all serious toxicity has yet been observed from prospective trials with less than 10 years follow-up.

Radiobiology of SBRT

Tumor biology

Classical understanding of radiobiology of tumor and normal tissue response was mostly derived from the administration of attainable dose per fraction. SBRT involves the administration of very high individual radiation doses. Because many of the fundamental tenets of classical radiobiology were derived and refined over decades through the study of small radiation doses, does SBRT stretch traditional radiation dose–response relationship concepts beyond their limits of applicability?

The most widely accepted means of describing the relationship between radiation dose and cell survival is the linear-quadratic (LQ) formula, shown and applied in a clinical example in the Pelvis/Retroperitoneum section below. Although this formula had served the field of radiobiology quite well for decades, Guerrero and Li have questioned whether it is applicable in the range of high doses applied with SBRT [13]. These authors have proposed modifying the linear-quadratic formula by incorporating features of the so-called lethal–potentially lethal (LPL) model [14]. The LPL model differs from the LQ model primarily insofar as it accounts for ongoing radiation repair processes that occur *during* the radiation exposure. The net result is a substantial difference in the predicted tumor cell kill at SBRT-level doses. For example, for a dose of approximately 20 Gy, the LQ model predicts, is that

the LQ model would predict several orders of magnitude greater cell kill than the LPL model [13].

This debate has practical clinical implications, because it is possible that different available techniques of SBRT will deliver the radiation at noticeably different dose rates, over quite variable lengths of total time. This problem of variable treatment delivery time for cranial radiosurgery has been evaluated experimentally by Benedict and colleagues, who evaluated clonogenic survival in vitro doses in the range of 12–18 Gy, using a glioma cell line [15]. For a dose of 18 Gy, increasing the length of treatment from approximately 1/2 to 2 hours corresponded to an order of magnitude decrement in cytotoxicity. Fowler and colleagues have reviewed this topic of loss of biological effect with length individual treatment delivery and concluded that any treatment administration that lasts more than half an hour might be associated with a clinically significant loss of cytotoxicity [16].

Normal tissue biology and tolerance

Within the lung itself, there are a variety of tissues that possess unique radiation tolerance characteristics, namely, the airways (both large and small functioning as serial structures), vascular trunks and pedicles following similar routes as the bronchial tree (functioning as serial structures), and the alveoli/capillary complexes (functioning as parallel structures) [17,18]. In addition, the thoracic cavity includes the serially functioning esophagus, serially functioning nerve tissue (e.g., phrenic nerves, brachial plexus, etc.), heart, pericardium, and pleura (all difficult to categorize as parallel or serial), and the bones and musculature of the chest wall. All of these structures will have a unique mechanism of injury and tolerance after SBRT.

Conventional radiotherapy commonly causes large serially functioning airway irritation, such as cough, but rarely dose limiting toxicity. In contrast, high-dose SBRT schemes may cause significant large airway damage by both mucosal injury and ultimate collapse of the airway. Along the routes of bronchial airways, a similar injury is experienced by blood vessels following a similar route. Altogether, this collective radiation injury appears to mostly affect oxygenation parameters including diffusing capacity for carbon monoxide (DLCO), arterial oxygen tension (pressure) on room air (PO_2), and supplemental oxygen requirements (FIO_2) [12]. Decline in spirometry indices, including FEV_1 and FVC, are less commonly observed. Because the degree of this airway injury toxicity is related to the proximity of the target to proximal trunks of the branching tubular lung structure, great care should be taken when considering treatment to tumors near the hilum or central chest.

While acute and sometimes severe esophageal toxicity is commonly seen after conventionally fractionated radiation for lung cancer, most of the injury is self-limiting and resolves after treatment. After high dose SBRT, esophageal strictures may form as a late effect. Another more unique toxicity from stereotactic body radiation therapy relates to pericardial injury. Pericardial effusions may result after treatment for tumors treated adjacent to the heart. Probably by a similar mechanism, pleural effusions commonly develop after SBRT treatment of tumors treated adjacent to the chest wall. Usually these fluid collections will reabsorb without intervention after several months of follow-up. Rarely, such fluid collections will need to be drained via thoracentesis in patients symptomatic with shortness of breath, pleurisy, or hypoxia.

Most reports of stereotactic body radiation therapy do not include long-term follow-up data. As such, there may be unexpected toxicities that need to be recognized, monitored, and evaluated. Particularly with large doses per fraction there may be unexpected injury related to nerve tissue and vascular tissue. Ideally, dose to brachial plexus, spinal cord, phrenic nerves, and intercostal nerves will be kept low via prudent treatment planning. Furthermore, avoiding large blood vessels in the central chest would be reasonable as well. Neurovascular calamities including aneurysms, fistulas with bleeding, or neuropathies (including phrenic or vagal nerve palsies) have rarely been reported but may only manifest after many years of follow-up.

Lung toxicity is correlated to target volume. Toxicity related to serially functioning tissues is more predominant in the central chest. Ideally, SBRT should demonstrate a high degree of conformality between the prescription dose and the target. Lung within the target exceeds tolerance and is no longer functional after high dose SBRT. A dose fall-off region exists outside of the target, the volume of which depends on the size of the target, the location of the target within the chest, the quality of the radiation dosimetry (e.g., number of beams, beam arrangements, radiation energy, etc.), and the type of radiation (e.g., photon versus proton, etc.). This dose fall-off region, also called the gradient region, constitutes unintended radiation exposure and should be kept as small as possible.

Defining SBRT

In 2004 after several years of planning, the lung committee of the Radiation Therapy Oncology Group (RTOG) finalized plans to carry out a multicenter trial of SBRT in patients with medically inoperable nonsmall cell lung cancer (NSCLC). As this was the first multicenter trial of its kind, the first step was to define the therapy. Previously, a working group from the American College of Radiology and American Society for Therapeutic Radiology and Oncology had formulated guidelines for the conduct of SBRT [1]. The guidelines described the following essential components collectively unique to its conduct:

1 Secure immobilization avoiding patient movement for the typical long treatment sessions.

2 Accurate repositioning of the patient from planning sessions to each of the treatment sessions.

3 Proper accounting of inherent internal organ motion including breathing motion consistently between planning and treatment.

4 Construction of dose distributions confidently covering tumor and yet falling off very rapidly to surrounding normal tissues. The dosimetry must be extremely conformal in relation to the prescription isodose line compared to the target outline but may allow very heterogeneous target dose ranges.

5 Registration of the patient's anatomy, constructed dosimetry, and treatment delivery to a 3D coordinate system as referenced to fiducials. Fiducials are "markers" whose position can be confidently correlated both to the tumor target and the treatment delivery device. A "stereotactic" treatment is one directed by such fiducial references.

6 Biologically potent dose prescriptions using a few (i.e., 1–5) fractions of very high dose (e.g., generally a minimum of 6 Gy per fraction but often as high as 20–30 Gy per fraction).

This therapy is used to treat well demarcated visible gross disease up to 5–7 cm in dimension. It is not used for prophylactic (adjuvant) treatment as the intent is to totally disrupt clonogenicity and likely disrupt all cellular functioning of the target tissues (i.e., the definition of an ablative therapy).

Effectively, SBRT is a treatment that can ablate or totally destroy that to which it is aimed. Such a treatment, properly directed would constitute a most potent form of cancer therapy. In turn, if misdirected or used too liberally, SBRT could lead to debilitating toxicity. Whether the potent SBRT dose can truly be placed primarily within tumor using stereotactic targeting, motion control, ideal immobilization and specialized dosimetry techniques remains to be proven in all clinical circumstances. At any rate, SBRT is not similar to CFRT in its conduct, toxicity, or ability to control cancer.

Immobilization and target motion issues related to SBRT

The geometry and dose distribution from the radiation therapy treatment plan should be a reasonably true characterization of what is actually delivered to the patient. With the typical large volume of treatment and homogeneous dose distributions characteristic of CFRT, such an emphasis on the proper correlation of the treatment plan and actual treatment is probably not so critical. However, for SBRT, claims regarding accuracy of equipment, quality of dose distributions, and dose tolerance should not be made based on the virtual computer simulation of the treatment plan; rather, on actual delivery of dose to treated patients. This is particularly true for predicting normal tissue toxicity from SBRT where both heterogeneous dose and differential volume effects may equally affect outcome.

Consistent and reproducible immobilization is one option for improving treatment accuracy. Body frames, vacuum pillows, thermal plastic restraints, and other equipment have been used to try to achieve relocalization similar to the position of simulation [19–32]. Other systems will effectively relocate a reference position within the patient prior to each treatment without the aid of frames or other immobilization devices (i.e., "frameless" systems) [33–36]. Both approaches have advantages and disadvantages and no clearly superior method has been identified in clinical practice. In the end, it is most critical to be practical. SBRT treatment sessions are longer than CFRT sessions. Hence, it is important that the positioning system be comfortable and avoid awkward positions or positions fighting against gravity. In addition, the system employed must be properly utilized. As such, staff training and properly administered quality assurance programs are more essential than using a particular brand of equipment.

Motion control devices fall into three general categories: (a) dampening, (b) gating, and (c) chasing. Within the category of dampening includes the systems of abdominal compression aimed at decreasing one of the largest contributors to respiratory motion related to the diaphragm [22,25,26,28,29,32]. Also included in this category are the systems employing breath hold maneuvers to "freeze" the tumor in a reproducible stage of the respiratory cycle (e.g., deep inspiration) [37–40]. Gating systems follow the respiratory cycle using a surrogate and employ an electronic beam activation trigger allowing irradiation to only occur during a specific segment (e.g., end expiration) [34,41–43]. Tracking systems literally move the radiation beam along the same path as the tumor from the beam's eye view [7,44–47]. Tracking may be accomplished by moving the entire accelerator, the aperture (e.g., with the multileaf collimator), or moving the patient on the couch counter to the motion of the tumor. In the case of gating and breath hold, the beam is triggered on and off constituting a duty cycle avoided by the other systems. In any case, the acquisition of planning information must include the same consideration for motion accounting as the treatment in order to achieve accuracy. Despite available motion control equipment, some uncertainty continues to require that planning treatment volume (PTV) is larger than gross tumor volume (GTV). In general for typical dose prescriptions, this enlargement should not be greater than 1.0 cm in the cranial caudal plane and 0.5 cm in the axial plane.

Physics and dosimetry of SBRT

SBRT requires extremely conformal dose distributions that fall off very rapidly, ideally in all directions, generally requires the use of multiple shaped beams [48–50]. Highly shaped beams are desired because high dose is best eliminated in normal tissues by sharp collimation of primary beam fluence attenuation outside of the target from the beam's-eye-view. Conversely, smaller nonshaped beams may be used to treat successive regions of the target [51]. Scatter dose is less easily controlled, even by highly shaped beams. Most modern SBRT treatments for lung and liver targets use around 10–12 highly collimated beams. In order to avoid overlap dose between entrance and exit trajectories, these beams are ideally nonopposing and have as large hinge angles between them as possible. In addition and in an effort to assure dose gradients fall off rapidly in all directions, the beams should generally be noncoplanar. Coplanar treatments such as is commonly utilized in CFRT particularly with IMRT results in low and intermediate dose "spillage" that surrounds the tumor in an annular fashion. Ideally, this spillage dose would be distributed in a geometry potentially capable of treating occult microscopic extension of tumor. Except perhaps for targets in the vertebral bodies of the spine, there is no reason based on anatomy, tissue function, or known patterns of tumor spread to construct such a predominantly axial dose distribution around the target. Collisions between the patient and accelerator head or the couch and accelerator head will limit the ability to create truly isotropically decreasing dose gradients around targets, but effort should be made to mimic such ideal distributions as much as possible [52,53].

For SBRT, it is assumed that the GTV is nearly identical to the clinical target volume (CTV) for conduct of the treatment. Because of target motion and setup inaccuracies, an additional margin must encompass the GTV/CTV target in order to avoid missing the intended target during part or all of the treatment session. This expanded target called the PTV constitutes the final target for high-dose conformal coverage. In addition to the PTV and its contents, ablation is likely to occur in the shell of normal tissue immediately outside of the target in the regions of intermediate to high dose. As such, side effects will or will not occur depending on: (1) how essential this inner shell of tissue is for normal function of the organ, and (2) the thickness or volume of this shell as it relates to the quality of the dosimetry. This *high dose spillage* is likely the culprit in most of the toxicity related to serially functioning tissues like tubular structures in the lung, GI tract, and liver causing obliteration of the lumen and subsequent downstream effects. Furthermore, the quality of the dose distribution will affect the volume and geometry of low to intermediate dose distributions. This *intermediate dose spillage* is characterized by the maximum dose at a defined distance away from the target (e.g., 2–3 cm) or by the volume of tissue encompassed by an intermediate isodose line (e.g., the 50% of prescription isodose line). *Intermediate dose spillage* can affect the organ more globally, similar to the historically large fields associated with CFRT damaging parallel functioning tissues, but may also cause focal organ injury if the prescription dose is high enough.

Prescription isodose conformality to the target volume is generally assessed by a conformality index. This index is the ratio of the prescription isodose volume to the PTV volume. Generally, this ratio should be kept below 1.2. Achieving this degree of conformality is easier with larger targets. While CFRT results in mostly homogeneous target dose distributions, SBRT may have dramatic heterogeneity of dose. It must be insured that regions within the PTV target is not underdosed relative to the minimum prescription dose; however, overdosage is probably of no consequence and may even be advantageous in centrally hypoxic tumors. It is critical, however, that high dose "hot spots" associated with this dose heterogeneity are not physically located outside of the PTV. This would be an extreme form of *high dose spillage* and can generally be avoided by using additional highly shaped beams with unique entrance angles.

Table 17.1 Normal tissue dose constraints for 3 fraction SBRT treatments to the lung.

Organ	Volume	Dose (cGy)
Spinal cord	Any point	18 Gy (6 Gy per fraction)
Esophagus	Any point	27 Gy (9 Gy per fraction)
Ipsilateral brachial plexus	Any point	24 Gy (8 Gy per fraction)
Heart/pericardium	Any point	30 Gy (10 Gy per fraction)
Trachea and ipsilateral bronchus	Any point	30 Gy (10 Gy per fraction)
Skin	Any point	24 Gy (8 Gy per fraction)

Organ exposure limits must be respected with SBRT. It has been known that radiation tolerance of specific organs is related to total dose (and fractionation), volume, and inherent radiosensitivity. However, most quoted tolerances are generally quantified as essentially dose limits. Such characterization is clearly inadequate for SBRT where toxicity is more often related to exceeding a specified volume of tissue receiving a given dose than the absolute dose level itself. Data are accumulating for dose–volume tolerances for specific organs affected by SBRT. At the present time, however, such tolerances are not available. Instead, most investigators are using limits converted from CFRT using linear quadratic modeling or applying limits based on limited experience in treated patients. Since volume effects are poorly understood, absolute point limits were implemented for critical organs like the spinal cord, esophagus, and major bronchial airways. These limits are subject to modification after further evaluation but the limits used in the RTOG lung cancer 3 fraction protocols are listed for reference in Table 17.1. These were implemented as part of a protocol that uses 60 Gy total in 3 fractions (20 Gy per fraction) for target prescription and would not necessarily apply to different fractionation schedules.

Many potential targets for SBRT will require beams to travel through tissues of variable electronic density en route to the target. Ideally, then, the planning system would include algorithms for accurate accounting of tissue heterogeneity effects as it relates to dose deposition from both attenuation and scattering events. Some planning systems do a good job of modeling these effects; however, some do a very poor job. Indeed, published reports show that using a primitive heterogeneity correction algorithm may lead to greater inaccuracies of dose representation at the edge of the PTV than using no correction at all [54]. As such, it seems most reasonable that either sophisticated heterogeneity corrections be implemented (e.g., collapsed cone) or that no heterogeneity corrections should be used for SBRT treatments in or near the lungs.

An example of typical SBRT dosimetry for treating a primary lung cancer is shown in Plate 17.1. The beam angles were chosen by first considering the realm of attainable beam angles for a tumor in this location avoiding collisions with the accelerator head. Within this subset of attainable beam angles, a beam weight optimization algorithm was used to select these particular 10 angles using the RTOG tolerances to construct avoidance structures. In the end, the beams are noncoplanar, nonopposing, and are separated by fairly large hinge angles. Beam weights are divided fairly equal between all beams so as to spread out entrance dose.

Treatment experience in nonsmall cell lung cancer

Medically inoperable stage I patients

Early experience using SBRT for NSCLC consisted of mostly uncontrolled retrospective reports as mentioned above in section under history. These experiences showed that tumor shrinkage early after therapy was very likely after SBRT, even with more modest dose prescriptions. There was wide variability of both the number of fractions and the dose prescribed per fraction, even within a single institution experience. Some reports had very small numbers followed short periods of time, yet made strong conclusions regarding adequacy of dose and late effects.

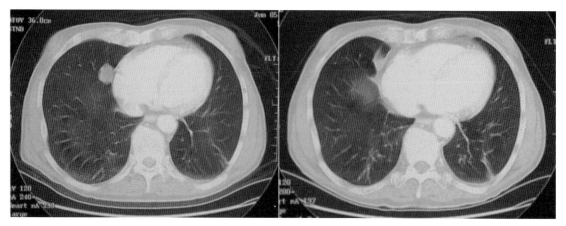

Figure 17.2 Patient with a solitary pulmonary nodule before and 2 years after treatment with SBRT. The tumor has dramatically reduced in size, but a remnant remains. The lung shows some focal fibrosis and the nearby pericardium is thicker in the posttreatment scan.

Tumor recurrence after an effective therapy will occur much later than after an ineffective therapy due to population growth kinetics. Furthermore, toxicity of high dose per fraction therapy will likely occur quite late after therapy. Therefore, it is most rational to investigate the role of SBRT in NSCLC using clearly defined selection, consistent treatment, strict quality assurance measures, and uniform follow-up policy. In addition, follow-up should make mandatory that all patients are assessed and published reports await mature evaluation of outcome data. Such constraints can only be met by regimented prospective testing.

Using the treatment process described above, researchers at Indiana University performed a formal phase I dose escalation toxicity study with 47 patients with medically inoperable lung cancer [12,55]. The starting dose was 8 Gy per fraction times three, 24 Gy total. All patients were treated with 3 fractions at all dose levels. Independent dose escalation trials were carried out in three separate patient groups: T_1 tumor patients, T_2 tumor <5 cm patients, and T_2 tumor 5–7 cm patients. There was no restriction regarding the location of the tumor in the lung as both central and peripheral tumors were treated. A total of seven dose levels were tested. The maximum tolerated dose (MTD) was never reached for T_1 tumors and T_2 tumors less than 5 cm despite reaching 60–66 Gy in 3 fractions. For the largest

tumors, dose was escalated all the way to 72 Gy in 3 fractions which proved to be too toxic. A characteristic tumor response for a patient is shown in Figure 17.2. Dose limiting toxicity in that subset included pneumonia and pericardial effusion. Therefore, the MTD for tumors 5–7 cm in diameter was 66 Gy in 3 fractions while the MTD for smaller tumors lies at an undetermined level beyond this dose. Classic radiation pneumonitis (fever, chest pain, shortness of breath, dry cough, and infiltrative X-ray findings), which had been erroneously predicted to be the dose-limiting toxicity, only occurred sporadically.

At the lower doses (i.e., 24–36 Gy in 3 fractions), very impressive tumor responses with little normal tissue effects were observed by 3 months. Unfortunately many of these patients ultimately had tumor recurrence. As the dose was escalated beyond 42–48 Gy, striking imaging changes began to appear near the treated tumor by around 6–12 months. This seemed to be related to a bronchial toxicity, which was not commonly described with CFRT. Radiographic changes by themselves were not considered dose limiting, and most of these imaging changes were asymptomatic. In many cases the radiographic changes mimic tumor recurrence. With no salvage therapy in this population, patients were followed without treatment. Repeat PET scans and biopsies showed no evidence of tumor recurrence in

Table 17.2 Local control in early-stage nonsmall cell lung cancer.

Author	Treatment	Local control	Single fraction equivalent dose (ref. [62])	Reference
North America/Europe				
Timmerman, 2006	20–22 Gy × 3	95% (2+ yr)	56–62 Gy	[56]
Baumann, 2006	15 Gy × 3	80% (3 yr)	41 Gy	[57]
Fritz, 2006	30 Gy × 1	80% (3 yr)	30 Gy	[58]
Nyman, 2006	15 Gy × 3	80% (crude)	41 Gy	[59]
Zimmermann, 2005	12.5 Gy × 3	87% (3 yr)	43.5 Gy	[60]
Timmerman, 2003	18–24 Gy × 3	90% (2 yr)	50–68 Gy	[12,55]
Asia				
Xia, 2006	5 Gy × 10	95% (3 yr)	32 Gy	[64]
Hara, 2006	30–34 Gy × 1	80% (3 yr)	30–34 Gy	[65]
Nagata, 2005	12 Gy × 4	94% (3 yr)	42 Gy	[63]

the large majority of patients treated at the higher dose levels. In the end, a dose of 60–66 Gy in 3 fractions was determined to be reasonably safe for enrolled medically inoperable NSCLC patients.

Upon completion of the phase I study finding a clearly potent dose for SBRT, the Indiana group embarked on a 70-patient phase II study in the same population. The phase II study was aimed at validating toxicity in a larger patient population and determining efficacy (local control or survival) using a total dose of 60 Gy in 3 fractions for the small tumors and 66 Gy in 3 fractions for the large tumors (35 patients for each group). The target control rate for the statistical power calculation was 80% which is dramatically higher than the typical 30–45% control seen with CFRT. All high-grade adverse events (e.g., emergency room visits, surgical procedures, hospitalizations, and deaths) were reviewed by an independent data safety monitoring panel to determine if the event was treatment related (i.e., treatment-related toxicity). In addition, this panel was responsible for final scoring of efficacy such as determining local recurrence.

The preliminary results of this phase II trial are in Timmerman *et al.* [56]. The actuarial 2-year local control for this potent dose regimen is 95%, and isolated hilar or mediastinal nodal relapse is extremely rare despite clinical staging. The overall 2-year survival for this frail population is poor at 56% with most of the deaths related to comorbid

illness rather than disease progression or toxicity. The protocol placed no time limits on scoring treatment-related toxicity and many late toxic events have been recorded. Fewer than 20% of patients have experienced high-grade toxicity confirming the phase I model. However, interim analysis showed that severe toxicity (grade 3–5) was significantly more likely in patients treated for tumors in the regions around the proximal bronchial tree or central chest region. In fact, the risk of severe toxicity is 11 times greater when treating central tumors as compared to peripheral tumors.

Similar experience has been reported in Europe and Japan. Active groups from Sweden, Denmark, Germany, the Netherlands, and Italy have reported rates of local control and toxicity similar to the Indiana experience at similar dose levels [57–60]. A variety of dose and fractionation schemes have been used, however, generally fewer than 5 total fractions have been employed. As with the Indiana group, Wulf and colleagues from Wurzburg have demonstrated a clear dose response relationship with better control at higher dose levels [61]. As shown in Table 17.2, clinical results are generally better with similar dose potency in Japan as opposed to North America/Europe [62–65]. As an example, Nagata and colleagues from Kyoto University published a series of 45 patients treated with a dose of 48 Gy in 4 fractions to the isocenter [63]. This dose is biologically less potent than the dose fractionation schemes used in prospective North American trials (60–66 Gy in 3 fractions) or and roughly equivalent to European trials (45 Gy in 3 fractions). Still, Nagata reported effectively no in-field local failures (100% local control) with this dose which is in contrast to the results published from North America and Europe where local control is only 70–80% with dose prescriptions in the this range. The techniques used by Nagata and colleagues for immobilization, targeting, dosimetry, and treatment conduct are essentially identical to what was used at Indiana University. This same dose prescription piloted at Kyoto University is being tested in the larger Japan Clinical Oncology Group 0403 trial for peripheral T1N0 stage I patients which is still accruing patients. A clue to the likely explanation for these conflicting results between experienced centers in North America and Asia may be found in the overall survival results. Two-year overall survival in the Nagata series was over 80% in striking contrast to the Indiana phase II study and European experiences where only around 50% of patients are alive. Indeed, the Nagata series survival for medically inoperable patients is quite comparable to series describing operable patients in North America. As such, it appears these are different populations indicating a striking difference in patient selection.

In 2004, after several years of planning, the lung committee of the RTOG finalized plans to carry out a multicenter trial of SBRT in patients with medically inoperable NSCLC. RTOG 0236 using SBRT for medically inoperable lung cancer in patients with peripherally situated tumors has completed its accrual of 52 patients. This trial was based on the preliminary data from Indiana University using 60 Gy in 3 fractions for T1, T2, and peripheral T3 tumors less than 5 cm in diameter. Extensive accreditation, conduct, and dosimetry constraints were developed in the RTOG Lung, Physics, and Image-Guided Therapy Committees in order to form a basis for meaningful quality assurance and consistent treatment for a multicenter trial. Three toxicity analyses were performed during the trial which showed no excessive toxicity warranting trial closure. Results from RTOG 0236 will not be available for some time. It will be followed by RTOG 0624, a trial giving adjuvant systemic therapy along with

SBRT in an effort to reduce the risk of patients at higher risk of systemic relapse. Another trial in patients with centrally situated tumors, RTOG 0633, is being planned that will use a more gentle fractionation scheme for medically inoperable patients.

RTOG 0618 is in the finalization process for patients with documented NSCLC who are medically suitable for surgical anatomical resection. This is a dramatic departure from previous trials in North America where only frail medically inoperable patients were enrolled onto SBRT trials. This trial, patterned after RTOG 0236, will include an early assessment for surgical salvage in people with less than ideal response. As such, SBRT is being studied in broader populations with early stage NSCLC building on the existing prospective testing.

Operable stage I patients

Patients deemed healthy enough for surgery have been treated with SBRT based on the patient's preference to avoid surgery. Most of the work in this population has been carried out in Japan. Onishi and colleagues performed a large retrospective chart review of patients treated at several Japanese centers using SBRT in early stage NSCLC [66]. While dose and number of fractions varied considerably, all patients were treated with small volumes under stereotactic guidance. This report included a large number of operable patients that were analyzed separately. For such patients who received dose levels such that the biological effective dose (BED) was greater than 100 [67], local control and survival rivaled best surgical series according to the authors. The 3-year overall survival in this group was 88%. This report has formed the basis for enrolling patient with operable tumors onto a separate arm of the Japan Clinical Oncology Group 0403 trial for peripheral T1N0 stage I patients.

In the United States, very few patients with operable stage I NSCLC have been treated on clinical trials. That situation will change with the enactment of RTOG 0618 for operable patients. Based on best surgical literature, it will be required that SBRT attain a local control rate of 90% or better in order to compete with lobectomy [68]. As such, very potent dose prescriptions will be required. As noted above, it is likely that higher dose levels will be required in the United States as opposed to Asia series in order to attain this high rate of local control. RTOG 0618 is modeled after RTOG 0236 except eligibility is for healthier patients capable of tolerating thoracotomy. The prescription dose is 60 Gy in 3 fractions and frequent tumor status assessments are made in order to identify failure early and attempt surgical salvage.

Summary

The technological developments surrounding the implementation of SBRT were the product of mostly engineering and physics research. However, they facilitate the exploitation of the more important biological determinants of local control [69]. Ablation of tumor using total dose or dose per fraction well beyond conventional radiation promises in the end to serve to improve outcome. This necessary collaboration between technical resource development and biological innovation holds considerable promise for patients with lung cancer.

As systemic treatments become more effective, radiotherapy will be used more selectively to target isolated deposits of gross disease [2]. Currently limited to treatment with curative intent in stage I–III disease, radiotherapy will likely be used more often in stage IV disease either as a measure for consolidation or to ablate cancer deposits resistant to systemic therapy. With exploitation of technology and biological understanding, this is an ideal role for radiotherapy as an effective and cost effective modality for local control of gross disease.

The goal of technical, biological, and clinical research in radiation oncology as well as in collaboration with surgical and medical oncologists is to facilitate adaptive therapy [70–72]. In this paradigm, pretreatment diagnostic information including imaging, staging, tissue samples (proteomic, genomics, etc), and other predictive assays are integrated to make therapy selection [73]. Having chosen the correct approach, the patient is started on therapy while monitoring progress. Early assessments relating to accuracy of delivery, tumor response, metabolic changes, tolerance, and others can be used to change the therapy appropriately during therapy [74–76]. Soon after treatment, imaging and metabolic assessment may direct the need for adjuvant therapies or avoid toxicity. Rather than a "one size fits all" cancer therapy, the adaptive process uses a tailored approach that constantly re-evaluates and responds to redirect the therapy toward a better outcome. Until this goal is achieved, patients will continue to be enrolled onto well-designed prospective trials such that SBRT might be refined to its optimal potential.

References

1 Potters L, Steinberg M, Rose C *et al.*, for American Society for Therapeutic Radiology and Oncology; American College of Radiology. American Society for Therapeutic Radiology and Oncology and American College of Radiology practice guideline for the performance of stereotactic body radiation therapy. *Int J Radiat Oncol Biol Phys* Nov 15, 2004; **60(4)**:1026–32.

2 Timmerman R, Papiez L. Review of Song *et al.*, re Stereotactic body radiation therapy: rationale, techniques, applications, and optimization of an emerging technology. *Oncology* 2004; **18(4)**:474–7.

3 Leksell L. The stereotaxic method and radiosurgery of the brain. *Acta Chir Scand* 1951; **102**:316–9.

4 Hamilton AJ, Lulu BA, Fosmire H, Stea B, Cassady JR. Preliminary clinical experience with linear accelerator-based spinal stereotactic radiosurgery. *Neurosurgery* 1995; **36(2)**:311–9.

5 Lax I, Blomgren H, Naslund I, Svanstrom R. Stereotactic radiotherapy of extracranial targets. *Z Med Phys* 1994; **4**:112–3.

6 Blomgren H, Lax I, Naslund I, Svanstrom R. Stereotactic high dose fraction radiation therapy of extracranial tumors using an accelerator. *Acta Oncol* 1995; **34(6)**:861–70.

7 Shirato H, Shimizu S, Tadashi S, Nishioka T, Miyasaka K. Real time tumour-tracking radiotherapy. *Lancet* 1999; **353**:1331–2.

8 Uematsu M, Shioda A, Tahara K *et al.* Focal, high dose, and fractionated modified stereotactic radiation therapy for lung carcinoma patients: a preliminary experience. *Cancer* Mar 15, 1998; **82(6)**:1062–70.

9 Herfarth KK, Debus J, Lohr F *et al.* Stereotactic single-dose radiation therapy of liver tumors: results of a phase I/II trial. *J Clin Oncol* Jan 1, 2001; **19(1)**:164–70.

10 Wulf J, Hadinger U, Oppitz U, Thiele W, Ness-Dourdoumas R, Flentje M. Stereotactic radiotherapy of targets in the lung and liver. *Strahlenther Onkol* Dec 2001; **177(12)**:645–55.

11 Nagata Y, Negoro Y, Aoki T *et al*. Clinical outcomes of 3D conformal hypofractionated single high-dose radiotherapy for one or two lung tumors using a stereotactic body frame. *Int J Radiat Oncol Biol Phys* Mar 15, 2002; **52(4)**:1041–6.

12 Timmerman R, Papiez L, McGarry R *et al*. Extracranial stereotactic radioablation: results of a phase I study in medically inoperable stage I non-small cell lung cancer. *Chest* Nov 2003; **124(5)**:1946–55.

13 Guerrero M, Li X. Extending the linear–quadratic model for large fraction doses pertinent to stereotactic radiotherapy. *Phys Med Biol* 2004; **49**:4825–35.

14 Curtis SB. Lethal and potentially lethal lesions induced by radiation–a unified repair model. *Radiat Res* 1986; **106**:252–70.

15 Benedict SH, Lin PS, Zwicker RD *et al*. The biological effectiveness of intermittent irradiation as a function of overall treatment time: development of correction factors for linac-based stereotactic radiotherapy. *Int J Radiat Oncol Biol Phys* 1997; **37**:765–9.

16 Fowler JF, Welsh JS, Howard SP. Loss of biological effect in prolonged fraction delivery. *Int J Radiat Oncol Biol Phys* May 1, 2004; **59(1)**:242–9.

17 Wolbarst AB, Chin LM, Svensson GK. Optimization of radiation therapy: integral-response of a model biological system. *Int J Radiat Oncol Biol Phys* 1982; **8**:1761–9.

18 Yeas RJ, Kalend A. Local stem cell depletion model for radiation myelitis. *Int J Radiat Oncol Biol Phys* 1988; **14**:1247–59.

19 Nevinny-Stickel M, Sweeney RA, Bale RJ, Posch A, Auberger T, Lukas P. Reproducibility of patient positioning for fractionated extracranial stereotactic radiotherapy using a double-vacuum technique. *Strahlenther Onkol* Feb 2004; **180(2)**:117–22.

20 Fuss M, Salter BJ, Rassiah P, Cheek D, Cavanaugh SX, Herman TS. Repositioning accuracy of a commercially available double-vacuum whole body immobilization system for stereotactic body radiation therapy. *Technol Cancer Res Treat* Feb 2004; **3(1)**:59–67.

21 Hof H, Herfarth KK, Munter M, Essig M, Wannenmacher M, Debus J. The use of the multislice CT for the determination of respiratory lung tumor movement in stereotactic single-dose irradiation. *Strahlenther Onkol* Aug 2003; **179(8)**:542–7.

22 Nagata Y, Negoro Y, Aoki T *et al*. Three-dimensional conformal radiotherapy for extracranial tumors using a stereotactic body frame. *Igaku Butsuri* 2001; **21(1)**:28–34.

23 Fairclough-Tompa L, Larsen T, Jaywant SM. Immobilization in stereotactic radiotherapy: the head and neck localizer frame. *Med Dosim* Fall 2001; **26(3)**:267–73.

24 Alheit H, Dornfeld S, Dawel M *et al*. Patient position reproducibility in fractionated stereotactically guided conformal radiotherapy using the BrainLab mask system. *Strahlenther Onkol* May 2001; **177(5)**:264–8.

25 Negoro Y, Nagata Y, Aoki T *et al*. The effectiveness of an immobilization device in conformal radiotherapy for lung tumor: reduction of respiratory tumor movement and evaluation of the daily setup accuracy. *Int J Radiat Oncol Biol Phys* 2001; **50(4)**:889–98.

26 Wulf J, Hadinger U, Oppitz U, Olshausen B, Flentje M. Stereotactic radiotherapy of extracranial targets: CT-simulation and accuracy of treatment in the stereotactic body frame. *Radiother Oncol* Nov 2000; **57(2)**:225–36.

27 Takacs II, Kishan A, Deogaonkar M *et al*. Respiration induced target drift in spinal stereotactic radiosurgery: evaluation of skeletal fixation in a porcine model. *Stereotact Funct Neurosurg* 1999; **73(1–4)**:70.

28 Herfarth KK, Debus J, Lohr F *et al*. Extracranial stereotactic radiation therapy: set-up accuracy of patients treated for liver metastases. *Int J Radiat Oncol Biol Phys* Jan 15, 2000; **46(2)**:329–35.

29 Lohr F, Debus J, Frank C *et al*. Noninvasive patient fixation for extracranial stereotactic radiotherapy. *Int J Radiat Oncol Biol Phys* Sep 1, 1999; **45(2)**:521–7.

30 Bale RJ, Sweeney R, Vogele M *et al*. Noninvasive head fixation for external irradiation of tumors of the head–neck area. *Strahlenther Onkol* Jul 1998; **174(7)**:350–4.

31 Lax I, Blomgren H, Larson D, Naslund I. Extracranial stereotactic radiosurgery of localized targets. *J Radiosurg* 1998; **1(2)**:135–48.

32 Lax I, Blomgren H, Naslund I, Svanstrom R. Stereotactic radiotherapy of malignancies in the abdomen: methodological aspects. *Acta Oncol* 1994; **33(6)**:677–83.

33 Takai Y, Mituya M, Nemoto K *et al*. Simple method of stereotactic radiotherapy without stereotactic body frame for extracranial tumors. *Nippon Igaku Hoshasen Gakkai Zasshi* Jul 2001; **61(8)**:403–7.

34 Wang LT, Solberg TD, Medin PM, Boone R. Infrared patient positioning for stereotactic radiosurgery of extracranial tumors. *Comput Biol Med* Mar 2001; **31(2)**:101–11.

35 Uematsu M, Shioda A, Suda A *et al*. Intrafractional tumor position stability during computed tomography (CT)-guided frameless stereotactic radiation therapy for lung or liver cancers with a fusion of CT and linear

accelerator (FOCAL) unit. *Int J Radiat Oncol Biol Phys* Sep 1, 2000; **48(2)**:443–8.

36 Uematsu M, Sonderegger M, Shioda A *et al.* Daily positioning accuracy of frameless stereotactic radiation therapy with a fusion of computed tomography and linear accelerator (focal) unit: evaluation of z-axis with a z-marker. *Radiother Oncol* 1999; **50(3)**:337–9.

37 Kimura T, Hirokawa Y, Murakami Y *et al.* Reproducibility of organ position using voluntary breath-hold method with spirometer for extracranial stereotactic radiotherapy. *Int J Radiat Oncol Biol Phys* Nov 15, 2004; **60(4)**:1307–13.

38 O'Dell WG, Schell MC, Reynolds D, Okunieff R. Dose broadening due to target position variability during fractionated breath-held radiation therapy. *Med Phys* Jul 2002; **29(7)**:1430–7.

39 Murphy MJ, Martin D, Whyte R, Hai J, Ozhasoglu C, Le QT. The effectiveness of breath-holding to stabilize lung and pancreas tumors during radiosurgery. *Int J Radiat Oncol Biol Phys* Jun 1, 2002; **53(2)**:475–82.

40 Yin F, Kim JG, Haughton C *et al.* Extracranial radiosurgery: immobilizing liver motion in dogs using high-frequency jet ventilation and total intravenous anesthesia. *Int J Radiat Oncol Biol Phys* Jan 1, 2001; **49(1)**:211–6.

41 Kini VR, Vedam SS, Keall PJ, Patil S, Chen C, Mohan R. Patient training in respiratory-gated radiotherapy. *Med Dosim* Spring 2003; **28(1)**:7–11.

42 Vedam SS, Keall PJ, Kini VR, Mohan R. Determining parameters for respiration-gated radiotherapy. *Med Phys* Oct 2001; **28(10)**:2139–46.

43 Hara R, Itami J, Aruga T *et al.* Development of stereotactic irradiation system of body tumors under respiratory gating. *Nippon Igaku Hoshasen Gakkai Zasshi* Mar 2002; **62(4)**:156–60.

44 Kuriyama K, Onishi H, Sano N *et al.* A new irradiation unit constructed of self-moving gantry-CT and linac. *Int J Radiat Oncol Biol Phys* Feb 1, 2003; **55(2)**: 428–35.

45 Kitamura K, Shirato H, Seppenwoolde Y *et al.* Tumor location, cirrhosis, and surgical history contribute to tumor movement in the liver, as measured during stereotactic irradiation using a real-time tumor-tracking radiotherapy system. *Int J Radiat Oncol Biol Phys* May 1, 2003; **56(1)**:221–8.

46 Sharp GC, Jiang SB, Shimizu S, Shirato H. Prediction of respiratory tumour motion for real-time image-guided radiotherapy. *Phys Med Biol* Feb 7, 2004 ; **49(3)**:425–40.

47 Schweikard A, Shiomi H, Adler J. Respiration tracking in radiosurgery. *Med Phys* Oct 2004; **31(10)**:2738–41.

48 Papiez L, Timmerman R, DesRosiers C, Randall M. Extracranial stereotactic radioablation: physical principles. *Acta Oncol* 2003; **42(8)**:882–94.

49 Liu R, Wagner TH, Buatti JM, Modrick J, Dill J, Meeks SL. Geometrically based optimization for extracranial radiosurgery. *Phys Med Biol* Mar 21, 2004; **49(6)**:987–96.

50 Cardinale RM, Wu Q, Benedict SH, Kavanagh BD, Bump E, Mohan R. Determining the optimal block margin on the planning target volume for extracranial stereotactic radiotherapy. *Int J Radiat Oncol Biol Phys* Sep 1, 1999; **45(2)**:515–20.

51 Papiez L. On the equivalence of rotational and concentric therapy. *Phys Med Biol* Feb 2000; **45(2)**:399–409.

52 Hadinger U, Thiele W, Wulf J. Extracranial stereotactic radiotherapy: evaluation of PTV coverage and dose conformity. *Z Med Phys* 2002; **12(4)**:221–9.

53 Papiez L, Moskvin V, Timmerman R. Dosimetry of stereotactic body radiation therapy treatments. In: *Stereotactic Body Radiation Therapy.* Baltimore, MD: Lippincott, Williams and Wilkins, 2005:57–68.

54 Mayer R, Williams A, Frankel T *et al.* Two-dimensional film dosimetry application in heterogeneous materials exposed to megavoltage photon beams. *Med Phys* 1997; **24(3)**:455–60.

55 McGarry RC, Papiez L, Williams M *et al.* Stereotactic body radiation therapy of early-stage non-small-cell lung carcinoma: phase I study. *Int J Radiat Oncol Biol Phys* 2005; **63**:1010–5.

56 Timmerman RD, McGarry R, Yiannoutsos C *et al.* Excessive toxicity when treating central tumors in a phase II study of stereotactic body radiation therapy for medically inoperable early-stage lung cancer. *J Clin Oncol* 2006; **24**:4833–9.

57 Baumann P, Nyman J, Lax I *et al.* Factors important for efficacy of stereotactic body radiotherapy of medically inoperable stage I lung cancer. A retrospective analysis of patients treated in the Nordic countries. *Acta Oncol* 2006; **45**:787–95.

58 Fritz P, Kraus HJ, Muhlnickel W *et al.* Stereotactic, single-dose irradiation of stage I non-small cell lung cancer and lung metastases. *Radiat Oncol* 2006; **1**: 30.

59 Nyman J, Johansson KA, Hulten U. Stereotactic hypofractionated radiotherapy for stage I non-small cell lung cancer—mature results for medically inoperable patients. *Lung Cancer* 2006; **51**:97–103.

60 Zimmermann FB, Geinitz H, Schill S *et al.* Stereotactic hypofractionated radiation therapy for stage I non-small cell lung cancer. *Lung Cancer* 2005; **48**:107–14.

61 Wulf J, Baier K, Mueller G *et al.* Dose–response in stereotactic irradiation of lung tumors. *Radiother Oncol* 2005; **77**:83–7.

62 Timmerman RD, Park C, Kavanagh BD. The North American experience with stereotactic body radiation

therapy in non-small cell lung cancer. *J Thorac Oncol* Jul 2007; **2(7, Suppl 3)**:S101–12.

63 Nagata Y, Takayama K, Matsuo Y *et al.* Clinical outcomes of a phase I/II study of 48 Gy of stereotactic body radiotherapy in 4 fractions for primary lung cancer using a stereotactic body frame. *Int J Radiat Oncol Biol Phys* 2005; **63**:1427–31.

64 Xia T, Li H, Sun Q *et al.* Promising clinical outcome of stereotactic body radiation therapy for patients with inoperable Stage I/II non-small-cell lung cancer. *Int J Radiat Oncol Biol Phys* 2006; **66**:117–25.

65 Hara R, Itami J, Kondo T *et al.* Clinical outcomes of single-fraction stereotactic radiation therapy of lung tumors. *Cancer* 2006; **106**:1347–52.

66 Onishi H, Araki T, Shirato H *et al.* Stereotactic hypofractionated high-dose irradiation for stage I non-small cell lung carcinoma: clinical outcomes in 245 subjects in a Japanese multiinstitutional study. *Cancer* 2004; **101**:1623–31.

67 Fowler JF. The linear-quadratic formula and progress in fractionated radiotherapy. *Br J Radiol* 1989; **62**:679–94.

68 Ginsberg RJ, Rubinstein LV. Randomized trial of lobectomy versus limited resection for T1 N0 non-small cell lung cancer. *Ann Thorac Surg* 1995; **60**:615–23.

69 Timmerman RD, Story M. Stereotactic body radiation therapy: a treatment in need of basic biological research. *Cancer J* Jan–Feb 2006; **12(1)**:19–20.

70 Martinez AA, Yan D, Lockman D *et al.* Improvement in dose escalation using the process of adaptive radiotherapy combined with three-dimensional conformal or intensity-modulated beams for prostate cancer. *Int J Radiat Oncol Biol Phys* Aug 1, 2001; **50(5)**:1226–34.

71 Bortfeld T, Paganetti H. The biologic relevance of daily dose variations in adaptive treatment planning. *Int J Radiat Oncol Biol Phys* Jul 1, 2006; **65(3)**:899–906.

72 Song W, Schaly B, Bauman G, Battista J, Van Dyk J. Image-guided adaptive radiation therapy (IGART): radiobiological and dose escalation considerations for localized carcinoma of the prostate. *Med Phys* Jul 2005; **32(7)**:2193–203.

73 Potti A, Mukherjee S, Petersen R *et al.* A genomic strategy to refine prognosis in early-stage non-small-cell lung cancer. *N Engl J Med* Aug 10, 2006; **355(6)**:570–80.

74 Yan D, Lockman D, Brabbins D, Tyburski L, Martinez A. An off-line strategy for constructing a patient-specific planning target volume in adaptive treatment process for prostate cancer. *Int J Radiat Oncol Biol Phys* Aug 1, 2000; **48(1)**:289–302.

75 Wu C, Jeraj R, Olivera GH, Mackie TR. Re-optimization in adaptive radiotherapy. *Phys Med Biol* Sep 7, 2002; **47(17)**:3181–95.

76 Brahme A. Biologically optimized 3-dimensional in vivo predictive assay-based radiation therapy using positron emission tomography-computerized tomography imaging. *Acta Oncol* 2003; **42(2)**:123–36.

CHAPTER 18

Proton Therapy

Joe Y. Chang, Alfred R. Smith, and James D. Cox

Introduction

Despite preventive care, early-detection methods, and therapeutic advances, lung cancer remains the leading cause of cancer death in both men and women. In 2006, the American Cancer Society estimated there would be 174,470 newly diagnosed patients with lung cancer and there would be 162,460 deaths [1]. Nonsmall cell lung cancer (NSCLC) accounts for 80% of all lung cancer cases. Only 20–25% of patients with NSCLC present with early-stage disease that can be surgically resected, and a substantial number of these patients are considered unable to tolerate surgery because of comorbidities. For this latter cohort, radiotherapy has been the standard treatment.

Approximately 50% of NSCLC patients present with locally advanced disease and require multimodality treatment, including radiotherapy. For patients with stage I disease, radiotherapy provides 2 years of local control with a survival rate of about 50% [2–4]. For patients with stage III disease, locoregional control with radiotherapy with or without chemotherapy results in a survival rate of <50%. Curran *et al.* [5], for instance, observed a median survival time of 17 months and an expected 4-year survival rate of 21% for patients with stage III disease.

Uncontrolled locoregional disease is a major source of continuous seeding to distant organs and is the eventual cause of treatment failure; thus, its

Lung Cancer, 3rd edition. Edited by Jack A. Roth, James D. Cox, and Waun Ki Hong. © 2008 Blackwell Publishing, ISBN: 978-1-4051-5112-2.

eradication is essential for cure. There is increasing clinical evidence suggesting a radiation dose–response relationship in both survival and local control in NSCLC patients [6–8]. However, higher radiation doses are associated with higher toxicity, particularly with concurrent chemotherapy [5,9].

The current standard dose of radiation for lung cancer is between 60 and 66 Gy, based on the Radiation Therapy Oncology Group (RTOG) 73-01 trial, which showed survival benefit with doses >60 Gy [10]. However, doses ranging from 60 to 66 Gy are substantially lower than the anticipated dose needed to achieve a local control rate of >50%. A review of published data showed that a local control rate as high as 90% could theoretically be achieved in NSCLC with a radiation dose of 80 Gy [11], although this projection was made with the assumptions that the imaging was accurate and the target volume was delineated with tumor motion consideration. The RTOG 83-11 trial, led by Cox *et al.* [12], showed that radiotherapy alone with a dose of 69.6 Gy with 1.2 Gy/fraction led to higher survival rates. However, the RTOG 94-10 trial indicated that treatment with 69.6 Gy and concurrent chemotherapy, compared with treatment with 60 Gy and concurrent chemotherapy, resulted in a higher toxicity level and no survival advantage [5].

Advances in diagnostic imaging in the 1980s led to more individualized radiation therapy based on the specific anatomy of individual patients rather than on anatomic atlases. Computed tomography (CT) and other tomographic scanning technologies permitted a three-dimensional (3D) display of tumors in relation to the surrounding normal anatomy. Accurate 3D radiation dose computations were developed, as were multileaf collimators in linear accelerators. These tools permitted a "beams-eye" view of tumors and a conformal delivery of radiation to them.

Commercial treatment-planning systems allowed 3D conformal radiation therapy (CRT) by the early 1990s. Computer simulations of dose distributions clearly showed that with 3D CRT, higher total doses could be delivered to the gross tumor volume than were possible with two-dimensional (2D) treatment. Also with 3D CRT, normal tissues could be avoided or at least be exposed to much lower doses than with 2D treatment. The rapid adoption of 3D CRT was based entirely on computer-generated treatment plans that showed a reduced volume of normal tissue irradiated with this method compared with 2D treatment plans and delivery. Recent clinical trials showed that using 3D CRT allowed a dose escalation from 63 to 74 Gy with concurrent chemotherapy in patients with stage III NSCLC [13,14].

The delivery of small X-ray beams with different intensities permitted further shaping of the high-dose volume. Physicists optimized the different intensities, and with use of dynamic multileaf collimators, intensity-modulated radiation therapy (IMRT) was fully realized. In contrast to the rather rapid adoption of 3D CRT, IMRT was appreciated and introduced more slowly [15]. Physicians, physicists, and dosimetrists had to devote much more time and effort to treatment planning with IMRT [16,17], but achieving reduced toxicity with this therapy was a worthy goal that has been realized [18]. Such precision in radiation delivery requires more careful target delineation, treatment planning, and quality assurance. Moreover, because of the risk of missing tumors that may move between daily fractions or during treatments (e.g., during respiration), imaging is needed with each treatment. Image-guided radiotherapy encompasses such daily imaging as well as 3D CRT and IMRT.

Although 3D CRT or IMRT have the potential to reduce normal tissue toxicity, the relatively high exit dose of photon X-ray therapy limits the possibility of dose escalation or acceleration. A proton beam, on the other hand, is made up of charged particles that have a well-defined range of penetration into tissues. As the proton beam penetrates the body, the particles slow down, and deposit a large fraction of their energy near the end of their range. The resultant central axis depth dose distribution is known as the Bragg peak. By modulating the Bragg peak in both energy and time, a full, localized, uniform dose can be delivered to the target while sparing the surrounding normal tissues. Proton beam treatment is ideal when organ preservation is a priority, particularly in patients with lung cancer and in pediatric patients. In this chapter, we review the rationale and the treatment planning and delivery of proton therapy for patients with lung cancer; the clinical outcome of these patients is discussed as well.

Relative biologic effectiveness and biological research

Protons have nearly the same relative biologic effectiveness (RBE) as photons. Paganetti *et al.* summarized the available data from numerous experiments with protons and concluded that the RBE of protons is approximately 1.1 [19]. By contrast, the RBE for carbon ions is approximately 3, similar to the RBE for neutrons. Higher RBE with carbon ions would seem advantageous for control of hypoxic tumors, but it is disadvantageous for normal tissues. Thus, more than a century of experience with X-rays and gamma rays provides the basis for understanding the biological effects of protons.

Future research of molecular biology to address mechanism of DNA damage/repair and signal transduction pathway induced by proton treatment might help us to identify optimal regimen and schema of proton therapy [20]. In addition, interaction of proton treatment with chemotherapy and/or molecular targeting therapy might open a new field of research aiming to further improve therapeutic ratio [21].

Rationale for proton therapy

Proton beams are essentially low linear energy transfer (LET) radiation. Their primary advantage for cancer therapy is their highly localized dose distribution, rather than an enhanced biological

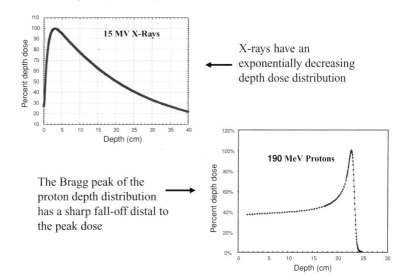

X-rays have an exponentially decreasing depth dose distribution

The Bragg peak of the proton depth distribution has a sharp fall-off distal to the peak dose

Figure 18.1 A typical proton dose distribution for a Bragg peak.

effect. A high dose of therapeutic proton beams can be safely delivered to the tumor/target volume while sparing adjacent normal tissues that are vulnerable to radiation injury, particularly, those tissues that are distal to the target volume in the beam direction. When similar complexities and treatment-delivery techniques have been used, protons have typically deposited one half or less of the integral dose that X-rays deposit to uninvolved normal tissues [22]. Higher doses should result in an increased probability of local tumor control [23,24].

The fundamental property of proton beams that provides a substantial advantage over X-ray beams is that protons can be made to stop within a few millimeters past the distal surface of the target volume, whereas X-rays deposit their dose in the healthy tissues and organs that lie in the beam path beyond the target volume and then exit the patient on the side opposite to the beam entrance. In addition, protons deposit a lower dose than do X-rays to normal tissues and organs that lie in the beam path between the surface of the patient and the target volume. For a given level of normal tissue toxicity, the maximum tolerated dose of proton radiotherapy is likely higher than that of conventional photon radiotherapy because of the physical characteristics of the proton beam (i.e., its Bragg peak). Therefore, proton radiotherapy may have an advantage over conventional photon therapy, including IMRT,

in attaining local tumor control and improving survival rates [25].

Physical characteristics of proton beams

As with all heavy charged particles (helium and carbon ions, negative pi-mesons, etc.), protons have a unique depth dose distribution, commonly referred to as the Bragg peak. The depth dose is characterized by a low entrance dose (about 30–40% of the maximum dose), followed by a relatively flat dose plateau, which rises sharply to a narrow peak (the Bragg peak) and then falls rather rapidly to zero dose immediately after the maximum dose is reached. The depth of the Bragg peak depends on the composition of the material being penetrated and the energy of the proton. A typical Bragg peak is shown in Figure 18.1.

The width of the Bragg peak is too narrow to allow treatment of any but the smallest of clinical targets, which typically range up to 20 cm deep. Generally, range modulation, i.e., adding Bragg peaks of sequentially lower energies and smaller weights (time duration), is used to produce an extended region of dose uniformity in depth called a spread-out Bragg peak (SOBP) (Figure 18.2). SOBPs can be achieved by placing either a range modulation wheel (for

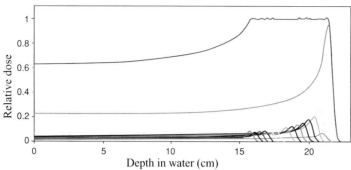

SOBP resulting from 16 beam energies and differential weights

Figure 18.2 Spread-out Bragg peak (SOBP).

dynamic modulation) or a ridge filter (for passive modulation) in the beam or by changing the energy in the accelerator or energy-selection system while adjusting the weight (time duration) of each individual Bragg peak. By appropriately selecting the range pullback and weight of each pristine Bragg peak, depth uniformity can be achieved that covers the tumor. To achieve lateral uniformity in the tumor target, the beam must also be spread laterally by either a passive, double scattering system or magnetically scanning a small spot beam in a uniform pattern. In general, SOBPs can be produced with different widths, customized to individual target volumes. It should be noted that as the width of the SOBP increases, the surface dose increases. A SOBP that extends to the surface (full modulation) would have a surface dose of 100%.

Proton therapy requires a source of protons in an energy range of about 70 to 230–250 MeV to achieve penetration in the patient from 7 to 30–37 cm. Dose rates should be approximately 2 Gy/min. Two types of hospital-based devices have been used to accelerate protons to energies and dose rates that are suitable for proton therapy: cyclotrons and synchrotrons.

Proton treatment planning and delivery

Passive scattering systems
Until recently, passive scattering systems were the standard method for spreading the proton beam laterally for therapeutic applications. In this sys-

tem, the proton beam is passed through a range-modulating wheel, which is often part of the first scatterer, a second scattering device, a range shifter, an aperture for shaping the beam laterally, and a customized compensator before it enters the patient. The double scattering system (use of the range-modulating wheel/first scatterer and the second scattering device) creates a broad flattened beam at the final aperture. The range shifter determines the maximum depth penetrated by the protons. The range-modulating wheel spreads the narrow Bragg peak, forming a uniform dose distribution that covers the target while sparing the surrounding normal tissue (the SOBP). The customized range compensator tailors the distal surface of the dose distribution to match the distal shape of the target volume with necessary margins and lateral smearing to allow for possible small misalignment of the compensator with the patient anatomy. In the design of the range compensator, the treatment planning system calculates the water equivalent path-lengths between the patient surface and the distal planning volume, thereby calculating the thickness of each point of range compensator in order to correct for the shape of the patient surface, all inhomogeneities between the patient surface and the planning target volume, and the shape of distal surface of the planning target volume.

The advantages of passive scattering systems are safety, simplicity, and a lower sensitivity to the time structure of the accelerator. Although these systems have well served their intended purpose, they have a number of disadvantages, the most serious being that they are only about 20–40% efficient and therefore waste a large number of protons in the scattering system and in the beam-limiting aperture. This substantial loss of protons can pose a problem for synchrotron-based proton therapy systems, in which the dose rate is more limited than in cyclotrons. Passive scattering systems also tend to be sensitive to variations in the beam position. Furthermore, when protons are stopped in the scattering system and aperture, they produce secondary neutrons, many of which can contribute to the whole-body dose of the patient. Neutrons have a high relative biological effectiveness and are thought to be the source of secondary cancers in some patients [26]. Another disadvantage of this system is that it produces a single SOBP for the entire target volume; thus, during treatment of large irregular target volumes with notable differences in their thickest and thinnest depths, the high-dose region is pulled back into normal tissues. For this reason, the dose-shaping properties of passive scattering techniques are often described as 2.5-dimensional. The solution to the disadvantages of passive scattering systems is found in dynamic spot scanning systems.

Dynamic spot scanning systems

In dynamic spot scanning, a narrow beam entering the treatment nozzle is magnetically scanned across the target cross-section and in depth to achieve the intended dose pattern. The beam can be either scanned continuously or stopped at predetermined positions for a specified time until the desired dose is delivered. In discrete spot scanning, the beam is then turned off and the currents in the magnets are adjusted so as to move the next beam spot to the desired position [27]. The deepest layer is scanned by selecting the appropriate energy, and when scanning of that layer is completed, the energy is decreased and the next layer is scanned. In this manner, the entire target volume can be irradiated either to deliver a uniform dose distribution for each field, much like the passive scattering method, or to deliver a nonuniform dose distribution for each field in such a way that when the doses from all fields are summed, the total dose distribution is uniform. This is called intensity-modulated proton therapy (IMPT). Plate 18.1 shows a typical dynamic spot scanning system [.28]. With continuous scanning, the intensity of the beam can be varied as the spot is moved to produce a nonuniform dose distribution. With discrete spot scanning, the time that the spot remains at each "voxel" can be varied to produce the nonuniform dose distribution.

The dynamic spot scanning has several advantages: it provides full 3D shaping of the dose distribution to the target volume; no devices such as dose-limiting apertures and range compensators are required; the efficiency is high because very few protons are wasted; and very few neutrons are produced. One disadvantage of dynamic spot scanning is the difficulty in delivering a desired dose to tumors that move during irradiation; however, beam gating techniques such as respiratory-gated proton beam radiotherapy (see the "tumor motion consideration" section) should decrease the uncertainty in such treatments. Another way to decrease the effect of target motion is to scan each layer multiple times—the dose error due to target motion decreases as the number of scans increases, although there is a practical limit to the number of times a layer can be rescanned. The time required to deliver IMPT should be comparable to that required for X-ray IMRT.

Comparison of proton therapy and photon therapy planning

As with X-rays and electrons, proton treatments use multiple treatment fields, often noncoplanar, to keep the skin dose at reasonable limits and to spare normal tissues in the beam path. However, treatment-planning strategies involving protons can be quite different from those involving X-rays and electrons because of the particular properties of proton beams. For example, in proton-based treatments, the rapid distal falloff of the proton dose distribution permits the planner to aim a proton beam directly at a critical normal structure, as opposed to X-ray-based and electron-based therapies, which may deliver toxic dose to critical structures due to significant exit dose. However, there is some uncertainty about distal edge of proton dose and possible increased RBE toward the end of SOBP. Caution should be taken to take these into consideration.

Therefore, proton-based therapies require a more critical understanding of the proton beam to reduce uncertainty. Specifically, the uncertainties associated with the exact stopping point of the proton beam, due to errors in the CT data and/or in the treatment planning and delivery process, can result in either the beam being stopped too quickly, under dosing the target, or the beam's being delivered for too long, overdosing a critical structure. A correlation between CT Hounsfield units and proton mass stopping powers, based on measurements of materials of known stopping powers on the CT scanner, is used to calculate proton ranges in tissue [29–31]. Uncertainty of RBE is another concern. Preliminary data showed that RBE of proton beam is dependent on tissue specificity, dose, dose rate, energy, and depth of penetration [19] but does not vary significantly from its nominal value.

Another important difference between X-ray and proton treatment planning is the use of margins to expand the clinical target volume to the planning target volume. Proton beams have essentially three edges, the two lateral penumbras resulting from coulomb multiple scattering and the distal falloff—resulting from range straggling. Since both multiple scattering and range straggling are range (energy) dependent, proton dose distributions have three sides with depth-dependent dose gradients. Also, the depth dependence of the lateral penumbra is stronger than that of X-rays for water equivalent depths over about 17 cm; for shallower depths the proton lateral penumbra is generally smaller than that for X-rays. In general, each treatment beam must have its own margins that are dependent on the distance traveled by the beam in tissue. Therefore, expanding the clinical target volume to the planning target volume is not a straightforward process and depends strongly upon the beam direction is, therefore, beam dependent. Indeed, the concept of the planning target volume for proton treatment planning is not useful.

The most severe limitation of the proton therapy plans for passive scattering arises from the uniform width of the SOBP throughout the target volume, which results in some high-dose spillover into adjacent normal tissues. However, this problem is greatly reduced by the use of multiple beams and is completely eliminated by the use of spot scanning techniques and intensity-modulated treatment planning. With the advent of dynamic spot scanning techniques, proton therapy has taken an important step forward. As stated earlier in this chapter, spot scanning allows the application of intensity-modulated techniques in treatment planning and delivery, which substantially improves the proton dose distribution, as has been the case for IMRT in X-ray therapy.

IMPT plans are optimized with an "inverse" treatment-planning system, which is similar to the inverse planning for IMRT [32,33]. However, there is additional complexity in IMPT because the energy of each proton pencil beam, in addition to the intensity and dose of each beam, can be varied, which increases the number of degrees of freedom for optimization and the dose-shaping potential of the IMPT plans, but at the cost of both computational and treatment complexity.

With equal complexity of treatment plans, the IMPT plans will always be superior to IMRT plans, especially in the sparing of normal tissues. The coverage of the target volume can be quite similar for IMPT and IMRT. On average, IMRT plans have twice the integral dose of IMPT plans, which results in substantial sparing of critical tissues and organs with the IMPT plans [22].

Image-guided proton delivery

Proton dose distributions are highly localized because of the SOBP high-dose region that is followed by an abrupt falloff of the dose to a zero value. However, much of this advantage (compared with X-rays) can be lost if the treatment-planning process, patient setup, or delivery is not optimized, appropriate, and accurate. An error in the calculated range of the proton beam can either cause a portion of the distal target volume to receive no dose (if the range is too short) or cause an overdose to a critical structure (if the range is too long). The accuracy of the patient setup for treatment and of the treatment delivery is usually ensured by the use of onboard imaging and extensive monitoring and by the quality assurance of the beam-delivery process.

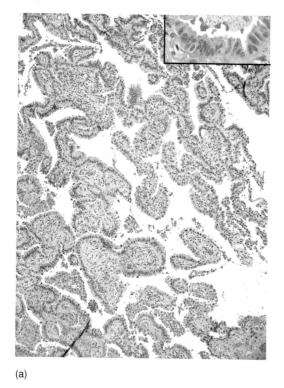

(a)

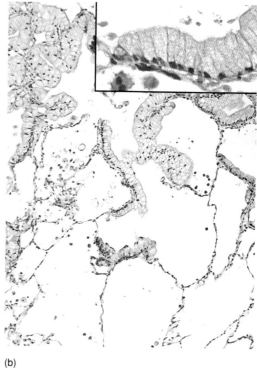

(b)

Figure 8.1 Bronchioloalveolar carcinoma. (a) Nonmucinous: There is some thickening of the alveolar septae but otherwise the alveolar architecture is intact. *Inset* shows tumor cell details at high magnification. The cells are columnar and eosinophilic cytoplasm and rounded apices.

(b) Mucinous: Mucinous tumor cells extend along the alveolar septae with preservation of alveolar architecture in a pattern referred to as "lepidic." *Inset* shows high magnification of tall columnar tumor cells with copious mucin in the apical cytoplasm.

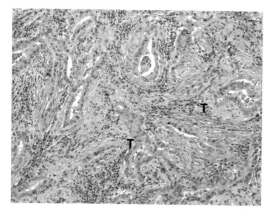

Plate 8.2 Complex microarchitecture of typical invasive carcinoma. Tubular structures (T) formed by tumor cells are surrounded by fibrous and plasmacytic stromal response.

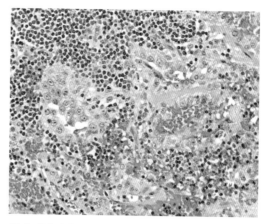

Plate 8.3 Adenocarcinoma surrounded and infiltrated by lymphocytes (tumor infiltrating lymphocytes, TIL).

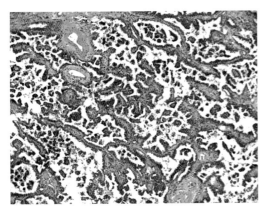

Plate 8.4 Low magnification photomicrograph depicting papillary carcinoma with complex papillae and epithelial tufts projecting into remnant alveolar spaces.

Plate 8.5 Mucinous carcinoma at low magnification showing a rim of epithelial cells on the edge of a fibrous band, all surrounding lakes of mucin.

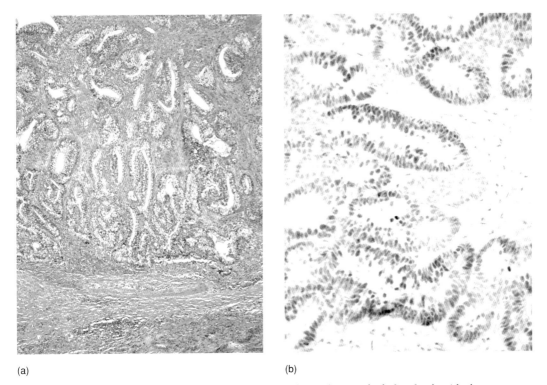

(a)   (b)

Plate 8.6 Low-grade fetal adenocarcinoma. H&E section (a) shows clusters of tubular glands with clear cytoplasm. The tumor is TTF-1 positive as indicated by the nuclear staining on the right (b).

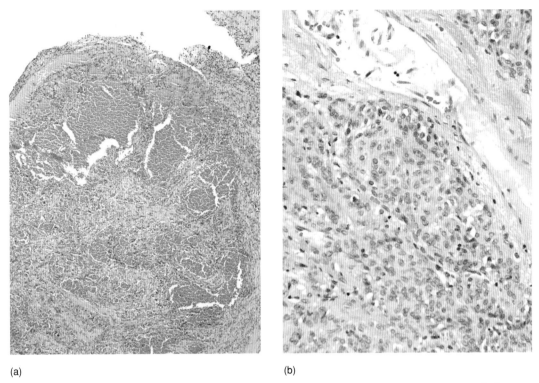

(a)

(b)

Plate 8.7 Sclerosing hemangioma. (a) Large blood filled spaces occupy a portion of the well-circumscribed mass along with (b) round to ovoid cells in solid centers of papillary clusters observed on the right that proved to be TTF-1 positive.

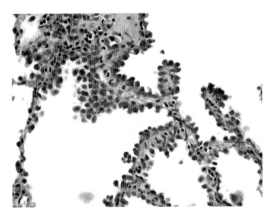

Plate 8.8 Atypical adenomatous hyperplasia. Low-grade type II-like cells line alveolar septae of small <5 mm lesion.

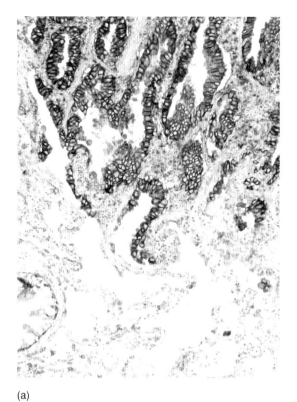

(a)   (b)

Plate 8.9 Candidate predictive markers for EGFR blockade in adenocarcinoma. (a) EGFR immunohistochemical
stain for EGFR produces heavy brown coloring of adenocarcinoma cells in upper part of frame. (b) EGFR FISH
image of pulmonary adenocarcinoma. Nuclei are shown
in blue (DAPI stain), centromeric probe for chromosome
7 is labeled in green and probe for the EGFR locus is labeled in red. Nuclei are large and adherent to each other
and contain large red clusters representing true amplification of the EGFR locus. Tumors with high levels of both
IHC and FISH markers are reported to have the greatest
survival benefit (see text). (Figure courtesy Dr Marileila
Varella-Garcia, University of Colorado, Denver, and Health
Sciences Center.)

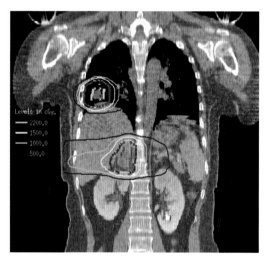

Plate 16.1 A 46-year-old with metastatic SCLC, s/p
five chemotherapy regimens, with persistent disease in
RLL and right adrenal. A single fraction of radiation
therapy to a dose of 22 Gy was delivered to these two
sites safely.

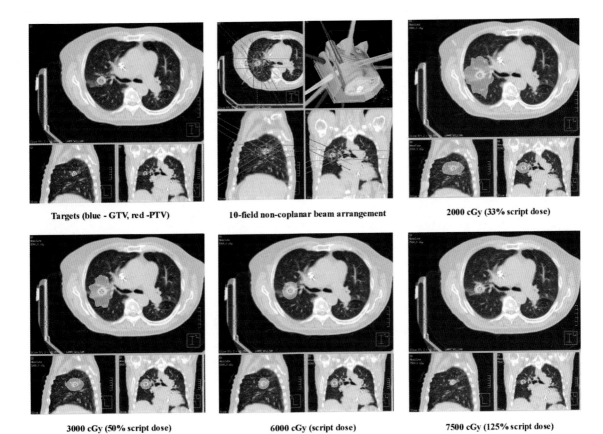

Targets (blue - GTV, red -PTV) **10-field non-coplanar beam arrangement** **2000 cGy (33% script dose)**

3000 cGy (50% script dose) **6000 cGy (script dose)** **7500 cGy (125% script dose)**

Plate 17.1 Targeting and dose construction for a typical SBRT treatment in the lung. Ten nonopposing and noncoplanar beams deliver radiation fluence to the demarcated tumor target with high dose delivery to the tumor and margin and rapid falloff in all directions.

118 MeV Proton Spot Beam used for IMPT

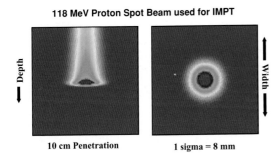

10 cm Penetration **1 sigma = 8 mm**

Plate 18.1 Typical dynamic spot scanning system.

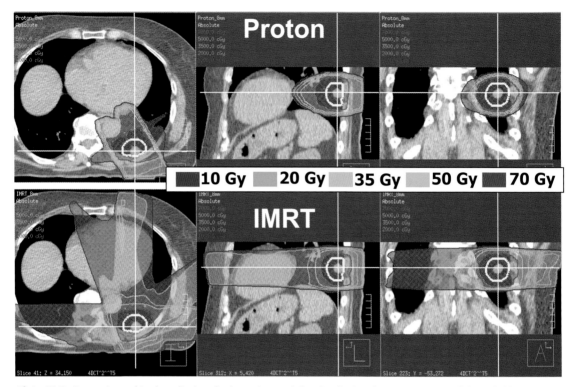

Plate 18.2 Comparison of isodose displays for intensity-modulated radiation therapy (IMRT) and three fields proton radiotherapy in a patient with stage I nonsmall cell lung cancer that was treated with 70 Gy. Orange contour: ITV.

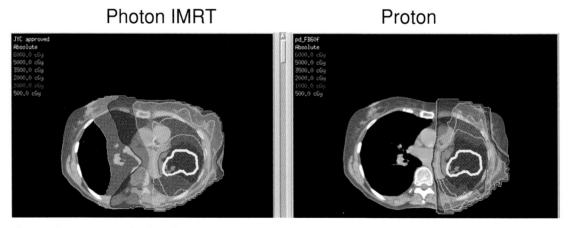

Plate 18.3 Comparison of isodose displays for photon intensity-modulated radiation therapy (IMRT) and three fields proton radiotherapy in a patient with stage III nonsmall cell lung cancer treated with 60 Gy. Orange contour: ITV.

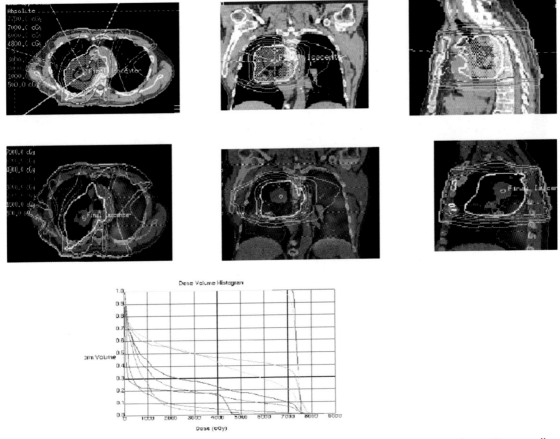

Plate 19.1 Typical dose–distribution and dose–volume histograms for use in planning treatment of stage III nonsmall cell lung cancer (NSCLC). Upper panel: intensity-modulated radiation therapy (IMRT) plan based on CT image; middle panel: IMRT plan based on lung SPECT image; lower panel: typical dose volume histogram.

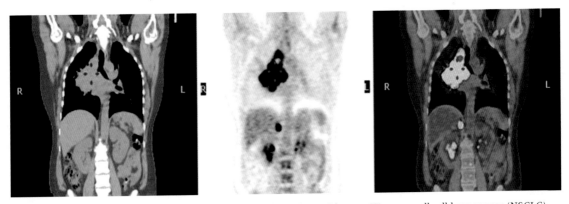

Plate 19.2 Positron emission tomography (PET) scans of a patient with stage IIIa nonsmall cell lung cancer (NSCLC). The scans incidentally demonstrate adrenal metastases

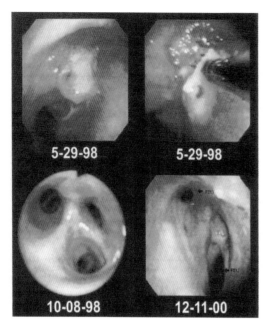

Plate 26.1 Right upper lobe tumor in a patient unable to be treated with surgery because of poor pulmonary function and ineligible for chemotherapy because of cardiac disease and obstructed bronchus (5/29/98). Patient was treated with three injections of *Ad-p53* (3 × 10^{11} viral particles) and radiation therapy (60 Gy) by bronchoscopy (5/29/98) with a complete response 3 months after completion of therapy (10/8/98) and no pathologic evidence of tumor 29 months after therapy (12/11/00). The patient died from a noncancer-related cause 2 years later.

Most proton treatment delivery systems contain three orthogonal imaging systems (X-ray tubes and flat-panel imagers), image analysis systems, and computerized couches with six degrees of freedom; with these technologies, stereotactic techniques can be used to accurately position the patient, correct for misalignments, and verify the treatment setup daily for each treatment field.

Substantially reduced normal tissue dose with proton therapy compared with 3D CRT and IMRT

As mentioned earlier, increasing evidence suggests that dose escalation of radiotherapy improves local disease control and survival rates in patients with NSCLC. Toxicity in normal tissues, especially in important organs such as the lungs, spinal cord, esophagus, and heart, limits the potential for dose escalation. In addition, secondary malignancy is another concern for patients whose lung cancer has been cured. As we know, 3D CRT, compared with 2D radiation therapy, has been shown to spare more normal tissues and to more effectively reduce toxicity in lung cancer patients. However, more improvement is needed to allow substantial dose escalation without increasing toxicity.

IMRT may offer the benefit of dose escalation without causing greater toxicity to surrounding normal tissue in selected patients with lung cancer [34–36]. The application of IMRT to the treatment of lung cancer, however, has been delayed because of general concerns and because IMRT may deliver low but damaging doses to a larger volume of normal lung tissue than would be affected by other treatments. The possible movement of a tumor due to respiration introduces another level of complexity to both the dosimetry and the technique used with IMRT [37,38]. However, our preliminary study showed that IMRT may allow greater dose escalation than 3D CRT without significantly increasing the incidence of adverse effects in selected patients with locally advanced disease and tumor motion of <5 mm [34,35,39,40].

We conducted a virtual clinical trial to compare dose–volume histograms (DVHs) in patients with either stage I or stage IIIA/B NSCLC treated with standard-dose 3D CRT or IMRT or with simple 3D (without IMPT) proton radiotherapy at standard or escalated doses [41]. We found that proton treatment improved the DVHs of all of the critical organs, particularly for the lungs, with about 10–20% absolute improvement. Proton treatment significantly reduced the dose to normal lungs, esophagus, spinal cord, and heart, even with dose escalation, compared with standard-dose photon therapy (Plates 18.2 and 18.3). In addition, there was a 33–60% absolute improvement of the nontarget integral dose with proton therapy. The reduction was more notable in stage I disease and in the contralateral lung. In stage I disease, proton therapy almost completely spared the contralateral lung and the heart, esophagus, and spinal cord (Plate 18.2). In stage III disease, after a dose escalation in photon 3D CRT from the conventional 63–74 Gy, 9 of 10 patients may have experienced considerable lung toxicity based on a lung V20 (the volume of total lung that received at least 20 Gy) of >35% or a mean total lung dose of >20 Gy [29–31]. In all patients receiving proton radiotherapy, however, even in patients in whom doses were escalated, the lung V20 was <35%. In both stage I and stage III disease, even when doses were escalated from 66 to 87.5 Gy for stage I and from 63 to 74 Gy for stage III, proton therapy improved normal tissue parameters, including the mean total lung V5, V10, V20, contralateral lung V5, integral dose, spinal cord maximum dose, and heart V40, compared with photon 3D CRT or IMRT at the conventional dose. This indicated that proton therapy with dose escalation and/or acceleration may translate to better local control and survival rates without increasing the toxicity in patients with NSCLC.

Another concern about IMRT is low-dose radiation exposure to normal lung. As our previous studies showed, IMRT increased the lung V5 in half of the patients we tested, compared with 3D CRT [34,35,40]. Our study demonstrated that proton therapy spared 15–17% of the total lung and that 19–23% of the contralateral lung received 5 Gy, compared with IMRT [41] (Plates 18.2 and 18.3). This finding shows that proton therapy, compared with IMRT, may substantially reduce lung toxicity.

Tumor motion consideration

Proton radiotherapy in lung cancer raises many important issues. Among the most challenging is tumor motion during treatment due to the patient's breathing [42–44]. The beating of the heart also causes tumor motion, but the magnitude is relatively small compared with the motion caused by respiration. Development of multislice detectors and faster imaging reconstruction has made it possible to image patients during breathing in real time and to assess organ motion using four-dimensional (4D) CT [42].

A more interesting and challenging application for 4D CT images is the planning of a 4D treatment, in which the actual dose distributions for free-breathing treatment can be calculated [45]. In this process, the dose distributions are calculated for each phase of the breathing cycle and then added by deformable image registration. Such composite dose distribution and DVHs demonstrate the actual dose that the patient receives from the treatment if the patient breathes in the same way as shown in the 4D CT images.

To ensure that all the cancer cells were adequately covered by the proton beam, we conducted 4D CT-based treatment planning to evaluate the proton dose volume distribution in target and in normal tissues. The internal target volume (ITV) was obtained by combining the gross tumor volumes at different phases of the respiratory cycle. We used the internal gross target volume (IGTV) created with maximal intensity projection (MIP) density for compensator design [43]. In our preliminary 4D treatment-planning study, the IGTV MIP density approach achieved a dose distribution similar to that actually delivered. Compared with the use of a large smearing margin in highly mobile lung tumors, as proposed by Moyers et al. [46], the IGTV MIP density approach achieved similar target coverage while sparing more normal tissue, since a uniformly large smearing margin was not used in the IGTV MIP density approach. Instead, individualized IGTV that was based on actual tumor motion was used for the compensator design [43]. This approach may slightly over-treat the normal tissues behind the tumor when the tumor moves out of the field, but it ensures that the whole tumor is treated adequately, no matter where it moves during the different breathing phases.

To reduce the effect of motion in proton therapy, particularly in IMPT, we conducted a 4D-based proton therapy virtual clinical study to determine the extent of improvement in normal tissue sparing with respiratory-gated proton beam radiotherapy compared with the free-breathing ITV approach in mobile lung cancers (Chang et al., October 2006 presentation at the Particle Therapy Co-operative Oncology Group, Houston). We found an approximate 25% relative reduction of total mean lung dose and a 5–7% absolute improvement of the V5, V10, and V20 in gated proton treatment compared with the ITV approach ($p < 0.002$). The maximal dose to the spinal cord, the esophageal V55, and the heart V40 were also significantly improved ($p < 0.03$). Patients treated with the respiratory-gating approach, especially those with substantial tumor motion (>10 mm), benefited more in normal tissue sparing than did those treated with the ITV approach. These data indicated that respiratory-gated proton radiotherapy, compared with the non-gated ITV approach, improved normal tissue sparing for the lung, heart, esophagus, and spinal cord. The gated treatment approach allows for further reduction in normal tissue toxicity and/or dose escalation or acceleration in patients with large tumor motion.

Clinical trials

Several proton radiotherapy clinical trials have been conducted in patients with NSCLC. These trials focused on dose-escalated or accelerated proton therapy in early-stage disease and showed promising clinical results that were comparable to surgical resection in stage IA cases.

Bush et al. [47] studied 68 patients with clinical stage I disease treated with 51 cobalt Gray equivalents (CGE) in 10 fractions over 2 weeks or with 60 CGE in 10 fractions over 2 weeks. No cases of symptomatic radiation pneumonitis or late esophageal or cardiac toxicity were seen. The 3-year local control and disease-specific survival rates were

74% and 72%, respectively. There was significant improvement in local tumor control in T1 (87%) and T2 (49%) tumors, with a trend toward improved survival rates. Local tumor control appeared to improve compared with historical results from conventional radiotherapy, with a good expectation of disease-specific survival 3 years after treatment. Currently, Bush *et al.* are conducting a phase I/II study with 70 CGE in 10 fractions in patients with stage I NSCLC.

Shioyama *et al.* [48] described 51 patients with NSCLC who were treated with proton therapy. The median fraction and total doses given were 3.0 Gy and 76.0 Gy, respectively. The 5-year overall survival rates were 70% for 9 stage IA patients and 16% for 19 stage IB patients ($p < 0.05$). The 5-year in-field local control rate was higher in patients with stage IA disease (89%) than in those with stage IB disease (39%). Forty-seven patients (92%) experienced acute lung toxicity of grade 1 or less; three had grade 2, one had grade 3, and none experienced grade 4 or higher toxicity. Patients in this study showed very little late toxicity.

Nihei *et al.* [49] recently reported the results from their preliminary study of 37 patients with stage I NSCLC who received 70–94 CGE delivered in 20 fractions. The 2-year progression-free survival and overall survival rates were 80% and 84%, respectively. The 2-year locoregional relapse-free survival rates in patients with stage IA and stage IB disease were 79% and 60%, respectively. No serious acute toxicity was observed, and only three patients developed grade 2/3 chronic lung toxicity.

These reported clinical studies indicated the safety and efficacy of proton therapy in early-stage NSCLC. However, the optimal regimen has not been well defined. In addition, simple 3D proton therapy was used in these studies; optimized proton therapy such as IMPT was not available, and image-guided radiotherapy was not strictly applied. Clinically, minimal data are available about proton therapy for patients with stage III NSCLC, the most common stage requiring radiotherapy.

At The University of Texas M. D. Anderson Cancer Center, we are conducting phase II clinical trials using image-guided proton radiotherapy for patients with NSCLC [40]. Twenty-three patients with medically inoperable stage I NSCLC and 56 patients with stage IIIA/B NSCLC will receive this therapy. Positron emission tomographic and CT studies will be used in all patients for both staging and treatment planning. We plan to deliver a total dose of 87.5 CGE in 2.5-CGE fractions for stage I disease and 74 CGE (2 CGE per fraction) with concurrent chemotherapy followed by adjuvant chemotherapy for stage III disease. In addition, a 4D CT study is required to plan for tumor motion and to decide on the treatment-delivery technique (free-breath ITV, breath-hold, or gated treatment). The IGTV MIP approach is being used for the compensator design.

We are studying the optimization of proton therapy with the appropriate management of uncertainties. Gated proton therapy and IMPT will be implemented soon. We plan to conduct randomized studies to compare IMRT with proton therapy using dose-escalated radiotherapy. In addition, stereotactic hypofractionated proton radiotherapy will be implemented for early stage NSCLC and will be compared with hypofractionated stereotactic photon-based body radiotherapy, particularly for centrally located early stage NSCLC.

Summary

The dose distributions of proton Bragg peaks led to superior treatment plans for proton therapy compared with X-ray therapy in reducing the radiation dose to normal tissues adjacent to the target, such as those of the esophagus, lung, heart, and spinal cord, and to intervening tissues in the path of the radiation beams. Preclinical and clinical research has supported the superiority of proton therapy. However, appropriate management of various sources of uncertainties in the planning and delivery of proton therapy is essential. Proton dose distributions may be perturbed more than photon dose distributions by anatomic variations and by organ or tumor motion. Radiobiological uncertainties may also play a greater role in proton therapy. Furthermore, in general, proton dose distributions for thoracic tumors may be substantially more inhomogeneous than photon dose distributions. Therefore, proton dose distributions are more challenging to optimize and evaluate.

Investigations of proton therapies such as IMPT may further improve the therapeutic ratio of proton treatment. For lung cancer, tumor motion must be considered and 4D CT planning is recommended. Gated proton treatment further improves normal tissue sparing. Onboard imaging such as cone beam CT will also be developed for proton treatment gantries and will lead to more accuracy in treatment delivery.

Because of the reductions in the "dose bath" and in the volume of normal tissues irradiated with proton therapy, patients' tolerance of radiation and/or chemoradiotherapy would be enhanced, allowing the delivery of higher doses of these treatments. These higher doses, combined with the increased accuracy in targeting and the greater avoidance of normal tissues, would lead to less toxicity and better local disease control and survival rates in patients with lung cancer. Combined proton therapy and novel systemic treatment such as molecular targeting treatment might bring a new future of lung cancer management.

References

1 Jemal A, Siegel R, Ward E *et al*. Cancer statistics. *CA Cancer J Clin* 2006; **56(2)**:106–30.

2 Kaskowitz L, Graham M, Emami B, Halverson K, Rush C. Radiation therapy alone for stage I non-small cell lung cancer. *Int J Radiat Oncol Biol Phys* 1993; **27**:517–23.

3 Dosoretz D, Katin M, Blitzer P *et al*. Medically inoperable lung carcinoma: the role of radiation therapy. *Semin Radiat Oncol* 1996; **6**:98–104.

4 Dosoretz D, Galmarini D, Rubenstein J *et al*. Local control in medically inoperable lung cancer: an analysis of its importance in outcome and factors determining the probability of tumor eradication. *Int J Radiat Oncol Biol Phys* 1993; **27**:507–16.

5 Curran W, Scott C, Langer C *et al*. Long term benefit is observed in a phae III comparison of sequential vs concurrent chemo-radiation for patients with unresectable NSCLC: RTOG 9410. *Proc ASCO* 2003; **22**:621a.

6 Rosenman J, Halle J, Socinski M *et al*. High-dose conformal radiotherapy for treatment of stage IIIA/IIIB non-small-cell lung cancer: technical issues and results of a phase I/II trial. *Int J Radiat Oncol Biol Phys* 2002; **54(2)**:348–56.

7 Kong F, Ten Haken R, Schipper M *et al*. High-dose radiation improved local tumor control and overall survival in patients with inoperable/unresectable non-small-cell lung cancer: long-term results of a radiation dose escalation study. *Int J Radiat Oncol Biol Phys* 2005; **63(2)**:324–33.

8 Choi N, Doucette J. Improved survival of patients with unresectable non-small-cell bronchogenic carcinoma by an innovated high-dose en-bloc radiotherapeutic approach. *Cancer*1981; **48**:101–9.

9 Bradley J, Paulus R, Graham M *et al*. Phase II trial of postoperative adjuvant paclitaxel/carboplatin and thoracic radiotherapy in resected stage II and III. A non-small-cell lung cancer: promising long-term results of the radiation therapy oncology group-RTOG 9705. *J Clin Oncol* 2005; **23(15)**:3480–7.

10 Perez C, Bauer M, Edelstein S, Gillespie B, Birch R. Impact of tumor control on survival in carcinoma of the lung treated with irradiation. *Int J Radiat Oncol Biol Phys* 1986; **12**:539–47.

11 Vijayakumar S, Myrianthopoulos L, Rosenberg I, Halpern H, Low N, Chen G. Optimization of radical radiotherapy with beam's eye view techniques for non-small cell lung cancer. *Int J Radiat Oncol Biol Phys* 1991; **21**:779–88.

12 Cox J, Azarnia N, Byhardt R, Shin K, Emami B, Pajak T. A randomized phase I/II trial of hyperfractionated radiation therapy with total doses of 60.0 Gy to 79.2 Gy: possible survival benefit with greater than or equal to 69.6 Gy in favorable patients with Radiation Therapy Oncology Group stage III non-small-cell lung carcinoma: report of Radiation Therapy Oncology Group 83-11. *J Clin Oncol* 1990; **8(9)**:1543–55.

13 Schild S, McGinnis W, Graham D *et al*. Results of a Phase I trial of concurrent chemotherapy and escalating doses of radiation for unresectable non-small-cell lung cancer. *Int J Radiat Oncol Biol Phys* 2006; **65(4)**:1106–11.

14 Belderbos J, Heemsbergen W, De Jaeger K, Baas P, Lebesque J. Final results of a Phase I/II dose escalation trial in non-small-cell lung cancer using three-dimensional conformal radiotherapy. *Int J Radiat Oncol Biol Phys* 2006; **66(1)**:126–34.

15 Mell L, Roeske J, Mundt A. A survey of intensity-modulated radiation therapy use in the United States. *Cancer* 2003; **98(1)**:204–11.

16 Miles E, Clark C, Urbano M *et al*. The impact of introducing intensity modulated radiotherapy into

routine clinical practice. *Radiother Oncol* 2005; **77(3)**: 241–6.

17 Bentzen S. Radiation therapy: intensity modulated, image guided, biologically optimized and evidence based. *Radiother Oncol* 2005; **77(3)**:227–30.

18 Lin A, Kim H, Terrell J, Dawson L, Ship J, Eisbruch A. Quality of life after parotid-sparing IMRT for head-and-neck cancer: a prospective longitudinal study. *Int J Radiat Oncol Biol Phys* 2003; **57(1)**:61–70.

19 Paganetti H, Niemierko A, Ancukiewicz M *et al.* Relative biological effectiveness (RBE) values for proton beam therapy. *Int J Radiat Oncol Biol Phys* 2002; **53(2)**:407–21.

20 Halperin E. Particle therapy and treatment of cancer. *Lancet Oncol* 2006; **7(8)**:676–85.

21 Baumann M. Keynote comment: radiotherapy in the age of molecular oncology. *Lancet Oncol* 2006; **7(10)**:786–7.

22 Lomax A, Bortfeld T, Goitein G *et al.* A treatment planning inter-comparison of proton and intensity modulated photon radiotherapy. *Radiother Oncol* 1999; **51(3)**:257–71.

23 Thames H, Schultheisis T, Henry J, Tucker S, Dubray B, Brock W. Can modest escalations of dose be detected as increased tumor control. *Int J Radiat Oncol Biol Phys* 1992; **22**:241.

24 Suit H, Goitein M, Munzenrider J *et al.* Increased efficacy of radiation therapy by use of proton beams. *Strahlentherapie* 1990; **166**:40–44.

25 Fowler J. What can we expect from dose escalation using protons beam? *Clin Oncol* 2003; **15(1)**:S10–5.

26 Hall E. Intensity-modulated radiation therapy, protons, and the risk of second cancers. *Int J Radiat Oncol Biol Phys* 2006; **65(1)**:1–7.

27 Kanai T, Kawachi K, Kumamoto Y *et al.* Spot scanning system for proton radiotherapy. *Med Phys* 1980; **7(4)**:365–9.

28 Goitein M, Lomax A, Pedroni E. Treating cancer with protons. *Phys Today* 2002; **55**:45–50.

29 Schneider U, Pedroni E, Lomax A. The calibration of CT Hounsfield units for radiotherapy treatment planning. *Phys Med Biol* 1996; **41**:111–24.

30 Kanematsu N, Matsufuji N, Kohno R, Minohara S, Kanai T. A CT calibration method based on the poly-binary tissue model for radiotherapy treatment planning. *Phys Med Biol* 2003; **48**:1053–64.

31 Chen G, Singh A. Treatment planning for heavy ion radiotherapy. *Int J Radiat Oncol Biol Phys* 1979; **5**:1809–19.

32 Oelfke U, Bortfeld T. Inverse planning for photon and proton beams. *Med Dosim* 2001; **26(2)**:113–24.

33 Bortfeld T. An analytical approximation of the Bragg curve for therapeutic proton beams. *Med Phys* 1997; **24**:2024–33.

34 Murshed H, Liu H, Liao Z *et al.* Dose and volume reduction for normal lung using intensity-modulated radiotherapy for advanced-stage non-small-cell lung cancer. *Int J Radiat Oncol Biol Phys* 2004; **58(4)**:1258–67.

35 Liu H, Wang X, Dong L *et al.* Feasibility of sparing lung and other thoracic structures with intensity-modulated radiotherapy for non-small-cell lung cancer. *Int J Radiat Oncol Biol Phys* 2004; **58(4)**: 1268–79.

36 Grills I, Yan D, Martinez A, Vicini F, Wong J, Kestin L. Potential for reduced toxicity and dose escalation in the treatment of inoperable non-small-cell lung cancer: a comparison of intensity-modulated radiation therapy (IMRT), 3D conformal radiation, and elective nodal irradiation. *Int J Radiat Oncol Biol Phys* 2003; **57(3)**:875–90.

37 Chui C, Yorke E, Hong L. The effects of intra-fraction organ motion on the delivery of intensity-modulated field with a multileaf collimator. *Med Phys* 2003; **30(7)**:1736–46.

38 Bortfeld T, Jokivarsi K, Goitein M, Kung J, Jiang S. Effects of intra-fraction motion on IMRT dose delivery: statistical analysis and simulation. *Phys Med Biol* 2002; **47(13)**:2203–20.

39 Yom SS, Liao Z, Hu C *et al.* Preliminary report of radiation pneumonitis (RP) in patients with non-small cell lung cancer (NSCLC) treated with intensity modulated radiotherapy (IMRT) and concurrent chemotherapy (ConChT). *Int J Radiat Oncol Biol Phys* 2005; **63(Suppl 1)**:S407.

40 Chang J, Liu H, Komaki R. Intensity modulated radiation therapy and proton radiotherapy for non-small cell lung cancer. *Curr Oncol Rep* 2005; **7**:255–9.

41 Chang J, Zhang X, Wang X *et al.* Significant reduction of normal tissue dose by proton radiotherapy compared with three-dimensional conformal or intensity-modulated radiation therapy in Stage I or Stage III non-small-cell lung cancer. *Int J Radiat Oncol Biol Phys* 2006; **65(4)**:1087–96.

42 Liu H, Wei X, Jang S. Impact of respiratory motion on dose distributions and DVHs of thoracic structures-evaluation using 4DCT. *Med Phys* 2005; **32(6)**:1924.

43 Kang Y, Zhang X, Wang H. Proton treatment planning for mobile lung tumors. *Med Phys* 2005; **32(6)**:2144.

44 Chang J, Dong L, Mohan R, Liao Z, Cox J, Komaki R. Image-guided proton radiotherapy for medically inoperable stage I non-small cell lung cancer. *Int J Radiat Oncol Biol Phys* 2005; **63(2)**:S41.

45 Engelsman M, Rietzel E, Kooy H. Four-dimensional proton treatment planning for lung tumors. *Int J Radiat Oncol Biol Phys* 2006; **64(5)**:1589–95.

46 Moyers M, Miller D, Bush D, Slater J. Methodologies and tools for proton beam design for lung tumors. *Int J Radiat Oncol Biol Phys* 2001; **49(5)**:1429–38.

47 Bush D, Slater J, Shin B, Cheek G, Miller D, Slater J. Hypofractionated proton beam radiotherapy for stage I lung cancer. *Chest* 2004; **126(4)**:1198–203.

48 Shioyama Y, Tokuuye K, Okumura T *et al.* Clinical evaluation of proton radiotherapy for non-small-cell lung cancer. *Int J Radiat Oncol Biol Phys* 2003; **56(1)**:7–13.

49 Nihei K, Ogino T, Ishikura S, Nishimura H. High-dose proton beam therapy for Stage I non-small-cell lung cancer. *Int J Radiat Oncol Biol Phys* 2006; **65(1)**:107–11.

CHAPTER 19

Combinations of Radiation Therapy and Chemotherapy for Nonsmall Cell Lung Carcinoma

Zhongxing Liao, Frank V. Fossella, and Ritsuko Komaki

Introduction

Many patients with nonsmall cell lung cancer (NSCLC) are unable to undergo surgical resection with curative intent. This has compelled oncologists to reconsider alternative treatment strategies. In many cases, palliative radiation therapy (RT) or chemotherapy or enrollment in clinical trials may be appropriate. For a select population, especially those patients who have no evidence of distant metastasis, few symptoms of disease (good performance status), and minimal weight loss, therapy with curative intent is appropriate.

What is the potential for cure in these cases? This is one of the most important questions for patients and physicians alike, and the answer is changing rapidly in light of findings from recent clinical trials of combination radiation therapy and chemotherapy.

Rationale for combining radiation therapy and chemotherapy

A thorough review of the preclinical evidence for combining chemotherapy and radiation therapy is

beyond the scope of this chapter. However, excellent reviews are provided by Hill and Bellamy [1] and John *et al.* [2]. The clinical relevance of the preclinical data is tenuous because of variations in dose–fractionation schedules (single versus multiple), treatment sequence, timing, drug dosage, drug delivery methods, and the duration of drug exposure in the clinical setting. Nonetheless, a few generalizations can be made. Of the four possible ways to improve therapeutic effect proposed by Steel *et al.* [3] (i.e., toxicity independence, normal tissue protection, spatial cooperation, and tumor response enhancement), only spatial cooperation and tumor response enhancement find consistent clinical expression in NSCLC. The virtues of spatial cooperation (i.e., radiation therapy for the local–regional tumor and chemotherapy for metastases) are obvious; those of tumor response enhancement, less so. Terms such as *radiation sensitization* may have different meanings for different investigators. We prefer the terminology suggested by Steel and Peckham [4] (Figure 19.1). Despite preclinical in vitro evidence that irradiated tumor cells become more resistant to certain drugs [5], this phenotype does not include multidrug resistance. The cellular responses to other drugs may remain unchanged, or sensitivity to them may be enhanced.

Clinically, the empirical rationale for combining radiation therapy and chemotherapy is the all-too-frequent failure of either modality to effect a cure

Lung Cancer, 3rd edition. Edited by Jack A. Roth, James D. Cox, and Waun Ki Hong. © 2008 Blackwell Publishing, ISBN: 978-1-4051-5112-2.

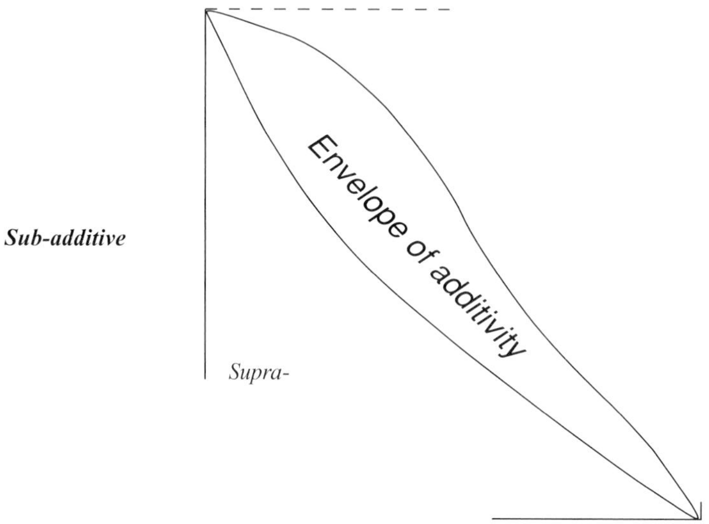

Figure 19.1 An *isobologram* is an isoeffect plot of the doses of two agents that together give a fixed biological effect. If dose–response curves are nonlinear, there is a region of uncertainty about the existence of "additivity." (Reproduced with permission of the *International Journal of Radiation Oncology, Biology, Physics*, from Steel and Peckham [4].)

when administered by itself. They do not fail for the same reasons. Radiation therapy alone often fails to treat distant subclinical metastases. Chemotherapy alone often fails to eradicate bulky, unresectable tumors. In the early days of cytotoxic chemotherapy, some had hoped that it would eventually become effective enough to eliminate both local and metastatic disease. However, in the case of far more sensitive tumors such as small cell lung cancer (SCLC) and strikingly chemosensitive diseases such as malignant lymphoma, it soon became apparent that maximum control of bulky tumors would require additional local treatment. Thus, chemotherapy alone is unlikely to adequately treat NSCLC.

In most patients with unresectable NSCLC, the actual cause of death is a local tumor that has been treated either inadequately or not at all. This is supported by strong clinical evidence. First, several studies have shown that tumor progression within the field of irradiation is associated with poorer survival among patients who receive RT alone as opposed to patients who receive RT after local tumor control has been achieved [6–8]. Second, patients who receive only palliative RT or single-agent chemotherapy die more frequently of intrathoracic disease than of extrathoracic metastasis [9], especially if the tumor is a squamous cell carcinoma. Third, as Saunders *et al.* discovered while studying

causes of death in patients whose localized but unresectable NSCLCs were treated with a few large fractions of radiation, many more patients died of local intrathoracic tumor complications than died of distant metastasis (72% versus 15%) [10]. Conversely, Perez *et al.* [11] showed that improved local tumor control was associated with an increased incidence of distant metastasis. Finally, as Schaake-Konning *et al.* have shown, concurrent chemotherapy and radiation therapy improves local tumor control, which in turn improves survival [12] (*vide infra*).

Induction chemotherapy before radiotherapy

Induction chemotherapy before RT has two attractive features. First, it permits the most immediate attack on all components of the tumor: both those evident clinically and those presumed to be present at subclinical levels. Second, if systemic chemotherapy elicits a response, then its continuation during or after RT is justified. Although overall survival in several prospective randomized clinical trials has been mixed, the overall survival has been favorable in three particular trials of cisplatin-based chemotherapy and continuous irradiation to total doses of 60 Gy or more (Table 19.1) [13–17].

Table 19.1 Trials of sequential chemotherapy and radiation therapy for locally advanced nonsmall cell lung cancer.

First author, year [ref.]	Number of patients	RT (Gy)	CT	MST (mo)	LRC (%) 3 yr	LRC (%) 5 yr	OS (%) 3 yr	OS (%) 5 yr
Dillman et al., 1996 [13]	77	60	—	9.7	6	5	11	7
	79	60	PV	13.8	18	6 ($p = 0.026$)	23	19 ($p = 0.012$)
Brodin et al., 1996 [14]	164	56 (SC)	—	N/R	N/R	3 (4 yr)	6	1.4
	163	56 (SC)	CE	N/R	N/R	7 (4 yr) ($p = 0.07$)	13	3 ($p = 0.16$)
Morton et al., 1991 [15]	58	60	—	9.6	N/R	N/R	N/R	7
	56	60	MACC	10.4	N/R	N/R	N/R	5
Le Chevalier et al., 1992 [16]	177	65	—	10.0	17 (1 yr)	N/R	4	3
	176	65	VCPC	12.0	15 (1 yr)	N/R	12	6 ($p < 0.02$)
Sause et al., 2000 [17]	149	60	—	11.4	N/R	N/R	11	5
	151	60	PV	13.2	N/R	N/R	17	8
	152	69.6 (bid)	—	12	N/R	N/R	14	6 ($p = 0.04$)

CT, chemotherapy; LRC, local–regional control; MACC, methotrexate, doxorubicin, cyclophosphamide, lomustine; MST, median survival time; N/R, not reported; OS, overall survival; PV, cisplatin, vinblastine; RT, radiation therapy; SC, split course; bid, 1.2 Gy twice daily; VCPC, vindesine, cyclophosphamide, cisplatin, lomustine.

Together, these three trials, whose results are discussed below, provide a basis for future trials.

The most well known of the three trials was reported by the Cancer and Leukemia Group B (CALGB) and showed a clear survival advantage for induction chemotherapy. Called CALGB 8433 [18], this trial compared two treatment regimens. Patients in one treatment arm received induction therapy with cisplatin (100 mg/m^2 on days 1 and 29) and vinblastine (5 mg/m^2 weekly for 5 weeks) followed by RT (2.0 Gy/fraction, 5 days/week, to a total dose of 60 Gy) beginning on day 50; those in the other treatment arm received only the RT from day 1. This trial was closed before the planned accrual was reached because the improvement in survival on the induction chemotherapy arm met the study's early stopping rules. Patients in the induction chemotherapy arm had superior median and 5-year survivals and continued to enjoy a survival benefit on long-term follow-up [13]. However, failure patterns in this trial have not been analyzed, and the CALGB has given no indication that local tumor control improved with induction chemotherapy.

The encouraging results of the CALGB trial were validated by a second trial conducted in 353 patients by Le Chevalier's French cooperative group [16,19,20]. As in the earlier CALGB trial, patients were randomly assigned to undergo either induction chemotherapy followed by RT or RT alone. Those in the induction chemotherapy arm received 3 monthly cycles of vindesine (1.5 mg/m^2 on days 1–2), cyclophosphamide (200 mg/m^2 on days 2–4), cisplatin (100 mg/m^2 on day 2), and lomustine (75 mg/m^2 on day 3) followed by RT (daily 2.5-Gy fractions, 4 days/week, to a total dose of 65 Gy) beginning on day 75–80; those in the other arm received only the RT. Survival improved on the induction chemotherapy arm. Moreover, the incidence of distant metastasis was significantly reduced, although there was no accompanying improvement in local tumor control. In fact, because of its policy of performing systematic fiberoptic bronchoscopy and biopsy at the site of the original lesions 3 months after the start of treatment, the French group was able to demonstrate high treatment failure rates at tumor sites (>80%) in both treatment arms and no advantage for induction chemotherapy in terms of local control.

These results led the Radiation Therapy Oncology Group (RTOG) and the Eastern Cooperative

Oncology Group (ECOG) to conduct a cooperative three-arm trial (RTOG 88-08, ECOG 4588) comparing survival rates of standard RT, sequential chemoradiation therapy (i.e., the CALGB regimen), and hyperfractionated radiotherapy (to a total dose of 69.6 Gy) [17,21]. Sequential chemoradiation therapy was found to be statistically significantly superior to both standard RT and hyperfractionated RT, while standard RT and hyperfractionated RT were found to be essentially similar in effect. Later, in a study of failure patterns among the patients in this trial [22], Komaki *et al.* found that control of distant metastasis improved only in patients who had squamous cell carcinomas chemotherapy and that chemotherapy had no influence of on the local tumor, a finding consistent with that of the French trial.

After completing their CALGB trial, Dillman and associates [13,18] later conducted a retrospective quality-control review of the trial data and found that, in a relatively large proportion of cases (23%), radiation fields failed to completely encompass the primary tumor. In addition, all of the induction chemotherapy-RT trials discussed above utilized two-dimensional (2D) radiation therapy for treatment planning.

In light of the induction chemotherapy-RT trials to date, several assumptions can be made. Chemotherapy is important to the success of such regimens [23]. Chemotherapy, perhaps selectively, can control the distant metastatic spread of squamous cell carcinoma. Primary tumor control within the field of irradiation is poorer than originally thought, and induction chemotherapy offers no further benefit in that regard.

Concurrent chemotherapy and radiation therapy

Further efforts to improve local control and reduce distant metastasis have led investigators to pursue other strategies including concurrent cisplatin-based chemotherapy and RT, combination of chemotherapy and hyperfractionated RT, and combination of new chemotherapeutic and molecular targeting agents with RT. The specific rationale for adding a single chemotherapeutic agent to RT is to increase local tumor control.

Concurrent single-agent chemotherapy and radiation therapy

Few, if any, advocates of single-agent chemotherapy would suggest that concurrent single-agent chemotherapy and RT is the best approach to controlling distant metastasis. Nevertheless, in a very important trial from the European Organization for Research and Treatment of Cancer (EORTC), Schaake-Konning *et al.* [12] compared RT alone, RT plus weekly cisplatin (30 mg/m^2), and RT plus daily cisplatin (6 mg/m^2). Two features of this trial are important to note. First, the same total dose of cisplatin was given in both arms of the study. Second, the RT fractionation schedule used (3.0 Gy in 10 fractions, 5 days/week, for 2 weeks; a 3- to 4-week interruption; and finally 2.5 Gy in 10 fractions, 5 fractions/week, for 2 weeks) would not be considered standard in the United States. In fact, in light of studies from the RTOG [24], the overall increase in time needed to deliver this total radiation dose might even be considered a disadvantage. Nonetheless, both of the cisplatin-containing regimens improved local tumor control, which was in turn reflected in significantly better overall survival (Figure 19.2).

Concurrent combination chemotherapy and radiation therapy

The most aggressive approach to treating unresectable NSCLC tumors is concurrent combination chemotherapy and RT. The rationale for this approach comes from a prospective randomized comparative trial conducted by the EORTC [12] and from a meta-analysis suggesting that only cisplatin-based regimens are beneficial in a combined approach [23].

The RTOG has conducted several pilot studies of the concurrent approach, using tolerance (hematologic and nonhematologic) and short-term survival as endpoints. The RTOG has not used response rates as an endpoint because (a) they do not predict survival in NSCLC and (b) they are meaningless in the context of concurrent therapy. Survival in the RTOG studies has varied widely in the face of

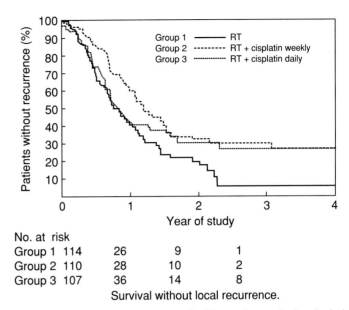

No. at risk
Group 1 114   26   9   1
Group 2 110   28   10   2
Group 3 107   36   14   8

Survival without local recurrence.

The time to local recurrence was significanty longer in the cisplatin groups (*p* = 0.015; overall). For the comparison of group 2 with group 1, *p* = 0.15; group 3 with group 1, *p* = 0.003; group 2 with group 3, *p* = 0.17; and group 1 with groups 2 and 3, *p* = 0.009

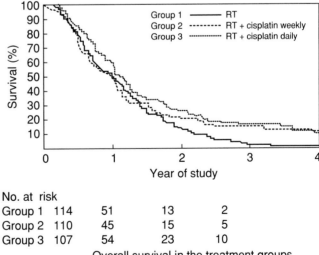

No. at risk
Group 1 114   51   13   2
Group 2 110   45   15   5
Group 3 107   54   23   10

Overall survival in the treatment groups.

The four-year point denotes survival as of May 1991, for which *p* = 0.054 overall. Kaplan–Meier analysis showed that for the comparison of group 2 with group 1, *p* = 0.36; group 3 with group 1, *p* = 0.009; group 2 with group 3, *p* = 0.20; and group 1 with groups 2 and 3, *p* = 0.04. RT denotes radiotherapy.

Figure 19.2 Survival without local recurrence (upper panel) and overall survival (lower panel) in a European Organization for Research and Treatment of Cancer (EORTC) trial comparing RT alone, RT plus weekly cisplatin, and RT plus daily cisplatin. (Reproduced with permission of the *New England Journal of Medicine*, from Schaake-Konning *et al*. [12].)

strongly determinant pretreatment prognostic factors. However, recursive partitioning analyses of the large RTOG database have helped to identify suitable groups of patients in which to compare outcomes across studies and thus select regimens for comparison in phase III trials, which provide the only rational basis on which to justify changes in standard practice in treating this disease. The major prognostic variables identified so far in RTOG studies are Karnofsky performance status [25], weight loss, and extent of nodal disease (N).

The first RTOG trial of concurrent combination chemotherapy and RT was reported by Byhardt *et al.* [26]. Designated RTOG 90-15, this trial combined the cisplatin-vinblastine regimen from the CALGB 8433 trial and a regimen of hyperfractionated RT (69.6 Gy delivered in 1.2-Gy fractions twice daily, 5 days/week) that had been chosen for its superiority in light of a recent dose-seeking study by Cox *et al.* [27]. Although few patients in the RTOG 90-15 trial had favorable prognostic factors, their median survival was an encouraging 12.2 months [26]. It should also be noted that, while the RTOG 90-15 trial was ongoing, this hyperfractionated RT regimen was simultaneously being compared with standard fractionation in the RTOG 88-08 and ECOG 4588 trials.

A successor trial to RTOG 90-15, designated RTOG 91-06, employed the same design but advanced the hypothesis that oral etoposide given daily during much of the RT period would be a more effective addition to cisplatin than vinblastine [28]. In brief, cisplatin (75 mg/m^2 IV on days 1 and 29) and etoposide (50 mg PO twice daily on days 1–14 and days 29–43) were given with hyperfractionated RT, also beginning on day 1. The toxicity of this combined regimen, especially to the esophagus, was considerable. However, its effect on survival was remarkable. For patients with favorable prognostic factors, the median survival was 21 months, and the 2-year survival rate was 42%. Corroborative results were obtained in a contemporary French trial, reported by Reboul *et al.* from Avignon [29], that employed a similar chemotherapy regimen but a more standard RT fractionation schedule.

To reduce the severity of the RTOG 91-06 regimen's acute effects, the chemotherapy schedule was slightly modified for use in a subsequent phase I/II trial designated RTOG 92-04 [30]. In brief, etoposide (50 mg PO) was omitted on the weekends, when irradiation was not given, thus reducing from 28 to 20 the total number of days on which etoposide was administered. The results were mixed. Although use of the modified chemotherapy regimen lowered the risk of chemotherapy-induced nonhematologic toxicity, it did so at the price of a higher in-field tumor progression rate. Moreover, median survival and 1-year survival rates did not significantly improve (15.5 mo versus 14.1 mo and 65% versus 58%, respectively).

Table 19.2 shows the results of five randomized phase III trials of concurrent chemotherapy and RT versus RT alone [12,31–34]. In three of them, concurrent therapy offered a survival advantage; 1-year survival rates were 73% in two of these three trials. However, toxicity was considerable. Approximately one third of the patients who received the concurrent therapy experienced grade ≥ 3 acute toxicity, including hematologic and gastrointestinal (esophageal) sequelae and pneumonitis [28,35]. In one of the trials, patients who were randomly assigned to an intensified regimen of hyperfractionated RT (to a total dose of 64.8 Gy) and weekly chemotherapy (carboplatin and VP-16) had a 5-year survival rate of 21% [35]. In light of the observed treatment toxicities, the benefit, if any, of adding hyperfractionated RT in this setting remains unclear.

Sequential versus concurrent chemotherapy and radiotherapy

The optimal sequence of treatment in patients with unresected stage III NSCLC but good performance status has been studied in six randomized trials to date (Table 19.3). Except for the RTOG 94-10 trial, whose results have only been reported in abstract form, all of these trials have been reported in full [36–41].

Three of these trials [36–38,40] employed cisplatin-based chemotherapy in their concurrent therapy regimen and demonstrated a significant survival benefit for that approach. One of these trials, the large RTOG 94-10 trial, evaluated combinations of cisplatin and vinblastine [37,42] in 611 patients randomly assigned to three chemoradiation

Table 19.2 Trials of concurrent chemotherapy and radiation therapy for locally advanced nonsmall cell lung cancer.

First author, year [ref.]	Number of patients	CT	RT (Gy)	MST (mo)	LRC (%) 3 yr	LRC (%) 5 yr	OS (%) 3 yr	OS (%) 5 yr
Trovo et al., 1992 [31]	88	—	45	10.3	11	N/R	8	N/R
	85	CDDP (weekly)	45	9.97	8	N/R	8	N/R
Blanke et al., 1995 [32]	111	—	60–65	11.5	67	N/R	3	2
	104	CDDP (weekly)	60–65	10.6	69	N/R	9	5 ($p = 0.25$)
Schaake-Konning et al., 1992 [12]	108	—	55	N/R	19 (2 yr)	N/R	2	N/R
	98	CDDP (weekly)	55	N/R	30 (2 yr)	N/R	13	N/R
	102	CDDP (daily)	55	N/R	31 (2 yr)	N/R	16 ($p = 0.009$)	N/R
Jeremic et al., 1996 [33]	56	—	64.8 (HF)	8	N/R	N/R	6.6	4.9
	78	CBP, VP-16 (weeks 1, 3, and 5)	64.8 (HF)	13	N/R	N/R	16	16
Groen et al., 2004 [34]	82	—	60	N/R	38 (2 yr)	N/R	28 (2 yr)	N/R
		CBP (daily)	60	N/R	35 (2 yr)	N/R	20 (2 yr)	N/R

CBP, carboplatin; CDDP, cisplatin; CT, chemotherapy; HF, hyperfractionated (1.2 Gy twice daily); LRC, local–regional control; MST, median survival time; N/R, not reported; OS, overall survival; RT, radiation therapy.

treatment arms: sequential chemotherapy and RT (the CALGB regimen), concurrent chemotherapy and daily fractionated RT, and concurrent chemotherapy and hyperfractionated RT [37]. The first two treatment arms called for cisplatin and vinblastine; the third treatment arm called for cisplatin and oral VP-16. The median survival times on the three treatment arms were 14.6, 17, and 15.6 months, respectively. Moreover, the 4-year survival rate was significantly better on the daily fractionated concurrent chemoradiation arm than on the hyperfractionated radiation arm (21% versus 12%; $p = 0.046$), thus favoring concurrent therapy with single daily fractions during early follow-up. Early acute toxicity was a problem, occurring more frequently on the two concurrent treatment arms and most frequently on the concurrent hyperfractionated treatment arm (30% versus 48% versus 62%). In contrast, late toxicity occurred with similar frequency on all three arms.

The second of these cisplatin-based trials, a Japanese multicenter trial reported by Furuse et al., employed a combination of mitomycin, vindesine, and cisplatin [36]. Patients were randomly assigned to receive (a) concurrent therapy involving two

cycles of MVP (mitomycin, vindesine, and cisplatin) every 28 days along with split-course RT (total dose of 56 Gy) or (b) sequential therapy involving two cycles of MVP followed by continuous-course RT (total dose of 56 Gy). (It should be noted that this trial was criticized by some for including split-course RT in the concurrent therapy and for using lower total doses of radiation.) The median survival times were 16.5 versus 13.3 months, and the 5-year survival rates were 19% versus 9% ($p = 0.04$) (Figure 19.3). In a subsequent report, Furuse et al. suggested that patterns of relapse may have differed between the two treatment arms (i.e., more frequent local recurrence only and distant recurrence with or without local recurrence on the sequential schedule and more frequent brain-only recurrence on the concurrent schedule) [43].

In the third cisplatin-based trial referred to above [38], 102 patients with stage IIIa/IIIb NSCLC were randomly assigned to receive (a) concurrent or (b) sequential therapy involving four cycles of cisplatin (80 mg/m^2 on day 1) and vinorelbine (25 mg/m^2 during the first and fourth cycles and 12.5 mg/m^2 during the second and third cycles) on days 1, 8, and 15 of a 28-day cycle combined with RT

Table 19.3 Randomized trials of sequential versus concurrent chemoradiation therapy.

First author, year [ref.]	Number of patients	CT	RT	Median survival (mo)	OS (%) 3 yr	OS (%) 5 yr
Furuse et al., 1999 [36]	158	MVP → RT	56 Gy	13	27.4	10.1
	156	MVP/RT	56 Gy (split)	17	34.6	17.9 ($p = 0.046$)
Fournel et al., 2005 [40]	101	CDDP/VNR → RT	66 Gy	14.5	18.6	14.2 (4 yr)
	100	CDDP/Etopo + RT → CDDP/VNR	66 Gy	16.3	24.8 ($p = 0.41$)	20.7 (4 yr)
Zatloukal et al., 2004 [38]	50	CDDP/Nav → RT	60 Gy	12.9	9.5	N/R
	52	CDDP/Nav/RT → CDDP/Nav	60 Gy	16.6	18.6 ($p = 0.0225$)	N/R
Belani et al., 2005 [41]	91	Paclitaxel/CBP → RT	63 Gy	13.0	17	N/R
	74	Paclitaxel/CBP → Paclitaxel/CBP/RT	63	12.7	15	N/R
	92	Paclitaxel/CBP/RT → Paclitaxel/CBP	63	16.3	17	N/R
Huber et al., 2006 [39]	115	Paclitaxel/CBP → RT	60	14.1	16.8	2*
Curran, 2005 [37]	205	CDDP/VBL → RT	60 Gy	14.6	31	N/R
	203	CDDP/VBL/RT	60 Gy	17	37	N/R
	203	CDDP/Etopo/RT	69.6 Gy (HFRT)	15.6	37	N/R

*Estimated from reported survival graphs.

CBP, carboplatin; CDDP, cisplatin; CT, chemotherapy; Etopo, etoposide; HFRT, hyperfractionated radiotherapy (1.2 Gy twice daily); MVP, mitomycin, vinidesine, cisplatin; Nav, navelbine; N/R, not reported; RT, radiation therapy; VBL, vinblastine; VNR, vinorelbine.

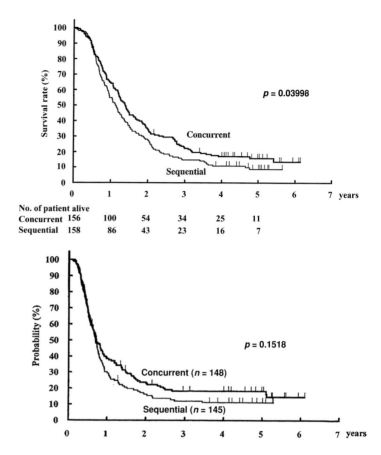

Figure 19.3 Overall (upper panel) and failure-free (lower panel) survival in patients with nonsmall cell lung cancer (NSCLC) according to treatment group. (Reproduced with permission of the *Journal of Clinical Oncology*, from Furuse *et al.* [36].)

(30 fractions to a total dose of 60 Gy). The main difference between treatment groups was that the concurrent group started RT on day 4 of cycle 2, while the sequential group started RT within 2 weeks after completion of chemotherapy. Overall, the concurrent therapy resulted in significantly better median survival time (16.6 mo versus 12.9 mo, $p = 0.023$), an especially notable improvement given the small number of patients studied, and significantly better median time to progression (11.9 mo versus 8.5 mo, $p = 0.024$). Unfortunately, concurrent therapy also markedly increased the frequency of grade ≥ 3 nausea or vomiting (39% versus 15%), leukopenia (53% versus 19%), and esophagitis (18% versus 4%).

A fourth cisplatin-based trial, a French multicenter study, employed a chemotherapy regimen of cisplatin and vinorelbine [40]. Two hundred five patients were randomly assigned to either sequential or concurrent therapy. The sequential treatment arm consisted of induction therapy with cisplatin (120 mg/m^2) on days 1, 29, and 57 and vinorelbine (30 mg/m^2/wk) on days 1–78, followed by thoracic RT (total dose of 66 Gy in 33 fractions of 2 Gy each, 5 fractions/week). The concurrent treatment arm consisted of the same RT regimen, starting on day 1; two concurrent cycles of cisplatin (20 mg/m^2/day) and etoposide (50 mg/m^2/day) given on days 1–5 and days 29–33; and consolidation therapy with cisplatin (80 mg/m^2) on days 78 and 106 and vinorelbine (30 mg/m^2/wk) from day 78 to 127. Three-year and 4-year survival rates improved on the concurrent treatment arm, though not significantly. However, early mortality was high on both treatment arms. The fact that most of these deaths were due to disease progression suggests that the trial may have included a negatively selected patient population. In addition, the excess of treatment-related deaths on the concurrent treatment arm was apparently due to massive pulmonary hemoptysis. As this specific toxicity was not observed in any of the other trials that used high radiation doses of approximately 65 Gy, this finding may have been due in part to differences in the pre-existing comorbidity profiles of the two treatment groups.

The other two trials of sequential versus concurrent chemotherapy and RT investigated a two-drug combination of carboplatin and the newer drug paclitaxel [39,41]. Neither trial showed any significant improvement in overall survival due to concurrent therapy.

Further support for the use of cisplatin-based chemoradiation therapy protocols comes from the randomized, multicenter North American Intergroup trial 0139 (INT 0139/RTOG 9309), a recently reported landmark study that has introduced this treatment strategy into broad clinical practice [44]. This trial confirmed the curative efficacy of a cisplatin-based chemoradiation protocol in a large, though selective, patient population.

Together, the evidence from these multicenter clinical trials warrants use of concurrent chemoradiation therapy protocols that include a cisplatin-based combination chemotherapy regimen. This approach gives the best 5-year survival results and is a curative treatment option for patients with inoperable stage IIIA or IIIB NSCLC.

Concurrent combination chemotherapy and radiation therapy followed by resection

Another concurrent approach of interest is induction chemotherapy and RT followed by surgical resection. This approach makes sense in patients whose disease might be considered resectable by one group of thoracic surgeons but unresectable by another and in patients who are willing to accept the operative risks. Unfortunately, most trials of this approach to date have not clearly defined the subsets of stage IIIA N2 NSCLC that might be

amenable to this approach, nor have they clearly defined eligibility criteria. There has been significant clinical heterogeneity in the size and number of lymph nodes involved, and some trial results suggest that patients with minimal mediastinal nodal involvement might be best treated with preoperative chemotherapy [45]. This has limited the applicability of trial results to wider clinical practice.

In a phase II study designated SWOG 8805 [46], the Southwest Oncology Group (SWOG) evaluated the three-modality approach in 126 carefully selected patients with stage IIIA or IIIB tumors and mediastinal lymph node metastasis documented by biopsy or percutaneous fine-needle aspiration. The trial regimen consisted of combination chemotherapy with cisplatin (50 mg/m^2 on days 1, 8, 29, and 36) and intravenous etoposide (50 mg/m^2 on days 1–5 and 29–33) and concurrent RT (45 Gy in 1.8-Gy fractions, 5 days/week) for 5 weeks, followed 2–4 weeks later by thoracotomy and resection. The median survival time was 15 months, and the 2-year survival was 40%. More than 50% of patients who had N2 disease before chemoradiation therapy had their tumors downstaged to N0 afterward. Yet, almost 40% of patients experienced a local recurrence, and most patients experienced distant metastasis. The overall 3-year survival was 27%. However, when classified by mediastinal disease status after chemoradiation therapy, the 3-year survival was significantly better in those patients whose disease was eradicated than in those whose disease persisted (44% versus 18%).

These encouraging results led to a randomized trial comparing the roles of surgery versus combination chemotherapy and RT in patients with stage N2 disease (RTOG 93-09 and ECOG, SWOG 9336, INT 0139) [44] (Figure 19.4). All patients underwent a 5-week regimen of induction chemotherapy and RT similar to that used in the SWOG 8805 study. Then, half of the patients were randomly assigned to undergo surgical exploration after an interval of 2–4 weeks, while the other half were randomly assigned to continue uninterrupted their chemotherapy and RT (total dose of 61.0 Gy in 33 fractions). For most patients on the surgical treatment arm (88%), surgery resulted in R0 resections. However, treatment-related mortality was higher than on the

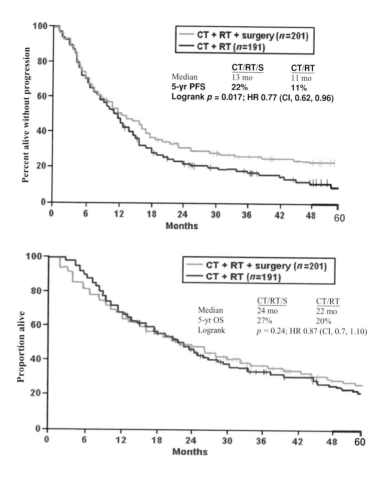

Figure 19.4 Progression-free survival (upper panel) and overall survival (lower panel) on protocol RTOG 93-09/INT-0139. There was a statistically significant difference in progression-free survival but not in overall survival. (Reproduced with permission of the *Journal of Clinical Oncology*, from Albain *et al.* [44].)

chemoradiation treatment arm (7% versus 1.6%), mainly as the result of a high rate of right-sided pneumonectomy. Also, surgery offered a significant improvement in 3-year disease-free survival (29% versus 19%; $p = 0.02$) but not in overall 3-year survival (38% versus 33%; $p = 0.51$). Downstaging of mediastinal disease to N0, regardless of T status, by chemoradiation was again predictive of survival; this subset of patients had a 3-year overall survival of 50% in patients who had a lobectomy [44].

Despite the negative survival results associated with the addition of surgery, some investigators remain enthusiastic its utility in patients with resectable N2 disease. The high mortality rates in the surgery treatment arm could have masked an overall survival benefit. However, there is concern that preoperative radiation may have increased

perioperative mortality. Two recent studies address this second question. In 2004, the German Lung Cancer Cooperative Group reported results of a phase III trial in which 558 patients were randomly assigned to receive neoadjuvant chemotherapy with RT delivered either before or after surgery [47]. There was no difference in treatment-related mortality (5.6% versus 5.3%), progression-free survival, or overall survival between groups [47]. A phase III intergroup trial (RTOG-0412) was developed in order to compare preoperative concurrent chemoradiotherapy and preoperative chemotherapy alone in patients with resectable N2 tumors (Figure 19.5) [42]. This trial was capitalizing on the encouraging results seen in the INT 0139/RTOG 93-09/SWOG-9336 trials and in another prior trial (SWOG-9504) by (a) maintaining cisplatin and

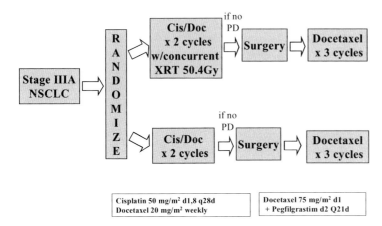

Figure 19.5 Intergroup trial of induction chemotherapy with or without radiation therapy for resectable stable IIIA N2 nonsmall cell lung cancer (NSCLC) [42].

substituting docetaxel for etoposide during induction and (b) having all patients receive consolidation therapy with docetaxel alone [48]. Patients were being randomly assigned to platinum-based chemotherapy alone or in combination with RT; those who experience no subsequent disease progression then undergo resection followed by three cycles of consolidation chemotherapy with docetaxel. The RTOG-0412 trial's main aim was to establish a standard of care for a common, well-defined subset of patients having resectable, limited N2-positive NSCLC. Other aims were to (a) define and further stratify the subsets of N2-positive NSCLC in order to clarify optimal treatment for this heterogeneous group, (b) assess the prognostic value of postinduction therapy positron emission tomography (PET) scanning, (c) evaluate differences in quality of life between the two induction approaches, and (d) incorporate the findings of groundbreaking proteomic and immunohistochemical correlative research into the treatment protocol. However, this trial was closed before meeting the accrual goal due to lack of interested participants.

Radiation therapy

Determination of treatment volumes and portal configurations

Several factors determine the volume to be treated and the configuration of the radiation portals to be used in treating NSCLC. These factors include the size and location of the primary tumor, the areas of lymphatic drainage in the hila and mediastinum, the histologic tumor type, and the equipment and beam energy available. Historically, treatment portals have been designed to encompass a 2-cm margin around any gross tumor seen on posteroanterior radiographs and approximately a 1-cm margin around any regional lymphatic drainage areas to be treated electively.

Two-dimensional radiotherapy

When traditional portals are designed to cover areas of potential lymphatic drainage, the following guidelines are suggested:

1 If the primary tumor is in an upper lobe, the ipsilateral supraclavicular region should be included in the treatment portal. The inferior margin of the portal should be 5–6 cm below the carina.

2 If the primary tumor is located in a middle or lower lobe and no mediastinal lymphadenopathy is present, the supraclavicular areas do not have to be included.

3 If there is a gross upper mediastinal tumor as demonstrated by computed tomography (CT) or established by mediastinoscopy, the ipsilateral supraclavicular area should be included.

4 The ipsilateral hilum is typically included in the irradiated volume; the contralateral hilum, never.

Reduced volumes are irradiated in order to deliver higher doses to the primary tumor or to grossly involved lymph nodes.

Three-dimensional conformal radiation therapy

With the advent of three-dimensional conformal radiation therapy (3DCRT), traditionally recommended portals, target volumes, and beam arrangements have come into question. Because of NSCLC's reportedly high local failure rates, one goal of 3DCRT is to increase the radiation dose delivered to the gross tumor while minimizing the radiation dose delivered to normal tissues. Three-dimensional conformal radiation therapy has several significant advantages over traditional RT techniques: improved delineation of tumor and normal tissue, image segmentation and display, accurate dose calculation, and the ability to manipulate beam geometry and weighting through forward planning. The importance of improved target delineation cannot be overemphasized. Once the patient is immobilized and can undergo CT in the treatment position, the radiation oncologist can delineate the tumor and adjacent tissues in three dimensions; choose beam angles that maximize tumor coverage, minimize the amount of normal tissue exposed to radiation, or both; alter beam weighting; and perhaps alter couch angles for noncoplanar beam delivery. This conformal technique also enables the fusion of complementary imaging modalities, such as PET to aid in tumor delineation and single photon emission computed tomography (SPECT) to choose beam angles. Purdy and colleagues have provided an excellent overview of 3DCRT [49].

Planning for 3DCRT in NSCLC has benefitted from the application of target-defining guidelines published by the International Commission on Radiation Units [50]. The gross tumor volume (GTV) is defined as the primary tumor and any grossly involved lymph nodes. The clinical tumor volume (CTV) is defined as the anatomically defined area thought to harbor micrometastases (hilar or mediastinal lymph nodes or a margin around the grossly visible disease). The planning target volume (PTV) accounts for physiologic organ motion during treatment and the uncertainties of daily setup for

fractionated therapy. When 3D treatment planning is done with the goals of conformal high-dose irradiation of the GTV and minimal irradiation of surrounding normal organs (especially lungs), unique portals, beam arrangements, and beam weights result.

In applying 3DCRT, it is extremely important not to exceed the maximum doses tolerated by sensitive and intrathoracic structures such as the lungs, spinal cord, and heart. Unfortunately, partial-volume normal tissue tolerances are not well understood. Special care should be taken to restrict the radiation dose to the normal lung (i.e., to >20 Gy, uncorrected for inhomogeneity) whenever possible. Dose–volume histograms (DVHs) for all normal thoracic organs should be evaluated for dose and volume of irradiation. Although DVH analysis is still a developing technique, preliminary results indicate that it can be used to predict complications such as pneumonitis and to improve treatment planning [51–55]. Plate 19.1 shows typical radiographic images used in planning 3CDRT for a stage T2N2 squamous cell carcinoma of the right upper lung.

The potential benefits of 3DCRT currently are being investigated in prospective trials.

Three-dimensional conformal radiation therapy clinical trial results

Several reports of recent 3DCRT trials have been published. The most recent is M. D. Anderson Cancer Center's experience with 3DCRT and concurrent chemotherapy in patients with predominantly stage III NSCLC [56]. Of 265 patients enrolled, 127 (48%) were initially treated with two or three cycles of dual-agent induction chemotherapy; most of those ($n = 121$) received platinum and taxane. However, all 265 patients received 3DCRT and concurrent chemotherapy (typically a weekly platinum- and taxane-based regimen). Radiation therapy typically targeted the GTV and involved lymph nodes. Uninvolved lymph nodes were not electively irradiated. The CTV was defined as the GTV plus an 8-mm margin, and the PTV was defined as the CTV plus a 10- to 15-mm margin. The radiation dose that was prescribed covered at least 95% of the PTV. Patients received radiation either daily in 1.8- or 2-Gy fractions ($n = 183$) or twice daily

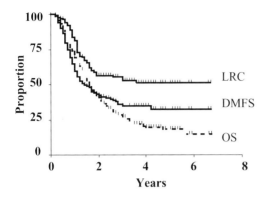

Figure 19.6 Overall survival (OS), distant metastasis-free survival (DMFS), and local regional control (LRC) rates for 265 patients who were treated with three-dimensional conformal radiation therapy and concurrent chemotherapy at a single institution. The 2-year OS, DMFS, and LRC rates for the entire group were 41%, 43%, and 57%, respectively; the 5-year rates, 19%, 33%, and 51%, respectively.

in 1.2-Gy fractions ($n = 82$), to a median dose of 63 Gy (range, 34.8–72 Gy). Nine patients who were unable to complete RT because of toxicity or disease progression and who thus received doses of >60 Gy were nevertheless included in the final analysis. The rates of overall survival, distant metastasis-free survival, and local regional control for the entire group of 265 patients were 41%, 43%, and 57%, respectively, at 2 years and 19%, 33%, and 51%, respectively, at 5 years (Figure 19.6).

Another trial of 3DCRT, reported by Bradley *et al.*, involved 207 patients with stage I–III inoperable bronchogenic carcinoma [57]. The overall survival at 1 and 2 years was 59% and 41%, respectively. On multivariate analysis, the most important prognostic factor was GTV; tumor, nodal, and overall stage were not significant factors at all. Tumor doses of ≥70 Gy resulted in improved local control and cause-specific survival rates but did not improve overall survival. Care must be taken, however, in interpreting the dose data from this trial. Larger tumors were often treated with lower doses to keep normal tissues within their tolerance limits. Nonetheless, 3D dose escalation data from other institutions support the notion that doses ≥60 Gy improve local control [58–62].

Elective nodal irradiation

In many respects, surgery and external-beam RT play similar roles in the treatment of lung cancer. The intent of both modalities is local control in the treated field. Thus, for many years and with only a few recent exceptions [59,63–67), standard RT practice in the United States was to deliver 40–50 Gy to electively irradiated regional lymph nodes (e.g., ipsilateral hilum, ipsilateral and contralateral mediastinum, supraclavicular fossa) and an additional 20 Gy to the primary tumor through reduced fields. This approach was based on pathologic data indicating a high incidence of hilar and mediastinal node metastases in patients with bronchogenic carcinoma. Indeed, up to 26% of patients with stage I NSCLC may have pathologically proven nodal metastases [68,69], and an estimated 25% of T1N0 tumors and 35% of T2N0 tumors are consistently upstaged on the basis of surgical and pathological findings [70,71]. Moreover, the risk of lymphatic metastasis increases with tumor size: from 0% at < 1.0 cm to 17% at 1.1–2.0 cm and 38% at >2.0 cm [72]. Poorly differentiated tumors have a higher rate of nodal micrometastasis, which in itself is an independent prognostic factor for survival [73,74]. In one trial, patients treated with lobectomy rather than with limited resection had significantly lower rates of local and regional failure and showed a trend toward improved survival, suggesting that the improvements were due to removal of both the primary tumor and the draining lymphatics [70]. This conclusion is supported by a recent meta-analysis of four randomized trials of systemic nodal dissection versus more limited mediastinal lymph node sampling, which revealed an association between more aggressive treatment of the mediastinal lymphatics and significantly better 5-year overall survival [75].

The principle that adequate surgical resection of a T1N0 tumor requires systematic removal of all hilar and mediastinal lymph nodes [70,72] suggests that radiation fields should encompass the draining nodal areas. In an analysis of protocol compliance among patients with radiographically negative lymph nodes in the RTOG 73-01 trial [76], Perez and associates observed better (but not significantly better [$p = 0.35$]) survival among patients

Table 19.4 Survival by adequacy of nodal field border in trials of elective nodal irradiation.

Nodal field border	Median survival (yr)	2-yr survival	p value
Mediastinal			
Adequate	1.3	23%	
Inadequate	1.2	37%	0.85
Contralateral hilar			
Adequate	1.3	36%	
Inadequate	1.1	35%	0.27
Ipsilateral hilar			
Adequate	1.2	35%	
Inadequate	1.3	37%	0.81
Supraclavicular			
Adequate	1.2	36%	
Inadequate	1.5	44%	0.32

whose treatment did not vary from the protocol and who had adequate coverage of the hilar/mediastinal lymph nodes. Together, such findings provide a rationale for elective nodal irradiation (ENI).

The major argument against ENI is the high rate of local recurrence within previously irradiated tumor volumes. If one cannot control gross disease, why enlarge the irradiated volumes to include areas that might harbor microscopic disease? Such concerns have been allayed by several major changes in lung cancer therapy since the RTOG 73-01 first established the standards for radiation doses and volumes: namely, the use of chemotherapy, the advent of 3DCRT, and the incorporation of PET into NSCLC staging protocols. Table 19.4 summarizes recent trials of ENI.

According to a review of the patterns of failure after definitive RT in early-stage NSCLC, isolated regional failure occurs in no more than 15% of cases [77,78]. This suggests the possibility of creating localized radiation fields without utilizing ENI.

In one trial, Zhang and colleagues [67] observed 3- and 5-year overall survival rates of 55% and 32%, respectively, in selected patients with bronchogenic carcinoma whose primary tumors were irradiated but whose lymphatics were not. In another trial, Dosoretz and associates [59] observed

no correlation between field size and treatment outcome, even after stratifying their data according to tumor size. In a third trial, Krol and colleagues [64] reported 3- and 5-year overall survival rates of 31% and 15%, respectively, in 108 patients with stage I lung cancer who underwent definitive RT encompassing the primary tumor but no ENI. More notably, the 3- and 5-year cancer-specific survival rates were 42% and 31%, respectively. These results are comparable to results achieved in trials of RT encompassing both traditional fields and regional lymphatics. They have also been confirmed by Senan and colleagues [66], who reported similarly low failure rates in untreated elective nodal areas in stage III patients.

Nevertheless, the results of ENI trials to date need to be examined carefully because of the significant radiation doses ($\geq$40 Gy) delivered electively to regions outside the intended CTV [53,65]. In their series of 171 patients in which involved field volumes were treated definitively with 3DCRT but without ENI, Rosenzweig and coworkers reported an overall elective nodal failure rate of only 6.4%, including 1% in the ipsilateral supraclavicular region, 3% in the contralateral supraclavicular region, 4% in the ipsilateral inferior mediastinal region, and 1% in the contralateral inferior mediastinal region [65]. However, these investigators also estimated that the ipsilateral superior mediastinum, inferior mediastinum, and subcarinal regions received incidental doses of at least 40 Gy (a median dose of 18 Gy to all elective regions) in 34%, 63%, and 41% of cases, respectively [65]. Similar analyses by others found that the ipsilateral hilum, subcarinal region, low paratracheal region, and contralateral hilum and AP window received incidental doses of at least 50 Gy in 100%, 97%, 59%, and 57% of cases, respectively [60,79]. It may be that these incidental doses were not delivered in standard fractions and that the biologically effective dose may not have been sufficient to control any disease that may have been present. Nevertheless, the impact of incidental radiation should be explored further before discounting its possible contribution to nodal failure. Dosimetric analyses (e.g., prospective analyses that correlate nodal failures with dose received) might be helpful in this regard.

There are at least two possible explanations for the lower-than-expected elective nodal failure rates observed in trials of ENI. First, incidental doses to the ipsilateral hilar, paratracheal, and subcarinal nodes approach 40–50 Gy when these regions are not intentionally irradiated [53]. Second, lung cancer patients face multiple competing causes of death (e.g., local failure, distant failure, or intercurrent illness) that may kill them without elective nodal failures ever being detected.

Role of positron emission tomography in nodal treatment planning

The efficacy of ENI may be improved upon by utilizing PET in lung cancer treatment planning. PET has been a major innovation in lung cancer imaging, mainly because of its ability to supplement the structural information provided by traditional anatomical imaging (e.g., CT scans) with functional information about the tumor cells themselves. PET images have added significantly to the accuracy of conventional imaging in estimating the true extent of NSCLC tumors [80]. More accurate clinical staging with PET may allow radiation oncologist to include involved hilar and mediastinal nodes that are not appreciated on the CT scan and reduce the probability of elective nodal failures. As more and more facilities acquire dedicated fluorodeoxyglucose (FDG)-PET scanners and, more specifically, combined PET-CT units, radiation oncologists will be better able to delineate PTVs. Accurate definition and delineation of nodal metastases are crucial for planning curative RT, particularly since routine ENI is no longer recommended in patients NSCLC [81]. Systematic review of the available evidence suggests that FDG-PET is superior to conventional mediastinal staging by CT and esophageal ultrasonography [80,82–84]. One recent modeling study suggests that treating only FDG-positive mediastinal areas would decrease the volumes of lung and esophagus exposed to radiation, thus allowing for radiation dose escalation and hence an improved radiotherapeutic ratio [85]. In one prospective clinical trial of this approach, the rate of isolated nodal failure was only 2% (1/44) [86]. However, in other trials, the rate of false-positive mediastinal nodes on

PET scans has ranged as high as 39% [87,88]. This suggests that histological confirmation of nodal failure is critical when it would have a major impact on the treatment. Plate 19.7 shows a PET scan of a right upper lobe tumor contiguous with a hilar mass, metastasis to an upper paratracheal node, and incidentally right-sided adrenal metastasis.

PET's potential role in planning RT for primary NSCLC is under investigation. PET scanning would certainly help to delineate the GTV in the presence of significant obstructive atelectasis. However, its relatively low spatial resolution (presently 6–8 mm and physically limited to approximately 2 mm) and the resulting blurring of tumor edges make PET-based contouring difficult. Autocontouring using predefined standard uptake value (SUV) thresholds has been reported [89,90]. However, at present, the threshold-defining criteria for contouring GTVs in NSCLC lack pathological correlates. One attractive area of research concerns the use of PET SUV thresholds in planning "metabolic boosts" (i.e., delivery of higher radiation doses to areas with high SUV thresholds while sparing "hypodense" regions identified on FDG-PET scans). However, there is little pathological evidence that "hypodense" regions represent exclusively sites of necrosis and/or atelectasis. Thus, before the concept of modulating radiation doses to tumor subvolumes can be tested rationally in clinical trials, there will have to be studies that correlate pathology with PET images and studies that correlate PET tracer uptake with the molecular characteristics of tumor cells.

Role of chemotherapy in treating microscopic and nodal disease

There is mounting evidence that chemotherapy can effectively control microscopic disease in NSCLC. In several trials, patients receiving chemotherapy for completely resected NSCLC derived an overall survival benefit [91–95]. In a randomized trial of sequential therapy (chemotherapy followed by RT) versus RT alone for unresectable lung cancer, microscopic control was achieved [19]. In a randomized RTOG trial of chemotherapy (vinblastine and cisplatinum) plus RT versus RT alone, analysis of failure patterns revealed a significant

Table 19.5 Normal tissue tolerance of therapeutic irradiation: traditional estimates.

Organ	Portion of organ irradiated			Selected end point
	1/3	2/3	3/3	
		$TD^*_{5/5}$		
Spinal cord	5000	5000	4700	—
Lung	4500	3000	1750	Pneumonitis
Heart	6000	4500	4000	Pericarditis
Esophagus	6000	5800	5500	Clinical stricture/perforation
Brachial plexus	6200	6100	6000	Clinically apparent nerve damage
Thyroid	—	—	—	Not included
		$TD^*_{50/5}$		
Spinal cord	7000	7000	—	—
Lung	6500	4000	2450	Pneumonitis
Heart	7000	5500	5000	Pericarditis
Esophagus	7200	7000	6800	Clinical stricture/perforation
Brachial plexus	7700	7600	7500	Clinically apparent nerve damage
Thyroid	—	—	—	Not included

*$TD_{5/5}$ and $TD_{50/5}$ represent the estimated dose for each organ volume or partial organ volume resulting in a 1–5% risk and a 50% risk, respectively, at 5 years.
Reproduced with permission of the *International Journal of Radiation Oncology, Biology, Physics*, from Emami *et al.* [96].

improvement in the rate of distant metastases for patients treated with the combination therapy ($p < 0.04$) [30]. However, the RT regimen used in both of these randomized trials included ENI and had no effect on local control even with the addition of chemotherapy. Now that combined chemotherapy and radiotherapy has become the established treatment of choice for patients with locally advanced NSCLC, it is reasonable to suggest that chemotherapy may adequately address regional disease and that ENI may not be necessary, particularly in patients whose tumors will be treated with a combination of chemotherapy and RT after CT and PET staging.

Radiation toxicity

For the last decade, partial-volume organ tolerances for irradiation have been defined according to parameters established by an NCI-designated task force [96]. These parameters were based on a re-

view of the literature and the clinical opinions of experienced radiation oncologists (Table 19.5). The toxicity endpoints for irradiated are a 5% complication rate at 5 years ($TD_{5/5}$) and a 50% complication rate at 5 years ($TD_{50/5}$). However, even at the time of their publication, the NCI task force acknowledged that the parameters, especially those regarding normal thoracic tissues, were based on "less than adequate" information compiled in an era before the advent of biologic modifiers and concurrent chemotherapy and 3D conformal radiation.

In lung cancer patients, the organs most prone to radiation exposure are the lung and esophagus. Both will be discussed here. The various parameters for predicting radiation pneumonitis, esophagitis, cardiac toxicity, and brachial plexopathy are more completely reviewed in a recent *Updates to Principles and Practice of Radiation Oncology* [97].

Lung toxicity
Radiation-induced lung injury is related to both dose and volume effects. The acute complication of

radiation-induced lung injury is treatment-related pneumonitis (TRP). The late complication is lung fibrosis. Both complications may be severely debilitating and even fatal.

The incidence of TRP ranges from 13 to 44%. This variance is due to inconsistencies in criteria used, heterogeneity in patient populations enrolled, and differences in treatment regimens and RT techniques employed [54,58,98–101]. Clinical factors thought to predict TRP include poor ECOG performance status [102], poor pulmonary function before RT, concurrent cigarette smoking [103,104], chronic obstructive pulmonary disease (COPD) [105], lower-lobe tumors [106], concurrent chemotherapy [106], high total radiation dose, and high radiation dose per fraction. Dosimetric factors thought to predict TRP include mean lung dose (MLD) [105,107–109] and percentage volume of lung receiving more than a threshold dose (V_{dose}) [52,101,103,107,109–111]. In most combined analyses of these clinical and dosimetric factors, many clinical factors lost their ability to predict TRP; the only ones that did not were concurrent smoking, history of COPD, and induction chemotherapy with mitomycin. However, most of those studies included patients who were treated with RT alone or with some combination of chemotherapy and RT; only in one small study were all patients treated with concurrent chemoradiation therapy [111]. Meanwhile, reports of other studies failed to describe important treatment details (e.g., whether patients received any kind of chemotherapy) [98,112]. This lack of information on important variables (chemotherapy) that might influence the occurrence of TRP has led to confusion in the definition, measurement, and prediction of TRP in radiation oncology clinics.

Predictive dosimetric parameters range from the simple to the complex. Mean lung dose is both simple and clinically useful. So are the volumes of total lung irradiated to doses of ≥ 20 Gy (V_{20}) and ≥ 30 Gy (V_{30}) [113]. All three of these parameters have the advantage of being easily calculated. Other parameters that involve more complicated calculations include DVH reduction (i.e., reduction of the DVH of an organ to a single effective uniform dose), effective lung dose (V_{eff}), normal tissue complication probability (NTCP) [114–116], and the func-

tional subunit model of Niemierko [117]. These more complicated parameters have not been clinically confirmed and are technically difficult to calculate.

Recently, in a single institution study in which 223 patients with NSCLCs of similar stage were uniformly treated with concurrent RT and chemotherapy [55], dosimetric factors were the only factors found to be associated with grade ≥ 3 TRP (as defined according to National Cancer Institute–Common Toxicity Criteria for Adverse Events [NCI-CTCAE] version 3.0.) Interestingly, the only significant factor associated with time to grade ≥ 3 TRP on multivariate analysis was the relative volume of total normal lung treated to 5 Gy (rV5). For rV5 $\leq 42\%$ and rV5 $> 42\%$, the 1-year actuarial incidence of grade ≥ 3 TRP was 3% and 40%, respectively ($p = 0.001$) (Figure 19.7). The frequent high correlation of dose–volume parameters suggests that the shape of the DVH may be more important than single points on the DVH curve (e.g., V20, rV5, or MLD) in predicting the probability of TRP (Table 19.6) [55]. It also suggests that delivery of even a small dose of radiation as low as 5 Gy to a large volume of lung is not safe. Normal lung tissue is highly sensitive to low doses of radiation. Therefore, whereas the probability of tumor control may be predicted by the high-dose distribution around the tumor target, the NTCP might be predicted by the dose–volume relationship in the low-dose region.

This finding is supported by findings of Gopal *et al.* [118], who observed a sharp loss in the carbon monoxide diffusing capacity of normal lung exposed to as little as 13 Gy. The investigators concluded that a small dose of radiation to a large volume of lung could be much more damaging than a large dose to a small volume. Yorke *et al.* [112] reported that the risk of complications rose steeply when the MLD exceeded 10 Gy, indicating the need to limit widespread irradiation of normal lung tissue even at low doses. In contrast, Willner *et al.* [109] reported a sharp increase in the risk of TRP at higher doses, as shown on logistic regression curves for V10, V20, V30, and V40, and concluded that a small dose (e.g., 10 Gy) to a large volume of normal lung is preferable to a large dose (e.g., 40 Gy) to a small volume. We believe that the volume of normal lung receiving

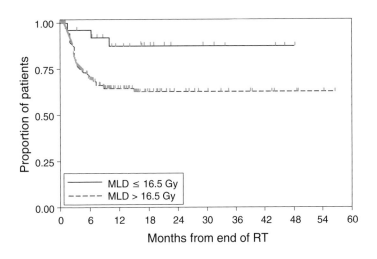

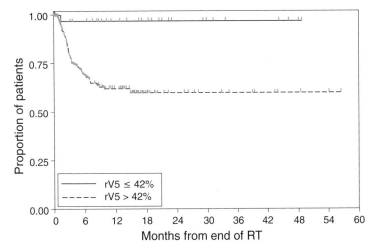

Figure 19.7 Effects of mean lung dose (MLD) (upper panel) and volume of lung receiving 5 Gy (lower panel) on freedom from grade ≥3 treatment-related pneumonitis (TRP) in 222 patients with stage III nonsmall cell lung cancer (NSCLC) after undergoing concurrent radiotherapy and chemotherapy. (Reproduced with permission of the *International Journal of Radiation Oncology, Biology, Physics,* from Wang [55].)

low-dose irradiation should be minimized to avoid severe TRP.

Mechanisms for reducing lung toxicity

The mechanisms for minimizing or avoiding radiation-induced lung toxicity can be broken down into improved radiation delivery, medical intervention to impede the normal lung's inflammatory response to irradiation, and the ability to predict inflammatory response on the basis of genetic predisposition.

Improved radiation delivery

The emerging technology of intensity-modulated radiation therapy (IMRT) is rapidly gaining in popularity [119]. Its increased conformality allows greater sparing of normal tissue at a number of sites [120]. This approach may be useful in boosting radiation doses to lung tumors or in re-treating previously irradiated sites [121,122] However, the clinical experience with IMRT has been limited to treating malignancies of the head and neck, brain, and pelvis; tumor excursion secondary to ventilatory and/or cardiac motion is considered problematic in IMRT for thoracic and abdominal malignancies. One planning study demonstrated a higher conformity index for IMRT than for 3DCRT in the definitive treatment of lung and esophageal cancers [123]. Another study comparing IMRT and 3DCRT

Table 19.6 Incidence of grade ≥3 treatment related pneumonitis in 222 NSCLC patients treated with concurrent radiation therapy and chemotherapy.

Variable	Number of patients	Median (range)	Group*	Incidence of RP at 1 yr (95% CI)	p value
MLD	30	22.4 Gy (5.1–44.6 Gy)	≤ 16.5Gy	13% (4–35%)	0.018
	193		>16.5 Gy	36% (28–44%)	
GTV	181	143 cc (1.5–1186 cc)	≤ 310cc	28% (21–36%)	0.003
	42		>310 cc	54% (37–73%)	
Lung volume	200	3349 cc (1639–7871 cc)	≤ 5040cc	35% (28–44%)	0.024
	23		>5040 cc	6% (1–33%)	
rV5	32	57% (12–98%)	≤ 42%	3% (<1–22%)	0.001
	191		>42%	38% (30–47%)	
rV10	25	47% (18–76%)	≤ 33%	5% (1–28%)	0.007
	198		>33%	37% (29–45%)	
rV15	26	43% (9–90%)	≤ 31%	4% (1–27%)	0.005
	197		>31%	37% (29–46%)	
rV20	30	38% (8–78%)	≤ 28%	4% (1–24%)	0.003
	193		>28%	37% (30–46%)	
rV25	33	34% (7–71%)	≤ 27%	3% (<1–22%)	0.001
	190		>27%	38% (30–47%)	
rV30	28	32% (7–66%)	≤ 22%	10% (3–35%)	0.014
	195		>22%	36% (28–44%)	
rV35	56	29% (6–59%)	≤ 24%	12% (5–28%)	<0.001
	167		>24%	39% (31–49%)	
rV40	54	27% (6–56%)	≤ 22%	12% (5–28%)	<0.001
	169		>22%	39% (31–48%)	
rV45	61	24% (1–52%)	≤ 20%	14% (6–28%)	<0.001
	162		>20%	39% (31–49%)	
rV50	35	21% (0–48%)	≤ 14%	15% (6–37%)	0.021
	188		>14%	36% (28–44%)	
rV55	75	18% (0–46%)	≤ 15%	16% (8–31%)	<0.001
	148		>15%	40% (31–50%)	
rV60	44	15% (0–45%)	≤ 10%	16% (7–35%)	0.018
	179		>10%	36% (29–45%)	
rV65	119	10% (0–43%)	≤ 11%	25% (17–36%)	0.021
	104		>11%	40% (30–52%)	
aV55	71	590 cc (0–2603 cc)	≤ 493cc	21% (12–34%)	0.046
	152		>493 cc	38% (29–47%)	

*Population subgroups were defined by univariate partitioning analysis of MLD, GTV, lung volume, and rV5 through rV65, and absolute volume of esophagus received 55 Gy (aV55).
Reproduced with permission of the *International Journal of Radiation Oncology, Biology, Physics*, from Wang *et al.* [126].

concluded that IMRT could be delivered at a 25–30% higher dose in node-positive patients while still meeting a conservative set of normal tissue constraints [124]. An initial analysis of TRP incidence in patients whose NSCLCs were treated with concurrent chemotherapy and either IMRT or 3DCRT suggested that IMRT significantly re-duced TRP incidence [125,126]. Indeed, despite a greater median GTV on the IMRT arm (194 mL [range, 21–911 mL] versus 142 mL [range, 1.5–1186 mL]) ($p = 0.002$), the rate of grade ≥3 TRP at 12 months was significantly lower (8% [95% CI, 4–19%)] versus 32% [95% CI, 26–40%]) ($p = 0.002$) (Figure 19.8) [125]. Interestingly, V5 (i.e., >70%)

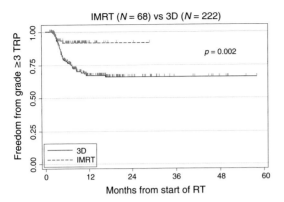

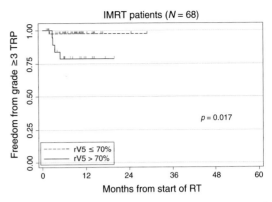

Figure 19.8 Freedom from grade ≥3 treatment-related pneumonitis (TRP) in patients with advanced nonsmall cell lung cancer (NSCLC) after undergoing concurrent chemotherapy and either three-dimensional conformal radiation therapy (3DCRT) or intensity-modulated radiation therapy (IMRT). (Reproduced with permission of the *International Journal of Radiation Oncology, Biology, Physics*, from Yom *et al.* [125].)

Figure 19.9 Freedom from high-grade treatment-related pneumonitis (TRP) in patients with advanced nonsmall cell lung cancer (NSCLC) after undergoing intensity-modulated radiation therapy (IMRT). Patients were stratified according to the relative volume of total normal lung treated to 5 Gy (rV5) (i.e., ≤70% versus >70%). (Reproduced with permission of the *International Journal of Radiation Oncology, Biology, Physics*, from Yom *et al.* [125].)

was again found to be significantly predictive of TRP (Figure 19.9).

Modification of inflammatory response

Attempts to modify the inflammatory response of irradiated lung are under investigation in various clinical trials. Tannehill and colleagues [127] have shown that treatment with amifostine before chemotherapy and RT lowers the expected incidence of esophagitis. In a laboratory model, Vujaskovic and associates have shown that the protection afforded by amifostine against lung parenchymal toxicities is separate from its protection against esophagitis [128].

In a Greek phase III trial of conventional RT with or without amifostine pretreatment [340 mg/m^2 IV] reported by Antonadou *et al.* [129], patients receiving amifostine had decreased rates of clinical pneumonitis, radiographic infiltrates, pulmonary fibrosis, and acute esophagitis. After completion of therapy, the amifostine treatment arm had lower rates of clinical grade ≥2 pneumonitis at 2 months (16% versus 49%) and 3 months (19% versus 52%), lower rates of fibrosis at 6 months (28% versus 58%), and significantly lower rates of esophagitis at 3–6 weeks. However, amifostine apparently had

no effect on complete or partial response rates at 32 months.

Also, in another smaller randomized phase III trial, Antonadou and associates [130] treated 68 patients with amifostine (300 mg/m^2) in conjunction with radiation plus paclitaxel, radiation plus carboplatin, or radiation. They found that amifostine reduced esophagitis and lung parenchymal toxicity in all patients who received chemoradiation.

In a randomized phase III trial from M. D. Anderson, Komaki and colleagues [131] compared complication rates following chemoradiation with or without amifostine in 60 patients with inoperable stage II or III NSCLC. All patients received fractionated RT (1.2-Gy fractions twice daily to a total dose of 69.6 Gy), oral VP-16, and IV cisplatin; in addition, half were randomly assigned to receive amifostine (500 mg IV) twice weekly before chemoradiation. Of 53 evaluable patients, those who received amifostine (*n* = 27) had lower rates of severe esophagitis (7% [2/27] versus 31% [8/26]) (*p* = 0.03) and acute severe pneumonitis (4% [1/27] versus 23% [6/26]) (*p* = 0.04) but a higher rate of hypotension (70%), although only one patient discontinued treatment because of hypotension. The incidence of nausea and vomiting was not reported. The amifostine group also had a higher complete response rate (26% [7/27] versus 7% [2/26]) ($p = 0.07$).

Prednisolone and prednisone have been shown to protect against the early phase of pneumonitis by reducing the inflammatory and exudative components of lung injury. When the steroid treatment is stopped, alveolitis reappears. In rats, D-penicillamine has been shown to inhibit collagen deposition and preserve pulmonary function. However, penicillamine has not been widely tested clinically because of the need for continuous administration. Preclinical studies in rats suggest that the angiotensin-converting enzyme inhibitor captopril may protect target endothelial cells from radiation-induced cell death by reducing endothelial dysfunction after irradiation and reducing radiation-induced lung fibrosis. In light of these exciting data, a clinical trial of captopril is being planned for lung cancer patients undergoing RT.

Identification of genetic predictors of inflammatory response

Clinically, there is wide variation in the degree of acute pneumonitis and lung fibrosis in patients who have been similarly treated. This suggests a wide variation in the lungs' radiosensitivity from person to person. One approach to increasing the probability of lung tumor control while maintaining an acceptable toxicity profile would be to identify sensitive patients before treatment. This might be done by identifying, before or during therapy, important cytokines or growth factors that correlate with the degree of pneumonitis or fibrosis. For example, prospective studies suggest that transforming growth factor-β may be a useful predictor of pulmonary fibrosis [101,132].

Esophageal toxicity

The radiotherapeutic management of thoracic malignancies often exposes the esophagus to high levels of ionizing radiation. After 2–3 weeks of conventionally fractionated RT, patients will often complain of acute reactions such as dysphagia, odynophagia, or both. These reactions can cause significant morbidity due to dehydration and weight loss that may necessitate treatment interruption.

Late reactions of the esophagus to radiation generally involve fibrosis that can lead to stricture. Patients may experience various degrees of dysphagia and may require endoscopic dilation. In rare instances, acute and late responses may both involve esophageal perforation or obstruction.

The clinical and dosimetric predictors of acute and late esophagitis are not well characterized. Emami and colleagues [96] have reported $TD_{5/5}$ and $TD_{50/5}$ values for stricture and perforation of the esophagus but have not addressed the issues of acute and late esophagitis. Moreover, these investigators have acknowledged that, even in light of the limited endpoints of stricture and perforation, "[the] data . . . are quite soft . . . , especially since few authors have attempted to define a dose volume relationship" [96].

The scarcity of data regarding the clinical and dosimetric predictors of acute and late esophagitis has become particularly important in the era of radiation dose escalation and combined chemoradiation therapy. Further intensification of these regimens will not be possible without further characterization of dose-limiting toxicities such as esophagitis.

Clinical studies of esophageal toxicity

Seaman and Ackerman noted that radiologic findings of esophagitis, though rare, usually appeared as luminal narrowing. These investigators also inferred that the esophagus can tolerate a radiation dose of up to 6000 rad, at a rate of 1000 rad per week. These figures are remarkably similar to those later suggested by Emami and associates [133–135].

Goldstein and colleagues [136] reported on 30 patients who developed esophagitis after thoracic RT. Most showed no abnormality on barium swallow esophagrams; those who did usually showed altered esophageal motility. Lepke and Libshitz [137] reported on 250 patients who received thoracic RT with or without chemotherapy. Forty patients had abnormal esophagrams. Patients treated with combined chemotherapy and RT had a nearly fivefold higher incidence of esophageal abnormalities than did those treated with RT alone (7.7% [10/132] versus 1.6% [1/63]).

Several large trials have shown that the esophagus can tolerate relatively high doses of conventionally fractionated radiation alone. Other trials suggest that platinum-based induction chemotherapy does not significantly lower esophageal tolerance. In a randomized trial of combination induction chemotherapy (vinblastine and cisplatin) and RT (total dose of 60 Gy) versus RT alone, Dillman and colleagues observed a similar incidence of severe esophageal toxicity (<1%) in both treatment arms [138]. These findings were similar to those of the comparable RTOG 88-08 trial [139].

Several trials have shown that adding concurrent chemotherapy to RT increases esophageal toxicity. In trials of concurrent chemotherapy and RT versus conventionally fractionated RT alone (i.e., daily fractions of 1.8–2 Gy to a total dose of <60 Gy), the concurrent regimen markedly increased the incidence of esophagitis [140,141]. Choy and colleagues reported a 46% incidence of acute grade 3–4 esophagitis in a trial of concurrent chemotherapy and RT consisting of weekly paclitaxel and carboplatin and daily 2-Gy fractions to a total dose of 66 Gy [139].

Byhardt and coworkers [140] reported on the toxicity results from five RTOG lung cancer trials of combined RT and cisplatin-based chemotherapy. The investigators segregated patients into three groups according to treatment: neoadjuvant chemotherapy and definitive radiation (group 1), neoadjuvant chemotherapy followed by concurrent chemoradiation (group 2), and concurrent chemotherapy and hyperfractionated radiation (group 3). The incidence of grade ≥3 acute esophagitis was significantly higher in group 3 than in either of the other two groups. Similarly, the incidence of late esophagitis in group 3 showed a trend toward significance (2% versus 4% versus 8%, $p = 0.077$).

Clinical and dosimetric studies of esophageal toxicity

There have been recent attempts to define the clinical and dosimetric predictors of esophagitis. In a recent report from M. D. Anderson, investigators noted a 20.5% incidence of grade 3 acute esophagitis in 215 NSCLC patients treated with concurrent 3DCRT and chemotherapy (Figure 19.10). They also identified three significant predictive factors on univariate analysis (i.e., mean esophageal

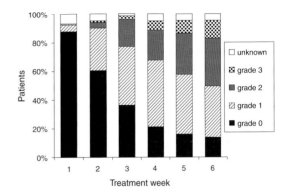

Figure 19.10 Incidence of acute esophagitis (grades 0–3) during each week of concurrent chemoradiotherapy. The incidence of severe acute esophagitis increased with time. (Reproduced with permission of the *International Journal of Radiation Oncology, Biology, Physics*, from Wei *et al.* [142].)

dose, absolute esophageal volume receiving 10–45 Gy, and relative esophageal volume receiving 10–45 Gy) (Figure 19.11) and one significant predictive factor on multivariate analysis (i.e., relative V20) [142]. In their report on 91 patients [141], Maguire and colleagues noted an 11% (10/91) incidence of acute grade ≥3 esophagitis and a 13% (12/91) incidence of late grade ≥3 esophagitis. In that study, 48% of patients received concurrent chemotherapy and 57% received hyperfractionated RT. Univariate analysis revealed no significant predictive factors for acute esophagitis but did identify one predictive factor for late esophagitis (i.e., length of 100% circumference receiving >50 Gy). In addition, multivariate analysis revealed two other predictive factors for late esophagitis (i.e., percentage of organ volume treated receiving >50 Gy and maximum percentage receiving >80 Gy).

Werner-Wasik and associates analyzed clinical and dosimetric predictors of esophagitis in 105 patients treated for lung cancer [143]. They noted that 55% (58/105) received concurrent chemotherapy and that 7% (7/105) received twice-daily fractionated RT. They found that concurrent chemotherapy and twice-daily fractionation were associated with higher grades and longer durations of acute esophagitis, but that the absolute length of esophagus exposed to radiation did not predict esophagitis.

Table 19.7 Published results for risk factors associated with grade ≥3 acute esophagitis.

First author, year [ref.]	Criteria used	Overall incidence (%)	Total number of patients	Incidence of CCT + RT (qd) (%)	Incidence of CCT + RT (bid) (%)	Risk factors identified
Belderbos et al., 2005 [145]	RTOG	6	156	27	N/A	CCT, V35
Qiao et al., 2005 [146]	RTOG	12	208	46	N/A	CCT, Dmax 60
Bradley et al., 2004 [147]	RTOG	5	166	N/A	N/A	CCT, A55, V60
Patel et al., 2004 [148]	RTOG	5	36	N/A	5	V50
Singh et al., 2003 [144]	RTPG	8	207	26	N/A	CCT, Dmax >58
Hirota et al., 2001 [149]	CTC 2.0	7	26	7	N/A	L45, V45
Werner-Wasik et al., 2000 [143]	RTOG	13	105	18	43	CCT, bid
Maguire et al., 1999 [141]	RTOG	11	91	N/A	N/A	Pre-RT dysphagia, bid
Werner-Wasik et al., 1999 [150]	RTOG	7	682	N/A	41	CCT

A55, esophageal area receiving radiation dose >55 Gy; bid, twice daily; CCT, concurrent chemotherapy; CTC 2.0, National Cancer Institute–Common Toxicity Criteria for Adverse Events version 2.0; Dmax 60, maximal dose to the esophagus treated with >60 Gy; Dmax >58, maximal dose to the esophagus treated with >58 Gy; N/A, not available; qd, daily; L45, esophageal length receiving radiation dose >45 Gy; RT, radiation therapy; RTOG, Radiation Therapy Oncology Group; V35, esophageal volume receiving radiation dose >35 Gy; V45, esophageal volume receiving radiation dose >45 Gy; V50, esophageal volume receiving radiation dose >50 Gy; V60, esophageal volume receiving radiation dose >60 Gy.

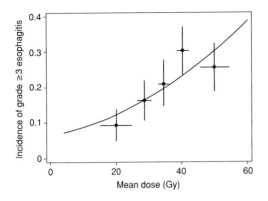

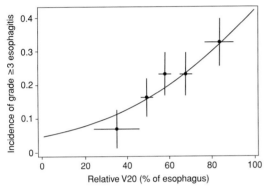

Figure 19.11 Effects of mean esophagus dose (upper panel) and volume of esophagus receiving 20 Gy (lower panel) on freedom from grade ≥3 acute esophagitis in 222 patients with stage III nonsmall cell lung cancer (NSCLC) after undergoing concurrent radiotherapy and chemotherapy. (Reproduced with permission of the *International Journal of Radiation Oncology, Biology, Physics,* from Wei *et al.* [142].)

In a Washington University study of 207 patients treated with definitive RT or chemoradiation therapy, multivariate analysis revealed concurrent chemotherapy to be the predominant factor in treatment-related esophagitis [144]. Overall, 8% of patients (16/207) in the study developed acute or late grade 3–5 esophagitis, and most of those ($n = 14$) had received concurrent chemoradiation therapy.

Again, as described earlier, patients in a multi-center Greek trial were randomly assigned to receive fractionated RT with or without amifostine pretreatment [129]. The incidence of grade ≥2 acute esophagitis on the amifostine treatment arm was significantly lower, most notably in the fourth week of radiotherapy (4% versus 42%). Also, toxicity attributable to amifostine was generally mild, causing nausea and vomiting in two patients and transient hypotension in five. However, amifostine had no effect on complete or partial response rates [129]. Table 19.7 summaries the published results for risk factors associated with grade ≥ acute esophagitis [141,143–150].

Conclusions

Although quite limited, the successes achieved to date by combining chemotherapy with RT for NSCLC warrant continuation of this strategy. Major issues still to be addressed are the sequence and timing of the two modalities and the contributory role of surgery in treating marginally resectable tumors. Progress in treating NSCLC continues to be hampered by the rush to follow up phase I studies of toxicity with phase II trials rather than with comparative, phase III trials. Moving newer and more effective drugs more quickly from phase I to phase III studies should help increase the pace of progress in treating NSCLC, while at the same time providing appropriate general standards for comparison and clinical practice.

References

1 Hill B, Bellamy A. *Antitumor Drug-Radiation Interactions.* Boca Raton, FL: CRC Press, 1990.
2 John M, Flam M, Legha S, Phillips T. *Chemoradiation: A Integrated Approach to Cancer Treatment.* Philadelphia: Lea & Febiger, 1993.
3 Steel G, Hill R, Peckham M. Combined radiotherapy–chemotherapy of Lewis lung carcinoma. *Int J Radiat Oncol Biol Phys* 1978; **4**:49–52.
4 Steel G, Peckham M. Exploitable mechanisms in combined radiotherapy–chemotherapy: the concept of additivity. *Int J Radiat Oncol Biol Phys* 1979; **5**:85–91.
5 Hill B. *In vitro* drug-radiation interactions using fractionated X-irradiation regimens. In: Hill B, Bellamy A (eds). *Antitumor Drug-Radiation Interactions.* Boca Raton, FL: CRC Press, 1990:207–24.

6 Eisert D, Cox J, Komaki R. Irradiation for bronchial carcinoma: reasons for failure. I. Analysis of local control as a function of dose, time, and fractionation. *Cancer* 1976; **37**:2665–70.

7 Bauer M, Birch R, Pajak T, Perez C, Weiner J. Prognostic factors in cancer of the lung. In: Cox J (ed). *Lung Cancer: A Categorical Course in Radiation Therapy*. Oak Brook, IL: Radiological Society of North America, 1985:87–112.

8 Perez C, Bauer M, Edelstein S, Gillespie B, Birch R. Impact of tumor control on survival in carcinoma of the lung treated with irradiation. *Int J Radiat Oncol Biol Phys* 1986; **12**:539–47.

9 Cox J, Yesner R, Mietlowski W, Petrovich Z. Influence of cell type on failure pattern after irradiation for locally advanced carcinoma of the lung. *Cancer* 1979; **44**:94–8.

10 Saunders M, Bennett M, Dische S, Anderson P. Primary tumor control after radiotherapy for carcinoma of the bronchus. *Int J Radiat Oncol Biol Phys* 1984; **10**:499–501.

11 Perez C, Pajak T, Rubin P *et al.* Long-term observations of the patterns of failure in patients with unresectable non-oat cell carcinoma of the lung treated with definitive radiotherapy. Report by the Radiation Therapy Oncology Group. *Cancer* 1987; **59(11)**:1874–81.

12 Schaake-Konning C, Van Den Bogaert W, Dalesio O *et al.* Effects of concomitant cisplatin and radiotherapy on inoperable non-small-cell lung cancer. *N Engl J Med* 1992; **326**:524–30.

13 Dillman RO, Herndon J, Seagren SL, Eaton WL, Green MR. Improved survival in stage III non-small-cell lung cancer: seven-year follow-up of cancer and leukemia group B (CALGB) 8433 trial. *J Natl Cancer Inst* 1996; **88**:1210–5.

14 Brodin O, Nou E, Mercke C *et al.* Comparison of induction chemotherapy before radiotherapy with radiotherapy only in patients with locally advanced squamous cell carcinoma of the lung. *Eur J Cancer* 1996; **32A**:1893–900.

15 Morton R, Jett J, McGinnis W *et al.* Thoracic radiation therapy alone compared with combined chemoradiotherapy for locally unresectable non-small cell lung cancer. A randomized, phase III trial. *Ann Inter Med* 1991; **115**:681–6.

16 Le Chevalier T, Arriagada R, Tarayre M *et al.* Significant effect of adjuvant chemotherapy on survival in locally advanced non-small-cell lung carcinoma. *J Natl Cancer Inst* 1992; **84**:58.

17 Sause W, Kolesar P, Taylor SIV *et al.* Final results of phase III trial in regionally advanced unresectable non-small cell lung cancer: radiation therapy oncology group, eastern cooperative oncology group, and southwest oncology group. *Chest* 2000; **117**:358–64.

18 Dillman RO, Seagren SL, Propert KJ *et al.* A randomized trial of induction chemotherapy plus high-dose radiation versus radiation alone in stage III non-small-cell lung cancer *N Engl J Med* 1990; **323**:940–5.

19 Le Chevalier T, Arriagada R, Quoix E *et al.* Radiotherapy alone versus combined chemotherapy and radiotherapy in nonresectable non-small-cell lung cancer: first analysis of a randomized trial in 353 patients. *J Natl Cancer Inst* 1991; **83**:417–23.

20 Arriagada R, Le Chevalier T, Quoix E *et al.* ASTRO (American Society for Therapeutic Radiology and Oncology) plenary: effect of chemotherapy on locally advanced non-small cell lung carcinoma: a randomized study of 353. *Int J Radiat Oncol Biol Phys* 1991; **20**:1183–90.

21 Sause WT, Scott C, Taylor S *et al.* Radiation Therapy Oncology Group (RTOG) 88-08 and Eastern Cooperative Oncology Group (ECOG) 4588: preliminary results of a phase III trial in regionally advanced, unresectable non-small-cell lung cancer. *J Natl Cancer Inst* 1995; **87**:198–205.

22 Komaki R, Scott CB, Sause WT *et al.* Induction cisplatin/vinblastine and irradiation vs. irradiation in unresectable squamous cell lung cancer: failure patterns by cell type in RTOG 88-08/ECOG 4588. Radiation Therapy Oncology Group. Eastern Cooperative Oncology Group. *Int J Radiat Oncol Biol Phys* 1997; **39**:537–44.

23 Non-small Cell Lung Cancer Collaborative Group. Chemotherapy in non-small cell lung cancer: meta-analysis using updated data on individual patients from 52 randomized clinical trials. *BMJ* 1995; **311**:899–909.

24 Cox J, Pajak T, Asbell S *et al.* Interruptions of high-dose radiation therapy decrease long-term survival of favorable patients with unresectable non-small cell carcinoma of the lung: analysis of 1244 cases from 3 Radiation Therapy Oncology Group (RTOG) trials. *Int J Radiat Oncol Biol Phys* 1993; **27**:493–8.

25 Karnofsky D, Burchenal J. The clinical evaluation of chemotherapeutic agents in cancer. In: MacLeod CM (ed). *Evaluation of Chemotherapeutic Agents, Symposium, Microbiology Section, New York Academy of Medicine*, Vol. 1. New York: Columbia University Press, 1949:191–205.

26 Byhardt R, Scott C, Ettinger D *et al.* Concurrent hyperfractionated irradiation and chemotherapy for unresectable nonsmall cell lung cancer. Results of radiation therapy oncology group 90-15. *Cancer* 1995; **75**:2337–44.

27 Cox JD, Azarnia N, Byhardt RW, Shin KH, Emami B, Pajak TF. A randomized phase I/II trial of hyperfractionated radiation therapy with total doses of 60.0 Gy to 79.2 Gy: possible survival benefit with greater than or equal to 69.6 Gy in favorable patients with Radiation Therapy Oncology Group stage III non-small-cell lung carcinoma: report of Radiation Therapy Oncology Group 83-11. *J Clin Oncol* 1990; **8**:1543–55.

28 Lee JS, Scott C, Komaki R *et al.* Concurrent chemoradiation therapy with oral etoposide and cisplatin for locally advanced inoperable non-small-cell lung cancer: radiation therapy oncology group protocol 91–06. *J Clin Oncol* 1996; **14**:1055–64.

29 Reboul F, Brewer Y, Vincent P, Chauvet B, Faure CF, Taulelle M. Concurrent cisplatin, etoposide, and radiotherapy for unresectable Stage III nonsmall cell lung cancer: a Phase II study. *Int J Radiat Oncol Biol Phys* 1996; **35**:343–50.

30 Komaki R, Scott C, Ettinger D *et al.* Randomized phase II study of chemotherapy/radiation therapy combinations for favorable patients with locally advanced inoperable nonsmall cell lung cancer: Radiation Therapy Oncology Group (RTOG) 92-04. *Int J Radiat Oncol Biol Phys* 1997; **38**:149–55.

31 Trovo M, Minatel E, Franchin G *et al.* Radiotherapy versus radiotherapy enhanced by cisplatin in stage III non-small cell lung cancer. *Int J Radiat Oncol Biol Phys* 1992; **24**:11–5.

32 Blanke C, Ansari R, Mantravadi R *et al.* Phase III trial of thoracic irradiation with or without cisplatin for locally advanced unresectable non-small-cell lung cancer: a Hoosier Oncology Group protocol. *J Clin Oncol* 1995; **13**:1425–9.

33 Jeremic B, Shibamoto Y, Acimovic L, Milisavljevic S. Hyperfractionated radiation therapy with or without concurrent low-dose daily carboplatin/etoposide for stage III non-small-cell lung cancer: a randomized study. *J Clin Oncol* 1996; **14**:1065–70.

34 Groen HJM, van der Leest AHW, Fokkema E *et al.* Continuously infused carboplatin used as radiosensitizer in locally unresectable non-small-cell lung cancer: a multicenter phase III study. *Ann Oncol* 2004; **15**:427–32.

35 Jeremic B, Shibamoto Y, Acimovic L, Djuric L. Randomized trial of hyperfractionated radiation therapy with or without concurrent chemotherapy for stage III non-small cell lung cancer. *J Clin Oncol* 1995; **13**:452–8.

36 Furuse K, Fukuoka M, Kawahara M *et al.* Phase III study of concurrent versus sequential thoracic radiotherapy in combination with mitomycin, vindesine, and cisplatin in unresectable stage III non-small cell lung cancer. *J Clin Oncol* 1999; **17**:2692–9.

37 Curran WJ. Treatment of locally advanced non-small cell lung cancer: what we have and have not learned over the past decade. *Semin Oncol* 2005; **32**:S2–5.

38 Zatloukal P, Petruzelka L, Zemanova M *et al.* Concurrent versus sequential chemoradiotherapy with cisplatin and vinorelbine in locally advanced non-small cell lung cancer: a randomized study. *Lung Cancer* 2004; **46**:87–98.

39 Huber R, Flentje M, Schmidt M *et al.* Simultaneous chemoradiotherapy compared with radiotherapy alone after induction chemotherapy in inoperable stage IIIA or IIIB non-small-cell lung cancer: study CTRT99/97 by the Bronchial Carcinoma Therapy Group. *J Clin Oncol* 2006; **24**:4397–404.

40 Fournel P, Robinet G, Thomas P *et al.* Randomized phase III trial of sequential chemoradiotherapy compared with concurrent chemoradiotherapy in locally advanced non-small-cell lung cancer: Groupe Lyon-Saint-Etienne d'Oncologie Thoracique-Groupe Francais de Pneumo-Cancerologie NPC 95-01 Study. *J Clin Oncol* 2005; **23**:5910–7.

41 Belani C, Choy H, Bonomi P *et al.* Combined chemoradiotherapy regimens of paclitaxel and carboplatin for locally advanced non-small-cell lung cancer: a randomized phase II locally advanced multi-modality protocol. *J Clin Oncol* 2005; **23**:5883–91.

42 PI-Werner-Waski M. Phase III randomized trial of preoperative chemotherapy versus preoperative concurrent chemotherapy and thoracic radiotherapy followed by surgical resection and consolidation chemotherapy in favorable prognosis patients with stage IIIA (N2) non-small cell lung cancer. Activated date: Apr 8, 2005; Closure date: Dec 15, 2006; Update date: Jan 26, 2006.

43 Furuse K. Impact of tumor control on survival in unresectable stage III non-small cell lung cancer (NSCLC) treated with concurrent thoracic radiotherapy (TRT) and chemotherapy CT. *Proc Am Soc Clin Oncol* 2000; **19**:1893.

44 Albain K, Swann R, Rusch V *et al.* Phase III study of concurrent chemotherapy and radiotherapy (CT/RT) vs CT/RT followed by surgical resection for stage

IIIA(pN2) non-small cell lung cancer (NSCLC): outcomes update of North American Intergroup 0139 (RTOG 9309). *Proc Am Soc Clin Oncol* 2005; **23**:624s.

45 Andre F, Grunenwald D, Pignon J. Survival of patients with resected N2 non-small cell lung cancer: evidence for a subclassification and implications. *J Clin Oncol* 2000; **18**:2981–9.

46 Albain KS, Rusch V, Crowley J *et al.* Concurrent cisplatin/etoposide plus chest radiotherapy followed by surgery for stages IIIA (N2) and IIIB non-small-cell lung cancer: mature results of Southwest Oncology Group phase II study 8805. *J Clin Oncol* 1995; **13**:1880–92.

47 Thomas M, Mach H, Ukena D. Cisplatin/etoposide (PE) followed by twice-daily chemoradiation (hfRT/CT) versus PE alone before surgery in stage III non-small cell lung cancer (NSCLC): a randomized phase III trial of the German Lung Cancer Cooperative Group (GLCCG). *Proc Am Soc Clin Oncol* 2004; **22**:618.

48 Gandara DR, Chansky K, Albain KS *et al.* Consolidation docetaxel after concurrent chemoradiotherapy in stage IIIB non-small-cell lung cancer: phase II southwest oncology group study S9504. *J Clin Oncol* 2003; **21**:2004–10.

49 Purdy J, Perez C, Klein E. *Three-Dimensional Conformal Radiation Therapy and Intensity Modulated Radiation Therapy: Practical Potential Benefits and Pitfalls.* New York: Lippincott, Williams & Wilkins, 2000.

50 ICRU Report 50. Prescribing, recording, and reporting photon beam. Bethesda, MD, 1993.

51 Graham M, Matthews J, Harms WS, Emami B, Glazer H, Purdy J. Three-dimensional radiation treatment planning study for patients with carcinoma of the lung. *Int J Radiat Oncol Biol Phys* 1994; **29**:1105–17.

52 Graham M, Purdy J, Emami B, Harms W, Bosch W, Lockett M. Clinical dose–volume histogram analysis for pneumonitis after 3D treatment for non-small cell lung cancer (NSCLC). *Int J Radiat Oncol Biol Phys* 1999; **45**:323–9.

53 Martel M, Strawderman M, Hazuka M, Turrisi A, Fraass B, Lichter A. Volume and dose parameters for survival of non-small cell lung cancer patients. *Radiother Oncol* 1997; **44**:23–9.

54 Martel M, Ten Haken R, Hazuka M. Dose–volume histogram and 3-D treatment planning evaluation of patients with pneumonitis. *Int J Radiat Oncol Biol Phys* 1994; **28**:575–81.

55 Wang S. Analysis of clinical and dosimetric factors associated with treatment related pneumonitis (TRP) in patients with non-small-cell lung cancer (NSCLC) treated with concurrent chemotherapy and three-dimensional conformal radiotherapy (3D-CRT). *Int J Radiat Oncol Biol Phys* 2006; **66(5)**:1399–1407.

56 Huang E, Liao Z, Cox J *et al.* Comparison of outcomes for patients with unresectable locally advanced non-small-cell lung cancer treated with induction chemotherapy followed by concurrent chemoradiation versus concurrent chemoradiation alone. *Int J Radiat Oncol Biol Phys* 2007; **68(3)**:779–85.

57 Bradley JD, Ieumwananonthachai N, Purdy JA *et al.* Gross tumor volume, critical prognostic factor in patients treated with three-dimensional conformal radiation therapy for non-small-cell lung carcinoma. *Int J Radiat Oncol Biol Phys* 2002; **52**:49–57.

58 Armstrong J, Raben A, Zelefsky M *et al.* Promising survival with three-dimensional conformal radiation therapy for non-small cell lung cancer. *Radiother Oncol* 1997; **44**:17–22.

59 Dosoretz D, Galmarini D, Rubenstein J *et al.* Local control in medically inoperable lung cancer: an analysis of its importance in outcome and factors determining the probability of tumor eradication. *Int J Radiat Oncol Biol Phys* 1993; **27**:507–16.

60 Hayman JA, Martel MK, Ten Haken RK *et al.* Dose escalation in non-small-cell lung cancer using three-dimensional conformal radiation therapy: update of a phase I trial. *J Clin Oncol* 2001; **19**:127–36.

61 Maguire P, Marks L, Sibley G *et al.* 73.6 Gy and beyond: hyperfractionated, accelerated radiotherapy for non-small-cell lung cancer. *J Clin Oncol* 2001; **19**:705–11.

62 Robertson J, Ten Haken R, Hazuka M *et al.* Dose escalation for non-small cell lung cancer using conformal radiation therapy. *Int J Radiat Oncol Biol Phys* 1997; **37**:1079–85.

63 Dosoretz DE, Katin MJ, Blitzer PH *et al.* Medically inoperable lung carcinoma: the role of radiation therapy. *Semin Radiat Oncol* 1996; **6**:98–104.

64 Krol A, Aussems P, Noordijk E, Hermans J, Leer J. Local irradiation alone for peripheral stage I lung cancer: could we omit the elective regional nodal irradiation? *Int J Radiat Oncol Biol Phys* 1996; **34**:297–302.

65 Rosenzweig K, Sim S, Mychalczak B, Braban L, Schindelheim R, Leibel S. Elective nodal irradiation in the treatment of non-small-cell lung cancer with three-dimensional conformal radiation therapy. *Int J Radiat Oncol Biol Phys* 2001; **50**:681–5.

66 Senan S, Burgers S, Samson M *et al.* Can elective nodal irradiation be omitted in stage III non-small-cell lung cancer? Analysis of recurrences in a phase II

study of induction chemotherapy and involved-field radiotherapy. *Int J Radiat Oncol Biol Phys* 2002; **54**:999–1006.

67 Zhang H, Yin W, Zhang L *et al*. Curative radiotherapy of early operable non-small cell lung cancer. *Radiother Oncol* 1989; **14**:89–94.

68 Conces DJJ, Klink JF, Tarver RD, Moak DG. T1B0JM0 lung cancer: evaluation with CT. *Radiology* 1989; **170**:643–6.

69 Heavey L, Glazer G, Gross B, Frances I, Orringer M. The role of CT in staging radiographic T1N0M0 lung cancer. *Am J Roentgenol* 1995; **146**:285–90.

70 Ginsberg R, Rubinstein L. Randomized trial of lobectomy versus limited resection for T1 N0 non-small cell lung cancer. Lung Cancer Study Group. *Ann Thorac Surg* 1995; **60**:908–13.

71 Naruke T, Goya T, Tsuchiya R, Suemasu K. Prognosis and survival in resected lung carcinoma based on the new international staging system. *J Thorac Cardiovasc Surg* 1988; **96**:440–7.

72 Ishida T, Yano T, Maeda K. Strategy for lymphadenopathy in lung cancer 3 cm or less in diameter. *Ann Thorac Surg* 1991; **50**:708–71.

73 Chen Z, Perez S, Holmes E *et al*. Frequency and distribution of occult micrometastases in lymph nodes of patients with non-small-cell lung carcinoma. *J Natl Cancer Inst* 1993; **85**:493–8.

74 Maruyama R, Sugio K, Mitsudomi T, Saitoh G, Ishida T, Sugimachi K. Relationship between early recurrence and micrometastases in the lymph nodes of patients with stage I non-small-cell lung cancer. *J Thorac Cardiovasc Surg* 1997; **114**:535–43.

75 Yang H, Wu Y, Yang X, Chen G. A meta-analysis of systematic lymph node dissection in resectable NSCLC [Abstract]. *J Clin Oncol* 2004; **22**:7190.

76 Perez C, Stanley K, Grundy G *et al*. Impact of irradiation technique and tumor extent in tumor control and survival of patients with unresectable non-oat cell carcinoma of the lung: report by the Radiation Therapy Oncology Group. *Cancer* 1982; **50**:1091–9.

77 Jeremic B, Classen J, Bamberg M. Radiotherapy alone in technically operable, medically inoperable, early-stage (I/II) non-small-cell lung cancer. *Int J Radiat Oncol Biol Phys* 2002; **54**:119–30.

78 Koto M, Miyamoto T, Yamamoto N, Nishimura H, Yamada S, Tsuji H. Local control and recurrence of stage I non-small cell lung cancer after carbon ion radiotherapy. *Radiother Oncol* 2004; **71**:147–56.

79 Martel M, Sahijdak W, Hayman JA, Ball D. Incidental doses to clinically negative nodes from conformal treatment fields for nonsmall cell lung can-

cer [Abstract 186]. *Proc Am Soc Clin Oncol* 1999; **45**: 244.

80 Dwamena BA, Sonnad SS, Angobaldo JO, Wahl RL. Metastases from non-small cell lung cancer: mediastinal staging in the 1990s—meta-analytic comparison of PET and CT. *Radiology* 1999; **213**:530–6.

81 Senan S, De Ruysscher D, Giraud P, Mirimanoff R, Budach V, on behalf of the Radiotherapy Group of the European Organization for Research and Treatment of C. Literature-based recommendations for treatment planning and execution in high-dose radiotherapy for lung cancer. *Radiother Oncol* 2004; **71**:139–46.

82 Fischer BMB, Mortensen J, Hojgaard L. Positron emission tomography in the diagnosis and staging of lung cancer: a systematic, quantitative review. *Lancet Oncol* 2001; **2**:659–66.

83 Gould MK, Kuschner WG, Rydzak CE *et al*. Test performance of positron emission tomography and computed tomography for mediastinal staging in patients with non-small-cell lung cancer: a meta-analysis. *Ann Inter Med* 2003; **139**:879–92.

84 Toloza EM, Harpole L, McCrory DC. Noninvasive staging of non-small cell lung cancer: a review of the current evidence. *Chest* 2003; **123**:137S–46S.

85 van der Wel A, Nijsten S, Hochstenbag M *et al*. Increased therapeutic ratio by 18FDG-PET-CT planning in patients with clinical CT stage N2/N3 M0 non-small cell lung cancer (NSCLC): a modelling study. *Int J Radiat Oncol Biol Phys* 2005; **61**:648–54.

86 De Ruysscher D, Wanders S, van Haren E *et al*. Selective mediastinal node irradiation on basis of the FDG-PET scan in patients with non-small cell lung cancer: a prospective clinical study. *Int J Radiat Oncol Biol Phys* 2005; **62(4)**:988–94.

87 Roberts PF, Follette DM, von Haag D *et al*. Factors associated with false-positive staging of lung cancer by positron emission tomography. *Ann Thorac Surg* 2000; **70**:1154–9.

88 Graeter TP, Hellwig D, Hoffmann K, Ukena D, Kirsch C-M, Schafers H-J. Mediastinal lymph node staging in suspected lung cancer: comparison of positron emission tomography with F-18-fluorodeoxyglucose and mediastinoscopy. *Ann Thorac Surg* 2003; **75**:231–6.

89 Paulino AC, Johnstone PAS. FDG-PET in radiotherapy treatment planning: Pandora's box? *Int J Radiat Oncol Biol Phys* 2004; **59**:4–5.

90 Caldwell CB, Mah K, Skinner M, Danjoux CE. Can PET provide the 3D extent of tumor motion for individualized internal target volumes? A phantom study

of the limitations of CT and the promise of PET. *Int J Radiat Oncol Biol Phys* 2003; **55**:1381–93.

91 Arriagada R, Bergman B, Dunant A, for The International Adjuvant Lung Cancer Trial Collaborative G. Cisplatin-based adjuvant chemotherapy in patients with completely resected non-small-cell lung cancer. *N Engl J Med* 2004; **350**:351–60.

92 Niiranen A, Niitamo-Korhonen S, Kouri M, Assendelft A, Mattson K, Pyrhonen S. Adjuvant chemotherapy after radical surgery for non-small-cell lung cancer: a randomized study. *J Clin Oncol* 1992; **10**:1927–32.

93 Wada H, Hitomi S, Teramatsu T. Adjuvant chemotherapy after complete resection in non-small cell lung cancer. *J Clin Oncol* 1996; **14**:1048–54.

94 Winton T, Livingston R, Johnson D, Rigas J, Cormier Y, Butts C, *et al*. A prospective randomized trial of adjuvant vinorelbine (VIN) and cisplatin (CIS) in completely resected stage 1B and II non small cell lung cancer (NSCLC) [Abstract]. *J Clin Oncol* 2004; **22**:7018.

95 Keller SM, Adak S, Wagner H *et al*. A randomized trial of postoperative adjuvant therapy in patients with completely resected stage II or IIIa non-small-cell lung cancer. *N Engl J Med* 2000; **343**:1217–22.

96 Emami B, Lyman J, Brown A *et al*. Tolerance of normal tissue to therapeutic irradiation. *Int J Radiat Oncol Biol Phys* 1991; **21**:109–22.

97 Bradley JD, Zoberi I, Wasserman TH. Normal tissue injury of thoracic organs to radiation therapy. In: Perez C, Brady L (eds). *Updates to Principles and Practice of Radiation Oncology*. Philadelphia: Lippincott, Williams & Wilkins, 2001.

98 Oetzel D, Schraube P, Hensley F, Sroka-Perez G, Menke M, Flentje M. Estimation of pneumonitis risk in three-dimensional treatment planning using dose–volume histogram analysis. *Int J Radiat Oncol Biol Phys* 1995; **33**:455–60.

99 Marks LB, Munley MT, Bentel GC *et al*. Physical and biological predictors of changes in whole-lung function following thoracic irradiation. *Int J Radiat Oncol Biol Phys* 1997; **39**:563–70.

100 Kwa S, Lebesque J, Theuws J *et al*. Radiation pneumonitis as a function of mean lung dose: an analysis of pooled data of 540 patients. *Int J Radiat Oncol Biol Phys* 1998; **42**:1–9.

101 Fu X, Huang H, Bentel G *et al*. Predicting the risk of symptomatic radiation-induced lung injury using both the physical and biologic parameters V(30) and transforming growth factor beta. *Int J Radiat Oncol Biol Phys* 2001; **50**:899–908.

102 Robnett TJ, Machtay M, Vines EF, McKenna MG, Algazy KM, McKenna WG. Factors predicting severe radiation pneumonitis in patients receiving definitive chemoradiation for lung cancer. *Int J Radiat Oncol Biol Phys* 2000; **48**:89–94.

103 Hernando ML, Marks LB, Bentel GC *et al*. Radiation-induced pulmonary toxicity: a dose–volume histogram analysis in 201 patients with lung cancer. *Int J Radiat Oncol Biol Phys* 2001; **51**:650–9.

104 Johansson S, Bjermer L, Franzen L, Henriksson R. Effects of ongoing smoking on the development of radiation-induced pneumonitis in breast cancer and oesophagus cancer patients. *Radiother Oncol* 1998; **49**:41–7.

105 Rancati T, Ceresoli GL, Gagliardi G, Schipani S, Cattaneo GM. Factors predicting radiation pneumonitis in lung cancer patients: a retrospective study. *Radiother Oncol* 2003; **67**:275–83.

106 Yamada M, Kudoh S, Hirata K, Nakajima T, Yoshikawa J. Risk factors of pneumonitis following chemoradiotherapy for lung cancer. *Eur J Cancer* 1998; **34**:71–5.

107 Claude L, PerolPérol D, Ginestet C *et al*. A prospective study on radiation pneumonitis following conformal radiation therapy in non-small-cell lung cancer: clinical and dosimetric factors analysis. *Radiother Oncol* 2004; **71**:175–81.

108 Kim TH, Cho KH, Pyo HR *et al*. Dose–volumetric parameters for predicting severe radiation pneumonitis after three-dimensional conformal radiation therapy for lung cancer. *Radiology* 2005; **235**:208–15.

109 Willner J, Jost A, Baier K, Flentje M. A little to a lot or a lot to a little? An analysis of pneumonitis risk from dose–volume histogram parameters of the lung in patients with lung cancer treated with 3-D conformal radiotherapy. *Strahlenther Onkol* 2003; **179**:548–56.

110 Armstrong J, Zelefsky M, Leibel S *et al*. Strategy for dose escalation using 3-dimensional conformal radiation therapy for lung cancer. *Ann Oncol* 1995; **6**:693–7.

111 Tsujino K, Hirota S, Endo M *et al*. Predictive value of dose–volume histogram parameters for predicting radiation pneumonitis after concurrent chemoradiation for lung cancer. *Int J Radiat Oncol Biol Phys* 2003; **55**:110–15.

112 Yorke ED, Jackson A, Rosenzweig KE *et al*. Dose–volume factors contributing to the incidence of radiation pneumonitis in non-small-cell lung cancer patients treated with three-dimensional conformal radiation therapy. *Int J Radiat Oncol Biol Phys* 2002; **54**:329–39.

113 Munley M, Marks L, Scarfone C *et al.* Multimodality nuclear medicine imaging in three-dimensional radiation treatment planning for lung cancer: challenges and prospects. *Lung Cancer* 1999; **23**:105–14.

114 Kutcher G, Burman C. Calculation of complication probability factors for non-uniform normal tissue irradiation: the effective volume method. *Int J Radiat Oncol Biol Phys* 1989; **23**:105–14.

115 Lyman J. Complication probability as assessed from dose–volume histograms. *Radiat Res* 1985; **8**:S13–9.

116 Seppenwoolde Y, Lebesque J, De Jaeger K *et al.* Comparing different NTCP models that predict the incidence of radiation pneumonitis. *Int J Radiat Oncol Biol Phys* 2003; **55**:724–35.

117 Niemierko A. Reporting and analyzing dose distributions: a concept of equivalent uniform dose. *Med Phys* 1997; **24**:103–10.

118 Gopal R, Tucker SL, Komaki R *et al.* The relationship between local dose and loss of function for irradiated lung. *Int J Radiat Oncol Biol Phys* 2003; **56**:106–13.

119 Mell L, Mehrotra A, Mundt A. Intensity-modulated radiation therapy use in the U.S., 2004. *Cancer* 2005; **104**:1296–303.

120 Hong L, Alektiar KM, Hunt M, Venkatraman E, Leibel SA. Intensity-modulated radiotherapy for soft tissue sarcoma of the thigh. *Int J Radiat Oncol Biol Phys* 2004; **59**:752–9.

121 Choi Y, Kim J, Lee H, Hur W, Chai G, Kang K. Impact of intensity-modulated radiation therapy as a boost treatment on the lung-dose distributions for non-small-cell lung cancer. *Int J Radiat Oncol Biol Phys* 2005; **63**:683–9.

122 Beavis A, Abdel-Hamid A, Upadhyay S. Re-treatment of a lung tumour using a simple intensity-modulated radiotherapy approach. *Br J Radiol* 2005; **78**:358–61.

123 Wu VWC, Sham JST, Kwong DLW. Inverse planning in three-dimensional conformal and intensity-modulated radiotherapy of mid-thoracic oesophageal cancer. *Br J Radiol* 2004; **77**:568–72.

124 Grills I, Yan D, Martinez A, Vicini F, Wong J, Kestin L. Potential for reduced toxicity and dose escalation in the treatment of inoperable non-small-cell lung cancer: a comparison of intensity-modulated radiation therapy (IMRT), 3D conformal radiation, and elective nodal irradiation. *Int J Radiat Oncol Biol Phys* 2003; **57**:875–90.

125 Yom S, Liao Z, Liu H *et al.* Initial evaluation of treatment-related pneumonitis in advanced-stage non-small cell lung cancer patients treated with concurrent chemotherapy and intensity-modulated radiation therapy. *Int J Radiat Oncol Biol Phys* 2007; **68(1)**:94–102.

126 Wang S, Liao Z, Wei X *et al.* Association between induction chemotherapy and increased risk of treatment related pneumonitis in esophageal cancer patients treated with concurrent chemoradiotherapy. *Int J Radiat Oncol Biol Phys* 2006; **66**:S261–2.

127 Tannehill S, Mehta M, Larson M *et al.* Effect of amifostine on toxicities associated with sequential chemotherapy and radiation therapy for unresectable non-small-cell lung cancer: results of a phase II trial. *J Clin Oncol* 1977; **15**:2850–7.

128 Vujaskovic Z, Feng QF, Rabbani ZN, Samulski TV, Anscher MS, Brizel DM. Assessment of the protective effect of amifostine on radiation-induced pulmonary toxicity. *Exp Lung Res* 2002; **28**:577–90.

129 Antonadou D, Coliarakis N, Synodinou M *et al.* Randomized phase III trial of radiation treatment +/− amifostine in patients with advanced-stage lung cancer. *Int J Radiat Oncol Biol Phys* 2001; **51**:915–22.

130 Antonadou D, Petridis A, Synodinou M *et al.* Amifostine reduces radiochemotherapy-induced toxicities in patients with locally advanced non-small cell lung cancer. *Semin Oncol* 2003; **6**:2–9.

131 Komaki R, Lee JH, Kaplan B. Randomized phase II-III study of chemoradiation + amifostine in patients with inoperable stage II–III non-small cell lung (NSCLC). *Proc Am Soc Clin Oncol* 2001; **20**:325.

132 Kong F, Anscher M, Sporn T *et al.* Loss of heterozygosity at the mannose 6-phosphate insulin-like growth factor 2 receptor (M6P/IGF2R) locus predisposes patients to radiation-induced lung injury. *Int J Radiat Oncol Biol Phys* 2001; **49**:35–41.

133 Englestad R. Uber die wikungender rontgenstrahlung auf osophagus und trchea. *Acta Radiol* 1934; **15**:608–14.

134 Phillips T, Ross G. Time–dose relationships in the mouse esophagus. *Radiology* 1974; **113**:435–40.

135 Northway M, Libshitz H, West J *et al.* The opossum as an animal model for studying radiation esophagitis. *Radiology* 1979; **131**:731–5.

136 Goldstein H, Rogers L, Fletcher G, Dodd G. Radiological manifestations of radiation-induced injury to the normal upper gastrointestinal tract. *Radiology* 1975; **117**:135–40.

137 Lepke R, Libshitz H. Radiation-induced injury of the esophagus. *Radiology* 1983; **148**:375–8.

138 Umsawasdi T, Valdivieso M, Barkley HJ *et al.* Esophageal complications from combined chemoradiotherapy (cyclophosphamide + Adriamycin +

cisplatin + XRT) in the treatment of non-small cell lung cancer. *Int J Radiat Oncol Biol Phys* 1985; **11**:511–9.

139 Choy H, Akerley W, Safran H *et al*. Multiinstitutional phase II trial of paclitaxel, carboplatin, and concurrent radiation therapy for locally advanced non-small-cell lung cancer. *J Clin Oncol* 1998; **16**:3316–22.

140 Byhardt R, Scott C, Sause W *et al*. Response, toxicity, failure patterns, and survival in five Radiation Therapy Oncology Group (RTOG) trials of sequential and/or concurrent chemotherapy and radiotherapy for locally advanced non-small-cell carcinoma of the lung. *Int J Radiat Oncol Biol Phys* 1998; **42**:469–78.

141 Maguire P, Sibley G, Zhou S *et al*. Clinical and dosimetric predictors of radiation-induced esophageal toxicity. *Int J Radiat Oncol Biol Phys* 1999; **45**:97–103.

142 Wei X, Liu HH, Tucker SL *et al*. Risk factors for acute esophagitis in non-small-cell lung cancer patients treated with concurrent chemotherapy and three-dimensional conformal radiotherapy. *Int J Radiat Oncol Biol Phys* 2006; **66**:100–7.

143 Werner-Wasik M, Pequignot E, Leeper D, Hauck W, Curran W. Predictors of severe esophagitis include use of concurrent chemotherapy, but not the length of irradiated esophagus: a multivariate analysis of patients with lung cancer treated with nonoperative therapy. *Int J Radiat Oncol Biol Phys* 2000; **48**:689–96.

144 Singh A, Lockett M, Bradley J. Predictors of radiation-induced esophageal toxicity in patients with non-small-cell lung cancer treated with three-dimensional conformal radiotherapy. *Int J Radiat Oncol Biol Phys* 2003; **55**:337–41.

145 Belderbos J, Heemsbergen W, Hoogeman M, Pengel K, Rossi M, Lebesque J. Acute esophageal toxicity in non-small cell lung cancer patients after high dose conformal radiotherapy. *Radiother Oncol* 2005; **75**:157–64.

146 Qiao W-B, Zhao Y-H, Zhao Y-B, Wang R-Z. Clinical and dosimetric factors of radiation-induced esophageal injury: radiation-induced esophageal toxicity. *World J Gastroenterol* 2005; **11**:2626–9.

147 Bradley J, Thorstad W, Mutic S *et al*. Impact of FDG-PET on radiation therapy volume delineation in non-small-cell lung cancer. *Int J Radiat Oncol Biol Phys* 2004; **59**:78–86.

148 Patel AB, Edelman MJ, Kwok Y, Krasna MJ, Suntharalingam M. Predictors of acute esophagitis in patients with non-small-cell lung carcinoma treated with concurrent chemotherapy and hyperfractionated radiotherapy followed by surgery. *Int J Radiat Oncol Biol Phys* 2004; **60**:1106–12.

149 Hirota S, Tsujino K, Endo M *et al*. Dosimetric predictors of radiation esophagitis in patients treated for non-small-cell lung cancer with carboplatin/paclitaxel/radiotherapy. *Int J Radiat Oncol Biol Phys* 2001; **51**:291–5.

150 Werner-Wasik M, Scott C, Graham ML *et al*. Interfraction interval does not affect survival of patients with non-small cell lung cancer treated with chemotherapy and/or hyperfractionated radiotherapy: a multivariate analysis of 1076 RTOG patients. *Int J Radiat Oncol Biol Phys* 1999; **44**:327–31.

CHAPTER 20

New Chemotherapeutic Agents in Lung Cancer

Anne S. Tsao

Introduction

Lung cancer is the leading cause of cancer-related death world wide. In the year 2007, it is estimated that 213,000 new cases of lung cancer will develop in the United States and that 160,390 patients will die from lung cancer [1]. Nonsmall cell lung cancer (NSCLC) comprises 85% of all lung cancers. The 5-year overall survival rate for all stages remains 15% and in patients with advanced unresectable or metastatic disease, the 5-year overall survival remains less than 1%. For the last several decades, before the era of targeted therapies, chemotherapy was the mainstay of palliative treatment.

In the 1960s–1970s, chemotherapy did not appear to provide substantial survival benefit. However, several agents (e.g., mitomycin, ifosfamide, cisplatin, and etoposide) were shown to improve quality of life and survival over placebo. In the 1990s, platinum-based doublets with third-generation chemotherapies became commonly used in the frontline treatment of advanced NSCLC with median survival times of 9 months and 1-year overall survival rate of 30–40%. These agents got approved by the Food and Drug Administration (FDA) for the treatment of patients with advanced NSCLC in the frontline and second-line settings (Figure 20.1). ECOG 1594 (see Table 20.1) compared four platinum-based regimens using

Lung Cancer, 3rd edition. Edited by Jack A. Roth, James D. Cox, and Waun Ki Hong. © 2008 Blackwell Publishing, ISBN: 978-1-4051-5112-2.

third-generation regimens and showed an improvement with these regimens in 1-year and 2-year overall survival rates of 33% and 11%, respectively [2]. The cisplatin versus carboplatin (CISCA) meta-analysis suggested some benefit of using cisplatin over carboplatin, especially in combination with third-generation chemotherapies [3]. Although platinum-based doublets appeared to be the standard of care for chemo-naïve patients with advanced NSCLC in the 1990s, within the last several years, additional large randomized trials and meta-analysis have shown that nonplatinum-based doublets with third-generation chemotherapies are as efficacious as platinum-based therapies [4,5]. It is therefore, the current standard of care in a good performance status patient to use a doublet combination regimen in the frontline setting of advanced NSCLC treatment, with nonplatinum containing regimens being used as an alternative to platinum-based combinations (Table 20.2) [6].

Despite numerous combinations, efforts to improve on survival outcomes with triplet regimens with the addition of other chemotherapies or novel targeted agents were unsuccessful until the year 2005 when the results of ECOG 4599 (see Table 20.1) were presented [2]. This trial showed improvement on median survival over chemotherapy with the addition of an antiangiogenic agent bevacizumab. Although a significant improvement was reported, the toxicities of bevacizumab preclude certain patients from receiving this regimen. Therefore, it remains the standard of care only for patients with nonsquamous cell histology, no brain

Table 20.1 Selected trials and comparison dosing regimens.

Frontline trials
ECOG 1594 [2]
  Cisplatin 75 mg/m^2 on day 2, Paclitaxel 135 mg/m^2 on day 1 over 24 h every 3 weeks
  Cisplatin 100 mg/m^2 on day 1, Gemcitabine 1000 mg/m^2 on days 1, 8, and 15 every 4 weeks
  Cisplatin 75 mg/m^2 on day 1, Docetaxel 75 mg/m^2 on day 1 every 3 weeks
  Carboplatin AUC 6 on day 1, Paclitaxel 225 mg/m^2 on day 1 over 3 h every 3 weeks
TAX 326 [7]
  Cisplatin 75 mg/m^2, Docetaxel 75 mg/m^2 every 3 weeks
  Carboplatin AUC 6, Docetaxel 75 mg/m^2 every 3 weeks
  Cisplatin 100 mg/m^2, Vinorelbine 25 mg/m^2/week every 4 weeks

Second-line trials
TAX 317 [8]
  Docetaxel 100 mg/m^2 every 3 weeks
  Docetaxel 75 mg/m^2 every 3 weeks
  Best supportive care
TAX 320 [9]
  Docetaxel 100 mg/m^2 every 3 weeks
  Docetaxel 75 mg/m^2 every 3 weeks
  Vinorelbine 30 mg/m^2 on days 1, 8, and 15 of each 3-week cycle or ifosfamide 2 mg/m^2/day on days 1 through 3
  of each 3-week cycle

---

metastasis, and no hemoptysis. The nonplatinum- or platinum-based doublet remains the standard of care for the frontline treatment of patients who cannot receive bevacizumab.

There have also been advances in the salvage setting of NSCLC. In the year 2000, docetaxel as a single agent was approved by the FDA for use in the treatment of advanced NSCLC after platinum failure. This was subsequently followed by FDA approval for pemetrexed and erlotinib (Table 20.3). Subset analyses of large randomized trials have shown that not all NSCLC patients are equal. A growing body of evidence indicates that individualized therapy, based on clinical and tumor biomarker prognostic factors, may provide the optimal treatment for the patients. Gender, ethnicity, and smoking status are some of the clinical factors that may predict response or better overall survival to particular agents. The remainder of this chapter will discuss the third-generation chemotherapy agents in detail and summarize the current treatment algorithms. Additional chapters will discuss the novel targeted therapies, mechanism of action, and trial development in further detail.

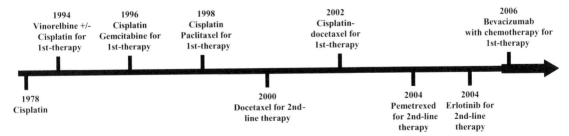

Figure 20.1 FDA approval for selected cytotoxic and biologic agents in the first- and second-line treatment of NSCLC.

Table 20.2 Commonly used regimens and schedules for frontline treatment of NSCLC.

Platinum doublets
Cisplatin (75 mg/m²) on day 2, Paclitaxel (135 mg/m²) on day 1 over 24 h every 3 weeks
Cisplatin (100 mg/m²) on day 1, Gemcilabine (1000 mg/m²) on days 1, 8, and 15 every 4 weeks
Cisplatin (75 mg/m²) on day 1, Docetaxel (75 mg/m²) on day 1 every 3 weeks
Cisplatin (100 mg/m²) on day 1, Vinorelbine (30 mg/m²/week) every 4 weeks
Cisplatin (50 mg/m²) on day 1 and 8, Vinorelbine (25 mg/m²/week) every 4 weeks

Carboplatin (AUC 6) on day 1, Paclitaxel (225 mg/m²) on day 1 over 3 h every 3 weeks
Carboplatin (AUC 6) on day 1, Paclitaxel (200 mg/m²) on day 1 over 3 h every 3 weeks
Carboplatin (AUC 5-6) on day 1, Gemcitabine (1000 mg/m²) on days 1 and 8 every 4 weeks

*Carboplatin (AUC 6), paclitaxel (200 mg/m²), bevacizumab (15 mg/kg) every 3 weeks for a
  maximum of 6 cycles of chemotherapy followed by maintenance bevacizumab every 3
  weeks until disease progression

Non-platinum doublets
Gemcitabine (1000 mg/m²) and Docetaxel (40 mg/m²) on days 1 and 8 every 3 weeks
Gemcitabine (1000 mg/m²) on days 1 and 8, Paclitaxel (200 mg/m²) on day 1 every 3 weeks
Gemcitabine (1000 mg/m²) and Vinorelbine (25 mg/m²) on days 1,8, and 15 every 4 weeks
Vinorelbine (25 mg/m²) on days 1 and 8, Docetaxel (60 mg/m²) on day 8 every 3 weeks

Single (Poor PS, elderly)
Vinorelbine (30 mg/m²) on days 1, 8, and 15 every 4 weeks

---

*ECOG 4599 regimen only for patients with nonsquamous NSCLC, no brain metastasis, no
hemoptysis, and no anticoagulation

Taxanes

Taxanes target the N-terminal of the β-subunit of microtubules, prevent tubulin depolymerization, stabilize the mitotic spindle complex, and thereby halt tumor cell proliferation [10]. The taxanes are administered intravenously and are hepatically metabolized and excreted in the stool. There is wide tissue distribution except into the central nervous system [10]. There are currently two commercially available taxoids, paclitaxel and docetaxel. A newer

Table 20.3 Commonly used agents in the salvage setting of NSCLC.

Docetaxel 75 mg/m² every 3 weeks with dexamethasone premedication

Pemetrexed 500 mg/m² every 3 weeks with vitamin B12 and folic acid supplementation, dexamethasone premedication

Erlotinib 150 mg oral daily dose

---

agent, paclitaxel poliglumex (PPX), is under investigation in phase III trials (Table 20.4). Doxetaxel has a longer intracellular half-life and a greater binding affinity to tubulin than paclitaxel [11].

Paclitaxel

Paclitaxel is extracted from the bark of the Pacific yew tree, *Taxus brevifolia* [14]. This agent promotes microtubule assembly and prevents disassembly, which leads to paralysis of the mitotic spindle apparatus. This agent is known to be an active agent in ovarian carcinoma, melanoma, breast cancer, and NSCLC. It is administered in conjunction with dexamethasone, Benadryl (diphenhydramine hydrochloride), and antihistamine agents as premedications. The main toxicity profile of paclitaxel includes myelosuppression, dose-dependent peripheral neuropathy (mostly sensory but also motor or autonomic), bradycardia, ventricular arrhythmias, mucositis (rare), diarrhea, nausea and vomiting, alopecia, transient elevations of liver function test values, and onycholysis [10]. The

Table 20.4 STELLAR trials [12,13].

Trial	n	Median OS (mo)	1-yr OS rate	2-yr OS rate
STELLAR 3				
PPX/carboplatin	199	7.8	31	13
Paclitaxel/carboplatin	201	7.9	31	11
STELLAR 4				
PPX	191	7.3	26	15
Gemcitabine or vinorelbine	190	6.6	26	10

dose-limiting toxicity is usually myelosuppression, specifically neutropenia [10]. In addition, there is the risk of acute hypersensitivity to the Cremophor vehicle, which presents as dyspnea, bronchospasm, skin flushing, urticaria, and hypotension [15]. As paclitaxel is hepatically metabolized, several drug interactions can occur. p450 enzyme inducers (i.e., phenytoin and phenobarbital) will accelerate paclitaxel metabolism and decrease therapeutic drug levels. Concomitant administration of cisplatin may also lower paclitaxel clearance rates and increase myelosuppression.

The efficacy of paclitaxel has primarily been seen in chemo-naïve NSCLC patients. The first trials in chemo-naïve patients showed significant single-agent efficacy in NSCLC, with doses ranging between 200 and 250 mg/m^2 given over 24 hours every 3 weeks and reported response rates of 21–24% [16,17]. Subsequently, paclitaxel was combined with cisplatin and demonstrated higher response rates and improved survival [10]. Paclitaxel is now commonly given in combination with a platinum agent in the frontline setting of advanced NSCLC. The large phase III trial, ECOG 1594, which defines the current standard of care clinical practice, used paclitaxel in two of the four treatment arms (combined with cisplatin and carboplatin) demonstrating equivalent efficacy between all four studied frontline platinum-based doublets [2]. However, the combination of carboplatin and paclitaxel had the least amount of toxicity compared to the other regimens and was therefore chosen to be the new ECOG reference standard for future clinical trials.

Single-agent trials in second-line therapy for NSCLC yield response rates between 0 and 30% [18–23]. Although several trials have evaluated different dosing regimens in the salvage setting, there is no schedule that appears more efficacious. Dosages given every 3 weeks (135–400 mg/m^2) have response rates between 0 and 3% [18,21–23]. Weekly paclitaxel (80 mg/m^2) in small trials report response rates of 8–37% [24,25]. Paclitaxel has also been studied in combination with carboplatin, hydroxyurea, gemcitabine, cisplatin, and vinorelbine in the salvage setting. The response rates in paclitaxel-containing combinations also range between 0 and 40% [16,26–29]. There is no significant survival improvement that is seen with the use of paclitaxel in the salvage setting.

Paclitaxel poliglumex

PPX is a macromolecule with a poly-L-glutamic acid backbone attached to paclitaxel [30]. This agent was designed to accumulate passively in tumor tissues leading to longer duration of exposure to the tumor but not systemic exposure. It also has a shorter infusion time than paclitaxel. The paclitaxel portion of PPX is released by lysosomal proteases, specifically cathepsin B. This enzyme is regulated by estrogen and it is suspected that hormonal status may affect treatment outcome with PPX [31]. PPX is administered intravenously as a 10- to 20-minute infusion once every 3 weeks. In the frontline setting of NSCLC, two large randomized phase III trials compared the efficacy of PPX to paclitaxel in performance status 2 patients (see Table 20.4). These trials were called the Selective Targeting for Efficacy in Lung Cancer, Lower Adverse Reactions (STELLAR) trials. STELLAR 3 compared PPX (210 mg/m^2)/carboplatin (AUC 6) to paclitaxel (225 mg/m^2)/carboplatin (AUC 6) every 3 weeks [12]. STELLAR 4 compared

PPX (175 mg/m^{2}Q3 weeks) to gemcitabine (1000 mg/m^2 on days 1, 8, 15) or vinorelbine (30 mg/m^2 on days 1, 8, 15) [13].

The survival analysis showed no significant difference between PPX and paclitaxel in combination with carboplatin in the frontline setting, nor as a single agent in comparison to gemcitabine or vinorelbine [12,13]. However, subset analysis in the trials showed that women who were premenopausal (i.e., higher estrogen levels) had a higher survival benefit with PPX [32]. The presumption is that estrogen cleaves cathepsin B and enables greater release of the paclitaxel agent in tumor cells. These results have led to the design of an additional phase III trial (Paclitaxel Poliglumex Investigating Outcomes in NSCLC; Establishing Estrogen Response) PIONEER, which specifically enrolls chemo-naïve women with advanced NSCLC and performance status 2 and randomizes them to either PPX 175 mg/m^2 or paclitaxel 175 mg/m^2 every 3 weeks [31]. The planned enrollment includes 300 patients per arm and all women will be stratified by stage, age, and geography. This trial will potentially validate the STELLAR subset analysis and may define a treatment, unique treatment algorithm, for women with advanced NSCLC. This trial will be the first large multinational NSCLC trial that only enrolls women.

Docetaxel

Docetaxel is a semisynthetic derivative from *Taxus brevifolia*, with the active antitumor component being a diterpenoid [33]. This agent stabilizes tubulin polymerization into microtubules, causes the cells to accumulate in the G$_2$M mitotic phase of the cell cycle, and enables apoptosis. Docetaxel has known clinical activity in breast, lung, head and neck, ovarian, bladder, testicular, and gastroesophageal cancers. The main toxicity is myelosuppression, with neutropenia as the dose-limiting toxicity [34–36]. Patients may also experience hypersensitivity reactions due to the carrier vehicle and it is mandatory to premedicate all patients with steroids before using docetaxel. Additional toxicities include a fluid-retention syndrome, rash, mild–moderate peripheral neuropathy, mucositis, general malaise, asthenia, and alopecia [10,37]. The risk of fluid accumulation increases with higher cumulative doses >400 mg/m^2 and often presents as edema, weight gain, pleural or pericardial effusion, and ascites.

Docetaxel is the only agent that is approved by the FDA for treatment in both frontline (in combination with a platinum agent) and in the second-line setting of advanced NSCLC. Several trials have evaluated docetaxel in chemo-naïve patients. ECOG 1594 compared cisplatin and docetaxel to three other platinum-based doublets and no significant survival difference between the arms was seen [2]. In this trial, there were more episodes of hypersensitivity reactions associated with the cisplatin–docetaxel regimen. TAX 326 (see Table 20.1) compared cisplatin–docetaxel to carboplatin–docetaxel and the reference regimen of cisplatin–vinorelbine in chemo-naïve patients [7]. This phase III trial enrolled 1218 patients. The docetaxel containing arms were more likely to have treatment delivery when compared to the control arm. The cisplatin–docetaxel regimen yielded the highest survival results with a response rate of 32% ($p = 0.029$), a median survival of 11.3 months, and 2-year overall survival rate of 21% ($p = 0.044$). Carboplatin–docetaxel had similar results in response rate and survival to cisplatin–vinorelbine. The cisplatin–vinorelbine regimen had more grade 3–4 anemia, nausea, and vomiting ($p < 0.01$). Patients enrolled on TAX 326 who received docetaxel reported better quality of life and symptom control [7]. The FDA therefore approved the combination regimen cisplatin (75 mg/m^2) and docetaxel (75 mg/m^2) for the use in frontline advanced NSCLC.

Additional phase III trials evaluating docetaxel with carboplatin have also shown reasonable efficacy with median survival range 7.9–9.2 months and 1-year survival rates between 32 and 36% [38–40]. Nonplatinum-based doublets with docetaxel in the frontline setting have used docetaxel in phase III trials. Docetaxel–gemcitabine appeared as efficacious as carboplatin–docetaxel with no difference in toxicity profiles [40].

In the second-line setting, several phase II clinical trials have evaluated docetaxel (100 mg/m^2 every 3 weeks) for NSCLC treatment. The response rates at these single institution studies have ranged from 15 to 22% with median survival between 5.8 and

11 months, and 1-year survival was 25–40% [41–44]. Two large randomized clinical trials, TAX 317 and TAX 320, compared docetaxel to best supportive care (BSC) and other chemotherapies (see Table 20.1) [8,9]. These two trials led to the FDA approval of docetaxel in the second-line setting for advanced NSCLC.

TAX 317 ($n = 103$) enrolled platinum-refractory patients onto three separate arms: docetaxel at 100 mg/m^2 and 75 mg/m^2, and BSC [8]. The docetaxel 75 mg/m^2 dose had the highest median survival at 7.5 months ($p = 0.01$) and 1-year overall survival of 37% ($p = 0.003$). This was in comparison to BSC with median survival at 4.6 months and 1-year overall survival rate of 11%. Twenty-two percent of patients on the docetaxel 100 mg/m^2 dose had febrile neutropenia with three associated deaths. Only one patient in the docetaxel 75 mg/m^2 arm died from febrile neutropenia. Patients who received chemotherapy reported better quality of life and similar nonhematologic toxicities (except for diarrhea) to BSC [8,40].

The TAX 320 phase III trial randomized 373 platinum-refractory patients to docetaxel (100 mg/m^2 every 3 weeks), docetaxel (75 mg/m^2 every 3 weeks), vinorelbine (30 mg/m^2 on days 1, 8, and 15 of each 3-week cycle) or ifosfamide (2 mg/m^2/day on days 1 through 3 of each 3-week cycle) [9]. Docetaxel at both doses were superior to vinorelbine and ifosfamide with response rates for docetaxel at 100 mg/m^2 and 75 mg/m^2 at 10.8% and 6.7%, respectively, and the vinorelbine and ifosfamide response rates at 0.8%. The median time to progression was equivalent between all arms of the study, although progression-free survival at 26 weeks was better in the docetaxel arms (19% for docetaxel 100 mg/m^2, 17% for 75 mg/m^2, and 8% in the vinorelbine/ifosfamide arm). The overall survival at 1-year was favored in the docetaxel 75 mg/m^2 arm (32% versus 19% vinorelbine/ifosfamide). Subset analysis revealed that prior exposure to paclitaxel therapy did not impact patient response to treatment with docetaxel and was not a prognostic factor. Docetaxel at 75 mg/m^2 given every 3 weeks was shown to improve tumor response, time to progression, and survival when compared to vinorelbine or ifosfamide and was ap-

proved by the FDA for second-line treatment in patients with NSCLC [9].

Summary taxanes

The current ASCO guidelines recommend a platinum-based or nonplatinum doublet in good performance status patients with advanced NSCLC in the frontline setting. Either paclitaxel or docetaxel can be used in combination with other third-generation agents or with either platinum agent. Commonly used regimens are displayed in Table 20.2. In the second-line setting, single-agent docetaxel 75 mg/m^2 given every 3 weeks is approved for use (see Table 20.3). Poliglumex paclitaxel is under investigation as an alternative in performance status 2 patients and may have benefited specifically in premenopausal women.

Antimetabolites

Antimetabolites are weakly acidic molecules that inhibit cellular metabolism. These agents are all cell cycle phase-specific and act as false substrates for DNA or RNA synthesis [45].

Gemcitabine

Gemcitabine is a fluorine-substituted analog of deoxycytidine that requires intracellular activation by deoxycytidine kinase to prevent DNA synthesis via inhibition of DNA polymerase [14,46]. This agent has a structure that is similar to cytarabine (ara-C) has been studied in several solid tumor types as a single agent and in combination with other therapies. This agent has demonstrated activity in cancers of the pancreas, lung, ovary, bladder, breast, and colon. Gemcitabine is metabolized in the liver, plasma, and peripheral tissues with most of the drug is excreted in the urine within 24 hours of administration. The dose-limiting toxicity is myelosuppression (neutropenia and thrombocytopenia) [14]. Common nonhematologic toxicities include a flu-like syndrome, nausea and vomiting, mild proteinuria or hematuria, and transient elevations in liver function test values. In rare situations, an infusion reaction (presents with acute dyspnea, flushing, facial swelling, headache, or hypotension) or even hemolytic–uremic syndrome has been reported [47,48].

In the chemo-naïve patients, gemcitabine was originally evaluated in early phase II trials as a single agent with response rates between 20 and 25%, median survival around 9 months, and 1-year survival between 30 and 40% [9]. These promising results led to combining gemcitabine with cisplatin in two large randomized trials, which led to FDA approval of the regimen as first-line therapy for advanced NSCLC patients [2,49]. The Hoosier Oncology Group enrolled 522 chemo-naïve patients compared cisplatin (100 mg/m^2) and gemcitabine (1000 mg/m^2 on days 1, 8, and 15) every 4 weeks to cisplatin (10 mg/m^2) alone every 4 weeks. The combination arm had superior response rates (30.4% versus 11.1%, $p < 0.0001$), median time to progression (5.6 mo versus 3.7 mo, $p = 0.0013$), and overall survival (9.1 mo versus 7.6 mo, $p = 0.004$) when compared to the cisplatin alone arm. There was more grade 4 neutropenia (35%) and thrombocytopenia (25.4%) in the combination arm, but no increase incidence of febrile neutropenia [2]. The second registration trial enrolled 135 chemo-naïve patients to either cisplatin (100 mg/m^2) combined with gemcitabine (1250 mg/m^2 on days 1 and 8) or cisplatin (100 mg/m^2) with etoposide (100 mg/m^2 on days 1–3) every 3 weeks [49]. The cisplatin–gemcitabine arm was superior to cisplatin–etoposide in response rate (40.6% versus 21.9%, $p = 0.02$) and time to progression (6.9 mo versus 4.3 mo, $p = 0.01$); but there was no significant difference in overall survival (8.7 mo versus 7.2 mo, $p = 0.18$). There were no major differences in quality of life or side effect profiles between the two arms.

Later on, the cisplatin–gemcitabine regimen was compared to other platinum-based regimens with conflicting results. ECOG 1594 compared the cisplatin–gemcitabine regimen to platinum–taxane containing arms in chemo-naïve patients, showing equivalent efficacy [2]. In ECOG 1594, cisplatin–gemcitabine had similar response rates but had a longer time to progression than cisplatin–paclitaxel and a trend toward improved 2-year survival. However, the toxicities were higher than carboplatin–paclitaxel and precluded the regimen being used as the ECOG reference standard. In contrast, a meta-analysis of 13 randomized trials with over 4500 patients comparing platinum–gemcitabine doublets to platinum-based comparator regimens showed that gemcitabine plus a platinum agent had better overall survival and progression-free survival [9,50]. However, this benefit was not as pronounced when compared to platinum-based regimens with other third-generation chemotherapies. Gemcitabine (1250 mg/m^2 on days 1 and 8 every 3 weeks) combined with carboplatin (AUC 5) has also been evaluated in phase III trials with response rates of 28–34%, time to progression of 5–6 months, median survival ranging between 7.6 and 11 months, and 1-year overall survival rates between 31 and 44% [4,5,51–53]. Gemcitabine has also been evaluated with nonplatinum agents in phase II trials with similar efficacy and appear to be feasible alternatives if patients cannot tolerate platinum therapy [4,5,9].

In the second-line setting for treatment of NSCLC, single-agent gemcitabine has shown modest activity after failure of platinum therapy. The most common regimen investigated is gemcitabine (1000 mg/m^2 on days 1, 8, and 15) in 4-week cycle, which yields overall response rates of 6–36% and 1-year overall survival rates of 22–45% [32,38,46,54,55]. There are conflicting results with regards to quality of life measurements. Additional trials have combined gemcitabine with other agents with no significant benefit. Hainsworth *et al.* reported no benefit to the addition of gemcitabine to docetaxel [56]. The Greek Cooperative Group also evaluated gemcitabine with docetaxel and growth factor support in a single-arm trial and reported 15.6% response rate, median time to progression 7 months, median survival 6.5 months, and 1-year survival 27.6% [57]. Gemcitabine has also been combined with vinorelbine, paclitaxel, etoposide with overall response rates ranging between 3 and 29% but no significant improvement in survival [28,58,59].

Topoisomerase inhibitors

Topoisomerase is an important nuclear protein that alleviates torsional stress and unwinds DNA for replication, recombination, and transcription [60].

In normal situations, topoisomerase I will unwind then rejoin the cleaved strand of DNA. Inhibitors of toposisomerase can stabilize the transient topoisomerase I-DNA complex, prevent religation of DNA, and when the replication fork is reached, can lead to irreversible double-strand breaks and apoptosis [61–64].

Topotecan

Topotecan is a semisynthetic camptothecin analogue derived from *Camptotheca acuminata* that targets topoisomerase I and is S-phase specific [60,65]. The efficacy of topotecan has been reported in human small cell lung, ovarian, prostate, brain, and hematologic cancers [66–68]. However, the most common setting that topotecan is used is in small cell lung and ovarian cancers. Topotecan is eliminated by the kidney and can be administered intravenously or orally. The dose-limiting toxicity for all administered forms of topotecan is neutropenia, which can frequently be associated with thrombocytopenia [61]. In addition, the most common symptoms include nausea, vomiting, fatigue, mucositis, flu-like symptoms with headache, fever, chills, malaise, transient elevation in serum transaminases, and skin rash [27,61,69].

There are several different dosing regimens for topotecan, but the one most frequently evaluated is a 30-minute infusion on 5 consecutive days given every 3 weeks. The phase I trials using this schedule established the maximum tolerated dose of topotecan at 1.5 mg/m^2/day [10,61,69–71]. The FDA has approved topotecan for use as second-line therapy for advanced ovarian and small cell lung cancers [72,73].

Topotecan has been investigated in chemo-naïve patients with NSCLC with single-agent response rates between 0 and 18%, median survival at 5.9–9 months, and 1-year overall survival rates between 30 and 39% [40,41,74,75]. Trials are ongoing with topotecan combined with platinum agents. In the salvage setting, an international phase III trial called Study 387 randomized 829 patients to oral topotecan 2.3 mg/m^2/day for 5 days or docetaxel 75 mg/m^2 every 3 weeks [8]. The response rate was similar between the two arms (5%) but median survival and 1-year overall survival favored docetaxel

(HR, 1.16 for topotecan; $p = 0.0568$). The median time to progression was 13.1 weeks in the docetaxel arm compared to topotecan at 11.3 weeks (HR, 1.19 for topotecan; $p = 0.0196$). There was more grade 3 thrombocytopenia and anemia in the topotecan arm and more cases of sepsis and neuropathy in the docetaxel arm. Based on this trial, topotecan is not commonly utilized in the treatment of salvage NSCLC.

Irinotecan

Irinotecan is a semisynthetic derivative of camptothecin, a plant alkaloid from *Camptotheca acuminata*. This agent has shown single-agent activity in colorectal, small cell lung, cervical, ovarian, gastric, esophageal cancer, and lymphoma malignancies. For irinotecan to be active, it requires passage through the hepatic system and activation by a carboxylesterase enzyme to form the SN-38 metabolite [27]. The dose-limiting toxicity is diarrhea (acute and delayed) or myelosuppression (with the 3-week schedule) [76,77]. Other common side effects include nausea and vomiting, transient elevations in transaminases, fatigue, and alopecia. Less frequent but serious adverse events include pneumonitis, arrythmias, and paralytic ileus [76,77].

In the frontline setting, irinotecan has been combined with platinums and taxanes. Cisplatin and irinotecan have been studied in several phase I–II trials with response rates ranging between 29 and 52%, median survival 8–11.6 months, and 1-year survival rates 33–46% [78–86]. The main toxicities seen include grade 3–4 neutropenia in half of the patients and grade 3–4 diarrhea in one third of patients. A phase III trial in the chemo-naïve Japanese population ($n = 398$) has evaluated cisplatin and irinotecan and compared it to cisplatin–vindesine and irinotecan alone [87]. This trial favored the cisplatin–irinotecan arm with a response rate of 44% and median overall survival time of 50 weeks [87]. This has yet to be validated in a Western clinical trial. Carboplatin and irinotecan report similar survival rates but lower response rates in the chemo-naïve setting [88]. A phase II trial evaluating irinotecan with paclitaxel had a response rate of 9% and median time to progression of 2.8 months, thereby leading to the recommendation to not study this regimen further [89]. The results with docetaxel were better with a phase II trial ($n = 39$) administering irinotecan 200 mg/m^2 and docetaxel 80 mg/m^2 with growth factor support every 3 weeks. This trial yielded a response rate of 23%, median time to progression 3 months, median overall survival 10.8 months, and 1-year overall survival rate 42% [90]. A 10% rate of grade 4 neutropenia, 23% grade 3–4 diarrhea, and 23.1% grade 2–3 fatigue were seen.

In second-line therapy, single-agent irinotecan was evaluated in two small trials at doses from 100 to 200 mg/m^2/week. In one trial, a 0% response rate was seen in 26 patients and in the other trial, 14% was seen [87,91]. Combination regimens in various stages of development have combined irinotecan with cisplatin, carboplatin, paclitaxel, docetaxel, and gemcitabine have been reported. Early trials using irinotecan with taxane combinations reported response rates of 38%, median survival 11 months, and 1-year survival of 47% [85]. However, recently, trials combining irinotecan with docetaxel in pretreated patients showed that irinotecan did not add any clinical benefit to docetaxel and only increased toxicity with neutropenia, febrile neutropenia, and diarrhea [92–95]. Similarly, the combination of gemcitabine with irinotecan has not been found to provide significant improvements in outcome [83,96,97].

Summary topoisomerase inhibitors

Currently, topotecan and irinotecan are not considered in the standard of care treatment algorithm in the United States. Efforts to improve on the efficacy and limit the side effects of this class of drug are ongoing, although early phase II trials using karenitecin, exatecan, and rubitecan were all negative for significant efficacy in NSCLC. Several novel agents that have enhanced binding capability to topoisomerase are in early phase I trials, including oral glimatecan, CKD-602, BAY 56-3722, MAG-CPT, CT-2106, polyethylene glycol-camptothecin, and DR-310 [98].

Vinka alkaloids

The class of vinca alkaloids includes vincristine, vinblastine, vindesine, and vinorelbine with vinorel-

bine being the newest agent. The vinca alkaloids bind tubulin, prevent tubulin dimer polymerization, and inhibit mitotic spindle apparatus formation leading to mitotic arrest and tumor cell apoptosis. The vinca alkaloids are metabolized in the liver by the cytochrome p450 system and are excreted in the biliary tract and stool [10]. Vinorelbine is an active agent in NSCLC and has been approved for use in the frontline and second-line setting as a single agent or in combination with chemotherapy. It is commonly given as adjuvant chemotherapy in earlier stage disease. However, the side effect profile and inconvenient weekly administration lead it to be used less commonly in the advanced frontline setting of NSCLC when compared to other doublet regimens.

Vinorelbine

Vinorelbine is a semisynthetic analogue of vinblastine derived from vinca rosea obtained from the *Mdagascar* periwinkle and blocks microtubule spindle formation during mitosis. It has known activity against nonsmall cell lung, breast, and head and neck cancers. The dose-limiting toxicity is myelosuppression with neutropenia the predominant feature. Other common side effects include nausea and vomiting, diarrhea, constipation, elevated transaminases, alopecia, peripheral neuropathy, and in rare cases SIADH. Vinorelbine is a vesicant and can induce severe phlebitis unless given quickly with rapid intravenous fluid flushing of the vein. Vinorelbine should also be administered with caution in the setting of concomitant medications that induce the p450 system [10]. The most common dosing schedule is weekly administration (25–30 mg/m^2) over 20 minutes.

In the chemo-naïve population, single-agent vinorelbine yields 12–29% response rate, 7–8 months median survival, and 25–30% 1-year overall survival [9,99,100]. One trial enrolled 211 patients and randomized them to either vinorelbine or 5-fluorouracil with leukovorin [9]. The vinorelbine arm had higher response rates, median survival, and 1-year overall survival rates compared to 5-fluorouracil. These results led to the FDA approval of vinorelbine as a single agent in chemo-naïve patients. A large European trial ($n = 612$) compared the combination of cisplatin (120 mg/m^2 on days 1 and 29 every 6 weeks) with vinorelbine (30 mg/m^2 weekly), to vinorelbine alone, and cisplatin with vindesine [100]. The cisplatin–vinorelbine arm had the highest response rates at 30% and a best median survival time at 9 months [100]. A North American trial, phase III trial SWOG 9308 ($n = 432$), compared cisplatin (100 mg/m^2 every 4 weeks) and vinorelbine (25 mg/m^2 weekly) to cisplatin alone (100 mg/m^2 every 4 weeks) and reported superior results for the combination arm with progression-free survival at 4 months, overall survival 8 months, and 1-year overall survival rate 36% [101]. Based on these two large phase III trials, vinorelbine with cisplatin is approved by the FDA for the frontline treatment of chemo-naïve patients with advanced NSCLC.

In single-agent studies of vinorelbine in second-line therapy, the response is modest in patients who have failed prior platinum therapy. Combination regimens with second-generation agents and vinorelbine have been widely studied in the salvage setting. Two multicenter phase II trials evaluated vinorelbine–ifosfamide (V-I) and vinorelbine–carboplatin (V-C) combinations in pretreated patients. The carboplatin–vinorelbine regimen yielded response rates of 16% with median survival 8.5 months and 1-year overall survival of 38% [102]. The vinorelbine–ifosfamide regimen did not show any significant efficacy. Vinorelbine has also been combined with the taxanes and gemcitabine. Weekly docetaxel (30 mg/m^2) was combined with vinorelbine 20 mg/m^2 (days 1, 8, and 15) but showed poor tolerance and accrual was terminated prematurely due to the toxicity and lack of tumor response [56]. The combination of gemcitabine and vinorelbine has been studied with various response rates ranging between 2.6 and 22.5% [59,103].

Multitargeted antifolate

Pemetrexed

Pemetrexed is a multitargeted antifolate that prevents purine and pyrimidine synthesis via inhibition of thymidylate synthase, dihydrofolate reductase, and glycinamide ribonucleotide formyltrans-

ferase. Pemetrexed must be administered with vitamin B12 supplementation (1000 mcg intramuscular every 9 weeks) and folic acid (400–800 mcg daily) to abbreviate myelosuppression and elevated homocysteine levels. Dexamethasone is also given as premedication to prevent allergic reactions and rash. The dose-limiting toxicity is myelosuppression and other common side effects include rash and fatigue.

In the chemo-naïve population, pemetrexed has been evaluated as a single-agent with response rates 16–23% and median overall survival rates 7.2–9.2 months [104,105]. Combination regimens have also been undertaken using the platinums and gemcitabine. Cisplatin–pemetrexed yields response rates between 39 and 45%, median survival 8.9–10 months, and 1-year overall survival rates around 50% [40,106]. Both carboplatin and oxaliplatin have been given with pemetrexed with response rates 27–32%, time to tumor progression 4.6–5.7 months, median overall survival 10.5–13.4 months, and 1-year survival 44–52% [46,107].

In the second-line setting, a phase III trial ($n = 571$) enrolled performance status 0–2 patients and compared docetaxel (75 mg/m^2 every 3 weeks) to pemetrexed (500 mg/m^2 every 3 weeks) [108]. Pemetrexed compared to docetaxel yielded response rates 9.1% versus 8.8% ($p = $ NS), median overall survival 8.3 months versus 7.9 months ($p = $ NS), and identical progression-free survival (2.9 mo) and 1-year overall survival rates (29.7%). There was more grade 3–4 neutropenia, febrile neutropenia, neutropenia with infections, incidence of hospitalizations, use of growth factor support, and more alopecia in the docetaxel arm compared to pemetrexed. The results of this trial led to the FDA approval of pemetrexed in the second-line setting for advanced NSCLC.

Summary pemetrexed

Pemetrexed is a new cytotoxic agent that has multiple targets in the folate pathway. It is FDA approved for the use in second-line therapy for NSCLC and in the frontline setting with cisplatin in malignant mesothelioma. Due to its promising activity in NSCLC, it is currently under investigation in the frontline therapy of NSCLC. A phase III trial is ongoing with an expected enrollment of

1700 chemo-naïve patients and randomization to cisplatin–pemetrexed versus cisplatin–gemcitabine [46].

Treatment of NSCLC—moving beyond cytotoxics

Chemotherapy treatments of NSCLC are primarily focused on platinum regimens in the frontline setting. In a trial led by Schiller *et al.*, ECOG 1594 demonstrated that platinum-containing doublet chemotherapies had no significant advantages over each other in advanced stage chemo-naïve patients [2]. The response rate was 19%, median survival was 7.9 months, 1-year survival 33% and 2-year survival 11%. Cisplatin–gemcitabine had a longer time to progression but caused more grade 3–5 renal toxicity. Later on, additional trials using nonplatinum-based doublets show similar efficacy and different toxicity profiles [4,5]. The current ASCO guidelines therefore recommend giving platinum-based doublets in the frontline setting but recommend the use of a nonplatinum doublet as an acceptable alternative if the patient cannot tolerate platinum therapy [6]. Despite multiple combinations with the newer third-generation chemotherapies, the survival benefit of cytotoxic treatment of chemo-naïve NSCLC patients appeared to reach a plateau in the early 2000s.

In 2005, the data from ECOG 4599 was presented at ASCO. This trial was the first study to show a significant survival improvement over chemotherapy doublets with the addition of a novel targeted agent, bevacizumab. Bevacizumab is a monoclonal antibody that targets vascular endothelial growth factor (VEGF) and prevents binding of VEGF to its receptor [2]. VEGF is an important angiogenic agent and inhibition of its effects can induce significant antitumor activity. Further details on bevacizumab and other antiangiogenic agents are provided in a subsequent chapter. ECOG 4599 randomized 878 patients with nonsquamous cell NSCLC, no brain metastasis, no prior hemptysis to either carboplatin (AUC 6) with paclitaxel (200 mg/m^2) or carboplatin–paclitaxel with bevacizumab (15 mg/kg every 3 weeks) [2]. Patients were given a maxi-

mum of six cycles of chemotherapy in each arm, and then continued on bevacizumab on the experimental arm until disease progression. There was no crossover allowed from the reference arm to bevacizumab. The response rate (27% versus 10%, $p < 0.0001$), progression-free survival (6.4 mo versus 4.5 mo, $p < 0.0001$), and overall survival (12.5 mo versus 10.2 mo) favored the bevacizumab containing arm. There was a higher incidence of grade 4–5 neutropenia, grade 3–4 hypertension, and grade 3–4 hemorrhage in the bevacizumab containing arm. There were more treatment-related deaths on the bevacizumab arm with (9 versus 2) with five patients dying from hemoptysis. However, given the significant survival benefit, this regimen has become the new ECOG reference standard for patients with nonsquamous NSCLC with no brain metastasis and no hemoptysis. This was the first trial using a triplet regimen with a novel targeted agent to show a survival in the frontline setting. Numerous other targeted therapies have been added to frontline chemotherapy in phase III trials with no impact on outcome [109–112].

The current treatment algorithm for second-line NSCLC has also become expanded to include targeted therapies. At this time, the FDA has approved cytotoxic agents docetaxel and pemetrexed for use as second-line therapy. However, erlotinib, an epidermal growth factor tyrosine kinase inhibitor, has also been approved for use in patients who have failed prior platinum-based chemotherapy. The BR.21 trial established that erlotinib was superior to placebo in terms of progression-free and overall survival and in symptom palliation [113,114].

Targeted therapies

Biological agents in combination with chemotherapies are a potential strategy in the future of lung cancer treatment. The two most advanced targets that have been successfully inhibited by agents that improve clinical outcome in NSCLC are VEGF and EGFR. Bevacizumab has been added to frontline chemotherapy in ECOG 4599 and erlotinib as a single agent is approved as a second- or third-line

agent in NSCLC (BR.21) [2,113]. The antiangiogenic agents and epidermal growth factor receptor
inhibitors will be discussed in greater detail in later
chapters. Although these two agents currently dom-
inate the commercial market, there are several other
classes of agents that inhibit other targets that are
under investigation and show promise in NSCLC
treatment. Additional novel targets in NSCLC include the retinoids, protein–kinase C-α, matrix
metalloproteinases, Ras oncogene, Raf-MEK-ERK
kinase, Src, glutathione-S-transferase (GST) P-1
pathway, histone deacetylase enzymes (SAHA), and
mTor (tesmirolimus) RAD001.

Proteosome

Proteosomes are important regulatory molecules
for cell survival and protein maintenance. Bortezomib, a proteasome inhibitor, has been evaluated
in SWOG trials in combination with chemotherapy
in the chemo-naïve and salvage populations with
promising survival rates [115,116]. Further details
on proteosome inhibitors will be included in a subsequent chapter.

Retinoids

The retinoids have been studied in depth in the
aerodigestive tract tumors both for therapy and
chemoprevention. Bexarotene, a synthetic analogue, binds to retinoid X receptor (RXR-α, -β, -γ),
and modulates cellular proliferation and differentiation. Bexarotene in combination with cisplatin–
gemcitabine appeared to be promising in a phase
II trial [54]. In chemo-naïve patients with NSCLC,
bexarotene (400 mg/m^2) was combined with frontline chemotherapy in two large phase III international trials, SPIRIT I (cisplatin–vinorelbine) and II
(carboplatin–paclitaxel) [117]. The main toxicities
encountered were hypertriglyceridemia and neutropenia. Unfortunately, there was no improvement
in efficacy and in fact, the bexarotene-containing
arms had lower median survival, PFS, and 2-year
survival rates. Despite the overall negative results,
subset analysis did reveal that patients who had
hypertriglyceridemia had better survival outcomes.
Further details on retinoid agents will be discussed
in detail in a subsequent chapter.

Protein kinase C

Protein kinase C is a downstream molecule of
transmembrane kinase receptors. It is activated by
diacylglycerol and has important functions with tumor cell proliferation. Aprinocarsen, a protein kinase C-α antisense oligonucleotide, was added to
gemcitabine–carboplatin with no survival benefit
[112]. Enzastaurin, a derivative of staurisporine, is
currently in clinical trials in both front- and second-
line NSCLC trials.

Raf kinase

Raf serine and threonine kinases regulate cell proliferation and survival through the Raf/mitogen
extracellular kinase/extracellular signal-related kinase pathway [118]. Several solid tumor types are
known to have activated Raf kinase. Sorafenib (BAY
43-9006) is an oral multikinase inhibitor that targets
Raf-1, wild-type B-Raf, and *b-raf* V600E, VEGFR-2,
VEGFR-3, PDGFR-β, Flt-3, and c-kit. It has been
recently approved by the FDA for treatment of advanced renal cell carcinoma [118]. In relapsed or
refractory NSCLC, sorafenib (400 mg oral BID) has
been evaluated in a phase II clinical trial ($n = 52$)
with a response rate of 0% [119]. However, this
trial reported a stable disease rate of 59% and median progression-free survival 11.9 weeks, and overall survival 29.3 weeks. The most common toxicities
encountered were diarrhea, hand–foot skin rash, fatigue, and nausea. Sorafenib is currently under investigation in a phase I/II clinical trial in combination with carboplatin–paclitaxel [3].

Matrix metalloproteinases

Matrix metalloproteinase (MMP) enzymes are
highly upregulated in carcinogenesis and function
by degrading all components of the extracellular
matrix thereby facilitating tumor angiogenesis,
invasion and metastasis [120]. Targeting MMPs
appeared to be a promising strategy with the
goal of cytostatic activity and several MMP inhibitors have been studied in clinical trials with
solid tumors. The early phase I trials revealed
the dose-limiting toxicity to be musculoskele-
tal pain and inflammation. Unfortunately, large
phase III clinical trials showed no significant activity of MMPs in NSCLC. Among these negative

trials include marimastat (stage IIIA/B patients), tanomastat (stage III patients—closed early due to possible worse survival), prinomastat (advanced stage patients with carboplatin–paclitaxel), BR.18 with neovastat (advanced stage patients, added to carboplatin–paclitaxel in chemo-naïve patients) [111,121].

Ras oncogene

Ras mutations are found in approximately 20% of NSCLC [122]. Farnesyl transferase inhibitors specifically target the posttranslational modification of Ras protein and prevent Ras from activating transmembrane receptors [123]. Farnesyl transferase inhibitors have dose-limiting toxicities of fatigue, neurotoxicity, and myelosuppression [122,123]. In chemo-naïve patients with NSCLC, R115777 and L-778,123, have been evaluated in phase II trials with no significant responses [122].

Src kinase

Src is an important tyrosine kinase that regulates tumor invasion and metastasis, angiogenesis, and proliferation. There are several Src inhibitors that have been created dasatinib, SU6656, AZD 0530, AP23846, SKI-606, and XL999 [124]. These agents often inhibit other targets in addition to Src as there is common homology of the adenosine-triphosphate-binding pocket between receptor and nonreceptor kinases. For example, dasatinib is a broad spectrum ATP-competative inhibitor of oncogenic tyrosine kinase/kinase families (BCR-ABL, Src, c-Kit, PDGFR-β, and ephrin receptor kinases) that has activity against NSCLC cell lines [125]. AZD0530 inhibits the tyrosine kinase activity of Src but also downregulates Bcl-X_L [124]. XL999 inhibits Src, VEGF receptor-2, PDGFR, fibroblast growth factor receptor, and FLT-3. Src small molecule inhibitors have preclinical efficacy and are ongoing in clinical trials [124].

Glutathione-S-transferase

Glutathione-S-transferase P1 is overexpressed in NSCLC and it suspected to have a role in multidrug resistance. TLK286 (Telcyta), a glutathione analogue, that is infused as prodrug then activated by tumor cells that have high levels of GST [126].

This thereby preferentially induces tumor cell apoptosis. Initial trials with single-agent TLK286 report a disease stabilization rate of 52% in patients refractory to chemotherapy and TLK286 is being evaluated in ongoing phase III trials [127].

Histone deacetylase enzymes

Histones are proteins that are integrated with genomic DNA and when acetylated, will alter chromatin structure and control gene transcription. Histone deacetylase enzymes (HDAC) regulate histone function via removal of the acetyl moiety and leads to local unfolding of the chromatin for gene transcription. De-acetylation will cause gene silencing and aberrant histone acetylation is associated with carcinogenesis. Some histone deacetylase inhibitors, suberoylanilide hydrozamic acid (SAHA), LAQ824, LBH589A, have been evaluated in early small studies in NSCLC [128]. SAHA is the most advanced in development and larger trials are ongoing to assess its efficacy in thoracic malignancies.

mTor

mTor is a serine/threonine kinase that regulates cell growth and proliferation. mTor is a downstream molecule of a few key regulatory molecules, specifically the growth factor receptors and PI3K/AKT pathway. There are several mTor inhibitors under investigation at this time, including rapamycin, CCI-779 (temsirolimus), RAD001 (everolimus), and AP23573 [129]. Everolimus is in phase II evaluation for NSCLC and is also being used in combination with epidermal growth factor receptor inhibitors.

References

1 Jemal A, Siegel R, Ward E et al. Cancer statistics. *CA Cancer J Clin* 2007; **57**:43–66.
2 Schiller JH, Harrington D, Belani CP et al. Comparison of four chemotherapy regimens for advanced non-small-cell lung cancer. *N Engl J Med* 2002; **346**:92–8.
3 Ardizzoni A, Tiseo M, Boni L et al. CISCA (cisplatin vs. carboplatin) meta-anaysis: an individual patient data meta-analysis comparing cisplatin versus carboplatin-based chemotherapy in first-line treatment of advanced non-small cell lung cancer

(NSCLC) [Abstract 7011]. *Proc Am Soc Clin Oncol* 2006; **24**:366S.

4 Treat J, Belani C, Edelman M *et al*. A randomized phase III trial of gemcitabine (G) in combination with carboplatin (C) or paclitaxel (P) versus paclitaxel plus carboplatin in advanced (Stage IIIB, IV) non-small cell lung cancer (NSCLC): update of the Alpha Oncology trial (A1-99002L) [Abstract 7025]. *J Clin Oncol, 2005 ASCO Annu Meet Proc* 2005; **23**:16S.

5 Kosmidis P, Kalofonos C, Syrigos K *et al*. Paclitaxel and gemcitabine vs carboplatin and gemcitabine. A multicenter, phase III randomized trial in patients with advanced inoperable non-small cell lung cancer (NSCLC) [Abstract 7000]. *J Clin Oncol, 2005 ASCO Annu Meet Proc* 2005; **23**:16S.

6 Pfister DG, Johnson DH, Azzoli CG *et al*. American Society of Clinical Oncology treatment of unresectable non-small-cell lung cancer guideline: update 2003. *J Clin Oncol* 2004; **22**:330–53.

7 Fossella F, Pereira JR, von Pawel J *et al*. Randomized, multinational, phase III study of docetaxel plus platinum combinations versus vinorelbine plus cisplatin for advanced non-small-cell lung cancer: the TAX 326 study group. *J Clin Oncol* 2003; **21**:3016–24.

8 Shepherd FA, Dancey J, Ramlau R *et al*. Prospective randomized trial of docetaxel versus best supportive care in patients with non-small-cell lung cancer previously treated with platinum-based chemotherapy. *J Clin Oncol* 2000; **18**:2095–103.

9 Fossella FV, DeVore R, Kerr RN *et al*., for The TAX 320 Non-Small Cell Lung Cancer Study Group. Randomized phase III trial of docetaxel versus vinorelbine or ifosfamide in patients with advanced non-small-cell lung cancer previously treated with platinum-containing chemotherapy regimens. *J Clin Oncol* 2000; **18**:2354–62.

10 Rowinsky EK. The taxanes: dosing and scheduling considerations. *Oncology (Huntingt)* 1997; **11**:7–19.

11 Diaz JF, Andreu JM. Assembly of purified GDP-tubulin into microtubules induced by taxol and taxotere: reversibility, ligand stoichiometry, and competition. *Biochemistry* 1993; **32**:2747–55.

12 Langer C, Socinski M, Ross H *et al*. Paclitaxel poliglumex (PPX)/carboplatin vs paclitaxel/carboplatin for the treatment of PS2 patients with chemotherapy-naïve advanced non-small cell lung cancer (NSCLC): a phase III study [Abstract 7011]. *J Clin Oncol, 2005 ASCO Annu Meet Proc* 2005; **23**:16S.

13 O'Brien M, Oldham F. Paclitaxel poliglumex vs gemcitabine or vinorelbine for the treatment

of performance status (PS) 2 patients with chemotherapy-naive advanced non-small cell lung cancer: the STELLAR 4 phase III study. *Eur J Cancer* 2005; **3(Suppl)**:324.

14 Ferrigno D, Buccheri G. Second-line chemotherapy for recurrent non-small cell lung cancer: do new agents make a difference? *Lung Cancer* 2000; **29**:91–104.

15 Goss PE, Ingle JN, Martino S *et al*. A randomized trial of letrozole in postmenopausal women after five years of tamoxifen therapy for early-stage breast cancer. *N Engl J Med* 2003; **349**:1793–802.

16 Chang AY, DeVore R, Johnson D. Pilot study of vinorelbine (navelbine) and paclitaxel in patients with refractory non-small cell lung cancer. *Semin Oncol* 1996; **23**:19–21.

17 Murphy WK, Fossella FV, Winn RJ *et al*. Phase II study of taxol in patients with untreated advanced non-small-cell lung cancer. *J Natl Cancer Inst* 1993; **85**:384–8.

18 Murphy W, Winn R, Huber M. Phase II study of Taxol in patients with non-small cell lung cancer who have failed platinum-containing chemotherapy. *Proc Am Soc Clin Oncol* 1994; **13**:363A.

19 Early Breast Cancer Trialists' Collaborative Group. Tamoxifen for early breast cancer: an overview of the randomised trials. *Lancet* 1998; **351**:1451–67.

20 Ruckdeschel J, Wagner H, Williams C. Second-line chemotherapy for resistant metastatic non-small cell lung cancer: the role of Taxol [Abstract 1200]. *Proc Am Soc Clin Oncol* 1994; **13**:357A.

21 Socinski M, Stageall A, Gillenwater H. Second-line chemotherapy with 96 hour infusional paclitaxel in refractory non-small cell lung cancer: report of a phase II trial. *Cancer Invest* 1999; **17**:181–8.

22 Hainsworth JD, Thompson DS, Greco FA. Paclitaxel by 1-hour infusion: an active drug in metastatic non-small-cell lung cancer. *J Clin Oncol* 1995; **13**:1609–14.

23 Sculier JP, Berghmans T, Lafitte JJ *et al*. A phase II study testing paclitaxel as second-line single agent treatment for patients with advanced non-small cell lung cancer failing after a first-line chemotherapy. *Lung Cancer* 2002; **37**:73–7.

24 Juan O, Albert A, Ordono F *et al*. Low-dose weekly paclitaxel as second-line treatment for advanced non-small cell lung cancer: a phase II study. *Jpn J Clin Oncol* 2002; **32**:449–54.

25 Socinski MA, Schell MJ, Bakri K *et al*. Second-line, low-dose, weekly paclitaxel in patients with stage IIIB/IV nonsmall cell lung carcinoma who fail

first-line chemotherapy with carboplatin plus pacli-taxel. *Cancer* 2002; **95**:1265–73.

26 Roa V, Conner A, Mitchell RB. Carboplatin and pacli-taxel for previously treated patients with non-small-cell lung cancer. *Cancer Invest* 1998; **16**:381–4.

27 Stewart DJ, Tomiak EM, Goss G *et al.* Paclitaxel plus hydroxyurea as second line therapy for non-small cell lung cancer. *Lung Cancer* 1996; **15**:115–23.

28 Georgoulias V, Kourousis C, Kakolyris S *et al.* Second-line treatment of advanced non-small cell lung cancer with paclitaxel and gemcitabine: a preliminary report on an active regimen. *Semin Oncol* 1997; **24**:S12-61-6.

29 Stathopoulos GP, Rigatos S, Malamos NA. Paclitaxel combined with cis-platin as second-line treatment in patients with advanced non-small cell lung cancers refractory to cis-platin. *Oncol Rep* 1999; **6**:797–800.

30 Singer JW, Shaffer S, Baker B *et al.* Paclitaxel poliglumex (XYOTAX; CT-2103): an intracellularly targeted taxane. *Anticancer Drugs* 2005; **16**:243–54.

31 Albain KS, Belani CP, Bonomi P *et al.* PIONEER: a phase III randomized trial of paclitaxel poliglumex versus paclitaxel in chemotherapy-naive women with advanced-stage non-small-cell lung cancer and performance status of 2. *Clin Lung Cancer* 2006; **7**:417–9.

32 Gridelli C, Perrone F, Gallo C *et al.* Single-agent gem-citabine as second-line treatment in patients with ad-vanced non small cell lung cancer (NSCLC): a phase II trial. *Anticancer Res* 1999; **19**:4535–8.

33 Douros J, Suffness M. New natural products under development at the National Cancer Institute. *Recent Results Cancer Res* 1981; **76**:153–75.

34 Pazdur R, Newman RA, Newman BM *et al.* Phase I trial of Taxotere: five-day schedule. *J Natl Cancer Inst* 1992; **84**:1781–8.

35 Bissett D, Setanoians A, Cassidy J *et al.* Phase I and pharmacokinetic study of taxotere (RP 56976) ad-ministered as a 24-hour infusion. *Cancer Res* 1993; **53**:523–7.

36 Burris H, Irvin R, Kuhn J *et al.* Phase I clinical trial of taxotere administered as either a 2-hour or 6-hour in-travenous infusion [Abstract 1116]. *J Clin Oncol* 1993; **11**:950–8.

37 Cortes JE, Pazdur R. Docetaxel. *J Clin Oncol* 1995; **13**:2643–55.

38 van Putten JW, Baas P, Codrington H *et al.* Activity of single-agent gemcitabine as second-line treatment after previous chemotherapy or radiotherapy in ad-vanced non-small-cell lung cancer. *Lung Cancer* 2001; **33**:289–98.

39 Lorigan P, Booton R, Ashcroft L *et al.* Randomized phase III trial of docetaxel/carboplatin vs MIC/MVP chemotherapy in advanced NSCLC—final results of a British Thoracic Oncology Group trial [Abstract 7066]. *Proc Am Soc Clin Oncol* 2004; **23**:629.

40 Shepherd FA, Fossella FV, Lynch T *et al.* Docetaxel (Taxotere) shows survival and quality-of-life benefits in the second-line treatment of non-small cell lung cancer: a review of two phase III trials. *Semin Oncol* 2001; **28**:4–9.

41 Fossella FV, Lee JS, Shin DM *et al.* Phase II study of docetaxel for advanced or metastatic platinum-refractory non-small-cell lung cancer. *J Clin Oncol* 1995; **13**:645–51.

42 Burris H, Eckardt J, Fields S *et al.* Phase II trials of Taxotere with non-small cell lung cancer [Abstract 1116]. *Proc Am Soc Clin Oncol* 1993; **12**:335a.

43 Gandara D, Vokes E, Green M *et al.* Docetaxel (Tax-otere) in platinum-treated non-small cell lung cancer: a confirmation of prolonged survival in a multicen-ter trial [Abstract 1632]. *Proc Am Soc Clin Oncol* 1997; **16**:454a.

44 Robinet G, Kleisbauer J, Thomas P *et al.* Phase II study of docetaxel (Taxotere) in first- and second-line NSCLC [Abstract 1726]. *Proc Am Soc Clin Oncol* 1997; **16**:480a.

45 Calabresi P, Chabner B. Chemotherapy of neoplastic disease. In: Gilman AG, Rall TW, Nies AS, Palmer T (eds). *Goodman and Gilman's the Pharmacological Basis of Therapeutics.* New York, NY: McGraw-Hill, 1990:1811.

46 Crino L, Mosconi AM, Scagliotti GV *et al.* Gemcitabine as second-line treatment for relapsing or refractory advanced non-small cell lung cancer: a phase II trial. *Semin Oncol* 1998; **25**:23–6.

47 Fung MC, Storniolo AM, Nguyen B *et al.* A review of hemolytic uremic syndrome in patients treated with gemcitabine therapy. *Cancer* 1999; **85**:2023–32.

48 Chu E, Mota A, Fogarasi M. Antimetabolites. In: De-Vita VHS, Rosenberg S (eds). *Cancer Principles and Prac-tice of Oncology.* Philadelphia, PA: Lippincott, Williams & Wilkins, 2001:388–415.

49 Cardenal F, Lopez-Cabrerizo MP, Anton A *et al.* Ran-domized phase III study of gemcitabine–cisplatin ver-sus etoposide–cisplatin in the treatment of locally ad-vanced or metastatic non-small-cell lung cancer. *J Clin Oncol* 1999; **17**:12–8.

50 Le Chevalier T, Scagliotti G, Natale R *et al.* Efficacy of gemcitabine plus platinum chemotherapy com-pared with other platinum containing regimens in advanced non-small-cell lung cancer: a meta-analysis of survival outcomes. *Lung Cancer* 2005; **47**:69–80.

51 Sederhorn C. Gemcitabine (G) compared with gemcitabine plus carboplatin (GC) in advanced non-small cell lung cancer (NSCLC): a phase III study by the Swedish Lung Cancer Study Group (SLUSG) [Abstract 1162]. *Proc Am Soc Clin Oncol* 2002; **21**:291a.

52 Rudd RM, Gower NH, Spiro SG *et al*. Gemcitabine plus carboplatin versus mitomycin, ifosfamide, and cisplatin in patients with stage IIIB or IV non-small-cell lung cancer: a phase III randomized study of the London Lung Cancer Group. *J Clin Oncol* 2005; **23**:142–53.

53 Grigorescu AC, Draghici IN, Nitipir C *et al*. Gemcitabine (GEM) and carboplatin (CBDCA) versus cisplatin (CDDP) and vinblastine (VLB) in advanced non-small-cell lung cancer (NSCLC) stages III and IV: a phase III randomised trial. *Lung Cancer* 2002; **37**:9–14.

54 Reddy G, Gandara D, Edelman M *et al*. Gemcitabine (GEM) in platinum (PLAT) treated non-small cell lung cancer (NSCLC) [Abstract 2007]. *Proc Am Clin Oncol* 1999; **18**:521a.

55 Sculier JP, Lafitte JJ, Berghmans T *et al*. A phase II trial testing gemcitabine as second-line chemotherapy for non small cell lung cancer. The European Lung Cancer Working Party. 101473.1044@compuserve.com. *Lung Cancer* 2000; **29**:67–73.

56 Hainsworth JD, Burris HA, III, Billings FT, III *et al*. Weekly docetaxel with either gemcitabine or vinorelbine as second-line treatment in patients with advanced nonsmall cell lung carcinoma: phase II trials of the Minnie Pearl Cancer Research Network. *Cancer* 2001; **92**:2391–8.

57 Kakolyris S, Papadakis E, Tsiafaki X *et al*. Docetaxel in combination with gemcitabine plus rhG-CSF support as second-line treatment in non-small cell lung cancer. A multicenter phase II study. *Lung Cancer* 2001; **32**:179–87.

58 Biesma B, Smit EF, Postmus PE. A dose and schedule finding study of gemcitabine and etoposide in patients with progressive non-small cell lung cancer after platinum containing chemotherapy. *Lung Cancer* 1999; **24**:115–21.

59 Pectasides D, Kalofonos HP, Samantas E *et al*. An out-patient second-line chemotherapy with gemcitabine and vinorelbine in patients with non-small cell lung cancer previously treated with cisplatin-based chemotherapy. A phase II study of the Hellenic co-operative Oncology Group. *Anticancer Res* 2001; **21**:3005–10.

60 Gupta M, Fujimori A, Pommier Y. Eukaryotic DNA topoisomerases I. *Biochim Biophys Acta* 1995; **1262**:1–14.

61 Garcia-Carbonero R, Supko JG. Current perspectives on the clinical experience, pharmacology, and continued development of the camptothecins. *Clin Cancer Res* 2002; **8**:641–61.

62 Stivers JT, Harris TK, Mildvan AS. Vaccinia DNA topoisomerase I: evidence supporting a free rotation mechanism for DNA supercoil relaxation. *Biochemistry* 1997; **36**:5212–22.

63 Champoux JJ. Mechanism of the reaction catalyzed by the DNA untwisting enzyme: attachment of the enzyme to 3′-terminus of the nicked DNA. *J Mol Biol* 1978; **118**:441–6.

64 Tsao YP, Russo A, Nyamuswa G *et al*. Interaction between replication forks and topoisomerase I-DNA cleavable complexes: studies in a cell-free SV40 DNA replication system. *Cancer Res* 1993; **53**:5908–14.

65 Tsao YP, D'Arpa P, Liu LF. The involvement of active DNA synthesis in camptothecin-induced G2 arrest: altered regulation of p34cdc2/cyclin B. *Cancer Res* 1992; **52**:1823–9.

66 Schiller JH. Future role of topotecan in the treatment of lung cancer. *Oncology* 2001; **61(Suppl 1)**:55–9.

67 Beran M, Kantarjian H, O'Brien S *et al*. Topotecan, a topoisomerase I inhibitor, is active in the treatment of myelodysplastic syndrome and chronic myelomonocytic leukemia. *Blood* 1996; **88**:2473–9.

68 Kantarjian HM, Beran M, Ellis A *et al*. Phase I study of Topotecan, a new topoisomerase I inhibitor, in patients with refractory or relapsed acute leukemia. *Blood* 1993; **81**:1146–51.

69 van Warmerdam LJ, Creemers GJ, Rodenhuis S *et al*. Pharmacokinetics and pharmacodynamics of topotecan given on a daily-times-five schedule in phase II clinical trials using a limited-sampling procedure. *Cancer Chemother Pharmacol* 1996; **38**:254–60.

70 Awada A, Eskens FA, Piccart M *et al*. Phase I and pharmacological study of the oral farnesyltransferase inhibitor SCH 66336 given once daily to patients with advanced solid tumours. *Eur J Cancer* 2002; **38**:2272–8.

71 Saltz L, Sirott M, Young C *et al*. Phase I clinical and pharmacology study of topotecan given daily for 5 consecutive days to patients with advanced solid tumors, with attempt at dose intensification using recombinant granulocyte colony-stimulating factor. *J Natl Cancer Inst* 1993; **85**:1499–507.

72 ten Bokkel Huinink W, Gore M, Carmichael J *et al.* Topotecan versus paclitaxel for the treatment of recurrent epithelial ovarian cancer. *J Clin Oncol* 1997; **15**:2183–93.

73 von Pawel J, Schiller JH, Shepherd FA *et al.* Topotecan versus cyclophosphamide, doxorubicin, and vincristine for the treatment of recurrent small-cell lung cancer. *J Clin Oncol* 1999; **17**:658–67.

74 Weitz J, Jung S, Marschke R *et al.* Randomized phase II trial of two schedules of Topotecan for the treatment of advanced stage non-small cell lung carcinoma (NSCLC): a North Central Cancer Treatment Group (NCCTG) Trial [Abstract 1053]. *Proc Am Soc Clin Oncol* 1995; **14**:348.

75 Kindler H, Kris M, Smith I *et al.* Continuous infusion topotecan as first-line therapy in patients with non-small cell lung cancer (NSCLC): a phase II study [Abstract 1697]. *Proc Am Soc Clin Oncol* 1997; **16**:472.

76 Nikolic-Tomasevic Z, Jelic S, Popov I *et al.* Colorectal cancer: dilemmas regarding patient selection and toxicity prediction. *J Chemother* 2000; **12**:244–51.

77 van Groeningen CJ, Van der Vijgh WJ, Baars JJ *et al.* Altered pharmacokinetics and metabolism of CPT-11 in liver dysfunction: a need for guidelines. *Clin Cancer Res* 2000; **6**:1342–6.

78 DeVore RF, Johnson DH, Crawford J *et al.* Phase II study of irinotecan plus cisplatin in patients with advanced non-small-cell lung cancer. *J Clin Oncol* 1999; **17**:2710–20.

79 Masuda N, Fukuoka M, Fujita A *et al.*, for CPT-11 Lung Cancer Study Group. A phase II trial of combination of CPT-11 and cisplatin for advanced non-small-cell lung cancer. *Br J Cancer* 1998; **78**:251–6.

80 Fukuoka M, Niitani H, Suzuki A *et al.* A phase II study of CPT-11, a new derivative of camptothecin, for previously untreated non-small-cell lung cancer. *J Clin Oncol* 1992; **10**:16–20.

81 Masuda N, Fukuoka M, Kudoh S *et al.* Phase I study of irinotecan and cisplatin with granulocyte colony-stimulating factor support for advanced non-small-cell lung cancer. *J Clin Oncol* 1994; **12**:90–6.

82 Devore R, III, Johnson D, Crawford J *et al.* Irinotecan plus cisplatin in patients with advanced non-small-cell lung cancer. *Oncology (Williston Park)* 1998; **12**:79–83.

83 Nakanishi Y, Takayama K, Takano K *et al.* Second-line chemotherapy with weekly cisplatin and irinotecan in patients with refractory lung cancer. *Am J Clin Oncol* 1999; **22**:399–402.

84 Kakolyris S, Kouroussis C, Kalbakis K *et al.* Salvage treatment of advanced non-small-cell lung cancer previously treated with docetaxel-based front-line chemotherapy with irinotecan (CPT-11) in combination with cisplatin. *Ann Oncol* 2000; **11**:757–60.

85 Langer CJ. Treatment of non-small-cell lung cancer in North America: the emerging role of irinotecan. *Oncology (Huntingt)* 2001; **15**:19–24.

86 Jagasia MH, Langer CJ, Johnson DH *et al.* Weekly irinotecan and cisplatin in advanced non-small cell lung cancer: a multicenter phase II study. *Clin Cancer Res* 2001; **7**:68–73.

87 Negoro S, Fukuoka M, Niitani H *et al.*, for CPT-11 Cooperative Study Group. A phase II study of CPT-11, a camptothecin derivative, in patients with primary lung cancer. *Gan To Kagaku Ryoho* 1991; **18**:1013–9.

88 Takeda K, Takifuji N, Uejima H *et al.* Phase II study of irinotecan and carboplatin for advanced non-small cell lung cancer. *Lung Cancer* 2002; **38**:303–8.

89 Murren JR, Andersen N, Psyrri D *et al.* Evaluation of irinotecan plus paclitaxel in patients with advanced non-small cell lung cancer. *Cancer Biol Ther* 2005; **4**:1311–5.

90 Ziotopoulos P, Androulakis N, Mylonaki E *et al.* Front-line treatment of advanced non-small cell lung cancer with irinotecan and docetaxel: a multicentre phase II study. *Lung Cancer* 2005; **50**:115–22.

91 Nakai H, Fukuoka M, Furuse K *et al.* An early phase II study of CPT-11 in primary lung cancer. *Gan To Kagaku Ryoho* 1991; **18**:607–12.

92 Wachters FM, Groen HJ, Biesma B *et al.* A randomised phase II trial of docetaxel vs docetaxel and irinotecan in patients with stage IIIb–IV non-small-cell lung cancer who failed first-line treatment. *Br J Cancer* 2005; **92**:15–20.

93 Grossi F, Fasola G, Rossetto C *et al.* Phase II study of irinotecan and docetaxel in patients with previously treated non-small cell lung cancer: an Alpe-Adria Thoracic Oncology Multidisciplinary group study (ATOM 007). *Lung Cancer* 2006; **52**:89–92.

94 Molina JR, Nikcevich D, Hillman S *et al.* A phase II NCCTG study of irinotecan and docetaxel in previously treated patients with non-small cell lung cancer. *Cancer Invest* 2006; **24**:382–9.

95 Pectasides D, Pectasides M, Farmakis D *et al.* Comparison of docetaxel and docetaxel–irinotecan combination as second-line chemotherapy in advanced non-small-cell lung cancer: a randomized phase II trial. *Ann Oncol* 2005; **16**:294–9.

96 Kosmas C, Tsavaris N, Syrigo K *et al.* A phase I–II study of bi-weekly gemcitabine and irinotecan as second-line chemotherapy in non-small cell lung cancer after prior taxane + platinum-based regimens. *Cancer Chemother Pharmacol* 2007; **59(1)**:51–9.

97 Georgoulias V, Kouroussis C, Agelidou A *et al.* Irinotecan plus gemcitabine vs irinotecan for the second-line treatment of patients with advanced non-small-cell lung cancer pretreated with docetaxel and cisplatin: a multicentre, randomised, phase II study. *Br J Cancer* 2004; **91**:482–8.

98 Wakelee HA, Sikic BI. Activity of novel cytotoxic agents in lung cancer: epothilones and topoisomerase I inhibitors. *Clin Lung Cancer* 2005; **7(Suppl 1)**:S6–12.

99 Depierre A, Lemarie E, Dabouis G *et al.* A phase II study of Navelbine (vinorelbine) in the treatment of non-small-cell lung cancer. *Am J Clin Oncol* 1991; **14**:115–9.

100 Le Chevalier T, Brisgand D, Douillard JY *et al.* Randomized study of vinorelbine and cisplatin versus vindesine and cisplatin versus vinorelbine alone in advanced non-small-cell lung cancer: results of a European multicenter trial including 612 patients. *J Clin Oncol* 1994; **12**:360–7.

101 Wozniak AJ, Crowley JJ, Balcerzak SP *et al.* Randomized trial comparing cisplatin with cisplatin plus vinorelbine in the treatment of advanced non-small-cell lung cancer: a Southwest Oncology Group study. *J Clin Oncol* 1998; **16**:2459–65.

102 Agelaki S, Bania H, Kouroussis C *et al.* Vinorelbine-based regimens as salvage treatment in patients with advanced non-small cell lung cancer: two parallel multicenter phase II trials. *Oncology* 2001; **60**:235–41.

103 Kosmas C, Tsavaris N, Panopoulos C *et al.* Gemcitabine and vinorelbine as second-line therapy in non-small-cell lung cancer after prior treatment with taxane + platinum-based regimens. *Eur J Cancer* 2001; **37**:972–8.

104 Clarke SJ, Abratt R, Goedhals L *et al.* Phase II trial of pemetrexed disodium (ALIMTA, LY231514) in chemotherapy-naive patients with advanced non-small-cell lung cancer. *Ann Oncol* 2002; **13**:737–41.

105 Rusthoven JJ, Eisenhauer E, Butts C *et al.*, for National Cancer Institute of Canada Clinical Trials Group. Multitargeted antifolate LY231514 as first-line chemotherapy for patients with advanced non-small-cell lung cancer: a phase II study. *J Clin Oncol* 1999; **17**:1194.

106 Manegold C, Gatzemeier U, von Pawel J *et al.* Front-line treatment of advanced non-small-cell lung cancer with MTA (LY231514, pemetrexed disodium, ALIMTA) and cisplatin: a multicenter phase II trial. *Ann Oncol* 2000; **11**:435–40.

107 Koshy S, Herbst R, Obasaju R *et al.* A phase II trial of pemetrexed (P) plus carboplatin (C) in patients (pts) with advanced non-small-cell lung cancer (NSCLC) [Abstract 7074]. *J Clin Oncol, 2004 ASCO Annu Meet Proc (Post-Meet Ed)* 2004; **22(145)**:70–74.

108 Hanna N, Shepherd FA, Fossella FV *et al.* Randomized phase III trial of pemetrexed versus docetaxel in patients with non-small-cell lung cancer previously treated with chemotherapy. *J Clin Oncol* 2004; **22**:1589–97.

109 Herbst RS, Shin DM. Monoclonal antibodies to target epidermal growth factor receptor-positive tumors: a new paradigm for cancer therapy. *Cancer* 2002; **94**:1593–611.

110 Blumenschein G, Khuri F, Gatzemeier U *et al.* A randomized phase III trial comparing bexarotene/carboplatin/paclitaxel versus carboplatin/paclitaxel in chemotherapy-naive patients with advanced or metastatic non-small cell lung cancer (NSCLC) [Abstract 7001]. *J Clin Oncol, 2005 ASCO Annu Meet Proc* 2005; **23**:16S.

111 Leighl NB, Paz-Ares L, Douillard JY *et al.* Randomized phase III study of matrix metalloproteinase inhibitor BMS-275291 in combination with paclitaxel and carboplatin in advanced non-small-cell lung cancer: National Cancer Institute of Canada–Clinical Trials Group Study BR.18. *J Clin Oncol* 2005; **23**:2831–9.

112 Paz-Ares L, Douillard JY, Koralewski P *et al.* Phase III study of gemcitabine and cisplatin with or without aprinocarsen, a protein kinase C-alpha antisense oligonucleotide, in patients with advanced-stage non-small-cell lung cancer. *J Clin Oncol* 2006; **24**:1428–34.

113 Shepherd FA, Rodrigues Pereira J, Ciuleanu T *et al.* Erlotinib in previously treated non-small-cell lung cancer. *N Engl J Med* 2005; **353**:123–32.

114 Bezjak A, Tu D, Seymour L *et al.* Symptom improvement in lung cancer patients treated with erlotinib: quality of life analysis of the National Cancer Institute of Canada Clinical Trials Group Study BR.21. *J Clin Oncol* 2006; **24**:3831–7.

115 Davies A, McCoy J, Lara P *et al.* Bortezomib + gemcitabine (Gem)/carboplatin (Carbo) results in encouraging survival in advanced non-small cell lung cancer (NSCLC): results of a phase II Southwest Oncology Group (SWOG) trial (S0339) [Abstract 7017]. *J Clin Oncol, 2006 ASCO Annu Meet Proc* 2006; **24**:18S.

116 Fanucchi M, Fossella F, Fidias P *et al.* Bortezomib ± docetaxel in previously treated patients with

advanced non-small cell lung cancer (NSCLC): a phase 2 study [Abstract 7034]. *J Clin Oncol, 2005 ASCO Annu Meet Proc* 2005; **23**:16S.

117 Tyagi P. Bexarotene in combination with chemotherapy fails to prolong survival in patients with advanced non-small-cell lung cancer: results from the SPIRIT I and II trials. *Clin Lung Cancer* 2005; **7**:17–9.

118 Gollob JA, Wilhelm S, Carter C *et al*. Role of Raf kinase in cancer: therapeutic potential of targeting the Raf/MEK/ERK signal transduction pathway. *Semin Oncol* 2006; **33**:392–406.

119 Gatzemeier U, Blumenschein G, Fossella F *et al*. Phase II trial of single-agent sorafenib in patients with advanced non-small cell lung carcinoma [Abstract 7002]. *J Clin Oncol, 2006 ASCO Annu Meet Proc* 2006; **24**:18S.

120 Coussens LM, Fingleton B, Matrisian LM. Matrix metalloproteinase inhibitors and cancer: trials and tribulations. *Science* 2002; **295**:2387–92.

121 Bonomi P. Matrix metalloproteinases and matrix metalloproteinase inhibitors in lung cancer. *Semin Oncol* 2002; **29**:78–86.

122 Johnson BE, Heymach JV. Farnesyl transferase inhibitors for patients with lung cancer. *Clin Cancer Res* 2004; **10**:4254s–7s.

123 Johnston SR. Farnesyl transferase inhibitors: a novel targeted therapy for cancer. *Lancet Oncol* 2001; **2**:18–26.

124 Lee D, Gautschi O. Clinical development of SRC tyrosine kinase inhibitors in lung cancer. *Clin Lung Cancer* 2006; **7**:381–4.

125 Johnson FM, Saigal B, Talpaz M *et al*. Dasatinib (BMS-354825) tyrosine kinase inhibitor suppresses invasion and induces cell cycle arrest and apoptosis of head and neck squamous cell carcinoma and non-small cell lung cancer cells. *Clin Cancer Res* 2005; **11**:6924–32.

126 Reddy G. Current data and ongoing trials in patients with recurrent non-small-cell lung cancer. *Clin Lung Cancer* 2004; **5(6)**:337–9.

127 Spicer J, Harper P. Targeted therapies for non-small cell lung cancer. *Int J Clin Pract* 2005; **59**:1055–62.

128 Aparicio A. The potential of histone deacetylase inhibitors in lung cancer. *Clin Lung Cancer* 2006; **7**:309–12.

129 Gomez-Martin C, Rubio-Viqueira B, Hidalgo M. Current status of mammalian target of rapamycin inhibitors in lung cancer. *Clin Lung Cancer* 2005; **7(Suppl 1)**:S13–8.

CHAPTER 21

Immunologic Approaches to Lung Cancer Therapy

Jay M. Lee, Steven M. Dubinett, and Sherven Sharma

Cancer immunosurveillance

Paul Ehrlich first proposed the concept of the immune system-mediated suppression of tumor growth of cancer cells nearly 100 years ago [1]. This idea was more thoroughly explored starting in the 1950s when seminal findings in immunology provided the conceptual framework to begin to understand this process. First, Sir Peter Medawar elucidated the central role for the cellular constituents of immunity in mediating allograft rejection [2]. Frank Macfarlane Burnet is credited with formulating the idea of cancer immunosurveillance with the introduction of the "clonal selection theory" in 1957 [3–5]. This concept suggested that the immune system recognized and destroyed clones of transformed cells before growth into clinically evident tumors [6]. A critical cornerstone of the cancer immunosurveillance hypothesis was subsequently demonstrated when mice were immunized against syngeneic tumor transplants that had been induced by chemical carcinogens or viruses [7]. Subsequent introduction of live tumor cells into the immunized mouse resulted in rejection of the tumor transplant. These studies were the initial findings that implied the existence of tumor-specific antigens. This hypothesis was eventually validated in a variety of more modern murine models in which immune deficiencies were noted to be associated with an in-

crease in spontaneous as well as induced neoplasms [8]. The evidence that cancer immunosurveillance may be operative in humans is exemplified in studies that document an increase in cancer incidence amongst immunosuppressed organ transplant recipients [7,9,10]. In a study of heart transplant recipients, Pham and colleagues reported a prevalence of lung cancer that was 25-fold higher than the general population [9]. Dickson *et al.* reported a 6.9% incidence of de novo primary lung cancer in the native lung in single-lung transplant recipients, which was characterized by an aggressive and frequently fatal course, and the history of tobacco-related lung disease significantly increased the risk of developing bronchogenic cancer after transplantation [10]. These results demonstrated that single-lung transplant patients had a significantly greater risk for developing lung cancer than the general nontransplanted population and double lung transplant recipients [10]. In addition, histopathologic evidence demonstrating the presence of inflammatory infiltrates in areas surrounding tumors and the finding of lymphocytic proliferation in tumor draining lymph nodes further support the existence of cancer immunosurveillance.

Cancer immunoediting

Although the hypothesis of cancer immunosurveillance is supported by a wealth of compelling evidence from murine and human studies [5–10], the process of cancer immunosurveillance has evolved

Lung Cancer, 3rd edition. Edited by Jack A. Roth, James D. Cox, and Waun Ki Hong. © 2008 Blackwell Publishing, ISBN: 978-1-4051-5112-2.

into a more current concept termed "immunoediting" by Schreiber and colleagues [5–8]. Given that immunocompetent individuals still develop malignancies despite the presence of an intact immune system and certain cancers are capable of escaping immune recognition and destruction, a complex interaction between the cancer cells and the host immune system may result in changing tumor immunogenicity. This is the fundamental basis of cancer immunoediting [5].

Prior to the detection of a clinically apparent lung cancer, there is an extensive interaction between the transformed cells and the host immune and inflammatory responses that may select for cancerous cells with the ability to survive in a competent immune environment. The ability of cancer cells to evade immune recognition may occur with acquisition of genetic mutations that facilitate the development of the malignant phenotype and subsequent tumor formation. These mutations may be critically linked to acquiring cellular properties associated with carcinogenesis, such as apoptosis resistance, unregulated proliferation, invasion, metastasis, and angiogenesis. Although both humoral (antibody) and cell-mediated immune (T lymphocyte) responses to the tumor have been demonstrated, the antitumor immune response has traditionally been understood as a cell-mediated process involving the presentation of tumor-associated antigens by antigen presenting cells (APC) to the T lymphocytes, resulting in the generation of immune effector cells with the ability to destroy cancerous cells [11]. Although antitumor humoral responses have been shown to exist in tumor bearing hosts, protection of the host from tumor progression has not been convincing [11]. As APC take up tumor antigens, the adaptive immune system may be alerted as the tumor antigen is presented to T cells. Investigators have detected tumor-specific humoral and cellular responses in patients with lung cancer indicating that the host immune system has recognized the tumor [12,13]. This immune recognition process through both humoral and cell-mediated mechanisms may result in the destruction of immunogenic tumor cells expressing a specific tumor antigen, and result in the selection of immune resistant and less immunogenic cancer cells. These re-

maining cells may possess properties to evade the immune system that include (1) failure to express major histocompatibility complex (MHC) which is required for immune effector cells to recognize processed tumor antigens and mediate cancer cell killing, (2) expression of poorly immunogenic antigen epitopes, or (3) production of immunosuppressive cytokines that suppress the antitumor immune responses. Thus, cancer immunoediting involves immunosurveillance via an immune-mediated tumor cell selection process that leads to alterations in the immunogenicity of the cancer, and this incomplete tumor destruction results in a population of cancer cells with the ability to evade the immune recognition and eradication [8]. Ultimately, these selected tumor cells resist immune and inflammatory responses, demonstrate the ability for progressive tumor growth, and result in a clinically detectable lung cancer.

Complicity of host cellular networks in lung tumorigenesis

Although the ability of the tumor cells to escape the immune effector contributes to cancer development, the pulmonary environment presents a unique milieu in which lung carcinogenesis proceeds in complicity with the host cellular network. The pulmonary diseases that are associated with the greatest risk for lung cancer are characterized by abundant and deregulated inflammation [14–16]. Pulmonary disorders such as chronic obstructive pulmonary disease (COPD)/emphysema and pulmonary fibrosis are characterized by profound abnormalities in inflammatory–fibrotic pathways [17–19]. For example, among the cytokines, growth factors, and mediators released in these lung diseases and the developing tumor microenvironment, IL-1β, PGE2, and TGF-β have been found to have deleterious properties that simultaneously pave the way for both epithelial mesenchymal transition (EMT) and destruction of specific host cell-mediated immune (CMI) responses against tumor antigens [20,21–24]. EMT is the developmental shift from a polarized, epithelial phenotype to a highly motile mesenchymal phenotype [25]. While this process is essential in embryogenesis and organ development, EMT is also critically involved in much adult pathology, including cancer, chronic inflammation, and fibrosis [25,26]. Although EMT is a tightly regulated process during embryonic development [27], in cancer progression, EMT is unregulated with selective elements of the process amplified and other aspects circumvented [28]. Thus, lung cancer develops in a host environment in which the deregulated inflammatory response both degrades CMI and promotes tumor progression. Investigators have attempted to reverse these events by stimulating host immune responses against tumor antigens in lung cancer.

Immunosuppression

It was originally hypothesized more than 30 years ago that specialized T cell subpopulations existed that functioned to suppress immune responses [29]. North and others pursued this avenue of investigation within the context of tumor immunity [30–33]. However, these early studies in the field of suppressor T cells were stymied by an inability to characterize the cellular and molecular mechanisms responsible for the observed suppressive phenomena. There has been a renewed interest in the study of T cell-mediated suppression of immunity that has been accompanied by the identification regulatory T cells. Although a variety of T regulatory (T reg) cells have been described [34], much attention has focused on the specific activities of those that have been referred to as "naturally occurring" CD4+CD25^{high} T reg cells [35,36], and hereafter refer to these as CD4+CD25+ T reg cells. Although investigators had pursued this topic for many years, the ground-breaking studies of Sakaguchi et al. [37] have been viewed as initiating a renaissance in T reg cell research; these as well as more recent results have led to the characterization of the CD4+CD25+ T cell population as "professional suppressor cells" [36]. These studies revealed that transfer of CD25-depleted CD4 cells to nude mice recipients resulted in the spontaneous development of autoimmune disease [37]. Reconstitution of CD4+CD25+ cells within

a limited period after transfer of CD4+CD25− cells prevented the autoimmune disease in a dose-dependent fashion. These initial studies indicated that CD4+CD25+ cells contribute to the maintenance of self-tolerance by downregulating immune response to self and nonself antigens; elimination or reduction of CD4+CD25+ cells ablated this general suppression, and thereby not only enhanced immune responses to nonself antigens, but also elicited autoimmune responses to certain self-antigens [37]. Subsequent studies have revealed that these cells are both hyporesponsive and suppressive and can act through an APC independent pathway [37–40]. The CD4+CD25+ cells were found to require TCR-dependent activation for induction of suppressor activity [38]. The thymic origin of CD4+CD25+ T reg cells has been documented [41,42]. As originally hypothesized by Shevach [43] and subsequently demonstrated by Jordan et al. [44], the derivation of T reg cells in the thymus appears to occur through a process referred to as "altered negative selection." More recently it has been appreciated that T reg cells can differentiate from activated human PBL CD4+CD25− cells in the periphery [45,46]. Although many aspects of this peripheral T reg cell differentiation pathway have not yet been defined, it may be pivotal in limiting immune responses to human cancer.

The active immune suppression induced by the tumor has been well documented in lung cancer and other malignancies [47]. Tumor-reactive T cells have been shown to accumulate in lung cancer tissues but fail to respond [48,49]. In fact, a high proportion of nonsmall cell lung cancer (NSCLC) tumor-infiltrating lymphocytes (TIL) are CD4+CD25^{high} T reg cells [50]. Tumor cells may contribute to promoting immune suppression by directing surrounding inflammatory cells to release suppressive cytokines in the tumor milieu, augmenting the trafficking of suppressor cells to the tumor site, and/or promoting differentiation of effector lymphocytes to a T reg cell phenotype [51,52]. Liu et al. recently demonstrated that tumor cells could directly convert CD4+CD25− T cells to T reg cells through the production of high levels of TGF-β, suggesting a possible mechanism through which tumor cells evade the immune system [53]. One major impediment to effective therapy is our inadequate understanding of how lung cancer cells escape immune surveillance and inhibit antitumor immunity [54]. In previous studies an immune suppressive network in NSCLC that is due to overexpression of tumor cyclooxygenase 2 (COX-2) has been defined. COX-2 isoenzyme activity is significantly increased in cancerous tissues compared to their normal counterparts in several malignancies and studies document this overexpression in human lung cancer [55]. In murine lung cancer models specific genetic or pharmacological inhibition of COX-2 in vivo led to significant tumor regression [56]. Although COX-2 metabolites have been identified as mediators of immunosuppression, the specific molecular and cellular pathways in the COX-2-dependent immune suppressive network are now being defined. Particular attention has recently focused on defining the pathways whereby COX-2 and its metabolite prostaglandin E2 (PGE2) inhibit immune responses in lung cancer by promoting T reg cell activity. PGE2 promotes the CD4+CD25+ T reg phenotype and increases the expression of the forkhead transcription factor FOXP3 that is known to program the development and function of T reg cells. This pivotal relationship is currently under investigation in the laboratory utilizing human cells in vitro as well as in patients with lung cancer. Based on the results of preclinical murine models [57] and human cells in vitro [20], clinical studies are now evaluating the optimal biological dose of a COX-2 inhibitor, celecoxib, to decrease FOXP3 and T reg function in patients with lung cancer.

Cancer immunotherapy

Although various methods of immune stimulation have been attempted for treatment of thoracic malignancies, none have proven to be reliably effective [58–60]. In contrast, immune-based therapies have proven more successful in melanoma and renal cell carcinoma [61,62], leading to the suggestion that thoracic malignancies are nonimmunogenic and will not be amenable to immunologic interventions. In groundbreaking studies, however, Boon and colleagues found that protective immunity could be generated against nonimmunogenic murine tumors [63,64]. These studies suggest that a tumor's apparent lack of immunogenicity is indicative of a failure to elicit an effective host response rather than a lack of tumor antigen expression [65,66]. Accordingly, a new paradigm emerged that focused on generating antitumor responses by therapeutic vaccination [67,68]. In this setting, vaccination refers to an intervention that unmasks tumor antigens leading to generation of specific host-immune responses against the tumor [69]. While there has been a multitude of lung cancer immunization studies, clinical trials focused on inducing a specific antitumor immune response can be categorized into (1) dendritic cell vaccines, (2) modified tumor cell vaccines, (3) tumor protein and peptide vaccines, (4) immune adjuvant vaccines, and (5) gene delivery vaccines.

Dendritic cell vaccines

The predominant mechanism of antitumor immunity is a cell (T lymphocyte)-mediated destruction of tumor cells. Specifically, the expansion of cytotoxic T lymphocytes (CTL) capable of recognizing antigens on cancerous cells presented in association with MHC molecules is the goal of most immunotherapy strategies. T cells can express clonally distributed antigen receptors in the context of MHC proteins. As a result, T cells have the capacity to recognize unique tumor antigens, such as those evolving from mutations or viral oncogenesis. These T cells may also recognize self-antigens, such as those derived from overexpression of proteins or aberrant expression of antigens that are normally developmentally or tissue restricted. APC appear to play a central role in T cell activation by presenting tumor antigens and providing essential costimulatory signals necessary for the production of CTL [70]. In optimal circumstances, APC can migrate and gain access to the tumor microenvironment, and overcome tumor-induced obstacles to have effective function. T cell activation results in the generation of CTL capable of recognizing and destroying cancer cells, and the production of cytokines, such as IFNγ and TNFα, which can suppress both tumor cell proliferation and induction of angiogenesis [71,72]. CTL can cause lysis of tumor cells mediated by perforin and/or Fas [71,73]. Therefore, therapeutic efforts have focused on identifying tumor antigens, providing the antigens in immunogenic contexts, manipulating T cell responses to increase the number of CTL, and thus augmenting these effector functions.

The numerous challenges that thwart the efficacy of cancer vaccines have been recently reviewed [74]. These obstacles include (1) correct identification of optimal antigens and immune adjuvants, (2) determination of the appropriate immune response to be generated, (3) elicitation of long-term antitumor memory, and (4) tumor-induced immunosuppression and immune evasion [74].

Investigators studying therapeutic vaccines have attempted to circumvent these problems by focusing on methods to restore tumor antigen presentation and antitumor effector activities in lung cancer patients by utilizing DC (dendritic cells)-based therapy [75–77]. DC are extremely potent APC that present tumor-associated antigens to T cells and thereby initiate tumor-specific immunity [78–81]. DC are bone marrow-derived leukocytes characterized by a high level of expression of MHC and costimulatory molecules [82]. As a result, they are capable of capturing antigens and producing large numbers of immunogenic MHC-peptide complexes [82]. Under the stimulation of maturation factors, such as inflammatory cytokines or CD40, DC can upregulate adhesion and costimulatory molecules to become terminally differentiated stimulators of T cell immunity [83]. They migrate to secondary lymphoid organs to select and stimulate antigen-specific T cells [84,85]. With the application of appropriate cytokines, one can generate large quantities of DC [86,87]. Human DC may be generated from proliferating CD34+ cells or from nonproliferating CD14+ progenitor cells. The production of DC from CD34+ cells requires GM-CSF and tumor necrosis factor alpha (TNF-α), whereas CD14+ cells require stimulation with GM-CSF and interleukin-4 (IL-4) to produce sufficient quantities of DC [88].

Because of the importance of DC in tumor immunity a variety of strategies have been used to exploit activated DC in cancer immunotherapy [84,89]. These strategies have included the use of DC pulsed with tumor antigen peptides [90–92], apoptotic tumor cells [93], or tumor lysates [90], or genetic modification of DC with genes encoding tumor antigens or total RNA from tumor cells [94,95]. Fully mature DC express the surface phenotype critical for effective antigen presentation, including MHC, adhesion molecules, and costimulatory molecules, such as B7.1 (CD80) and B7.2 (CD86) [84]. In the immature state, DC exist in tissue sites where they efficiently engulf antigens. Antigen uptake can serve to advance DC maturation and mobilization [96]. The maturation process includes heightened expression of MHC and accessory molecules but concomitant downregulation of antigen uptake capacities. In previous studies in which antigen pulsing of DC occurred ex vivo, it seemed that mature DC were optimal for administration. However, the inclusion of immature DC might heighten the efficacy of therapeutic vaccination due to more effective antigen capture. We have found that bone marrow-derived DC pulsed with tumor antigens are capable of inducing protective immunity [97].

Many clinical trials are addressing the feasibility and safety of DC-based strategies [98–102]. DC have recently been investigated as a delivery mechanism for tumor-associated antigens. Both whole cell and peptide strategies have been reported. Hirschowitz *et al.* used autologous DC pulsed with apoptotic bodies of an allogeneic NSCLC cell line that overexpressed five known antigens (Her2/*neu*, CEA, WT1, MAGE2, and survivin) [101]. The DC vaccines were administered intradermally two times, 1 month apart to 16 individuals with stage IA to IIIB NSCLC treated with surgery, chemoradiation, or multimodality therapy [101]. Vaccines were well tolerated with no unanticipated or serious adverse events. IFN-γ elispot assays demonstrated that immunologic responses to vaccines were independent of stage, histology, and prior treatment modality [101]. Eleven of 16 patients had immunological responses, 6 of 16 of which were specific to the antigens in the vaccine [101]. Due to the small sample size and patient heterogeneity, meaningful statistical analysis could not be performed for clinical outcomes, and immunologic responses did not appear to correlate with clinical events. A summary of clinical outcomes included five individuals with documented disease recurrence or progression and clinical benefit from vaccination could not be confirmed [101]. One of the limitations of this study is the selection of antigens used may not be optimal to all enrolled patients.

Kontani *et al.* studied autologous DC pulsed with either MUC-1 peptides in patients with MUC-1 positive tumors (9) or autologous tumor lysates in patients with MUC-1 negative tumors (5) in a total of 14 patients with locally advanced or metastatic lung (8 patients) or breast cancer (6 patients) [102]. After vaccination, all the MUC-1positive patients demonstrated MUC-1 antigen-specific immune responses whereas only one case with MUC-1 negative cancer showed an immune response [102]. Clinical response including reduction in tumor size, tumor marker level, or disappearance of malignant pleural effusion was seen in 7 of the 9 patients with MUC-1 expressing tumors [102]. Patients with tumors that were MUC-1 negative did not respond to the DC vaccine, with the exception of one case with MAGE3-positive lung cancer [102]. MUC-1 positive patients receiving peptide pulsed DC had significantly prolonged survival in comparison to MUC-1 negative patients receiving DC pulsed with autologous tumor lysates (mean survival: 16.75 mo versus 3.80 mo, $p = 0.01$) [102]. This study suggested that MUC-1 antigen is sufficiently immunogenic to induce a measurable antitumor immune response and that DC vaccines targeting MUC1 may have clinical benefit.

Antonia *et al.* reported on a vaccination strategy that entailed autologous DC transfected with an adenovirus containing wild-type p53 [100]. The tumor suppressor gene, p53, has a critical involvement as a regulator of the cell cycle and differentiation, and loss of p53 function compromises genetic homeostasis in cells exhibiting deregulated DNA replication and/or DNA damage [103]. p53 mutation is one of the most common mutations in lung cancer [104]. This trial exemplifies the concept of using adenovirus as a gene delivery tool into DC resulting in high production of the chosen protein [105,106]. Twenty-nine patients with previously treated extensive stage small cell lung cancer (SCLC) were vaccinated repeatedly at 2-week intervals [100]. Most of the patients received three immunizations [100]. Sixteen of the 28 tested patients (57%) demonstrated an immunological response to

vaccination by IFN-γ elispot assays [100]. Out of the 29 treated patients, 1 patient achieved a partial response, 7 had stable disease, and 21 patients developed progressive disease [100]. An objective clinical response (partial and complete responses) was seen in 62% of the 21 patients who received second-line chemotherapy [100]. Objective response to second-line chemotherapy in platinum resistant extensive stage SCLC is 2–5% [100]. Despite more than half of the patients exhibiting induction of p53 antigen-specific immunity, there was only one patient with a clinical objective outcome after vaccination therapy, but most of the vaccinated patients had objective clinical responses with second-line chemotherapy, suggesting a chemosensitizing effect following vaccination.

Insights into cellular and molecular events that lead to recruitment and activation of immune cells suggest that obstacles present at tumor sites might be bypassed and tumor immunity initiated by providing selected cytokines and/or chemokines at sites of solid tumors [107]. Although our knowledge of how to harness therapeutic chemoattractants and activators is still rudimentary, expression of molecules such as secondary lymphoid-tissue chemokine from gene-modified dendritic cells and intratumoral administration have shown efficacy in preclinical murine tumor models [76,77,108]. Activating DC within the lung tumor site may be a particularly effective approach. A correlation exists between the number of tumor-infiltrating DC and survival [109]. Thus, this approach achieves tumor antigen presentation by utilizing the tumor as an in vivo source of antigen for DC. In contrast to in vitro immunization with purified peptide Ag, autologous tumor has the capacity to provide the activated DC administered at the tumor site access to the entire repertoire of available antigens in situ. This may increase the likelihood of a response and reduce the potential for tumor resistance due to phenotypic modulation. A phase 1 trial to evaluate the intratumoral injection of CCL21-adenoviral gene-modified dendritic cells (DC-AdCCL21) in patients with advanced NSCLC will begin at UCLA in 2007. The trial will be a dose escalation of DC-AdCCL21 administered intratumorally in patients with advanced NSCLC.

Modified tumor cell vaccines

Tumors differ fundamentally from their normal cell counterparts in antigenic makeup and biologic behavior, and a defining component of carcinogenesis is genetic instability [110]. The culmination of genetic mutations in cancer cells is the generation of new antigens as tumors develop and progress [110]. As a result, autologous and allogeneic tumors are a rich source for tumor antigens in vaccine trials.

The advantage of autologous tumor vaccines is the ability to generate patient-specific immune responses and avoidance of identifying the tumor cell antigenic phenotype. However, this is weighed by the limitation in availability and amount of the patient's own tumor, and vaccine trials based on this concept are restricted to enrolling patients undergoing surgical resection. The utility of gene-modified tumor cell vaccines has been well established from several preclinical tumor models. The cytokine GM-CSF promotes immune memory, and prevents tumor recurrence and metastasis. GM-CSF is a mediator of proliferation, maturation, and migration of DC and enhances antitumor immunity [111,112]. Autologous, irradiated NSCLC cells engineered to secrete GM-CSF were tested in patients with metastatic NSCLC in a phase I clinical trial [113]. Resected metastases were processed and infected with a replication-defective adenoviral vector encoding GM-CSF [113]. In 18 of 25 assessable patients there was accumulation of immune cellular (DC, macrophage, granulocyte, and lymphocyte) infiltrates [113]. Delayed-type hypersensitivity reactions to irradiated, autologous, nontransfected tumor cells occurred in 18 of 22 patients [113]. Perhaps the most compelling evidence to support antitumor immunity after vaccination was demonstrated in the 3 of 6 patients with surgical excision of metastases that showed tumor necrosis and lymphocytic infiltrates [113]. With respect to clinical outcomes, 5 patients showed stable disease and 2 patients with no evidence of disease (NED) after surgery at enrollment remain free of disease at 43 and 42 months [113].

In an effort to remove the need for viral transduction of autologous tumors, a vaccine (GVAX) composed of the combination of autologous tumor cells and an allogeneic GM-CSF secreting cell line has been utilized in clinical trials [114,115]. In a phase I/II trial, Nemunaitis *et al.* evaluated 49 patients with advanced NSCLC (stage IIIA–IV) vaccinated 3–12 times biweekly with GVAX [115]. Analysis of the immune response was measured by DTH reactions to irradiated autologous tumor cells and induction of tumor reactive antibodies. DTH reactions were detected in prevaccination in 13% and postvaccination in 34% of patients [115]. Antibodies reactive against autologous tumor cells were seen in 31% of patients [115]. No patients demonstrated a partial or complete response to vaccination, and seven (14%) patients demonstrated stable disease [115]. Due to the lack of efficacy from GVAX in advanced NSCLC, this vaccine has transferred its use to other malignancies.

Allogeneic antigens are attractive sources of tumor antigens in vaccine trials given that they eliminate the need for patient tumor procurement. Tumor cell lines can serve as an allogeneic whole cell vaccine. Malignant cells often change the cell surface phenotype by lacking costimulatory signals required for the generation of effective antitumor immunity [116]. The most critical molecules involved in costimulation are CD80/CD86 and CD40L [116]. Lung cancer cells have been shown to downregulate MHC molecule expression on the cell surface [11,69,117,118]. As a result, several studies have embarked on genetic manipulation of tumor cell lines to express necessary costimulatory and MHC molecules necessary for induction of antitumor immunity [119,120]. Raez *et al.* who conducted a phase I trial in stage IIIB and IV NSCLC patients with a vaccine therapy comprised of a human lung adenocarcinoma cell line transfected with B7.1 (CD80) and HLA A1 or A2 (MHC I molecules) [120]. Nineteen patients received up to nine immunizations [120]. The vaccine was well tolerated, with four serious adverse events believed to be unrelated to the vaccine. All but one patient had a measurable CD8 T cell response after three immunizations [120]. Clinically, one patient had a partial response and five patients demonstrated stable disease [120]. Although allogeneic cell lines provide a convenient alternative to autologous patient tumors, a major limitation with the use of this strategy is the fundamental assumption that lung tumor antigens expressed on the cell line are common with the patient's unique tumor and this antigenic phenotype is also shared among different patients.

Tumor protein and peptide vaccines

Activated protooncogenes, inactivated tumor suppressor genes, and genetic mutations have been linked to molecular events involved in lung cancer tumorigenesis and has led to the identification of tumor associated antigens ideal for vaccine strategies. These allogeneic antigens in the form of proteins or peptides are another source of tumor antigens that addresses the inability or unfeasibility to access a patient's tumor in adequate quantities for autologous tumor vaccine production. Proteins and peptides are processed via MHC molecules and presented by APC on the cell surface to T lymphocytes resulting in the generation of a specific immune response [121]. Only a short segment of peptide sequences from the original tumor protein are immunogenic, and these peptide sequences, called epitopes, are presented by MHC molecules according to a complex set of cellular rules [121]. Peptides are smaller than proteins, readily produced, and generate reproducible immune responses by readily available immune assays. However, peptides are restricted to specific HLA types for presentation, which may not allow universal application to all patients [121].

In response to cellular stress such as DNA damage, hypoxia, or oncogene activation, the tumor suppressor protein p53 has a pivotal role in defining the cell's fate into short-term cell cycle arrest to allow cell repair (temporary cell arrest), senescence (permanent cell arrest), or apoptosis (programmed cell death) [122,123]. Abnormal or disrupted p53 activation pathways are present >50% of human tumors and has been implicated to be an important determining factor in the prevention of tumor development [122,123]. p53 mutation is one of the most common changes in lung cancer carcinogenesis and is highest in small cell and squamous cell carcinomas [124]. K-ras is a protooncogene critical in the downstream signaling pathway of several molecules, and genetic alterations of this gene may lead to growth stimulation and tumor development [125]. K-ras mutations are found in 15–30% of NSCLC tumors [126,127]. Mutations of p53 and

K-ras are frequent and often result in the generation of novel protein sequences that are overexpressed in tumor cells bearing these mutations [128–133]. Novel protein sequences generated by point mutations expressed intracellularly can be processed and presented on the cell surface in the context of MHC class I, and thus become accessible to cytotoxic T cells [131–134].

Carbone *et al.* conducted a phase I clinical trial immunizing patients with several types of cancers (lung, colon, breast, ovarian, head and neck, pancreatic, esophageal, gastric, and others) with mutant p53- and K-ras-derived peptides [135]. Patients in varying stages of disease underwent genetic analysis for mutations in K-ras and p53 [135]. Thirty-nine patients were enrolled of which 10 patients had lung cancer [135]. Peptides corresponding to the genetic mutations were custom synthesized, and baseline immunity was assessed for CTL response and IFN-γ release from mutant peptide-primed lymphocytes [135]. The peripheral blood mononuclear cells (PBMC) from patients were pulsed with the corresponding peptide, and administered intravenously every 2 months for a total of four immunizations [135]. Patients were observed for CTL response, cytokine expression (IFN-γ, interleukin (IL)-2, IL-5, and GM-CSF), treatment-related toxicity, and clinical tumor response [135]. The results indicated that no toxicity was observed [135]. Ten (26%) of 38 patients had detectable CTL against mutant p53 or K-ras, and 2 patients were positive for CTL at baseline [135]. Positive IFN-γ responses occurred in 16 patients (42%) after vaccination, whereas 4 patients had positive IFN-γ reaction before vaccination [135]. Of the 29 patients with clinically evident measurable disease, 5 had stable disease and 24 patients demonstrated disease progression [135]. Median survival times of 393 days versus 98 days for a positive versus negative CTL response ($p = 0.04$), respectively, and 470 days versus 88 days for a positive versus negative IFN-γ response ($p = 0.02$), respectively, were detected [135]. The results of this study indicated that custom-made peptide vaccination is feasible without toxicity, immune responses specific to a given mutation can be induced or enhanced with peptide vaccines, and induction of specific immunity to mutant p53 and K-ras peptides is associated with longer survival [135]. Of the 276 patients who were evaluated and screened for p53 and K-ras mutations, only 39 patients (14%) were eligible to be entered into the study and subsequently received immunizations [135]. The need for identification of the specific epitope in lung cancer and corresponding specific genetic mutation of the peptide is an obvious limitation in extending this strategy as a broad clinical approach to many patients.

The WT1 gene was initially isolated as a gene responsible for Wilms' tumor, and characterized as transcription factor involved in cell proliferation and differentiation, apoptosis, and organ development [136]. Furthermore, WT1 is overexpressed in leukemias and various types of solid tumors [136]. Oka *et al.* performed a phase I/II trial in patients with lung or breast cancer, myelodysplastic syndrome, and acute myeloid leukemia who were intradermally vaccinated with an HLA-A2402-restricted WT1 peptide and Montanide ISA51 immune adjuvant at 2-week intervals [136]. Of the 26 patients who enrolled into the study and received WT1 peptide vaccinations, 10 patients had lung cancer [136]. Toxicity consisted only of local erythema at the WT1 vaccine injection sites in all patients and no other toxicity was noted in the lung cancer patients [136]. In 3 of the 10 patients with lung cancer, a decrease in tumor markers was observed at WT1 vaccination [136]. The efficacy of WT1 vaccination could be assessed in 8 of the 10 lung cancer patients and showed reduction in tumor size in 2 patients, stable disease in 1 patient, and progression of disease in 4 patients [136]. A clear correlation was observed between an increase in the frequencies of WT1-specific CTL after vaccination and clinical responses. The study demonstrated that WT1 peptide vaccination could induce peptide-specific immunity and result in clinical cancer regression.

Epidermal growth factor (EGF) is a growth factor with a significant role in the regulation of apoptosis, cell survival, and cell proliferation [137]. Binding to its cell surface receptor, EGF activates an extensive network of signal transduction pathways that activate or inhibit transcription factors, which in turn regulate the expression of proteins integral to inducing or inhibiting apoptosis [137]. EGF-signaling pathways are often dysfunctional in cancer cells and promote cell survival and proliferation [137,138]. In NSCLC, EGFR expression has been shown to correlate with tumor metastasis and poor prognosis [139–141]. Ramos *et al.* reported the results of a phase I trial in 43 patients with advanced NSCLC (stage IIIB or IV) who received an EGF vaccine [142]. Patients were randomized to receive a single or double dose of the EGF vaccine composed of human recombinant EGF conjugated to a carrier protein (P64K *Neisseria meningitides* recombinant protein), weekly for 4 weeks, and monthly thereafter [142]. No significant toxicity was seen after vaccination [142]. Fifteen patients (39%) developed a good antibody response against EGF and these patients with a good humoral response had a significantly better survival when compared to poor responders [142]. An inverse correlation between anti-EGF antibody titers and EGF concentration was seen after immunization [142]. Patients who received the double dose of treatment showed a trend toward increased survival in comparison with patients who received the single dose [142]. The results of this study confirmed that EGF vaccination can achieve tumor protein-specific immunity in advanced stage NSCLC, resulted in reducing serum EGF levels, and antibody titers and serum EGF levels appear to correlate with patient survival [142]. Other EGF-based vaccine trials have also demonstrated acceptable safety and induction of specific immunogenicity to EGF in NSCLC [143–145].

The expression of the melanoma-associated antigen (MAGE) genes is silent in all normal cells except germ cells [146]. There has been more than 50 related MAGE genes identified thus far, and have been shown to play an important role physiologically and pathologically during embryogenesis, germ cell development, cell cycle progression, and apoptosis [146]. Nearly 75% of SCLC and approximately 40% of NSCLC express MAGE-3 and as a result this testis cancer antigen has received attention as an immunotherapy target [147]. Atanackovic *et al.* reported on the successful induction of humoral and specific cell-mediated immunity in early stage NSCLC (I and II) patients vaccinated with MAGE-3 protein [148]. Seventeen patients with MAGE-3 expressing NSCLC were analyzed in two groups, one receiving MAGE-3 protein alone and the other receiving MAGE-3 protein with adjuvant AS02B [148]. Of the 9 patients in the first cohort, 3 patients developed marginal Ab titers and another patient had a CD8 T cell response to HLA-A2-restricted peptide MAGE-3 271–279 [148]. In contrast, of 8 patients from the second cohort vaccinated with MAGE-3 protein and adjuvant, 7 patients developed antibody high titers to MAGE-3, and 4 had a strong concomitant CD4 T cell response to HLA-DP4-restricted peptide 243–258 [148]. One patient simultaneously developed CD8 T cells to HLA-A1-restricted peptide 168–176 [148]. Although the clinical relevance of the immune responses was not addressed, this study demonstrated the importance of CD4 T cell-mediated immunity that correlated with antibody production following vaccination, in addition to the traditionally understood involvement of antigen-specific CD8 T cell response. Moreover, this study provides the foundation for further evaluating integrated humoral and cell-mediated immune responses in vaccine strategies and also to pursue the relevance of this approach in clinical outcomes.

Immune adjuvant vaccines

Transforming growth factor-β (TGF-β) is a protein that inhibits proliferation and induces apoptosis in normal and neoplastic cells classifying it as a tumor suppressor gene, and regulates angiogenesis [149–151]. The accumulation of mutations in the TGF-β receptor or Smad genes inactivates the TGF-β receptor–Smad pathway favoring tumor growth [149,150]. All human tumors overproduce TGF-β whose actions promote tumor cell invasiveness and metastasis, and thus induce EMT [149]. TGF-β suppresses the proliferation and differentiation of lymphocytes including cytolytic T cells, natural killer cells, macrophages, and dendritic cells providing a mechanism of tumor-mediated immune evasion [149,151]. Elevated TGF-ß2 levels have been linked to immunosuppression in cancer patients [152], and TGF-ß2 levels have inversely correlated to prognosis of patients with NSCLC [153]. Current clinical approaches aim at establishing novel cancer drugs whose mechanisms target the TGF-β pathway.

Nemunaitis *et al.* performed a phase II study of belagenpumatucel-L, a TGF-ß2 antisense gene-modified allogeneic tumor cell line vaccine, in patients with stages II–IV NSCLC [154]. Each patient received belagenpumatucel-L on a monthly or every other month schedule to a maximum of 16 injections [154]. A dose-related survival difference was demonstrated in patients who received $\geq 2.5 \times 10^7$ cells/injection ($p = 0.0069$) [154]. In the 61 patients with advanced stage (IIIB and IV), a 15% partial response rate was seen [154]. The estimated survival at 1 and 2 years was 68% and 52%, respectively, for the higher dose groups combined, and 39% and 20%, respectively, for the low-dose group [154]. The induction of an immune response was evaluated in the 61 advanced stage patients. Increased cytokine production was observed among clinical responders at week 12 compared with patients with progressive disease (IFN-γ, $p = 0.006$; interleukin [IL]-6, $p = 0.004$; IL-4, $p = 0.007$) and elevated antibody-mediated response to vaccine HLA was demonstrated ($p = 0.014$) [154]. The study showed that belagenpumatucel-L was well tolerated, and the survival advantage justified pursuit for a phase III evaluation. Given that upregulation of the immune responses correlated to favorable clinical outcomes, this trial supports the concept that correct selection of allogeneic tumor cell lines that have shared immunodominant tumor antigens with the patient's tumor may be an effective antitumor strategy. Combining this approach with targeting the TGF pathway may add to this beneficial effect.

Anti-idiotypic monoclonal antibodies (Mab) can mimic both protein and nonprotein antigenic epitopes and induce immune responses against tumor antigens [155]. Anti-idiotypic antibody-based vaccines are ideal when the antigen is not readily available in sufficient quantities or when the antigen is not a protein [155]. SCLC is of neuroectodermal origin, and as a result, has a unique number of differentiation antigens as potential immune targets due to its specific embryonic basis [156]. Bec2 is an anti-idiotypic antibody that mimics GD3, a ganglioside antigen of neuroectodermal origin expressed on the surface of tumor cells, and are involved in numerous functions including cell–cell recognition, cell matrix attachment, and cell differentiation [156,157]. Giaccone *et al.* conducted a phase III trial immunizing Bec2 in combination with Bacille

Calmette-Guerin (BCG), in patients with limited-disease SCLC after a major response to chemotherapy and chest radiation [157]. Five hundred fifteen patients were randomly assigned to receive five vaccinations of Bec2/BCG vaccine over a 10-week period or follow-up [157]. The primary toxicities of immunization were transient skin ulcerations and mild flu-like symptoms [157]. In the patients who received the vaccine, there was no improvement in survival, progression-free survival, or quality of life [157]. The median survival from randomization was 16.4 and 14.3 months in the observation and vaccination arms ($p = 0.28$), respectively [157]. In summary, this study revealed that vaccination with Bec2/BCG had no impact on clinical outcome of patients with limited-disease SCLC responding to chemotherapy and radiation therapy. The anti-idiotypic antibody vaccine is the only phase III study in lung cancer. A series of other trials have established the immunogenicity of several keyhole limpet hemocyanin conjugate vaccines relevant to SCLC, including GM2, Globo H, fucosyl GM1, and polysialic acid [156].

Gene delivery vaccines

Gene transfer vectors have been utilized as drug delivery systems to provide high level expression of a protein of interest intracellularly or secretion into the local milieu of the tumor [158,159]. MUC1 is a glycoprotein normally found on the surface of mucin secreting epithelial cells [160], and its expression has been shown to be increased in breast, lung, ovary, and colon carcinomas suggesting that MUC1 aberrant expression is common to adenocarcinomas [161]. Humoral response to this protein has been detected in patients with NSCLC, and found to have prognostic significance [162]. Mennecier *et al.* reported a phase II trial with TG4010, a recombinant vaccinia vector (MVA) containing DNA sequences for the human MUC1 antigen and interleukin-2 (IL-2), in advanced NSCLC cancer patients [163]. A multicenter randomized trial was conducted in 65 stage IIIB and IV patients with either upfront TG4010 in combination with cisplatin and vinorelbine (arm 1) or TG4010 alone followed by both chemotherapeutic agents upon disease progression [163]. In arm 1, a partial response was seen

in 68% (24/35) patients [163]. In arm 2, two patients had stable disease, and in subsequent combination with chemotherapy, a partial response was seen in 3 of 14 patients [163]. TG4010 was well tolerated with the injection site reaction being the most common drug-related adverse event [163]. In this preliminary report, the combination of TG4010 with standard chemotherapy for NSCLC demonstrated encouraging results.

Conclusion

The challenge for immunotherapy is to use advances in cellular and molecular immunology to develop strategies that effectively and safely augment antitumor responses. This can be achieved through understanding the complex issues surrounding cancer immunosurveillance, cancer immunoediting, complicity of host cellular networks in lung tumorigenesis, and tumor-mediated immunosuppression. The numerous challenges that pose obstacles to cancer vaccine efficacy include (1) correct identification of optimal antigens and immune adjuvants, (2) determination of the appropriate immune response to be generated, (3) elicitation of long-term antitumor memory, and (4) tumor induced immunosuppression and immune evasion. When developing vaccine strategies, the requirements for (1) immune cell activation, homing, and accumulation at tumor sites, (2) disruption of the regulatory mechanisms that limit immune responses, and (3) the ability to direct a coordinated and effective attack against tumors engaging multiple components of the immune system should evolve in parallel. Ultimately, vaccination refers to an intervention that unmasks tumor antigens leading to the generation of specific host-immune responses against the tumor. While there has been a multitude of lung cancer immunization studies, clinical trials focused on inducing a specific antitumor immune response can be categorized into the following: (1) dendritic cell vaccines, (2) modified tumor cell vaccines, (3) tumor protein and peptide vaccines, (4) immune adjuvant vaccines, and (5) gene delivery vaccines. It is clear that effective antitumor responses require the complex interaction of APC, lymphocyte, and NK cells. As we unravel and elucidate the mechanisms of these combined approaches there will be additional opportunity for the development of effective immunotherapy for lung cancer.

References

1 Schwartz RS. Paul Erhlich's magic bullets. *NEJM* 2004; **350(11)**:1079–80.

2 Simpson E. Reminiscences of Sir Peter Medawar: in hope of antigen-specific transplantation tolerance. *Am J Transplant* 2004; **4(12)**:1937–40.

3 Fenner F, Ada G. Frank MacFarlane Burnet: two personal views. *Nat Immunol* 2007; **8**:111–3.

4 Burnet FM. *The Clonal Selection Theory of Acquired Immunity*. London: Cambridge University Press, 1959.

5 Dunn GP, Old LJ, Schreiber RD. The Immunobiology of cancer immunosurveillance and immunoediting. *Immunity* 2004; **21(2)**:137–48.

6 O'Mahony D, Kummar S, Gutierrez ME. Non-small-cell lung cancer vaccine therapy: a concise review. *J Clin Oncol* 2005; **23(35)**:9022–8.

7 Dunn GP, Old LJ, Schreiber RD. The three Es of cancer immunoediting. *Annu Rev Immunol* 2004; **22**:329–60.

8 Dunn GP, Bruce AT, Ikeda H, Old LJ, Schreiber RD. Cancer immunoediting: from immunosurveillance to tumor escape. *Nat Immunol* 2002; **3**:991–8.

9 Pham SM, Kormos RL, Landreneau RJ *et al*. Solid tumors after heart transplantation: lethality of lung cancer. *Ann Thorac Surg* 1995; **60**:1623–6.

10 Dickson R, Davis R, Rea J, Palmer S. High frequency of bronchogenic carcinoma after single-lung transplantation. *J Heart Lung Transplant* 2006; **25(11)**:1297–301.

11 Korst RJ, Crystal RG. Active, specific immunotherapy for lung cancer: hurdles and strategies using genetic modification. *Ann Thorac Surg* 2003; **76(4)**:1319–26.

12 Glassy MC, Yasutomi J, Koda K. Lessons learned about the therapeutic potential of the natural human immune response to lung cancer. *Expert Opin Investig Drugs* Jul 1999; **8(7)**:995–1006.

13 Ichiki Y, Takenoyama M, Mizukami M *et al*. Simultaneous cellular and humoral immune response against mutated p53 in a patient with lung cancer. *J Immunol* Apr 15, 2004; **172(8)**:4844–50.

14 Rennard SI. Chronic obstructive pulmonary disease: linking outcomes and pathobiology of disease modification. *Proc Am Thorac Soc* 2006; **3**:276–80.

15 O'Donnell R, Breen D, Wilson S, Djukanovic R. Inflammatory cells in the airways in COPD. *Thorax* 2006; **61**:448–54.

16 Sevenoaks MJ, Stockley RA. Chronic obstructive pulmonary disease, inflammation and co-morbidity – a common inflammatory phenotype? *Respir Res* 2006; **7**:70.

17 Reynolds PR, Cosio MC, Hoidal JR. Cigarette smoke-induced Egr-1 upregulates pro-inflammatory cytokines in pulmonary epithelial cells. *Am J Respir Cell Moll Biol* 2006; **35**:314–9.

18 Tan RJ, Fattman CL, Niehouse LM *et al*. Matrix metalloproteinases promote inflammation and fibrosis in asbestos-induced lung injury in mice. *Am J Respir Cell Mol Biol* 2006; **35**:289–97.

19 Soberman RJ, Christmas P. Revisiting prostacyclin-new directions in pulmonary fibrosis and inflammation. *Am J Physiol Lung Cell Mol Physiol* 2006; **291**:L142–3.

20 Baratelli F, Lin Y, Zhu L *et al*. Prostaglandin E2 induces FOXP3 gene expression and T regulatory cell function in human CD4+ T cells. *J Immunol* 2005; **175**:1483–90.

21 Dohadwala M, Yang SC, Luo J *et al*. Cyclooxygenase-2-dependent regulation of E-cadherin: prostaglandin E2 induces transcriptional repressors ZEB1 and Snail in non-small cell lung cancer. *Cancer Res* 2006; **66**:5338–45.

22 Charuworn B, Dohadwala M, Krysan K *et al*. Inflammation-mediated promotion of EMT in NSCLC: IL-1b mediates a MEK/Erk- and JNK/SAPK-dependent downregulation of E-cadherin. Abstract: American Thoracic Society 2006. *Am J Respir Crit Care Med* 2006; Abstracts Issue.

23 Keshamouni VG, Michailidis G, Grasso CS *et al*. Differential protein expression profiling by iTRAQ-2DLC-MS/MS of lung cancer cells undergoing epithelial-mesenchymal transition reveals a migratory/invasive phenotype. *J Proteome Res* 2006; **5**:1143–54.

24 Leng Q, Bentwich Z, Borkow G. Increased TGF-β, Cbl-b and CTLA-4 levels and immunosuppression in association with chronic immune activation. *Int Immunol* 2006; **18**:637–44.

25 Huber MA, Kraut N, Beug H. Molecular requirements for epithelial-mesenchymal transition during tumor progression. *Curr Opin Cell Biol* 2005; **17**:548–58.

26 Lee JM, Dedhar S, Kalluri R, Thompson EW. The epithelial–mesenchymal transition: new insights in signaling, development, and disease. *J Cell Biol* Mar 27, 2006; **172(7)**:973–81.

27 Thiery JP. Epithelial–mesenchymal transitions in development and pathologies. *Curr Opin Cell Biol* 2003; **15**:740–6.

28 Dasari V, Gallup M, Lemjabbar H, Maltseva I, McNamara N. Epithelial-mesenchymal transition in lung

cancer: is tobacco the "smoking gun"? *Am J Respir Cell Mol Biol* 2006; **35(1)**:3–9.

29 Gershon RK, Kondo K. Cell interactions in the induction of tolerance: the role of thymic lymphocytes. *Immunology* 1970; **18**:723.

30 Rakhmilevich AL, North RJ. Elimination of CD4+ T cells in mice bearing an advanced sarcoma augments the antitumor action of interleukin-2. *Cancer Immunol Immunother* 1994; **38**:107.

31 DiGiacomo A, North RJ. T cell suppressors of antitumor immunity. The production of Ly-1-,2+ suppressors of delayed sensitivity precedes the production of suppressors of protective immunity. *J Exp Med* 1986; **164**:1179.

32 Berendt MJ, North RJ. T-cell-mediated suppression of anti-tumor immunity. An explanation for progressive growth of an immunogenic tumor. *J Exp Med* 1980; **151**:69.

33 Dye ES, North RJ. T cell-mediated immunosuppression as an obstacle to adoptive immunotherapy of the P815 mastocytoma and its metastases. *J Exp Med* 1981; **154**:1033.

34 Antony PA, Restifo NP. Do CD4+ CD25+ immunoregulatory T cells hinder tumor immunotherapy? *J Immunother* 2002; **25**:202.

35 Maloy KJ, Powrie F. Regulatory T cells in the control of immune pathology. *Nat Immunol* 2001; **2**:816.

36 Shevach EM. Certified professionals: CD4(+) CD25(+) suppressor T cells. *J Exp Med* 2001; **193**:F41.

37 Sakaguchi S, Sakaguchi N, Asano M, Itoh M, Toda M. Immunologic self-tolerance maintained by activated T cells expressing IL-2 receptor alpha-chains (CD25). Breakdown of a single mechanism of self-tolerance causes various autoimmune diseases. *J Immunol* 1995; **155**:1151.

38 Thornton AM, Shevach EM. CD4+CD25+ immunoregulatory T cells suppress polyclonal T cell activation in vitro by inhibiting interleukin 2 production. *J Exp Med* 1998; **188**:287.

39 Takahashi T, Kuniyasu Y, Toda M et al. Immunologic self-tolerance maintained by CD25+CD4+ naturally anergic and suppressive T cells: induction of autoimmune disease by breaking their anergic/suppressive state. *Int Immunol* 1998; **10**:1969.

40 Thornton AM, Shevach EM. Suppressor effector function of CD4+CD25+ immunoregulatory T cells is antigen nonspecific. *J Immunol* 2000; **164**:183.

41 Papiernik M, de Moraes ML, Pontoux C, Vasseur F, Penit C. Regulatory CD4 T cells: expression of IL-2R

alpha chain, resistance to clonal deletion and IL-2 dependency. *Int Immunol* 1998; **10**:371.

42 Itoh M, Takahashi T, Sakaguchi N et al. Thymus and autoimmunity: production of CD25+CD4+ naturally anergic and suppressive T cells as a key function of the thymus in maintaining immunologic self-tolerance. *J Immunol* 1999; **162**:5317.

43 Shevach EM. Regulatory T cells in autoimmunity. *Annu Rev Immunol* 2000; **18**:423.

44 Jordan MS, Boesteanu A, Reed AJ et al. Thymic selection of CD4+CD25+ regulatory T cells induced by an agonist self-peptide. *Nat Immunol* 2001; **2**:301.

45 Walker MR, Kasprowicz DJ, Gersuk VH et al. Induction of FoxP3 and acquisition of T regulatory activity by stimulated human CD4+CD25− T cells. *J Clin Invest* 2003; **112**:1437.

46 Sakaguchi S. The origin of FOXP3-expressing CD4+ regulatory T cells: thymus or periphery. *J Clin Invest* 2003; **112**:1310.

47 Sogn JA. Tumor immunology: the glass is half full. *Immunity* 1998; **9**:757.

48 Batra RK, Lin Y, Sharma S et al. Non-small cell lung cancer-derived soluble mediators enhance apoptosis in activated T lymphocytes through an I kappa B kinase-dependent mechanism. *Cancer Res* 2003; **63**:642.

49 Yoshino I, Yano T, Murata M et al. Tumor-reactive T-cells accumulate in lung cancer tissues but fail to respond due to tumor cell-derived factor. *Cancer Res* 1992; **52**:775.

50 Woo EY, Yeh H, Chu CS et al. Cutting edge: regulatory T cells from lung cancer patients directly inhibit autologous T cell proliferation. *J Immunol* 2002; **168**:4272.

51 Huang M, Sharma S, Mao JT, Dubinett SM. Non-small cell lung cancer-derived soluble mediators and prostaglandin E$_2$ enhance peripheral blood lymphocyte IL-10 transcription and protein production. *J Immunol* 1996; **157**:5512.

52 Alleva DG, Burger CJ, Elgert KD. Tumor-induced regulation of suppressor macrophage nitric oxide and TNF-alpha production: role of tumor-derived IL-10, TGF-beta and prostaglandin E2. *J Immunol* 1994; **153**:1674.

53 Liu VC, Wong LY, Jang T et al. Tumor evasion of the immune system by converting CD4+CD25− T Cells into CD4+CD25+ T regulatory cells: role of tumor-derived TGF-beta. *J Immunol* Mar 1, 2007; **178(5)**:2883–92.

54 Dubinett S, Sharma S, Huang M, Mao J, Batra R. Lung cancer and immune dysfunction. In: Finke J, Bukowski R (eds). *Current Clinical Oncology: Cancer*

Immunotherapy at the Crossroads: How Tumors Evade Immunity and What Can be Done, Vol. 18. Totowa, NJ: Human Press, 2004:335.

55 Huang M, Stolina M, Sharma S *et al*. Non-small cell lung cancer cyclooxygenase-2-dependent regulation of cytokine balance in lymphocytes and macrophages: up-regulation of interleukin 10 and down-regulation of interleukin 12 production. *Cancer Res* 1998; **58**:1208.

56 Stolina M, Sharma S, Lin Y *et al*. Specific inhibition of cyclooxygenase 2 restores antitumor reactivity by altering the balance of IL-10 and IL-12 synthesis. *J Immunol* 2000; **164**:361.

57 Sharma S, Yang SC, Zhu L *et al*. Tumor cyclooxygenase-2/prostaglandin E2-dependent promotion of FOXP3 expression and CD4+ CD25+ T regulatory cell activities in lung cancer. *Cancer Res* Jun 15, 2005; **65(12)**:5211–20.

58 O'Reilly EM, Ilson DH, Saltz LB, Heelan R, Martin L, Kelsen DP. A phase II trial of interferon -2 and carboplatin in patients with advanced malignant mesothelioma. *Cancer Invest* 1999; **17**:195–200.

59 Sterman DH, Kaiser LR, Albelda SM. Advances in the treatment of malignant pleural mesothelioma. *Chest* 1999; **116**:504–20.

60 Dubinett SM. The immune response of lung tumors and the effects of cytokine administration on pulmonary immune cells. In: Kradin R, Robinson B (eds). *Immunopathology of Lung Disease*. Boston, MA: Butterworth-Heinemann, 1996:469–90.

61 Kugler A, Stuhler G, Walden P *et al*. Regression of human metastatic renal cell carcinoma after vaccination with tumor cell–dendritic cell hybrids. *Nat Med* 2000; **6**:332–6.

62 Thurner B, Haendle I, Roder C *et al*. Vaccination with mage-3A1 peptide-pulsed mature, monocyte-derived dendritic cells expands specific cytotoxic T cells and induces regression of some metastases in advanced stage IV melanoma. *J Exp Med* 1999; **190**:1669–78.

63 Van Pel A, Boon T. Protection against a nonimmunogenic mouse leukemia by an immunogenic variant obtained by mutagenesis. *Proc Natl Acad Sci USA* 1982; **79**:4718–22.

64 Boon T, Old L. Cancer tumor antigens. *Curr Opin Immunol* 1997; **9**:681–3.

65 Boon T, Gajewski TF, Coulie PG. From defined human tumor antigens to effective immunization? *Immunol Today* 1995; **16**:334–6.

66 Boon T, van der Bruggen P. Human tumor antigens recognized by T lymphocytes. *J Exp Med* 1996; **183**:725–9.

67 Pardoll D. Cancer vaccines. *Nat Med* 1998; **4(Suppl)**:525–31.

68 Dubinett SM, Miller PW, Sharma S, Batra RK. Gene therapy for lung cancer. *Hematol Oncol Clin North Am* 1998; **12**:569–94.

69 Dubinett SM, Batra RK, Miller PW, Sharma S. Tumor antigens in thoracic malignancy. *Am J Respir Cell Mol Biol* May 2000; **22(5)**:524–7.

70 Huang AYC, Golumbek P, Ahmadzadeh M, Jaffee E, Pardoll D, Levitsky H. Role of bone marrow-derived cells in presenting MHC class I-restricted tumor antigens. *Science* 1994; **264**:961–5.

71 Peng L, Krauss JC, Plautz GE, Mukai S, Shu S, Cohen PA. T cell-mediated tumor rejection displays diverse dependence upon perforin and IFN-gamma mechanisms that cannot be predicted from in vitro T cell characteristics. *J Immunol* Dec 15, 2000; **165(12)**:7116–24.

72 Poehlein CH, Hu HM, Yamada J *et al*. TNF plays an essential role in tumor regression after adoptive transfer of perforin/IFN-gamma double knockout effector T cells. *J Immunol* Feb 15, 2003; **170(4)**:2004–13.

73 Seki N, Brooks AD, Carter CR *et al*. Tumor-specific CTL kill murine renal cancer cells using both perforin and Fas ligand-mediated lysis in vitro, but cause tumor regression in vivo in the absence of perforin. *J Immunol* Apr 1, 2002; **168(7)**:3484–92.

74 Finn OJ. Cancer vaccines: between the idea and the reality. *Nat Rev Immunol* 2003; **3**:630–41.

75 Miller PW, Sharma S, Stolina M *et al*. Intratumoral administration of adenoviral interleukin 7 gene-modified dendritic cells augments specific antitumor immunity and achieves tumor eradication. *Hum Gene Ther* 2000; **11**:53–65.

76 Yang SC, Hillinger S, Riedl K *et al*. Intratumoral administration of dendritic cells overexpressing CCL21 generates systemic antitumor responses and confers tumor immunity. *Clin Cancer Res* 2004; **10**:2891–901.

77 Yang SC, Batra RK, Hillinger S *et al*. Intrapulmonary administration of CCL21 gene-modified dendritic cells reduces tumor burden in spontaneous murine bronchoalveolar cell carcinoma. *Cancer Res* 2006; **66**:3205–13.

78 Knight SC, Hunt R, Dore C, Medawar PB. Influence of dendritic cells on tumor growth. *Proc Natl Acad Sci U S A* 1985; **82**:4495–7.

79 Aragoneses-Fenoll L, Corbi AL. Dendritic cells: still a promising tool for cancer immunotherapy. *Clin Transl Oncol* Feb 2007; **9(2)**:77–82.

80 Fong L, Engleman EG. Dendritic cells in cancer immunotherapy. *Annu Rev Immunol* 2000; **18**:245–73.

81 Banchereau J, Palucka AK. Dendritic cells as therapeutic vaccines against cancer [Review]. *Nat Rev Immunol* Apr 2005; **5(4)**:296–306.

82 Pardoll DM. Spinning molecular immunology into successful immunotherapy. *Nat Rev Immunol* 2002; **2**:227–38.

83 van Kooten C, Banchereau J. Functions of CD40 on B cells, dendritic cells and other cells. *Curr Opin Immunol* 1997; **9**:330–7.

84 Banchereau J, Steinman RM. Dendritic cells and the control of immunity. *Nature* 1998; **392**:245–52.

85 Austyn JM. New insights into the mobilization and phagocytic activity of dendritic cells. *J Exp Med* 1996; **183**:1287–92.

86 Szabolcs P, Moore MA, Young JW. Expansion of immunostimulatory dendritic cells among the myeloid progeny of human CD34+ bone marrow precursors cultured with c-kit ligand, granulocyte-macrophage colony-stimulating factor, and TNF-alpha. *J Immunol* 1995; **154**:5851–61.

87 Strunk D, Rappersberger K, Egger C *et al.* Generation of human dendritic cells/Langerhans cells from circulating CD34+ hematopoietic progenitor cells. *Blood* 1996; **87**:1292–302.

88 Bender A, Sapp M, Schuler G, Steinman RM, Bhardwaj N. Improved methods for the generation of dendritic cells from nonproliferating progenitors in human blood. *J Immunol Methods* 1996; **196**:121–35.

89 Timmerman JM, Levy R. Dendritic cell vaccines for cancer immunotherapy. *Annu Rev Med* 1999; **50**:507–29.

90 Nestle FO, Alijagic S, Gilliet M *et al.* Vaccination of melanoma patients with peptide- or tumor lysate-pulsed dendritic cells. *Nat Med* 1998; **4**:328–32.

91 Itoh T, Ueda Y, Kawashima I *et al.* Immunotherapy of solid cancer using dendritic cells pulsed with the HLA-A24-restricted peptide of carcinoembryonic antigen. *Cancer Immunol Immunother* 2002; **51**:99–106.

92 Ueda Y, Itoh T, Nukaya I *et al.* Dendritic cell-based immunotherapy of cancer with carcinoembryonic antigen-derived, HLA-A24-restricted CTL epitope: clinical outcomes of 18 patients with metastatic gastrointestinal or lung adenocarcinomas. *Int J Oncol* 2004; **24**:909–17.

93 Goldszmid RS, Idoyaga J, Bravo AI, Steinman R, Mordoh J, Wainstok R. Dendritic cells charged with apoptotic tumor cells induce long-lived protective CD4+ and CD8+ T cell immunity against B16 melanoma. *J Immunol* 2003; **171**:5940–7.

94 Boczkowski D, Nair SK, Snyder D, Gilboa E. Dendritic cells pulsed with RNA are potent antigen-presenting cells in vitro and in vivo. *J Exp Med* 1996; **184**:465–72.

95 Boczkowski D, Nair SK, Nam JH, Lyerly HK, Gilboa E. Induction of tumor immunity and cytotoxic T lymphocyte responses using dendritic cells transfected with messenger RNA amplified from tumor cells [in process citation]. *Cancer Res* 2000; **60**:1028–34.

96 Watts C. Capture and processing of exogenous antigens for presentation on MHC molecules. *Annu Rev Immunol* 1997; **15**:821–50.

97 Sharma S, Stolina M, Lin Y *et al.* T cell-derived IL-10 promotes lung cancer growth by suppressing both T cell and APC function. *J Immunol* 1999; **163**:5020–8.

98 Nair SK, Hull S, Coleman D, Gilboa E, Lyerly HK, Morse MA. Induction of carcinoembryonic antigen (CEA)-specific cytotoxic T-lymphocyte responses in vitro using autologous dendritic cells loaded with CEA peptide or CEA RNA in patients with metastatic malignancies expressing CEA. *Int J Cancer* 1999; **82**:121–4.

99 Sharma S, Miller P, Stolina M *et al.* Multi-component gene therapy vaccines for lung cancer: effective eradication of established murine tumors in vivo with Interleukin 7/Herpes Simplex Thymidine Kinase-transduced autologous tumor and ex vivo-activated dendritic cells. *Gene Ther* 1997; **4**:1361–70.

100 Antonia SJ, Mirza N, Fricke I *et al.* Combination of p53 cancer vaccine with chemotherapy in patients with extensive stage small cell lung cancer. *Clin Cancer Res* 2006; **12**:878–87.

101 Hirschowitz EA, Foody T, Kryscio R, Dickson L, Sturgill J, Yannelli J. Autologous dendritic cell vaccines for non-small-cell lung cancer. *J Clin Oncol* 2004; **22**:2808–15.

102 Kontani K, Taguchi O, Ozaki Y *et al.* Dendritic cell vaccine immunotherapy of cancer targeting MUC1 mucin. *Int J Mol Med* Oct 2003; **12(4)**:493–502.

103 Bouchet BP, de Fromentel CC, Puisieux A, Galmarini CM. p53 as a target for anti-cancer drug development. *Crit Rev Oncol Hematol* Jun 2006; **58(3)**:190–207.

104 Campling BG, El-Deiry WS. Clinical implication of p53 mutation in lung cancer [Review]. *Mol Biotechnol* Jun 2003; **24(2)**:141–56.

105 Humrich J, Jenne L. Viral vectors for dendritic cell-based immunotherapy. *Curr Top Microbiol Immunol* 2003; **276**:241–59.

106 Gamvrellis A, Leong D, Hanley JC, Xiang SD, Mottram P, Plebanski M. Vaccines that facilitate antigen entry into dendritic cells. *Immunol Cell Biol* 2004; **82**:506–16.

107 Homey B, Muller A, Zlotnik A. Chemokines: agents for the immunotherapy of cancer? *Nat Rev Immunol* 2002; **2**:175–84.

108 Sharma S, Stolina M, Luo J *et al.* Secondary lymphoid tissue chemokine mediates T cell-dependent antitumor responses in vivo. *J Immunol* 2000; **164**:4558–63.

109 Zeid NA, Muller HK. S100 positive dendritic cells in human lung tumors associated with cell differentiation and enhanced survival. *Pathology* 1993; **25**:338–43.

110 Pardoll D. Does the immune system see tumors as foreign or self? *Annu Rev Immunol* 2003; **21**:807–39.

111 Dranoff G, Jaffee E, Lazenby A *et al.* Vaccination with irradiated tumor cells engineered to secrete murine granulocyte-macrophage colony-stimulating factor stimulates potent, specific, and long-lasting anti-tumor immunity. *Proc Natl Acad Sci USA* 1993; **90**:3539–43.

112 Miller PW, Sharma S, Stolina M *et al.* Dendritic cells augment granulocyte-macrophage colony-stimulating factor (GM-CSF)/herpes simplex virus thymidine kinase-mediated gene therapy of lung cancer. *Cancer Gene Ther* 1998; **5**:380–9.

113 Salgia R, Lynch T, Skarin A *et al.* Vaccination with irradiated autologous tumor cells engineered to secrete granulocyte-macrophage colony-stimulating factor augments antitumor immunity in some patients with metastatic non-small-cell lung carcinoma. *J Clin Oncol* 2003; **21**:624–30.

114 Nemunaitis J, Sterman D, Jablons D *et al.* Granulocyte-macrophage colony-stimulating factor gene-modified autologous tumor vaccines in non-small-cell lung cancer. *J Natl Cancer Inst* 2004; **96**:326–31.

115 Nemunaitis J, Jahan T, Ross H *et al.* Phase 1/2 trial of autologous tumor mixed with an allogeneic GVAX((R)) vaccine in advanced-stage non-small-cell lung cancer. *Cancer Gene Ther* Jun 2006; **13(6)**:555–62.

116 Singh NP, Yolcu ES, Taylor DD *et al.* A novel approach to cancer immunotherapy tumor cells decorated with CD80 generate effective antitumor immunity. *Cancer Res* July 15, 2003 **63**:4067–73.

117 Korkolopolulou P, Kaklamanis L, Pezzella F, Harris AL, Gatter KC. Loss of antigen-presenting molecules (MHC class I and TAP-1) in lung cancer. *Br J Cancer* 1996; **73**:148–53.

118 Chen HL, Gabrilovich D, Tampé R, Girgis KR, Nadaf S, Carbone DP. A functionally defective allele of TAP1 results in loss of MHC class I antigen presentation in a human lung cancer. *Nat Genet* Jun 1996; **13(2)**:210–3.

119 Raez LE, Cassileth PA, Schlesselman JJ *et al.* Induction of CD8 T-cell-Ifn-gamma response and positive clinical outcome after immunization with gene-modified allogeneic tumor cells in advanced non-small-cell lung carcinoma. *Cancer Gene Ther* 2003; **10**:850–8.

120 Raez LE, Cassileth PA, Schlesselman JJ *et al.* Allogeneic vaccination with a B7.1 HLA-A gene-modified adenocarcinoma cell line in patients with advanced non-small-cell lung cancer. *J Clin Oncol* July 15, 2004; **22(14)**:2800–7.

121 Ribas A, Butterfield LH, Glaspy JA, Economou JS. Current developments in cancer vaccines and cellular immunotherapy. *J Clin Oncol* Jun 15; 2003; **21(12)**:2415–32.

122 Levesque AA, Eastman A. p53-based cancer therapies: is defective p53 the Achilles heel of the tumor? *Carcinogenesis* 2007; **28(1)**:13–20.

123 Haupt S, Haupt Y. Importance of p53 for cancer onset and therapy. *Anticancer Drugs* 2006; **17**:725–32.

124 Campling BG, El-Deiry WS. Clinical implication of p53 in lung cancer. *Mol Biotechnol* 2003; **24(2)**:141–56.

125 Campbell SL, Khosravi-Far R, Rossman KL, Clark GJ, Der CJ. Increasing complexity of Ras signaling. *Oncogene* 1998; **17**:1395–413.

126 Huncharek M, Muscat J, Geschwind JF. K-ras oncogene mutation as a prognostic marker in non-small cell lung cancer: a combined analysis of 881 cases. *Carcinogenesis* 1999; **20**:1507–10.

127 Camps C, Sirera R, Bremnes R *et al.* Is there a prognostic role of K-ras point mutations in the serum of patients with advanced non-small cell lung cancer? *Lung Cancer* Dec 2005; **50(3)**:339–46.

128 Johnson L, Mercer K, Greenbaum D *et al.* Somatic activation of the K-ras oncogene causes early onset lung cancer in mice. *Nature* 2001; **410**:1111–6.

129 Takahashi T, Nau MM, Chiba I *et al.* p53: a frequent target for genetic abnormalities in lung cancer. *Science* 1989; **246**:491–4.

130 Slebos RJ, Kibbelaar RE, Dalesio O *et al.* K-ras oncogene activation as a prognostic marker in adenocarcinoma of the lung. *N Engl J Med* 1990; **323**:561–5.

131 Peace DJ, Smith JW, Chen W *et al.* Lysis of ras oncogene-transformed cells by specific cytotoxic T lymphocytes elicited by primary in vitro immunization with mutated ras peptide. *J Exp Med* 1994; **179**:473–9.

132 Gnjatic S, Cai Z, Viguier M, Chouaib S, Guillet JG, Choppin J. Accumulation of the p53 protein allows recognition by human CTL of a wild-type p53

epitope presented by breast carcinomas and melanomas. *J Immunol* 1998; **160**:328–33.

133 Yanuck M, Carbone DP, Pendleton CD *et al.* A mutant p53 tumor suppressor protein is a target for peptide-induced CD8+ cytotoxic T-cells. *Cancer Res* 1993; **53**:3257–61.

134 Ciernik IF, Berzofsky JA, Carbone DP. Induction of cytotoxic T lymphocytes and antitumor immunity with DNA vaccines expressing single T cell epitopes. *J Immunol* 1996; **156**:2369–75.

135 Carbone DP, Ciernik IF, Kelley MJ *et al.* Immunization with mutant p53- and K-ras-derived peptides in cancer patients: immune response and clinical outcome. *J Clin Oncol* Aug 1, 2005; **23(22)**:5099–107.

136 Oka Y, Tsuboi A, Taguchi T *et al.* Induction of WT1 (Wilms' tumor gene)-specific cytotoxic T lymphocytes by WT1 peptide vaccine and the resultant cancer regression. *Proc Natl Acad Sci USA* Sep 21, 2004; **101(38)**:13885–90.

137 Henson ES, Gibson SB. Surviving cell death through epidermal growth factor (EGF) signal transduction pathways: implications for cancer therapy. *Cell Signal* Dec 2006; **18(12)**:2089–97.

138 Arteaga CL. EGF receptor mutations in lung cancer: from humans to mice and maybe back to humans. *Cancer Cell* Jun 2006; **9(6)**:421–3.

139 Pavelic K, Banjac Z, Pavelic J *et al.* Evidence for a role of EGF receptor in the progression of human lung carcinoma. *Anticancer Res* 1993; **13**:1133–7.

140 Veale D, Kerr N, Gibson GJ *et al.* The relationship of quantitative epidermal growth factor receptor expression in non-small cell lung cancer to long term survival. *Br J Cancer* 1993; **68**:162–5.

141 Rusch V, Baselga J, Cordon-Cardo C *et al.* Differential expression of the epidermal growth factor receptor and its ligands in primary non-small cell lung cancers and adjacent benign lung. *Cancer Res* 1993; **53**:2379–85.

142 Ramos TC, Vinageras EN, Ferrer MC *et al.* Treatment of NSCLC patients with an EGF-based cancer vaccine: report of a Phase I trial. *Cancer Biol Ther* Feb 2006; **5(2)**:145–9.

143 Gonzalez G, Crombet T, Catala M *et al.* A novel cancer vaccine composed of human-recombinant epidermal growth factor linked to a carrier protein: report of a pilot clinical trial. *Ann Oncol* 1998; **9**:431–5.

144 Gonzalez G, Crombet T, Torres F *et al.* Epidermal growth factor-based cancer vaccine for non-small-cell lung cancer therapy. *Ann Oncol* 2003; **14**:461–6.

145 Gonzalez G, Crombet T, Neninger E, Viada C, Lage A. Therapeutic vaccination with epidermal growth factor (EGF) in advanced lung cancer: analysis of pooled data from three clinical trials. *Hum Vaccine* Jan–Feb 2007; **3(1)**:8–13.

146 Tsai JR, Chong IW, Chen YH *et al.* Differential expression profile of MAGE family in non-small-cell lung cancer. *Lung Cancer* 2007; **56(2)**:185–92.

147 Weynants P, Lethé B, Brasseur F, Marchand M, Boon T. Expression of MAGE genes by non-small-cell lung carcinomas. *Int J Cancer* 1994; **56**:826–9.

148 Atanackovic D, Altorki NK, Stockert E *et al.* Vaccine-induced CD4+ T cell responses to MAGE-3 protein in lung cancer patients. *J Immunol* Mar 1, 2004; **172(5)**:3289–96.

149 Pardali K, Moustakas A. Actions of TGF-beta as tumor suppressor and pro-metastatic factor in human cancer. *Biochim Biophys Acta* Jan 2007; **1775(1)**:21–62.

150 Levy L, Hill CS. Alterations in components of the TGF-beta superfamily signaling pathways in human cancer. *Cytokine Growth Factor Rev* Feb-Apr 2006; **17(1–2)**:41–58.

151 Gajewski TF, Meng Y, Harlin H. Immune suppression in the tumor microenvironment. *J Immunother* 2006; **29**:233–40.

152 Constam DB, Philipp J, Malipiero UV, ten Dijke P, Schachner M, Fontana A. Differential expression of transforming growth factor-beta 1, -beta 2, and -beta 3 by glioblastoma cells, astrocytes, and microglia. *J Immunol* 1992; **148**:1404–10.

153 Kong F, Jirtle RL, Huang DH, Clough RW, Anscher MS. Plasma transforming growth factor-beta1 level before radiotherapy correlates with long term outcome of patients with lung carcinoma. *Cancer* 1999; **86**:1712–9.

154 Nemunaitis J, Dillman RO, Schwarzenberger PO *et al.* Phase II study of belagenpumatucel-L, a transforming growth factor beta-2 antisense gene-modified allogeneic tumor cell vaccine in non-small-cell lung cancer. *J Clin Oncol* 2006; **24**:4721–30.

155 Chapman PB. Anti-idiotypic monoclonal antibody cancer vaccines. *Semin Cancer Biol* Dec 1995; **6(6)**:367–74.

156 Krug LM. Vaccine therapy for small cell lung cancer. *Semin Oncol* Feb 2004; **31(1, Suppl 1)**:112–6.

157 Giaccone G, Debruyne C, Felip E *et al.* Phase III study of adjuvant vaccination with Bec2/bacille Calmette-Guerin in responding patients with limited-disease small-cell lung cancer (European Organisation for Research and Treatment of Cancer 08971-08971B; Silva Study). *J Clin Oncol* 2005; **23**:6854–64.

158 Toloza EM, Morse MA, Lyerly HK. Gene therapy for lung cancer. *J Cell Biochem* Sep 1, 2006; **99(1)**:1–22.

159 Hege KM, Carbone DP. Lung cancer vaccines and gene therapy. *Lung Cancer* Aug 2003; **41(Suppl 1)**:S103–13.

160 Peat N, Gendler SJ, Lalani N, Duhig T, Taylor-Papadimitriou J. Tissue-specific expression of a human polymorphic epithelial mucin (MUC1) in transgenic mice. *Cancer Res* 1992; **52**:1954–60.

161 Ho SB, Niehans GA, Lyftogt C *et al.* Heterogeneity of mucin gene expression in normal and neoplastic tissues. *Cancer Res* 1993; **53**:641–51.

162 Hirasawa Y, Kohno N, Yokoyama A, Kondo K, Hiwada K, Miyake M. Natural autoantibody to MUC1 is a prognostic indicator for non-small cell lung cancer. *Am J Respir Crit Care Med* Feb 2000; **161(2, Pt 1)**:589–94.

163 Mennecier B, Ramlau R, Rolski J *et al.* Phase II study evaluating clinical efficacy of TG 4010 (MVA - MUC1-IL 2) in association with cisplatin and binorelbine in a patient with non small cell lung cancer. *Lung Cancer* 2006; **49**:S373.

CHAPTER 22

Epidermal Growth Factor Receptor Inhibitors

Lecia V. Sequist and Thomas J. Lynch

Introduction

For the last decade, combination platinum-based chemotherapy has been the primary modality and most efficacious treatment for advanced stage non-small cell lung cancer (NSCLC). However, the survival benefit of chemotherapy is modest, averaging only 2 months, and efforts to improve the outcome with additional modern chemotherapy agents have been largely unsuccessful [1–4]. As a result, a major focus of clinical research in NSCLC treatment has shifted toward "targeted therapy," meaning novel agents that are designed specifically to hit a molecular target known to occur more frequently on cancer cells or known to be an integral part of the cancer cell biology. The epidermal growth factor receptor (EGFR) is one of the most important of these targets in NSCLC. This chapter will (1) provide a brief overview of the molecular biology of EGFR in NSCLC as a background to understanding its importance as a therapeutic target; (2) summarize recent clinical trials evaluating agents that target EGFR; and (3) discuss the discovery of molecular markers that have launched the process of dividing and categorizing this heterogeneous disease into clinically and therapeutically relevant subgroups.

Lung Cancer, 3rd edition. Edited by Jack A. Roth, James D. Cox, and Waun Ki Hong. © 2008 Blackwell Publishing, ISBN: 978-1-4051-5112-2.

The molecular biology of EGFR

EGFR, also known as ErbB-1, is a member of the ErbB family of transmembrane receptors, along with ErbB-2/HER-2, ErbB-3, and ErbB-4. These four receptors share a basic structure, consisting of an extracellular ligand-binding domain, a single transmembrane domain, and a highly conserved intracellular catalytic domain with tyrosine kinase (TK) activity (see Figure 22.1). The four ErbB receptors translate growth factor signals from outside the cell to diverse and amplified intracellular signals through their redundant and multilayered network [5,6]. Each ErbB receptor binds a panel of activating ligands, with the exception of ErbB-2/HER-2, which has no known ligand and acts primarily as a dimerization partner for other ErbB receptors [7]. Upon ligand binding, ErbB receptors become activated by forming homo- or heterodimers with each other, and undergoing reciprocal TK phosphorylation, with the exception of ErbB-3, which lacks intrinsic TK activity but can nonetheless transmit a potent signal following heterodimerization with ErbB-2/HER-2 [8]. Phosphorylation of the receptors' TK domain creates docking sites for the recruitment of effector proteins, leading to the generation of intracellular signal transduction cascades. The panel of possible cellular responses to EGFR and ErbB family signaling is mediated by phosphorylation of distinct tyrosine residues within the TK domains, each of which can recruit diverse effector proteins leading to differential activation of downstream signaling cascades [5,6]. Hence, the

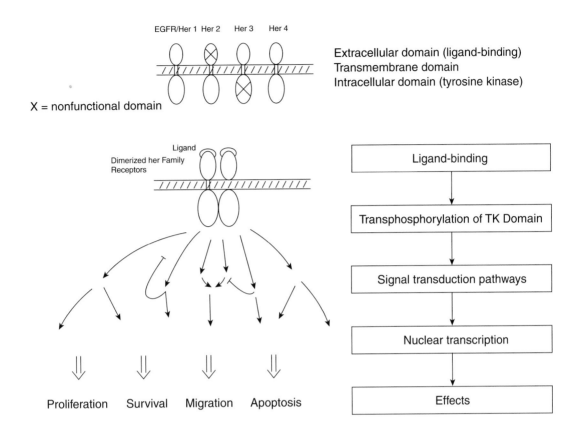

Figure 22.1 Schematic of the EGFR family of receptors and their multilayered downstream signaling network.

specific biologic endpoint of the EGFR signaling cascade is flexible and depends on the cellular context, including the stimulating ligand, the receptor dimerization partner, and the kinetics of the signaling pathways within the cell.

The EGFR pathway is a key regulator of many of the functions considered crucial for oncogenic transformation, including proliferation, survival (antiapoptosis), and metastasis [9]. Dysregulation and abnormal activation of the EGFR pathway have been implicated in several different types of cancer. Mechanisms of aberrant EGFR signaling in NSCLC include mutation or amplification of EGFR and other ErbB receptors, autocrine secretion of ligand by tumor cells, and paracrine production of ligand by surrounding stromal cells [6,10–13]. The central role of the EGFR signaling network makes it ideally suited as a target for the development of novel anticancer agents.

First-generation EGFR TKIs: gefitinib and erlotinib

Two basic strategies for therapeutically inhibiting EGFR signaling have been extensively studied to date: small molecule tyrosine kinase inhibitors and monoclonal antibodies. Monoclonal antibodies will be discussed later in the chapter. Small molecule tyrosine kinase inhibitors (TKIs) are orally bioavailable compounds that inhibit EGFR signal transduction by binding at the adenosine triphosphate (ATP) binding site within the TK domain of the receptor. By mitigating ATP binding, they prohibit receptor activation and decrease EGFR network signaling. We will begin our review with the so-called "first generation" of EGFR TKIs to be developed, consisting of gefitinib and erlotinib. Since both drugs have been evaluated in similar types of clinical trials, our discussion will focus on one clinical setting at a time, comparing the performance of the two compounds.

Single-agent phase I and II clinical trials

Gefitinib (also known as Iressa® and ZD1839) is an EGFR TKI that competes with ATP for receptor binding and suppresses downstream signaling of the EGFR network [14–17]. Phase I studies in patients with advanced solid tumors showed gefitinib to be well tolerated, with dose-limiting toxicities of acneiform rash and diarrhea at doses greater than 700–1000 mg/day [18–20]. Since 150 mg/day was found to be sufficient to suppress EGFR signaling in skin biopsy specimens, and since doses above 500 mg were associated with increased toxicity, daily doses of 250 mg and 500 mg were recommended for further study [19].

Gefitinib was examined as monotherapy for refractory NSCLC in two large phase II studies called the IDEAL trials, in which subjects were randomized to 250 mg or 500 mg of daily gefitinib [21,22]. The results were encouraging in that outcome with single-agent gefitinib was similar to what might be expected with single-agent chemotherapy in this population (see Table 22.1). Efficacy did not differ between dose levels but toxicity was greater at 500 mg, though was overall manageable and consisted primarily of rash and diarrhea. Due to the paucity of available treatment options for refractory NSCLC patients, the Food and Drug Administration (FDA) approved gefitinib (250 mg/day) as salvage third-line therapy for NSCLC in May 2003, based on the IDEAL trial results.

A pivotal observation from the IDEAL trials was that although responses occurred in only a minority of patients, they were often dramatic, accompanied by rapid symptom improvement. Furthermore, responses were more common among patients with specific characteristics. For example, the IDEAL-1 trial was performed in Japan, Europe, Australia, and South Africa. The response rate among Japanese subjects in this study was >2.5 times higher than in non-Japanese subjects (27% versus 10%, $p = 0.002$). In addition, multivariable analyses showed higher response rates in females compared to males (odds ratio [OR] 2.65; 95% confidence interval [CI], 1.19–5.91) and in patients with adenocarcinoma compared to other histological types (OR, 3.45; 95% CI, 1.29–11.02). As large expanded access programs for gefitinib opened during the FDA review process, it became increasingly apparent that specific subgroups of patients tended to respond more vigorously to EGFR TKI treatment [23–25]. Higher response rates were consistently observed in women, patients with well-differentiated adenocarcinoma and bronchioloalveolar carcinoma (BAC) and never smokers. These clinical observations would later serve as the stimulus for the discovery of molecular predictors of response to TKI agents.

To assess the efficacy of gefitinib in a population more narrowly defined by these clinical characteristics, the Southwest Oncology Group performed a phase II study of gefitinib therapy in BAC patients (see Table 22.1) [26]. At the time of the design of this study, the final dose of 250 mg had not yet been chosen, so this trial employed a dose of 500 mg/day. In addition, because of the historically low response of BAC to chemotherapy, newly diagnosed patients were allowed onto this trial, using gefitinib as a first-line modality; in fact, 72% of enrolled patients were treatment-naïve. Survival was prolonged in this trial compared to the IDEAL trials, perhaps because so many patients were treatment-naïve and/or because BAC portends a somewhat better prognosis than standard NSCLC [27]. Subgroup analyses revealed that median survival was prolonged in females compared with males (19 mo versus 8 mo, $p = 0.025$); in those that developed a rash compared with those that did not (16 mo versus 5 mo, $p = 0.003$); and in never smokers compared with former or current smokers (26 mo versus 10 mo, $p = 0.049$).

Erlotinib (also known as Tarceva®, OSI-774), like gefitinib, is an orally active reversible competitor for binding at the ATP pocket of the EGFR TK domain [28–30]. In a phase I study of erlotinib in patients with advanced solid tumors, diarrhea and rash were again the observed dose limiting toxicities and could now be attributed as a class effect of EGFR TKI agents [31]. The maximally tolerated dose of 150 mg/day was recommended for further study. A single-arm phase II study of erlotinib in refractory NSCLC patients demonstrated that the drug was well tolerated, with primary toxicities of rash and diarrhea, and with outcomes quite similar to

Table 22.1 Clinical trial results of single-agent gefitinib and erlotinib in NSCLC patients.

Trial name, author	Trial description	Arm, number of patients	Objective response rate (%)	Median time to disease progression (mo)	Median overall survival (mo)	p value
IDEAL-1, Fukuoka [21]	Phase 2 gefitinib in refractory patients, randomized to dose	250 mg n = 103	18	2.7	7.6	
		500 mg n = 106	19	2.8	8.0	
IDEAL-2, Kris [22]	Phase 2 gefitinib in refractory patients, randomized to dose	250 mg n = 106	12	—	7	
		500 mg n = 115	9	—	6	
S0126, West [26]	Phase 2 gefitinib in BAC patients, analyzed by prior treatment	500 mg, treatment naïve n = 104	12	4	13	
		500 mg, previously treated, n = 41	2	3	13	
Perez-Soler [32]	Phase 2 erlotinib in refractory patients, single-arm study	150 mg, n = 57	23	2.1	8.4	
ISEL, Thatcher [40]	Phase 3 randomized gefitinib/placebo	250 mg n = 1129	—	3.0	5.6	0.09
		Placebo n = 563	—	2.6	5.1	
BR.21, Shepherd [41]	Phase 3 randomized erlotinib/placebo	150 mg n = 488	8.2	2.2	6.7	<0.001
		Placebo n = 243	0.7	1.8	4.7	

—, not available or not published.

those observed with gefitinib in this setting (see Table 22.1) [32]. Interestingly, as in the trial of gefitinib in BAC patients, this trial found that development of a rash following treatment with erlotinib was predictive of improved survival, with subjects free from rash having a median survival of 1.5 months compared with 8.5 and 19.6 months for patients with a maximum of grade 1 rash and grade 2/3 rash, respectively. Rash has been correlated with response to EGFR-targeted therapy in other cancers as well, including colon cancer [33].

The mechanisms and biological implications of this phenomenon are not yet elucidated, but are under active investigation [33,34].

Combination chemotherapy and EGFR TKIs as first-line treatment

After confirmation of its single-agent activity in NSCLC, and given its lack of significant overlapping toxicity with traditional chemotherapy, gefitinib was examined in combination with first-line chemotherapy for advanced NSCLC in two large randomized phase III trials, known as the IN-TACT trials [35,36]. Similarly, erlotinib was combined with first-line chemotherapy in two large randomized clinical trials known as TRIBUTE and TALENT [37,38]. The general enthusiasm about the potential of the oral EGFR TKI agents led to the rapid accrual of over 4000 patients to these international randomized trials. Lamentably, all four studies failed to show a survival benefit for the addition of targeted therapy to chemotherapy, resulting in significant despair among investigators, clinicians and patients alike. It was hypothesized that perhaps chemotherapy and EGFR TKIs antagonized each other when given concurrently, or alternatively, that these four trials did not appropriately select the patient population most likely to benefit from the addition of EGFR-targeted therapy, either by clinical criteria or by molecular criteria (discussed below) [39]. As in the single-agent TKI studies, there was a hint that particular subgroups of patients might benefit from the strategy of EGFR TKIs with chemotherapy. Most notably, a subgroup analysis of the TRIBUTE study (utilizing chemotherapy with erlotinib or placebo) revealed that patients who reported that they had never smoked had an impressive prolongation in survival with erlotinib treatment (22.5 mo) compared to placebo treatment (10.1 mo, $p = 0.01$) [37].

Randomized trials of second- and third-line EGFR TKIs versus placebo

The ISEL trial evaluated the role of second-line gefitinib therapy in NSCLC, with 1692 chemotherapy-refractory patients randomized in a 2:1 fashion to gefitinib (250 mg/day) or placebo (see Table 22.1) [40]. The trial had a negative result, with no survival benefit seen compared to placebo. In June 2005, based on these results, the FDA restricted the use of gefitinib to patients participating in a clinical trial or continuing to benefit from treatment already initiated. This has effectively removed gefitinib from the US market, although the drug continues to be an important agent in several countries outside of the United States. Subgroup analyses were planned as part of the trial, given the substantial evidence in earlier phase trials that patients with certain characteristics were more likely to benefit from treatment.

These revealed no survival advantage of gefitinib in adenocarcinoma or female patients. Never smokers did achieve a survival benefit with gefitinib (hazard ratio [HR], 0.67; 95% CI, 0.49–0.92), as did patients of Asian origin (HR, 0.66; 95% CI, 0.48–0.91).

The BR.21 study examined the effectiveness of second-line erlotinib therapy [41]. It enrolled 731 patients who were randomized in a 2:1 fashion to salvage erlotinib at 150 mg/day or placebo (see Table 22.1). In contrast to the analogous ISEL trial, BR.21 demonstrated a survival advantage of 2 months for EGFR-targeted therapy in the salvage setting and became the first study to show a survival benefit for a targeted therapy in NSCLC. Based on the BR.21 results, the FDA-approved erlotinib for second- and third-line treatment of advanced NSCLC in November 2004 and it is currently used for this indication in the United States.

As has been discussed, the compounds gefitinib and erlotinib performed nearly identically in preclinical models, in single-arm clinical trials, and in randomized trials of first-line treatment with chemotherapy. It is therefore not clear why the BR.21 trial was able to demonstrate a survival benefit with second-line erlotinib treatment while the ISEL trial failed to show such benefit with second-line gefitinib, but several possibilities exist. Recall, erlotinib was dosed at its maximally tolerated dose while gefitinib was dosed at only one third to one-half its maximally tolerated dose. Perhaps the maximally tolerated dose of gefitinib would have demonstrated a survival benefit if compared to placebo.

Differences in the entry criteria may have also affected the results. For example, the ISEL study required that patients were refractory or intolerant to their previous chemotherapy regimen. Here, refractory was defined as having progressive disease during or within 90 days of their last chemotherapy treatment. This criterion yielded a study population in which only 18% of the patients had ever achieved a response to prior chemotherapy. This is important because response to first-line therapy is a significant predictor of response and survival with second-line therapy in NSCLC [41,42]. Contrast this population with the BR.21, in which no such entry criterion for refractory disease was present and 38% of the study population had achieved a prior response to chemotherapy, and it appears likely that the populations participating in these trials were different. Perhaps molecular characteristics associated with responsive disease, which will be discussed below, also differed between the two study populations and influenced the results. Because neither trial required its subjects to provide tissue for molecular analysis, analyses can only be performed in the subset of subjects with sufficient tissue. As a result, we cannot fully understand the molecular characteristics of the two trial populations and how they may have differed.

Finally, one must also consider the possibility that inherent and true differences in the effectiveness of the drugs led to the success of BR.21 and the failure of ISEL, and conversely that the drugs are equivalent and it was mere chance that produced different results.

Molecular predictors of benefit from gefitinib and erlotinib

EGFR mutations

NSCLC clinical studies using the EGFR TKI agents gefitinib and erlotinib repeatedly suggested that patients with adenocarcinoma, a low or absent smoking history, Asian origin and female gender benefited from treatment more than other patients. In 2004, two independent studies discovered somatic mutations in the *EGFR* TK domain underlying these associations [43,44]. Our own group tested the possibility that the dramatic drug responses observed in rare patients might be associated with mutational alterations in the drug target, and indeed found that 8 of 9 responsive cases harbored an *EGFR* mutation, compared with 0 of 7 unresponsive cases ($p < 0.001$) [43]. When transfected into NSCLC cell culture models, the somatic mutations preserved the ligand-dependence of the receptor, but imparted increased and prolonged EGFR TK domain phosphorylation compared to wild-type *EGFR*. In a screen for kinase mutations in untreated NSCLC cases, Paez *et al.* observed *EGFR* mutations predominantly in tumors from Asian patients and found mutations in 5 of 5 gefitinib-responsive cases [44]. Using three-dimensional conformation models of the

EGFR protein, they demonstrated that the mutations affected critical residues clustered around the TKI drug-binding site. Pao and coworkers extended these findings to erlotinib-responsive cases [45], and several other groups from around the world have since corroborated the presence of *EGFR* mutations in about 10% of North American and European NSCLC patients and 25–50% of Asian NSCLC patients [46–67].

Approximately 90% of *EGFR* mutations affect a few specific amino acids. Nearly 50% are a series of closely-related in-frame deletions in exon 19 centered about codons 746–750 (the LREA regions), while another 35–45% of mutations are the single missense mutation leucine to arginine at codon 858 (L858R) in exon 21 [46–49]. The recurrent nature of the somatic mutations implies specific "gain-of-function" properties mediated by the alterations.

The functions potentially gained by harboring an *EGFR* mutation have been partially elucidated with the discovery that mutations lead to preferential activation of intracellular signaling pathways involved in cell survival (via Akt), while having minimal effect on proliferative signals (via MAPK/ERK) [68]. *EGFR* mutations are thus transforming, meaning that they can lead to the development of the neoplastic phenotype in several in vitro model systems [68–73]. Constant exposure to survival signaling conditions, cells that harbor a mutation to become dependent on, or "addicted to," EGFR signaling [68]. Once cells become addicted to EGFR signaling pathways, they are rendered exquisitely sensitive to cell killing by TKI agents because the inactivation of EGFR signaling eliminates the primary promoter of survival and leads to apoptosis. This is clinically relevant, because complete abrogation of signaling is likely achieved at relatively low doses of TKI treatment in cases with mutated *EGFR*, whereas complete suppression of the wild-type receptor may require higher plasma drug levels.

Not surprisingly, patients that harbor an *EGFR* mutation derive significant clinical benefit from TKI treatment, manifested as an increased response rate and improved survival, see Figure 22.2 for an example [43–48,50–66]. A weighted-average composite analysis of all published series in mid-2006 showed

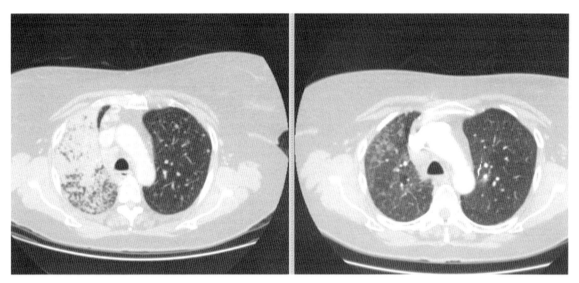

Figure 22.2 Dramatic response to gefitinib therapy in an NSCLC patient harboring an *EGFR* exon 19 deletion mutation. The left panel radiograph was taken just before the initiation of therapy and the right panel radiograph was 4 weeks after initiation

that the RR to TKI treatment among mutation-positive patients was 77% (range 30–100%, with most series reporting RR > 60%), compared to 10% in mutation-negative cases (range 0–33%) [74]. Similarly, five retrospective studies have demonstrated significantly prolonged survival in *EGFR* mutation-positive patients (up to 30 mo) compared to wild-type patients treated with EGFR TKIs [55–58,62]. There may be an outcome difference between types of mutation, as two groups have found that in mutation-positive patients treated with EGFR TKIs, those with an exon 19 deletion have a median survival double that of patients with an L858R substitution mutation [75,76]. As a result of these analyses, the benefit of TKI agents as first-line treatment for advanced NSCLC patients harboring a mutation has been tested in single-arm trials. Two Japanese groups have demonstrated that among patients with either an exon 19 deletion or an L858R mutation, the response rate to first-line gefitinib is 75% with a median progression-free survival of 9–10 months [77,78]. A Spanish group has reported similar results with erlotinib therapy [79], and our group has recently completed a US-based study using gefitinib, with results expected soon. An important caveat to these retrospective

and single-arm studies is that *EGFR* mutations seem to overall portend a better prognosis, complicating the conclusions drawn without a control group [80].

EGFR gene amplification

Another molecular marker that has been correlated with improved response and survival after EGFR TKI treatment is increased *EGFR* gene copy number as determined by fluorescent in situ hybridization (FISH) [51,64]. The two articles that established the potential of this biomarker were published by the same group of investigators and defined the "FISH+" designation as a composite endpoint that included chromosomal gene amplification (≥2 copies of *EGFR* within chromosome 7 in ≥10% of cells), extra-chromosomal gene amplification (≥15 copies of *EGFR* per cell in ≥10% of cells), or high-level polysomy (≥4 copies in ≥40% of cells) [51,64]. In retrospective analyses of NSCLC patients treated with single-agent gefitinib therapy, FISH+ status was associated with a response to treatment in 26–36% of patients and a median survival of 18 months. A considerable challenge in interpreting this data is that in some tumors a single *EGFR* allele undergoes simultaneous mutation and amplification [44,45,49,50,52–54,59,66,81]. This necessitates concurrent analyses of gene mutation and copy number to identify independent associations with clinical outcome, and few such studies have been reported. In fact, increased *EGFR* gene copy number, defined by the composite definition above, seems to describe a similar but larger population of patients than does *EGFR* mutation testing [51,62,82,83]. The unanswered question of great clinical interest is which of these biomarkers is a stronger predictor of clinical benefit.

Comparison of EGFR biomarkers

Direct comparison of the predictive ability of *EGFR* amplification and mutation status has been undertaken in several publications and is currently an area of great debate in the field (see Table 22.2) [51,62–64,82–84]. Gene copy number has been evaluated by both the FISH method described above and by quantitative real-time PCR (qPCR), which is a less subjective measure of the degree of gene amplification and does not account for polysomy. Evaluations have included retrospective case compilations as well as subset analyses of the available tumor specimens from the large randomized placebo-controlled trials with erlotinib (BR.21 trial) and gefitinib (ISEL trial). In the BR.21 analysis, FISH+ status was predictive of improved survival with erlotinib (HR 0.44; 95% CI, 0.23–0.82); however, no molecular markers were predictive of survival in a multivariable analysis [63]. The *EGFR* mutational analysis in this trial has come under significant criticism on technical grounds [85]. Mutations were initially reported in 23% of tumors and did not correlate with drug response; and while the extensive literature on *EGFR* mutations has confirmed that 80–90% of mutations arise within a small number of "hot spots," as many as half of the mutations reported in the BR.21 cohort were novel variants of unknown significance, suggestive of PCR artifacts. Subsequent data reanalysis, including the <20 tumors with the classical exon 19 deletions and L858R mutations, failed to show a survival benefit with erlotinib treatment over wild-type cases, but it is difficult to draw firm conclusions from such a small subgroup analysis [80]. The molecular subgroup analysis of the ISEL trial was recently reported and

did not reach any statistically significant endpoints, but did demonstrate a trend toward improved survival in FISH+ patients treated with gefitinib (HR 0.61; 95% CI, 0.36–1.04) [83]. Survival analysis for the *EGFR* mutation-positive patients was not possible because there were too few deaths in this cohort at the time of analysis.

Takano and colleagues from Japan used qPCR to evaluate gene copy number and found that in a multivariable analysis corrected for demographics and tumor characteristics that *EGFR* mutation status significantly predicted increased response and prolonged survival with TKI treatment, though increased gene copy number did not [62]. In this series, all tumors with high-level gain ($\geq$6 copies/cell) were found to have amplification of a mutant allele, suggesting that the gene amplification component of the FISH composite endpoint may be describing much the same population as *EGFR* mutations. Han and colleagues from Korea attempted to confirm the results reported with the composite FISH endpoint, but found that in a multivariable analysis, only *EGFR* mutation status was independently predictive of response to TKI treatment or survival [82]. The differences in results across these multiple studies have yet to be reconciled. It may be that geographic location (i.e., Asian versus North American/European origin) will be an important variable in gene copy number analyses, as it has been in *EGFR* mutational analyses. It is also noteworthy that all of the biomarker studies to date have been performed using banked available patient tumor tissue. The only definitive way to understand the true predictive ability of *EGFR* biomarkers going forward is to design clinical trials that require all participating patients have banked tissue available for subsequent analyses.

Resistance to EGFR TKIs and second-generation compounds

As discussed above, the response rate to EGFR TKI therapy ranges from 10 to 20%, meaning that the majority of patients treated with these agents are primarily resistant. Furthermore, even patients that do respond to EGFR TKIs eventually acquire

Table 22.2 Comparison of *EGFR* biomarkers.

Phase II trials or retrospective analyses in which all patients received TKI

Lead author	Study type	Number in analysis (mutation, GCN)	Mutations: TKI response rate (%)	Mutations: median survival (mo)	GCN: TKI response rate (%)	GCN: median survival (mo)	GCN method
Capuzzo	R	102, 102	54 vs. 5 $p <$ 0.001	20.8 vs. 8.4, $p = 0.09$	36 vs. 3, $p < 0001$	18.7 vs. 7.0, $p = 0.03$	FISH
Hirsch	SGA	81, 81	NA	NA	26 vs. 11, $p = 0.14$	NR vs. 8, $p = 0.042$	FISH
Han	R	69, 69	53 vs. 15, $p = 0.0005$	NR vs. 7.4, $p = 0.0001$	32 vs. 11, $p = 0.04$	12.3 vs. 8.4, $p = 0.49$	FISH
Takano	R	66, 66	82 vs. 11, $p < 0.0001$	20.4 vs. 6.9, $p = 0.0001$	72 vs. 38, $p = 0.005$	NA	qPCR
Bell/IDEAL	SGA	79, 90	46 vs. 10, $p = 0.005$	NS	29 vs. 15, $p = 0.319$	NS	qPCR

Randomized trials of TKI versus placebo

Lead author	Study type	Number in analysis (mutation, GCN)	Mutations: TKI response rate (%)	Mutations: hazard ratio for death on TKI (95% CI)	GCN: TKI response rate (%)	GCN: hazard ratio for death on TKI (95% CI)	GCN method
Bell/INTACT	SGA	312, 453	72 vs. 55, $p = 0.2$	1.77 (0.50–6.23)	56 vs. 53, $p = $ NS	2.03 (0.67–6.13)	qPCR
Tsao	SGA	177, 125	16 vs. 7, $p = 0.37$	0.77 (0.40–1.50)	20 vs. 2, $p = 0.03$	0.44 (0.23–0.82)	FISH
Hirsh	SGA	215, 370	37.5 vs. 2.6, $p = $ NA	Not enough events to assess	16.4 vs. 3.2, $p = $ NA	0.61 (0.36–1.04)	FISH

Shaded boxes represent statistically significant findings. All comparisons for mutations are mutation-positive versus mutation-negative, all comparisons for GCN are increased GCN versus nonincreased GCN; the exception to this is for hazard ratios for death which refer to the mutation-positive or GCN-positive groups and their risk of death on TKI treatment versus placebo treatment.

R, retrospective collection; SGA, subgroup analysis of a prospective trial; TKI, tyrosine kinase inhibitor; GCN, gene copy number; NR, not reached; NA, information not available in the original report; NS, reported as not significant but exact numbers not given; qPCR, quantitative polymerase chain reaction; FISH, fluorescent in situ hybridization; INTACT, a randomized phase III studies of chemotherapy with or without gefitinib; IDEAL, a phase II studies of single-agent gefitinib.

resistance to treatment and progress. The mechanisms of primary and secondary resistance are not yet elucidated in most cases; however, the general principles of signaling via parallel redundant pathways, constitutive activation of downstream mediators, altered receptor trafficking, efflux of the drug from the cell, and mutation of the drug target itself have been implicated as contributing factors [86–90]. Mutations in exon 2 of *KRAS*, a downstream component of the EGFR signaling network, have been associated with primary resistance to EGFR TKIs and have also been shown to be mutually exclusive with *EGFR* mutations and related to increased tobacco history [46,47,91–93]. This suggests the possibility of two distinct oncogenic pathways to NSCLC, specifically a *KRAS*-mutated lung cancer more common in smokers and an *EGFR*-mutated lung cancer more common in nonsmokers. However, *KRAS* mutations do not explain all cases of primary resistance.

A secondary point mutation in exon 20 of *EGFR* leading to a threonine to methionine substitution at codon 790 (T790M) has been described in up to 50% of cases with secondary EGFR TKI resistance [86,87]. The T790M mutation was discovered through examination of cases with an activating *EGFR* mutation and an initial response to EGFR TKI therapy, followed eventually by clinical progression and repeat biopsy of tumor tissue. Three-dimensional modeling suggests that the bulky methionine residue introduced by the T790M mutation impedes TKI binding, which is analogous to acquired resistance mutations found in *KIT* and *BCR-ABL* in gastrointestinal stromal tumors and chronic myelogenous leukemia, respectively [86,90,94]. Introduction of T790M into TKI-sensitive cell lines confers TKI-resistance but not all cells with acquired resistance have an identifiable T790M mutation [87]. However, a recent study indicates that T790M may be difficult to detect in tumors with amplified EGFR, suggesting that the current literature likely underrepresents the importance of this mutation in acquired EGFR TKI resistance [95].

In order to circumvent the clinical problems of primary and secondary EGFR TKI resistance, a second generation of TKI compounds is under development. The two most commonly employed strategies these agents use to overcome resistance are the introduction of covalent (irreversible) binding to the drug target and the broadening of receptor tyrosine kinase targets within the cell. The first-generation drugs gefitinib and erlotinib join to their target, the catalytic site in the EGFR TK domain, through classic competitive binding with ATP [15,96]. In contrast, many of the second-generation compounds form covalent, and therefore permanent, bonds with their target, which should theoretically increase their effectiveness by prolonging the inhibition of EGFR signaling to the entire lifespan of the drug-bound receptor molecule. In cell culture systems, such irreversibly-binding TKIs can effectively kill cells that have acquired resistance to first-generation TKIs [88].

The other design strategy common among many second-generation EGFR TKIs is kinase multitargeting. Gefitinib and erlotinib are both fairly selective for the EGFR TK domain [18,31]. Solitary blockade of the EGFR molecule itself likely promotes the emergence of resistant clones that bypass the inhibited receptor, given the divergent and redundant nature of the downstream signaling network [90]. Blocking multiple signaling pathways with either a combination of agents or a single multitargeted drug has been synergistic in preclinical models [97–100]. Second-generation EGFR TKIs are being developed that, in addition to blocking EGFR signaling, target additional members of the Erb-B family such as Her-2 or other downstream or parallel pathways such as the vascular endothelial growth factor receptor (VEGFR) pathway.

Many of the novel second-generation EGFR TKIs have been proven safe in cancer patients via the phase I clinical trial mechanism, including EKB-569, an irreversible EGFR inhibitor, HKI-272, an irreversible dual EGFR and Her-2 inhibitor, CI-1033, an irreversible pan-ErbB inhibitor, and ZD6474, a dual kinase inhibitor that primarily inhibits VEGFR-2, but also has moderate anti-EGFR activity [101–105]. Although evaluations of the clinical activity of these agents in patients with acquired resistance to first-generation EGFR TKIs have not yet been reported, a published case report has described two patients participating in a phase I trial of EKB-569 that each harbored an *EGFR* mutation at baseline and had acquired gefitinib resistance and then exhibited a clinical responses to treatment with EKB-569 [106].

Of the second-generation EGFR TKIs, ZD6474 is the furthest along in clinical NSCLC development. It was evaluated in parallel with gefitinib in a population of 168 previously treated NSCLC patients on a randomized phase II study with the option to crossover to the other drug at the time of progression [107]. The response rate was 8% in the ZD6474 arm and 1% in the gefitinib arm, with progression-free survivals prolonged on the ZD6474 arm compared to the gefitinib arm (11 weeks versus 8.1 weeks, respectively; $p = 0.03$). No survival difference was noted, perhaps because of the crossover design. A similar trial comparing ZD6474 and erlotinib is ongoing. Given the successful outcome of combining the anti-VEGF agent bevacizumab with chemotherapy in NSCLC patients [108], a second randomized phase II trial was performed using ZD6474 or placebo in combination with docetaxel chemotherapy in 127 previous treated NSCLC patients [109]. Progression-free survival was increased with ZD6474 compared to placebo (18.7 weeks versus 12.0 weeks, respectively; $p = 0.07$ which was interpreted as significant because they had a priori established a p value of <0.2 as significant enough to warrant further study). A phase II trial of ZD6474 in combination with carboplatin and paclitaxel for first-line treatment of NSCLC and a randomized phase III trial of docetaxel with ZD6474 or placebo for previously treated NSCLC patients are currently enrolling patients. Results of these and other clinical studies utilizing second-generation EGFR TKI agents in the general NSCLC population as well as specific subgroups defined by either clinical or molecular characteristics are anxiously awaited.

Monoclonal antibodies to EGFR

Antibodies directed to the extracellular portion of EGFR have also been developed. The primary compound from this class developed in NSCLC thus far is cetuximab (also known as Erbitux® and C225),

which is a chimeric IgG1 antibody directed against the ligand-binding domain of EGFR that competes with endogenous ligand for receptor binding, leads to receptor internalization, and inhibits cell cycle progression [110]. The primary toxicities of cetuximab are rash and antibody reactions. Cetuximab is FDA approved for the treatment of other solid tumors, in combination with chemotherapy (in colorectal cancer) or radiation therapy (in head and neck cancer) [111,112].

In NSCLC, single-agent cetuximab as a salvage therapy has minor activity, with a response rate of 3% and a disease stabilization rate of 28% in a phase II trial [113]. Analysis of *EGFR* mutations was performed in available tumor specimens from patients on this trial but only two responding patients had evaluable tissue and neither harbored a mutation, making it difficult to draw conclusions [114]. A phase II trial of single-agent salvage cetuximab with mandatory *EGFR* mutation analysis in all patients is ongoing; however, preclinical evidence suggests that *EGFR* mutations are not likely to be helpful in predicting response to EGFR-directed antibodies [115].

Cetuximab has also been studied in combination with chemotherapy for NSCLC. In first-line regimens, cetuximab with carboplatin/paclitaxel or with cisplatin/vinorelbine yields approximately a 25–35% response rate, 5-month median time to progression and 8- to 11-month median survival in phase II clinical trials, similar to expected results with platinum-based chemotherapy [116,117]. Two large phase III trials of chemotherapy with or without cetuximab as first-line NSCLC treatment are ongoing. Cetuximab is also under evaluation in combination with second-line chemotherapy, with radiation and chemotherapy for stage III disease, and with EGFR TKIs [114,118]. An identifiable subgroup of patients that benefit from cetuximab treatment has not yet emerged from these studies, as defined either by clinical characteristics or molecular biomarkers. Newer monoclonal antibodies against EGFR are under development, including matuzumab and panitumumab, both of which are less likely than cetuximab to induce human antimurine antibody responses and are therefore purported to be somewhat safer.

Conclusion

In conclusion, EGFR has proven to be an important "target" for novel therapies in NSCLC treatment. The most significant findings to date are (1) erlotinib, an EGFR TKI, can prolong survival compared to placebo in NSCLC patients previously treated with chemotherapy and (2) *EGFR* mutations define a subgroup of NSCLC patients whose tumors are addicted to EGFR signaling and these patients likely gain significant clinical benefit from treatment with EGFR TKIs.

The paradigm for developing novel-targeted therapies is not as simple as designing an agent that inhibits a molecule known to be commonly overexpressed in a given type of cancer. Rather, it is now clear that carcinomas are heterogeneous and molecularly-defined subgroups of patients have been or will likely be defined in the future that divide each disease into many more categories than historical pathologic nomenclature. Furthermore, due to the complex and redundant nature of the vital signaling pathways in cancer cells, to be successful we will likely need treatment regimens that combine multiple-targeted agents, simultaneously blocking a host of diverse intracellular signals.

In order to hasten the era of genotype-directed targeted therapy, it is important to move toward "smarter" clinical trials that evaluate novel agents and incorporate well-designed molecular correlative studies. Mandatory collection of tissue specimens from all patients is imperative to ensure that as new discoveries are made, complete cohorts of patients can be evaluated for the presence or absence of critical biomarkers. This type of paradigm change will help move us closer to the day when cancer therapies are individualized from patient to patient.

References

1 Non-small Cell Lung Cancer Collaborative Group. Chemotherapy in non-small cell lung cancer: a meta-analysis using updated data on individual patients from 52 randomised clinical trials. *BMJ* Oct 7, 1995; **311(7010)**:899–909.

2 Spiro SG, Rudd RM, Souhami RL *et al.* Chemotherapy versus supportive care in advanced non-small cell lung cancer: improved survival without detriment to quality of life. *Thorax* Oct 2004; **59(10)**:828–36.

3 Schiller JH, Harrington D, Belani CP *et al.* Comparison of four chemotherapy regimens for advanced non-small-cell lung cancer. *N Engl J Med* Jan 10, 2002; **346(2)**:92–8.

4 Delbaldo C, Michiels S, Syz N, Soria JC, Le Chevalier T, Pignon JP. Benefits of adding a drug to a single-agent or a 2-agent chemotherapy regimen in advanced non-small-cell lung cancer: a meta-analysis. *JAMA* Jul 28, 2004; **292(4)**:470–84.

5 Yarden Y, Sliwkowski MX. Untangling the ErbB signalling network. *Nat Rev Mol Cell Biol* Feb 2001; **2(2)**:127–37.

6 Mendelsohn J, Baselga J. Status of epidermal growth factor receptor antagonists in the biology and treatment of cancer. *J Clin Oncol* Jul 15, 2003; **21(14)**:2787–99.

7 Klapper LN, Glathe S, Vaisman N *et al.* The ErbB-2/HER2 oncoprotein of human carcinomas may function solely as a shared coreceptor for multiple stroma-derived growth factors. *Proc Natl Acad Sci USA* Apr 27, 1999; **96(9)**:4995–5000.

8 Guy PM, Platko JV, Cantley LC, Cerione RA, Carraway KL, III. Insect cell-expressed p180erbB3 possesses an impaired tyrosine kinase activity. *Proc Natl Acad Sci USA* Aug 16, 1994; **91(17)**:8132–6.

9 Mendelsohn J. Targeting the epidermal growth factor receptor for cancer therapy. *J Clin Oncol* Sep 15, 2002; **20(Suppl 18)**:1S–13S.

10 Holbro T, Civenni G, Hynes NE. The ErbB receptors and their role in cancer progression. *Exp Cell Res* Mar 10, 2003; **284(1)**:99–110.

11 Salomon DS, Brandt R, Ciardiello F, Normanno N. Epidermal growth factor-related peptides and their receptors in human malignancies. *Crit Rev Oncol Hematol* Jul 1995; **19(3)**:183–232.

12 Hirsch FR, Scagliotti GV, Langer CJ, Varella-Garcia M, Franklin WA. Epidermal growth factor family of receptors in preneoplasia and lung cancer: perspectives for targeted therapies. *Lung Cancer* Aug 2003; **41(Suppl 1)**:S29–42.

13 Normanno N, De Luca A, Bianco C *et al.* Epidermal growth factor receptor (EGFR) signaling in cancer. *Gene* Jan 17, 2006; **366**:2–16.

14 Barker AJ, Gibson KH, Grundy W *et al.* Studies leading to the identification of ZD1839 (IRESSA): an orally active, selective epidermal growth factor receptor tyrosine kinase inhibitor targeted to the

treatment of cancer. *Bioorg Med Chem Lett* Jul 23, 2001; **11(14)**:1911–14.

15 Wakeling AE, Guy SP, Woodburn JR *et al*. ZD1839 (Iressa): an orally active inhibitor of epidermal growth factor signaling with potential for cancer therapy. *Cancer Res* Oct 15, 2002; **62(20)**:5749–54.

16 Ciardiello F, Caputo R, Bianco R *et al*. Antitumor effect and potentiation of cytotoxic drugs activity in human cancer cells by ZD-1839 (Iressa), an epidermal growth factor receptor-selective tyrosine kinase inhibitor. *Clin Cancer Res* May 2000; **6(5)**:2053–63.

17 Ciardiello F, Caputo R, Bianco R *et al*. Inhibition of growth factor production and angiogenesis in human cancer cells by ZD1839 (Iressa), a selective epidermal growth factor receptor tyrosine kinase inhibitor. *Clin Cancer Res* May 2001; **7(5)**:1459–65.

18 Ranson M, Hammond LA, Ferry D *et al*. ZD1839, a selective oral epidermal growth factor receptor-tyrosine kinase inhibitor, is well tolerated and active in patients with solid, malignant tumors: results of a phase I trial. *J Clin Oncol* May 1, 2002; **20(9)**:2240–50.

19 Baselga J, Rischin D, Ranson M *et al*. Phase I safety, pharmacokinetic, and pharmacodynamic trial of ZD1839, a selective oral epidermal growth factor receptor tyrosine kinase inhibitor, in patients with five selected solid tumor types. *J Clin Oncol* Nov 1, 2002; **20(21)**:4292–302.

20 Herbst RS, Maddox AM, Rothenberg ML *et al*. Selective oral epidermal growth factor receptor tyrosine kinase inhibitor ZD1839 is generally well-tolerated and has activity in non-small-cell lung cancer and other solid tumors: results of a phase I trial. *J Clin Oncol* Sep 15, 2002; **20(18)**:3815–25.

21 Fukuoka M, Yano S, Giaccone G *et al*. Multi-institutional randomized phase II trial of gefitinib for previously treated patients with advanced non-small-cell lung cancer (The IDEAL 1 Trial) [corrected]. *J Clin Oncol* Jun 15, 2003; **21(12)**:2237–46.

22 Kris MG, Natale RB, Herbst RS *et al*. Efficacy of gefitinib, an inhibitor of the epidermal growth factor receptor tyrosine kinase, in symptomatic patients with non-small cell lung cancer: a randomized trial. *JAMA* Oct 22, 2003; **290(16)**:2149–58.

23 Janne PA, Gurubhagavatula S, Yeap BY *et al*. Outcomes of patients with advanced non-small cell lung cancer treated with gefitinib (ZD1839, "Iressa") on an expanded access study. *Lung Cancer* May 2004; **44(2)**:221–30.

24 Veronese ML, Algazy K, Bearn L *et al*. Gefitinib in patients with advanced non-small cell lung cancer (NSCLC): the expanded access protocol experience at the University of Pennsylvania. *Cancer Invest* 2005; **23(4)**:296–302.

25 Mohamed MK, Ramalingam S, Lin Y, Gooding W, Belani CP. Skin rash and good performance status predict improved survival with gefitinib in patients with advanced non-small cell lung cancer. *Ann Oncol* May 2005; **16(5)**:780–5.

26 West HL, Franklin WA, McCoy J *et al*. Gefitinib therapy in advanced bronchioloalveolar carcinoma: Southwest Oncology Group Study S0126. *J Clin Oncol* Apr 20, 2006; **24(12)**:1807–13.

27 Barkley JE, Green MR. Bronchioloalveolar carcinoma. *J Clin Oncol* Aug 1996; **14(8)**:2377–86.

28 Grunwald V, Hidalgo M. Development of the epidermal growth factor receptor inhibitor OSI-774. *Semin Oncol* Jun 2003; **30(3, Suppl 6)**:23–31.

29 Moyer JD, Barbacci EG, Iwata KK *et al*. Induction of apoptosis and cell cycle arrest by CP-358,774, an inhibitor of epidermal growth factor receptor tyrosine kinase. *Cancer Res* Nov 1, 1997; **57(21)**:4838–48.

30 Pollack VA, Savage DM, Baker DA *et al*. Inhibition of epidermal growth factor receptor-associated tyrosine phosphorylation in human carcinomas with CP-358,774: dynamics of receptor inhibition in situ and antitumor effects in athymic mice. *J Pharmacol Exp Ther* Nov 1999; **291(2)**:739–48.

31 Hidalgo M, Siu LL, Nemunaitis J *et al*. Phase I and pharmacologic study of OSI-774, an epidermal growth factor receptor tyrosine kinase inhibitor, in patients with advanced solid malignancies. *J Clin Oncol* Jul 1, 2001; **19(13)**:3267–79.

32 Perez-Soler R, Chachoua A, Hammond LA *et al*. Determinants of tumor response and survival with erlotinib in patients with non-small-cell lung cancer. *J Clin Oncol* Aug 15, 2004; **22(16)**:3238–47.

33 Perez-Soler R, Saltz L. Cutaneous adverse effects with HER1/EGFR-targeted agents: is there a silver lining? *J Clin Oncol* Aug 1, 2005; **23(22)**:5235–46.

34 Perez-Soler R, Delord JP, Halpern A *et al*. HER1/EGFR inhibitor-associated rash: future directions for management and investigation outcomes from the HER1/EGFR inhibitor rash management forum. *Oncologist* May 2005; **10(5)**:345–56.

35 Giaccone G, Herbst RS, Manegold C *et al*. Gefitinib in combination with gemcitabine and cisplatin in advanced non-small-cell lung cancer: a phase III trial–INTACT 1. *J Clin Oncol* Mar 1, 2004; **22(5)**:777–84.

36 Herbst RS, Giaccone G, Schiller JH *et al*. Gefitinib in combination with paclitaxel and carboplatin in advanced non-small-cell lung cancer: a phase III trial–INTACT 2. *J Clin Oncol* Mar 1, 2004; **22(5)**:785–94.

37 Herbst RS, Prager D, Hermann R *et al.* TRIBUTE: a phase III trial of erlotinib hydrochloride (OSI-774) combined with carboplatin and paclitaxel chemotherapy in advanced non-small-cell lung cancer. *J Clin Oncol* Sep 1, 2005; **23(25)**:5892–9.

38 Gatzemeier U, Pluzanska A, Szczesna A *et al.* Results of a phase III trial of erlotinib (OSI-774) combined with cisplatin and gemcitabine (GC) chemotherapy in advanced non-small cell lung cancer (NSCLC). Paper presented at American Society of Clinical Oncology, 2004, New Orleans, LA.

39 Gandara DR, Gumerlock PH. Epidermal growth factor receptor tyrosine kinase inhibitors plus chemotherapy: case closed or is the jury still out? *J Clin Oncol* Sep 1, 2005; **23(25)**:5856–8.

40 Thatcher N, Chang A, Parikh P *et al.* Gefitinib plus best supportive care in previously treated patients with refractory advanced non-small-cell lung cancer: results from a randomised, placebo-controlled, multicentre study (Iressa Survival Evaluation in Lung Cancer). *Lancet* Oct 29–Nov 4, 2005; **366(9496)**:1527–37.

41 Shepherd FA, Rodrigues Pereira J, Ciuleanu T *et al.* Erlotinib in previously treated non-small-cell lung cancer. *N Engl J Med* Jul 14, 2005; **353(2)**:123–32.

42 Shepherd FA, Dancey J, Ramlau R *et al.* Prospective randomized trial of docetaxel versus best supportive care in patients with non-small-cell lung cancer previously treated with platinum-based chemotherapy. *J Clin Oncol* May 2000; **18(10)**:2095–103.

43 Lynch TJ, Bell DW, Sordella R *et al.* Activating mutations in the epidermal growth factor receptor underlying responsiveness of non-small-cell lung cancer to gefitinib. *N Engl J Med* May 20, 2004; **350(21)**:2129–39.

44 Paez JG, Janne PA, Lee JC *et al.* EGFR mutations in lung cancer: correlation with clinical response to gefitinib therapy. *Science* Jun 4, 2004; **304(5676)**:1497–500.

45 Pao W, Miller V, Zakowski M *et al.* EGF receptor gene mutations are common in lung cancers from "never smokers" and are associated with sensitivity of tumors to gefitinib and erlotinib. *Proc Natl Acad Sci USA* Sep 7, 2004; **101(36)**:13306–11.

46 Shigematsu H, Lin L, Takahashi T *et al.* Clinical and biological features associated with epidermal growth factor receptor gene mutations in lung cancers. *J Natl Cancer Inst* Mar 2, 2005; **97(5)**:339–46.

47 Marchetti A, Martella C, Felicioni L *et al.* EGFR mutations in non-small-cell lung cancer: analysis of a large series of cases and development of a rapid and sensitive method for diagnostic screening with potential implications on pharmacologic treatment. *J Clin Oncol* Feb 1, 2005; **23(4)**:857–65.

48 Mitsudomi T, Kosaka T, Endoh H *et al.* Mutations of the epidermal growth factor receptor gene predict prolonged survival after gefitinib treatment in patients with non-small-cell lung cancer with postoperative recurrence. *J Clin Oncol* Apr 10, 2005; **23(11)**:2513–20.

49 Kosaka T, Yatabe Y, Endoh H, Kuwano H, Takahashi T, Mitsudomi T. Mutations of the epidermal growth factor receptor gene in lung cancer: biological and clinical implications. *Cancer Res* Dec 15, 2004; **64(24)**:8919–23.

50 Taron M, Ichinose Y, Rosell R *et al.* Activating mutations in the tyrosine kinase domain of the epidermal growth factor receptor are associated with improved survival in gefitinib-treated chemorefractory lung adenocarcinomas. *Clin Cancer Res* Aug 15, 2005; **11(16)**:5878–85.

51 Cappuzzo F, Hirsch FR, Rossi E *et al.* Epidermal growth factor receptor gene and protein and gefitinib sensitivity in non-small-cell lung cancer. *J Natl Cancer Inst* May 4, 2005; **97(9)**:643–55.

52 Tokumo M, Toyooka S, Kiura K *et al.* The relationship between epidermal growth factor receptor mutations and clinicopathologic features in non-small cell lung cancers. *Clin Cancer Res* Feb 1, 2005; **11(3)**:1167–73.

53 Huang SF, Liu HP, Li LH *et al.* High frequency of epidermal growth factor receptor mutations with complex patterns in non-small cell lung cancers related to gefitinib responsiveness in Taiwan. *Clin Cancer Res* Dec 15, 2004; **10(24)**:8195–203.

54 Kim KS, Jeong JY, Kim YC *et al.* Predictors of the response to gefitinib in refractory non-small cell lung cancer. *Clin Cancer Res* Mar 15, 2005; **11(6)**:2244–51.

55 Han SW, Kim TY, Hwang PG *et al.* Predictive and prognostic impact of epidermal growth factor receptor mutation in non-small-cell lung cancer patients treated with gefitinib. *J Clin Oncol* Apr 10, 2005; **23(11)**:2493–501.

56 Cortes-Funes H, Gomez C, Rosell R *et al.* Epidermal growth factor receptor activating mutations in Spanish gefitinib-treated non-small-cell lung cancer patients. *Ann Oncol* Jul 2005; **16(7)**:1081–6.

57 Chou TY, Chiu CH, Li LH *et al.* Mutation in the tyrosine kinase domain of epidermal growth factor receptor is a predictive and prognostic factor for gefitinib treatment in patients with non-small cell lung cancer. *Clin Cancer Res* May 15, 2005; **11(10)**:3750–7.

58 Zhang XT, Li LY, Mu XL *et al.* The EGFR mutation and its correlation with response of gefitinib in previously

treated Chinese patients with advanced non-small-cell lung cancer. *Ann Oncol* Aug 2005; **16(8)**:1334–42.

59 Mu XL, Li LY, Zhang XT *et al*. Gefitinib-sensitive mutations of the epidermal growth factor receptor tyrosine kinase domain in Chinese patients with non-small cell lung cancer. *Clin Cancer Res* Jun 15, 2005; **11(12)**:4289–94.

60 Tomizawa Y, Iijima H, Sunaga N *et al*. Clinicopathologic significance of the mutations of the epidermal growth factor receptor gene in patients with non-small cell lung cancer. *Clin Cancer Res* Oct 1, 2005; **11(19, Pt 1)**:6816–22.

61 Rosell R, Ichinose Y, Taron M *et al*. Mutations in the tyrosine kinase domain of the EGFR gene associated with gefitinib response in non-small-cell lung cancer. *Lung Cancer* Oct 2005; **50(1)**:25–33.

62 Takano T, Ohe Y, Sakamoto H *et al*. Epidermal growth factor receptor gene mutations and increased copy numbers predict gefitinib sensitivity in patients with recurrent non-small-cell lung cancer. *J Clin Oncol* Oct 1, 2005; **23(28)**:6829–37.

63 Tsao MS, Sakurada A, Cutz JC *et al*. Erlotinib in lung cancer – molecular and clinical predictors of outcome. *N Engl J Med* Jul 14, 2005; **353(2)**:133–44.

64 Hirsch FR, Varella-Garcia M, McCoy J *et al*. Increased epidermal growth factor receptor gene copy number detected by fluorescence in situ hybridization associates with increased sensitivity to gefitinib in patients with bronchioloalveolar carcinoma subtypes: a Southwest Oncology Group Study. *J Clin Oncol* Oct 1, 2005; **23(28)**:6838–45.

65 Kondo M, Yokoyama T, Fukui T *et al*. Mutations of epidermal growth factor receptor of non-small cell lung cancer were associated with sensitivity to gefitinib in recurrence after surgery. *Lung Cancer* Dec 2005; **50(3)**:385–91.

66 Yang SH, Mechanic LE, Yang P *et al*. Mutations in the tyrosine kinase domain of the epidermal growth factor receptor in non-small cell lung cancer. *Clin Cancer Res* Mar 15, 2005; **11(6)**:2106–10.

67 Yatabe Y, Kosaka T, Takahashi T, Mitsudomi T. EGFR mutation is specific for terminal respiratory unit type adenocarcinoma. *Am J Surg Pathol* May 2005; **29(5)**:633–9.

68 Sordella R, Bell DW, Haber DA, Settleman J. Gefitinib-sensitizing EGFR mutations in lung cancer activate anti-apoptotic pathways. *Science* Aug 20, 2004; **305(5687)**:1163–7.

69 Tracy S, Mukohara T, Hansen M, Meyerson M, Johnson BE, Janne PA. Gefitinib induces apoptosis in the EGFRL858R non-small-cell lung cancer cell line H3255. *Cancer Res* Oct 15, 2004; **64(20)**:7241–4.

70 Jiang J, Greulich H, Janne PA, Sellers WR, Meyerson M, Griffin JD. Epidermal growth factor-independent transformation of Ba/F3 cells with cancer-derived epidermal growth factor receptor mutants induces gefitinib-sensitive cell cycle progression. *Cancer Res* Oct 1, 2005; **65(19)**:8968–74.

71 Greulich H, Chen TH, Feng W *et al*. Oncogenic transformation by inhibitor-sensitive and -resistant EGFR mutants. *PLoS Med* Nov 2005; **2(11)**:e313.

72 Sato M, Vaughan MB, Girard L *et al*. Multiple oncogenic changes (K-RAS(V12), p53 knockdown, mutant EGFRs, p16 bypass, telomerase) are not sufficient to confer a full malignant phenotype on human bronchial epithelial cells. *Cancer Res* Feb 15, 2006; **66(4)**:2116–28.

73 Nagatomo I, Kumagai T, Yamadori T *et al*. The gefitinib-sensitizing mutant epidermal growth factor receptor enables transformation of a mouse fibroblast cell line. *DNA Cell Biol* Apr 2006; **25(4)**:246–51.

74 Sequist LV, Bell DW, Lynch TJ, Haber DA. Molecular predictors of response to EGFR antagonists in non-small cell lung cancer. *J Clin Oncol* Feb 10, 2007; **25(5)**:587–95.

75 Jackman DM, Yeap BY, Sequist LV *et al*. Exon 19 deletion mutations of epidermal growth factor receptor are associated with prolonged survival in non-small cell lung cancer patients treated with gefitinib or erlotinib. *Clin Cancer Res* Jul 1, 2006; **12(13)**:3908–14.

76 Riely GJ, Pao W, Pham D *et al*. Clinical course of patients with non-small cell lung cancer and epidermal growth factor receptor exon 19 and exon 21 mutations treated with gefitinib or erlotinib. *Clin Cancer Res* Feb 1, 2006; **12(3, Pt 1)**:839–44.

77 Asahina H, Yamazaki K, Kinoshita I *et al*. A phase II trial of gefitinib as first-line therapy for advanced non-small cell lung cancer with epidermal growth factor receptor mutations. *Br J Cancer* Oct 23, 2006; **95(8)**:998–1004.

78 Inoue A, Suzuki T, Fukuhara T *et al*. Prospective phase II study of gefitinib for chemotherapy-naive patients with advanced non-small-cell lung cancer with epidermal growth factor receptor gene mutations. *J Clin Oncol* Jul 20, 2006; **24(21)**:3340–6.

79 Pas-Ares L, Sanchez JM, Garcia-Velasco A *et al*. Prospective phase II trial of erlotinib in advanced non-small cell lung cancer (NSCLC) patients (p) with mutations in the tyrosine kinase (TK) domain of the epidermal growth factor receptor (EGFR). Paper

presented at American Society of Clinical Oncology, 2006, Atlanta, GA.

80 Shepherd FA, Tsao MS. Unraveling the mystery of prognostic and predictive factors in epidermal growth factor receptor therapy. *J Clin Oncol* Mar 1, 2006; **24(7)**:1219–20; author reply 1220–21.

81 Eberhard DA, Johnson BE, Amler LC *et al*. Mutations in the epidermal growth factor receptor and in KRAS are predictive and prognostic indicators in patients with non-small-cell lung cancer treated with chemotherapy alone and in combination with erlotinib. *J Clin Oncol* Sep 1, 2005; **23(25)**:5900–9.

82 Han SW, Kim TY, Jeon YK *et al*. Optimization of patient selection for gefitinib in non-small cell lung cancer by combined analysis of epidermal growth factor receptor mutation, K-ras mutation, and Akt phosphorylation. *Clin Cancer Res* Apr 15, 2006; **12(8)**:2538–44.

83 Hirsch FR, Varella-Garcia M, Bunn PA, Jr *et al*. Molecular predictors of outcome with gefitinib in a phase III placebo-controlled study in advanced non-small-cell lung cancer. *J Clin Oncol* Nov 1, 2006; **24(31)**:5034–42.

84 Bell DW, Lynch TJ, Haserlat SM *et al*. Epidermal growth factor receptor mutations and gene amplification in non-small-cell lung cancer: molecular analysis of the IDEAL/INTACT gefitinib trials. *J Clin Oncol* Nov 1, 2005; **23(31)**:8081–92.

85 Marchetti A, Felicioni L, Buttitta F. Assessing EGFR mutations. *N Engl J Med* Feb 2, 2006; **354(5)**:526–8; author reply 526–8.

86 Kobayashi S, Boggon TJ, Dayaram T *et al*. EGFR mutation and resistance of non-small-cell lung cancer to gefitinib. *N Engl J Med* Feb 24, 2005; **352(8)**:786–92.

87 Pao W, Miller VA, Politi KA, Riely GJ, Somwar R, Zakowski MF. Acquired resistance of lung adenocarcinomas to gefitinib or erlotinib is associated with a second mutation in the EGFR kinase domain. *PLoS Med* Feb 22, 2005; **2(3)**:e73.

88 Kwak EL, Sordella R, Bell DW *et al*. Irreversible inhibitors of the EGF receptor may circumvent acquired resistance to gefitinib. *Proc Natl Acad Sci USA* May 24, 2005; **102(21)**:7665–70.

89 Camp ER, Summy J, Bauer TW, Liu W, Gallick GE, Ellis LM. Molecular mechanisms of resistance to therapies targeting the epidermal growth factor receptor. *Clin Cancer Res* Jan 1, 2005; **11(1)**:397–405.

90 Rubin BP, Duensing A. Mechanisms of resistance to small molecule kinase inhibition in the treatment of solid tumors. *Lab Invest* Oct 2006; **86(10)**:981–6.

91 Pao W, Wang TY, Riely GJ *et al*. KRAS mutations and primary resistance of lung adenocarcinomas to gefitinib or erlotinib. *PLoS Med* Jan 2005; **2(1)**:e17.

92 Soung YH, Lee JW, Kim SY *et al*. Mutational analysis of EGFR and K-RAS genes in lung adenocarcinomas. *Virchows Arch* May 2005; **446(5)**:483–8.

93 Tam IY, Chung LP, Suen WS *et al*. Distinct epidermal growth factor receptor and KRAS mutation patterns in non-small cell lung cancer patients with different tobacco exposure and clinicopathologic features. *Clin Cancer Res* Mar 1, 2006; **12(5)**:1647–53.

94 Carter TA, Wodicka LM, Shah NP *et al*. Inhibition of drug-resistant mutants of ABL, KIT, and EGF receptor kinases. *Proc Natl Acad Sci USA* Aug 2, 2005; **102(31)**:11011–6.

95 Engelman JA, Mukohara T, Zejnullahu K *et al*. Allelic dilution obscures detection of a biologically significant resistance mutation in EGFR-amplified lung cancer. *J Clin Invest* Oct 2006; **116(10)**:2695–706.

96 Stamos J, Sliwkowski MX, Eigenbrot C. Structure of the epidermal growth factor receptor kinase domain alone and in complex with a 4-anilinoquinazoline inhibitor. *J Biol Chem* Nov 29, 2002; **277(48)**:46265–72.

97 Shaheen RM, Ahmad SA, Liu W *et al*. Inhibited growth of colon cancer carcinomatosis by antibodies to vascular endothelial and epidermal growth factor receptors. *Br J Cancer* Aug 17, 2001; **85(4)**:584–9.

98 Yokoi K, Thaker PH, Yazici S *et al*. Dual inhibition of epidermal growth factor receptor and vascular endothelial growth factor receptor phosphorylation by AEE788 reduces growth and metastasis of human colon carcinoma in an orthotopic nude mouse model. *Cancer Res* May 1, 2005; **65(9)**:3716–25.

99 Zhou Y, Brattain MG. Synergy of epidermal growth factor receptor kinase inhibitor AG1478 and ErbB2 kinase inhibitor AG879 in human colon carcinoma cells is associated with induction of apoptosis. *Cancer Res* Jul 1, 2005; **65(13)**:5848–56.

100 Zhou Y, Li S, Hu YP *et al*. Blockade of EGFR and ErbB2 by the novel dual EGFR and ErbB2 tyrosine kinase inhibitor GW572016 sensitizes human colon carcinoma GEO cells to apoptosis. *Cancer Res* Jan 1, 2006; **66(1)**:404–11.

101 Erlichman C, Hidalgo M, Boni JP *et al*. Phase I study of EKB-569, an irreversible inhibitor of the epidermal growth factor receptor, in patients with advanced solid tumors. *J Clin Oncol* May 20, 2006; **24(15)**:2252–60.

102 Wong KK, Fracasso PM, Bukowski RM *et al*. HKI-272, an irreversible pan erbB receptor tyrosine kinase

inhibitor: preliminary phase 1 results in patients with solid tumors. *J Clin Oncol* 2006; **24(18S)**:3018.

103 Calvo E, Tolcher AW, Hammond LA *et al*. Administration of CI-1033, an irreversible pan-erbB tyrosine kinase inhibitor, is feasible on a 7-day on, 7-day off schedule: a phase I pharmacokinetic and food effect study. *Clin Cancer Res* Nov 1, 2004; **10(21)**:7112–20.

104 Nemunaitis J, Eiseman I, Cunningham C *et al*. Phase 1 clinical and pharmacokinetics evaluation of oral CI-1033 in patients with refractory cancer. *Clin Cancer Res* May 15, 2005; **11(10)**:3846–53.

105 Holden SN, Eckhardt SG, Basser R *et al*. Clinical evaluation of ZD6474, an orally active inhibitor of VEGF and EGF receptor signaling, in patients with solid, malignant tumors. *Ann Oncol* Aug 2005; **16(8)**:1391–7.

106 Yoshimura N, Kudoh S, Kimura T *et al*. EKB-569, a new irreversible epidermal growth factor receptor tyrosine kinase inhibitor, with clinical activity in patients with non-small cell lung cancer with acquired resistance to gefitinib. *Lung Cancer* Mar 2006; **51(3)**:363–8.

107 Natale RB, Bodkin D, Govindan R *et al*. ZD6474 versus gefitinib in patients with advanced NSCLC: final results from a two-part, double-blind, randomized phase II trial. Paper presented at American Society of Clinical Oncology, 2006, Atlanta, GA.

108 Sandler A, Gray R, Brahmer J *et al*. Randomized phase II/III trial of paclitaxel (P) plus carboplatin (C) with or without bevacizumab (NSC #704865) in patients with advanced non-squamous non-small cell lung cancer (NSCLC): an Eastern Cooperative Oncology Group (ECOG) Trial – E4599. Paper presented at American Society of Clinical Oncology, 2005, Orlando, FL.

109 Heymach JV, Johnson BE, Prager D *et al*. A phase II trial of ZD6474 plus docetaxel in patients with previously treated NSCLC: Follow-up results. Paper presented at American Society of Clinical Oncology, 2006, Atlanta, GA.

110 Mendelsohn J. Epidermal growth factor receptor inhibition by a monoclonal antibody as anticancer therapy. *Clin Cancer Res* Dec 1997; **3(12, Pt 2)**:2703–7.

111 Cunningham D, Humblet Y, Siena S *et al*. Cetuximab monotherapy and cetuximab plus irinotecan in irinotecan-refractory metastatic colorectal cancer. *N Engl J Med* Jul 22, 2004; **351(4)**:337–45.

112 Bonner JA, Harari PM, Giralt J *et al*. Radiotherapy plus cetuximab for squamous-cell carcinoma of the head and neck. *N Engl J Med* Feb 9, 2006; **354(6)**:567–78.

113 Lilenbaum R, Bonomi P, Ansari R *et al*. A phase II trial of cetuximab as therapy for recurrent non-small cell lung cancer (NSCLC): final results. Paper presented at American Society of Clinical Oncology, 2005, Orlando, FL.

114 Lilenbaum RC. The evolving role of cetuximab in non-small cell lung cancer. *Clin Cancer Res* Jul 15, 2006; **12(14, Pt 2)**:4432s–5s.

115 Mukohara T, Engelman JA, Hanna NH *et al*. Differential effects of gefitinib and cetuximab on non-small-cell lung cancers bearing epidermal growth factor receptor mutations. *J Natl Cancer Inst* Aug 17, 2005; **97(16)**:1185–94.

116 Thienelt CD, Bunn PA, Jr, Hanna N *et al*. Multicenter phase I/II study of cetuximab with paclitaxel and carboplatin in untreated patients with stage IV non-small-cell lung cancer. *J Clin Oncol* Dec 1, 2005; **23(34)**:8786–93.

117 Rosell R, Daniel C, Ramlau R *et al*. Randomized phase II study of cetuximab in combination with cisplatin (C) and vinorelbine (V) vs. CV alone in the first-line treatment of patients (pts) with epidermal growth factor receptor (EGFR)-expressing advanced non-small-cell lung cancer (NSCLC). Paper presented at American Society of Clinical Oncology, 2004, New Orleans, LA.

118 Naret CL, Ramalingam S, Beattie L *et al*. Total blockade of the epidermal growth factor receptor with the combination of cetuximab and gefitinib: a phase I study for patients with recurrent non-small cell lung cancer (NSCLC). Paper presented at American Society of Clinical Oncology, 2006, Atlanta, GA.

CHAPTER 23

Tumor Angiogenesis: Biology and Therapeutic Implications for Lung Cancer

Emer O. Hanrahan, Monique Nilsson, and John V. Heymach

Tumor angiogenesis

Angiogenesis, the formation of new blood vessels from a preexisting vascular supply, occurs during physiological processes such as development, wound healing, and reproduction [1]. Early experiments using isolated organ perfusion and other systems demonstrated that tumors did not grow beyond 1 mm^3 in the absence of neovascularization, but were able to grow rapidly upon acquisition of a vascular supply [2,3]. As is true for normal cells, the survival and growth of tumor cells is dependent on an adequate supply of oxygen and nutrients. The diffusion limit for oxygen is approximately 100 μm, and tumor cells beyond this distance from a blood vessel are apoptotic or necrotic [4,5]. Based on these and other observations, it was proposed that tumor growth is angiogenesis-dependent and that tumor angiogenesis may be a therapeutic target in cancer [6]. Since these initial publications, a large body of data has been generated supporting the critical role of angiogenesis in tumor progression. Furthermore, the process of metastasis is angiogenesis dependent. For tumor cells to metastasize, they must penetrate the vasculature, survive the circulation, arrest in a capillary bed at a distant site, extravasate into the target organ, and proliferate [7,8].

Lung Cancer, 3rd edition. Edited by Jack A. Roth, James D. Cox, and Waun Ki Hong. © 2008 Blackwell Publishing, ISBN: 978-1-4051-5112-2.

Angiogenesis in lung cancer

Vascular density has been demonstrated to be an important prognostic factor in many solid malignancies. Lung cancer is no exception. Numerous prospective and retrospective studies have shown that tumor microvessel density (MVD) correlates with disease stage and patient survival [9–13].

Regulators of angiogenesis

Angiogenesis is controlled by the balance between positive and negative regulators produced by both tumor and stromal cells. Some of the potential regulators that have been implicated in tumor angiogenesis in lung cancer are listed in Table 23.1. For a tumor to switch to an angiogenic phenotype, it must shift this balance toward an excess of proangiogenic factors [14–16]. Once angiogenesis is initiated, endothelial cells elaborate proteases that degrade the basement membrane, proliferate, migrate to form capillary tubes, and become positioned to form new blood vessels that will perfuse the tissue [17]. Proangiogenic molecules including basic fibroblast growth factor (bFGF), platelet-derived endothelial cell growth factor (PDGF), and vascular endothelial growth factor (VEGF) are produced by lung cancer cells and are associated with an increased vascular density in human lung tumors [18–24]. High vascular density [9,10,25], as well as increased expression of VEGF [26–31], bFGF [16,32], and interleukin-8

369

Table 23.1 Potential regulators of angiogenesis in NSCLC.

Proangiogenic molecules	Antiangiogenic molecules	Transcription factors, oncogenes, and other regulators
Vascular endothelial growth factor (VEGF)	Thrombospondin	Hypoxia inducible factor 1-α
Transforming growth factor-α	Interferon-α, β, γ	Nuclear factor - κB
Epidermal growth factor	Angiopoietin 2	Ras
Platelet-derived growth factor	Tissue inhibitors of MMPs	p53
Basic fibroblast growth factor	Endostatin	Epidermal growth factor receptor
Angiogenin	Angiostatin	
Interleukin-8	Interleukin-12	
Interleukin-6		
Matrix metalloproteinases (MMPs)		

(IL-8) [29], has been shown to correlate with decreased survival time and/or increased risk of relapse in retrospective and prospective studies of nonsmall cell lung cancer (NSCLC) patients. Furthermore, high expression of VEGF mRNA is associated with an early postoperative relapse [28].

Tumor cell expression of proangiogenic molecules is regulated by multiple factors. Hypoxia is a primary driving force in the expression of angiogenic molecules through stabilization of the transcription factor hypoxia-inducible factor 1 (HIF-1α) [33]. Among NSCLC patients, elevated expression of HIF-1α is associated with shorter disease-free survival [34,35]. Additionally, oncogenic Ras, activated epidermal growth factor receptor (EGFR), and loss of wild-type p53, all of which have been well documented in NSCLC, promote tumor progression, in part, thought upregulation of proangiogenic molecules including VEGF [10,36–39].

The VEGF pathway

VEGF is thought to be the foremost mediator of angiogenesis, and is the prototypic member of a family of homodimeric growth factors that includes placental-growth factor (PlGF)-1 and 2, VEGF-B, VEGF-C, VEGF-D, and VEGF-E [40–42]. VEGF ligands exert their biological effects through interactions with several receptor tyrosine kinases including VEGFR-1 (Flt-1), VEGFR-2 (Flk-1, KDR), and VEGFR-3 (Flt-4). VEGF-mediated vascular permeability, endothelial cell proliferation, migration, and

survival occurs via VEGFR-2, which is expressed on nearly all endothelial cells [40]. Signal transduction through VEGFR-1, which binds VEGF, VEGF-B, PlGF-1, and -2, facilitates the recruitment of endothelial progenitors and monocyte migration, whereas VEGFR-3 expression is thought to be limited to lymphatic endothelium [43].

Therapeutic approaches to inhibiting angiogenesis

Because angiogenesis is necessary for tumor growth and metastatic spread, much effort has been directed toward the development of therapies targeting the vascular component of this disease. Various strategies have been utilized to target the VEGF pathway including monoclonal antibodies (i.e., bevacizumab) and proteins that bind VEGF such as VEGF-Trap, a fusion protein comprised of the VEGFR extracellular domain and the Fc portion of immunoglobulin (Ig) G1 [42]. Other agents developed to block VEGF signal transduction include antibodies that block the receptor (IMC-1121b) and small molecule inhibitors of the receptor tyrosine kinase (RTKIs) such as ZD6474, sunitinib, and sorafenib (Figure 23.1).

Clinical trials of antiangiogenic agents in the treatment of NSCLC

NSCLC is the leading cause of cancer-related mortality in the United States [44]. About two thirds

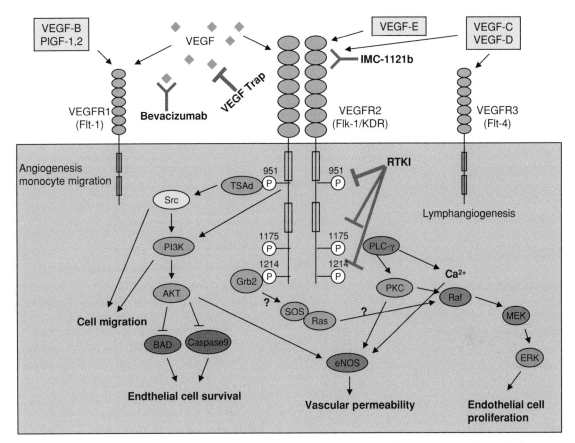

Figure 23.1 VEGF signal transduction and strategies for pathway inhibition. Following ligand binding to VEGFR2, signal transduction molecules including phospholipase C-γ (PLC-γ), PI3K, Akt, Ras, Src, and MAPK are activated which subsequently regulated endothelial cell proliferation, migration, survival, and vascular permeability. Strategies to inhibit VEGF signaling include monoclonal antibodies (bevacizumab) or other proteins (VEGF Trap) directed at the VEGF protein, antibodies directed against the receptor (IMC-1121b), and RTKIs. (Adapted from [42].)

of patients present with locally advanced, inoperable or metastatic disease. Chemotherapy in these patients improves survival compared to supportive care, but even with modern regimens, the median survival is only 8–10 months [45,46]. The addition of a third cytotoxic agent to doublet chemotherapy regimens generally has resulted in increased toxicity, but not an improvement in clinical outcome.

In order to enhance the efficacy of chemotherapy without significantly increasing its toxicities, recent efforts have focused on combinations of chemotherapy with targeted agents. EGFR tyrosine kinase inhibitors (TKIs), gefitinib and erlotinib, were among the earliest targeted agents tested. Although single-agent erlotinib was shown in a randomized trial to improve survival relative to supportive care for refractory stage IIIB/IV NSCLC, gefitinib in a similar trial did not [47,48]. Despite their activity as monotherapy, these agents did not improve survival in combination with first-line chemotherapy [49–52]. Results with combinations with antiangiogenic therapies have been more promising. In a landmark study, the median survival of patients with nonsquamous, advanced-stage NSCLC treated first-line with a combination of bevacizumab and standard doublet chemotherapy was significantly superior to patients treated with chemotherapy

Table 23.2 Examples of drugs targeting the VEGF pathway in clinical trials for NSCLC.

Target	Agent	Mechanism	Phase of development in NSCLC
VEGF ligand	Bevacizumab	Monoclonal antibody	Phase III–IV FDA approved for CRC and NSCLC
	VEGF Trap	Soluble receptor-based protein that binds VEGF-A, VEGF-B, and PIGF	Phase II
VEGFR extracellular domain	IMC-1121B	Monoclonal anti-VEGFR-2 antibody	Phase I in solid tumors
VEGFR TK domain	Sunitinib	RTKI of VEGFR-1, 2, 3; PDGFR, c-Kit, and Flt-3	Phase II
	ZD6474	RTKI of VEGFR-2, EGFR, and RET	Phase III
	AZD2171	RTKI of VEGFR-1,2,3, PDGFR and c-Kit	Phase II/III
	Axitinib	RTKI of VEGFR-1,2,3, PDGFR, and c-Kit	Phase II
Multiple levels	Sorafenib	RTKI of VEGFR-2, VEGFR-3, and PDGFR-β. Also inhibits the serine-threonine kinase of Raf-1	Phase III

TK, tyrosine kinase; EGFR, Epidermal growth factor receptor; NSCLC, nonsmall cell lung cancer; PDGFR, platelet-derived growth factor receptor; RTKI, small molecule receptor tyrosine kinase inhibitor; VEGF, vascular endothelial growth factor; VEGFR, vascular endothelial growth factor receptor.

alone, as discussed below [53]. This has given great impetus to the study of antiangiogenic agents in NSCLC, both as monotherapy and in combination regimens with either chemotherapy or other targeted agents. Further roles for bevaciuzmab in the management of NSCLC are being explored, and other antiangiogenic agents, particularly tyrosine kinase inhibitors of the VEGF receptors, are in various stages of clinical development (Table 23.2).

Antiangiogenic agents in combination with chemotherapy as first-line therapy for advanced NSCLC

In 2004, bevacizumab became the first clinically available antiangiogenic agent when it received Food and Drug Administration (FDA) approval for first-line use with 5-fluorouracil-based chemotherapy for metastatic colorectal cancer based on improved survival in a randomized, phase III trial [54]. Since then, bevacizumab with 5-fluorouracil-based chemotherapy has also been shown to improve survival in the second-line setting [55]. Furthermore, bevacizumab in combination with chemotherapy has recently demonstrated improved outcomes for first-line treatment of metastatic breast can-

cer (MBC) and advanced nonsquamous NSCLC, and it received FDA approval for nonsquamous NSCLC on the basis of the ECOG4599 trial discussed below [53].

The application of bevacizumab in NSCLC was first assessed in a randomized phase II study involving 99 patients with chemonaive stage IIIB (with pleural effusion; "wet") or IV NSCLC. The standard chemotherapy doublet of carboplatin (AUC = 6) and paclitaxel (200 mg/m^2) every 3 weeks was compared with the same regimen combined with either low-dose (7.5 mg/kg) or high-dose bevacizumab (15 mg/kg), also every 3 weeks [56]. Treatment with chemotherapy plus high-dose bevacizumab resulted in a higher response rate than either chemotherapy with either low-dose bevacizumab or chemotherapy alone (40% versus 21.9% and 31.3%, respectively), longer median time to progression (TTP; 7.0 mo versus 4.1 and 5.9 mo) and increased survival (17.7 mo versus 11.6 and 14.9 mo). This study also revealed an unanticipated and concerning side effect: severe pulmonary hemorrhage, which occurred in six patients who had received bevacizumab, and was fatal in four cases. Tumor characteristics associated with significant hemoptysis were

Table 23.3 Results from recent randomized trials of agents targeting the VEGF pathway in advanced stage NSCLC.

Reference	Phase	Line	Endpt	SCC*	Treatment arms	N	ORR (%)	PFS (mo)	OS (mo)
Sandler et al. [53]	II/III	1st	OS	No	PC	433	10	4.5	10.3
					PC + BV	417	27	6.4	12.3[†]
Heymach et al. [70]	II	2nd+	PFS	Yes	Doc + placebo	41	12	2.8	13.4
					Doc + ZD6474 100 mg	42	26	4.3[‡]	13.1
					Doc + ZD6474 300 mg	44	18	3.9	7.9
Natale et al. [115]	II	2nd+	PFS	Yes	Gefitinib	85	1	1.9	
					ZD6474 300 mg	83	8	2.5[§]	
Fehrenbacher et al. [94]	II	2nd+	PFS	No	Doc/Pem[‖] + placebo	41	12	3	NR
					Doc/Pem[‖] + BV	40	12	4.8	
					Erlotinib + BV	39	18	4.4	

*Whether patients with squamous cell carcinoma were eligible.
[†] $p = 0.007$.
[‡] $p = 0.074$; trial was designed with prespecified significance level for PFS was 0.2, so trial met its primary endpoint.
[§] $p = 0.011$; trial had crossover design to other treatment so survival cannot be compared between arms.
[‖] Chemotherapy was treating physician's choice of pemetrexed or docetaxel.
PC, paclitaxel and carboplatin; BV, bevacizumab, doc, docetaxel; pem, pemetrexed; ORR, objective response rate; PFS, median progression-free survival; OS, median overall survival; mo, months, endpt, primary endpoint; NR, not reported.

central location, proximity to major blood vessels, necrosis and cavitation before or during therapy, and squamous histology. Since squamous cell tumors are more commonly located centrally and have a greater tendency to cavitate than adenocarcinomas, it is unclear whether histology alone is the primary risk factor for hemoptysis, or simply a surrogate for other risk factors.

Based on the promising outcomes with high-dose bevacizumab in this phase II trial, a follow-up randomized, phase III trial was conducted by the Eastern Cooperative Oncology Group (ECOG), E4599, comparing standard carboplatin and paclitaxel for six cycles with or without bevacizumab (15 mg/kg) as first-line treatment for stage IIIB ("wet") or IV nonsquamous NSCLC. Due to concerns about life-threatening hemorrhage, patients with squamous histology, history of gross hemoptysis or brain metastases were excluded. There were 850 eligible patients treated on this trial, and the results of a planned second interim analysis have been reported [53]. Median survival (12.3 mo versus 10.3 mo, hazard ratio 0.79, $p = 0.003$), progression free survival (PFS, 6.2 mo versus 4.5 mo, hazard ratio 0.66, $p < 0.001$) and response rate (35% versus 15%, $p < 0.001$) were all superior in the bevacizumab-containing arm (Table 23.3). The main grade 3

or higher toxicities associated with bevacizumab were bleeding (4.4% versus 0.7% in the standard chemotherapy arm) and hypertension (7% versus 0.7%). Fifteen of seventeen reported treatment-related deaths occurred in the bevacizumab arm; five due to hemoptysis, two from gastrointestinal bleeding, five from neutropenic fever two from cerebrovascular events, and one from probable pulmonary embolis. This means that the rate of fatal hemoptysis with bevacizumab when squamous histology was excluded was approximately 1%. This may be considered an acceptable risk in light of the absolute improvements in survival of 7% and 8% at 1 and 2 years, respectively.

This was the first randomized phase III study in NSCLC that has shown superior survival when targeted therapy is combined with standard chemotherapy. Many oncologists regard this regimen as a new standard of care for patients with nonsquamous NSCLC, but others prefer to await a confirmatory trial. This may come from an ongoing phase III trial of gemcitabine and cisplatin with or without bevacizumab. Interestingly, a recently presented unplanned subset analysis of survival by gender in E4599 found that the survival benefit was confined primarily to male participants, although females did benefit in terms of response and PFS

[57]. The reason for this apparent gender-based difference in benefit is unclear.

Attempts are being made to extend the benefits of bevacizumab to patients with squamous NSCLC. A phase II study of radiotherapy followed by combination therapy with paclitaxel, carboplatin, and bevacizumab as first-line treatment in patients with advanced stage squamous NSCLC is being conducted. It is hoped that administration of radiotherapy to the main pulmonary lesion before systemic therapy will prevent the rapid cavitation that can occur and lead to major hemoptysis during bevacizumab-based therapy.

One promising VEGFR TKI for NSCLC is ZD6474, an orally administered RTKI that also inhibits EGFR (Table 23.2). It is administered orally and has a long half-life (in excess of 100 h) making it compatible with once-daily dosing [58]. ZD6474 was evaluated in two phase I studies of patients with refractory solid tumors; one involving a Western population [58] patients, and the other in Japan [59]. Therapy was well tolerated at doses of ≤300 mg/day. The main reported side effects were facial flushing, facial rash, fatigue, diarrhea, and asymptomatic QTc interval prolongation. Over 40% of patients in the Western study had stable disease of at least 8 weeks duration, and in the Japanese study tumor regression was observed in four of nine patients (44%) with NSCLC. A number of phase II studies of ZD6474 alone or in combination with chemotherapy for previously treated NSCLC have subsequently been conducted, with promising results and favorable toxicity (see below). A randomized, phase II, multicenter study of ZD6474 alone or in combination with standard carboplatin and paclitaxel as first-line treatment for patients with locally advanced, metastatic or recurrent NSCLC has been conducted [60]. Patients with squamous histology and treated brain metastases were eligible. This trial has recently completed accrual, and results are expected in 2007.

Sorafenib is another orally bioavailable RTKI that is under study in NSCLC (Table 23.2). Phase I studies of sorafenib identified 400 mg twice daily as the recommended phase II dose [61,62]. The toxicity profile of this agent is favorable and usually manageable. It has recently gained FDA approval for use in advanced RCC based on significant improvements in PFS in phase II (randomized discontinuation design) and phase III trials [63–65]. This agent is currently being investigated in advanced NSCLC. Data from 15 patients with advanced, progressive NSCLC participating in a phase I trial of sorafenib combined with carboplatin/paclitaxel were recently reported by Schiller *et al.* [66]. Carboplatin (AUC = 6) and paclitaxel (225 mg/m^2) were administered on day 1, and sorafenib (100, 200, or 400 mg twice daily by mouth) on days 2–18 of each 21-day cycle. Among 14 evaluable patients, the disease control rate was 79%, consisting of a partial response in 29% and stable disease in 50% of patients. The median PFS was 34 weeks. A randomized, phase III trial in chemonaive patients with stage IIIB–IV NSCLC is currently being conducted comparing standard carboplatin plus paclitaxel for six cycles with or without sorafenib (400 mg twice daily) as first-line therapy. Patients with squamous histology are eligible, but patients with significant hemoptysis within the preceding 4 weeks are excluded. The planned accrual is for 900 patients from more than 150 sites in North America, South America, Europe, and the Asia Pacific region, and overall survival is the primary endpoint.

AZD2171 is also an orally bioavailable RTKI (Table 23.2). In phase I studies, it has been well tolerated at doses ≤45 mg/day [67,68]. AZD2171 has recently been studied in combination with paclitaxel (200 mg/m^2) and carboplatin (AUC = 6) chemotherapy in patients with advanced NSCLC (any histologic subtype) [69]. A total of 20 patients participated. AZD2171 at a dose of 30 mg/day (cohort 1, 9 patients) or 45 mg/day (cohort 2, 11 patients) was commenced on day 2 of cycle 1 and continued until disease progression or dose-limiting toxicity (DLT) occurred. Overall, toxicities were manageable, and included fatigue, anorexia, mucositis, diarrhea, and hypertension. Of 15 evaluable patients, there were six partial responses and eight patients with stable disease. Tumor cavitation was also observed. A phase II/III trial of carboplatin and paclitaxel with or without AZD2171 for first-line treatment in stage IIIB–IV NSCLC is currently being conducted by the National Cancer Institute of Canada Clinical Trials Group. All NSCLC histologic subtypes will be allowed, but patients with a central thoracic lesion with cavitation or clinically relevant hemoptysis within the preceding 4 weeks will be excluded.

Antiangiogenic agents in combination with chemotherapy as second-line therapy for advanced NSCLC

A randomized, placebo-controlled phase II trial was conducted to evaluate the dual VEGFR/EGFR inhibitor ZD6474 in combination with chemotherapy for advanced-stage NSCLC patients previously treated with platinum-containing chemotherapy. One hundred twenty-seven patients were randomized to receive docetaxel 75 mg/m^{2}intravenously every 21 days with either placebo, ZD6474 100 mg or ZD6474 300 mg once daily [70]. Patients with squamous cell histology and previously treated brain metastases were eligible. Toxicities commonly associated with antiepidermal growth factor therapy, such as diarrhea and rash, were most common with the 300 mg dose of ZD6474. This study met its primary endpoint of prolonged median PFS in the ZD6474 100 mg arm (19 weeks with 100 mg + doc; 17 weeks with 300 mg + doc; 12 weeks in the placebo + doc control arm) (Table 23.3). There was no significant difference in survival between the treatment arms. An international, randomized, phase III trial of docetaxel combined with ZD6474 100 mg or placebo as first-line therapy for locally advanced or metastatic NSCLC is underway, and plans to accrue 1240 patients. Patients with squamous histology are included.

Antiangiogenic agents as monotherapy for advanced NSCLC

Although bevacizumab has improved survival in metastatic CRC and NSCLC in combination with chemotherapy, it has generally not been effective as a single agent in solid tumors. In fact, the phase III trial of FOLFOX and bevacizumab for second-line treatment of metastatic CRC had a bevacizumab monotherapy arm that was closed at a planned interim analysis due to lack of efficacy [55]. In the phase II trial of chemotherapy with or without bevacizumab for NSCLC described above, 19 patients

in the control arm received high-dose, single-agent bevacizumab on progression, and although five had disease stabilization, there were no objective responses [56]. On the other hand, there is considerable data from phase I–II trials suggesting that the VEGFR TKIs have marked activity in terms of response, disease stabilization, and/or PFS as single agents in NSCLC, although there are no results yet from large, randomized trials to determine if they will improve overall survival. Presumably this apparent difference in efficacy between VEGFR TKIs and bevacizumab as monotherapy relates to their differences in mechanisms of action. Bevacizumab is thought to be highly specific for the VEGF ligand itself (one of several ligands that binds to VEGF receptors), while most anti-VEGFR TKIs have a wider spectrum of activity and, therefore, have a higher likelihood of exerting antitumor activity through non-VEGF-mediated mechanisms. Although the exact mechanism of action of bevacizumab is unclear, it is thought that it both inhibits new vessel formation in tumors and may "normalize" the existing vasculature, allowing chemotherapy to better permeate tumors (i.e., making vessels less leaky, so that the interstitial fluid pressure is lower, and allowing more homogenous blood flow through tumors) [71]. This theory would be consistent with the limited efficacy of single-agent bevacizumab in most tumor types other than renal cell carcinoma [72].

Despite the low activity of single-agent bevacizumab, another anti-VEGF agent, VEGF Trap, is currently being assessed as a single agent in NSCLC (Table 23.2). It binds VEGF and neutralizes all VEGF-A isoforms with higher affinity than bevacizumab [73]. It also neutralizes other VEGF family members including VEGF-B. Phase I trials of single-agent VEGF Trap in patients with advanced solid tumors have shown it to be well tolerated, and one trial reported a disease stabilization rate of about 47% among 30 patients [74,75]. A phase II trial of single-agent VEGF Trap in locally advanced or metastatic platinum- and erlotinib-resistant, nonsquamous NSCLC is ongoing [76].

ZD6474 has demonstrated significant single-agent antitumor activity in a phase II randomized, double-blind, multicenter trial involving

168 patients with locally advanced or metastatic, platinum-refractory NSCLC (all histologic subtypes allowed). Patients were allocated to receive either daily oral ZD6474 (300 mg) or gefitinib (250 mg) until disease progression or limiting toxicity (part A) [77]. Upon progression, patients had the option to crossover to the alternative therapy after a 4-week wash-out period (part B). The primary endpoint was PFS in part A. There was a statistically significant improvement in median PFS with ZD6474 compared to gefitinib (11.0 weeks versus 8.1 weeks, $p = 0.011$) (Table 23.3). The disease control rate (response or stable disease for more than 8 weeks) with ZD6474 was 53% (8% response), and was 35% (1% response) with gefitinib. In part B, stable disease for longer than 8 weeks was achieved in 16 of 37 patients (43%) who switched from gefitinib to ZD6474 and in 7 of 29 (24%) who switched from ZD6474 to gefitinib.

Sorafenib has also shown evidence of single-agent activity in advanced NSCLC. In a recent single arm, multicenter phase II trial, 52 patients with advanced NSCLC and one to two prior treatments received sorafenib 400 mg twice daily [78]. Thirty-one percent had squamous cell carcinoma. Although there were no objective responses by RECIST criteria among 51 evaluable patients, four patients had central cavitation of their tumors. Furthermore, 59% of patients had stable disease. The median PFS for all patients was 2.7 months. There were four drug-related episodes of bleeding; three patients with epistaxis, and one patient with squamous cell carcinoma and a central cavitary lesion who died from pulmonary hemorrhage 30 days after stopping sorafenib. Based on these results, the ECOG is conducting a phase II randomized discontinuation study of sorafenib in patients with refractory NSCLC (E2501).

Sunitinib is another oral, multitargeted receptor TKI that is currently under study in advanced NSCLC with encouraging early results. It has activity against VEGFR-1, VEGFR-2, PDGFR-β, c-Kit, and Flt-3 (Table 23.2). Phase I clinical studies identified sunitinib 50 mg orally, once daily for 4 out of every 6 weeks/cycle as the dosing schedule of choice [79,80]. Sunitinib has already gained FDA approval in January 2006 for the treatment of advanced renal cell carcinoma (RCC) based on high clinical benefit rates (>60%) in two phase II trials in metastatic RCC

progressing postcytokine therapy, and a recently reported phase III trial of sunitinib versus interferon-α as first-line treatment that found that response rates and median PFS were significantly improved with sunitinib [81–83]. Sunitinib was also shown to significantly prolong median TTP and overall survival in imatinib-resistant gastrointestinal stromal tumor, and it has also gained FDA approval for that purpose [84].

Sixty-three patients received single-agent sunitinib (50 mg once daily for 4 out of every 6 weeks) on a phase II trial in previously treated (including a platinum) stage IIIB/IV NSCLC. Squamous histology was allowed, but patients with recent grade 3 hemorrhage or gross hemoptysis were excluded. Preliminary results have been reported [85]. Grade 3–4 toxicities included fatigue (21%), nausea (7%), vomiting (7%), abdominal pain (7%), and hypertension (5%). Two of the 22 participants with squamous histology died from pulmonary hemorrhage. Another patient with adenocarcinoma died from cerebral hemorrhage, which was subsequently found to be related to a brain metastasis. Of 47 patients with evaluable disease, there were six partial responses (9.5%), and stable disease in 12 patients (19.0%) [85].

Vatalanib is an oral small molecule TKI of VEGFR-1,-2,-3, PDGFR, c-Kit and c-Fms. A single-arm phase II study of vatalanib (1250 mg once daily) in patients with platinum-refractory advanced stage NSCLC is underway in Europe. The primary objective is to assess the efficacy of vatalanib monotherapy as second-line treatment in patients with stage IIIB/IV NSCLC. Like the other trials involving VEGFR TKIs, squamous histology is allowed. Preliminary data on the first 54 patients reported one patient with a partial response (2%) and 17 patients with stable disease (31%) after 12 weeks on study [86]. One patient with adenocarcinoma had a fatal pulmonary hemorrhage.

Axitinib (AG-013736) is another oral VEGFR TKI, with activity against all known VEGFRs, as well as PDGFR-β, and c-Kit (Table 23.1) [87]. In a phase I trial in 36 patients with advanced solid tumors, there were three confirmed partial responses (two in patients with RCC) and three minor responses [87]. Two patients with NSCLC had cavitation of their lung tumors, suggesting activity of this drug in this disease. A phase II trial open in multiple centers in Germany and the USA is currently evaluating single-agent axitinib as second-line or later therapy in stage IIIB/IV NSCLC [76].

Antiangiogenic agents in combination with other targeted therapies for NSCLC

The molecular pathways involved in the proliferation of cancer cells and tumor angiogenesis are highly complex, and inhibiting a single step in these pathways is unlikely to obtain long-term disease control, and experience thus far suggests that therapeutic resistance inevitably develops. Consequently, combining agents with different targets may obtain additional therapeutic benefit. EGFR and VEGFR share common downstream signaling pathways. There is evidence that VEGF is downregulated by EGFR inhibition, and also that blockade of VEGF-signaling may inhibit EGFR autocrine signaling [88,89]. Therefore, it has been hypothesized that dual blockade of these molecular targets would have additive or synergistic antitumor effects, and a number of preclinical studies support this theory [90–93]. Phase I and II clinical trials combining agents that target both VEGF and EGF signaling are already showing some promising results in solid tumors, including NSCLC.

A phase I/II study by Herbst *et al.* assessed erlotinib and bevacizumab in 40 patients with non-squamous stage IIIB/IV NSCLC, previously treated with one or more chemotherapy regimens [50]. There were 8 patients (20%) with partial responses and 26 patients (65%) had stable disease as their best response. The median overall survival and PFS for the patients treated at the phase II dose were 12.6 months and 6.2 months, respectively. In a randomized phase II trial, this combination compared favorably with chemotherapy alone (docetaxel or pemetrexed) or chemotherapy with bevacizumab (Table 23.3) [94]. Two phase III multicenter, placebo-controlled, randomized trials incorporating this therapeutic approach have opened in the USA [76]. The first is a study of erlotinib with or without bevacizumab in patients with NSCLC that progressed during or after first-line chemotherapy or chemoradiotherapy. Patients with squamous histology are only allowed to participate if they have

no intrathoracic disease or only small peripheral lesions. In the other study, previously untreated patients with locally advanced or metastatic NSCLC receive four cycles of standard chemotherapy plus bevacizumab, followed by "maintenance" with either bevacizumab plus erlotinib or bevacizumab plus placebo. Squamous histology is allowed, but patients with gross hemoptysis within 3 months prior to enrollment are excluded.

A number of ongoing early phase studies are considering combinations of TKIs of VEGFR and EGFR in solid tumors, and some of these trials are confined to NSCLC. Preliminary data have been reported on the first 32 participants in a phase I study examining the safety and efficacy of sorafenib and gefitinib combination in patients with refractory or recurrent NSCLC [95]. Nine patients were treated with gefitinib 250 mg orally once daily and sorafenib 200 mg orally twice daily, and 23 patients received the same gefitinib dose and a higher sorafenib dose of 400 mg twice daily. The most common drug-related adverse events were fatigue, diarrhea, elevated alanine aminotransferase (ALT) and/or aspartate aminotransferase (AST), rash/desquamation, and anorexia, and were predominantly grade 1–2. Drug-related serious adverse events were seen in four patients and consisted of diarrhea, elevated ALT, and elevated AST at the sorafenib 200 mg dose, and dyspnea at the 400 mg dose. Although there was only one patient with a partial response (8 mo duration), 20 patients (63%) had stable disease and the median PFS was 18 weeks. A recently opened randomized phase II trial is evaluating a similar regimen of erlotinib with or without sunitinib in patients with advanced NSCLC who have received previous treatment with a platinum-based regimen[76].

Antiangiogenic therapy in the neoadjuvant and adjuvant setting for operable NSCLC

Based on the improved outcomes with the addition of bevacizumab to standard chemotherapy for the treatment of advanced NSCLC, clinical trials are underway to determine if such an approach may also benefit patients with operable disease. Bevacizumab combined with chemotherapy in the neoadjuvant or adjuvant settings is being evaluated. One such trial is the phase II BEACON study (Bevacizumab and Chemotherapy for Operable NSCLC) at Memorial Sloan Kettering Cancer Center, involving patients with stage IB–IIIA resectable NSCLC [76]. The primary aim of this trial is to determine if the addition of bevacizumab to a cisplatin-based chemotherapy in the neoadjuvant setting for nonsquamous cell carcinomas improves the rate of pathologic downstaging. A recently approved phase III randomized ECOG trial (E1505) will assess four cycles of adjuvant platinum-based chemotherapy with or without bevacizumab for fully resected stage IB–IIIA NSCLC, including squamous histology.

Antiangiogenic agents in combination with radiotherapy for NSCLC

Based on the success of bevacizumab added to chemotherapy in stage IIIB and IV NSCLC, the potential for such antiangiogenic agents to improve outcome if added to chemoradiation for locally advanced NSCLC is being investigated.

Preclinical studies have demonstrated that antiangiogenic agents can synergize with or potentiate the effects of radiotherapy [96–100]. There are several potential explanations for this effect. Because hypoxia induces radiation resistance, there were initial concerns that antiangiogenic agents might have a negative impact on the efficacy of radiotherapy. However, it has been proposed that antiangiogenic agents "normalize" the disorganized and hyperpermeable vasculature in tumors, resulting in reduced intratumoral interstitial pressure and allowing more homogenous blood flow through tumors [101]. This in turn would allow greater delivery of oxygen to the tumor tissue, and could enhance radiation-induced cytotoxicity in part by increasing the formation of oxygen free radicals. This theory also suggests that prolonged use of antiangiogenic agents could eventually also reduce the "normalized" vessels in tumors, and that there would then be an inadequate amount of vasculature, such that the tumors would again be relatively hypoxic with reduced radiationsensitivity. This model has received experimental support from studies in mouse xenografts that supports the existence of a period of time ("normalization window")

during which radiation therapy used in conjunction with an antiangiogenic agent is most effective [102].

It was long thought that radiotherapy exacted its antitumor effect only through a direct action on cancer cells. However, evidence has emerged recently that radiotherapy may also act through the induction of endothelial cell apoptosis [103]. VEGFRs are expressed predominantly on vascular endothelial cells [104]. Therefore, using an anti-VEGF signaling agent in combination with radiotherapy may constitute a dual attack on the developing tumor vasculature. Furthermore, VEGF expression is induced by radiation and can contribute to radioresistance by blocking radiation-induced endothelial cell apoptosis [105,106]. Consequently, agents targeting the VEGF pathway may help sensitize endothelial cells to radiation.

The first antiangiogenic agent to be assessed in a phase III trial in combination with chemoradiotherapy was AE-941 (Neovastat). AE-941 is a naturally occurring antiangiogenic agent derived from shark cartilage. Its proposed mechanism(s) of action include inhibition of a number of matrix metalloproteinases, VEGF binding to endothelial cells and VEGF-dependent tyrosine phosphorylation [107]. AE-941 demonstrated superior antitumor activity compared to cisplatin in the Lewis lung carcinoma murine model, and a phase I/II clinical trial in advanced stage NSCLC patients showed that the agent was well tolerated and suggested that single agent, high-dose AE-941 improves disease stability and survival [107,108]. Based on these encouraging results, a phase III, double-blind, placebo-controlled trial of platinum-based chemotherapy and radiotherapy with or without AE-941 in locally advanced NSCLC was conducted. An interim report of toxicity data on the first 351 patients found no excess or differential toxicity between the AE-941 and placebo arms [109]. The trial has completed accrual and results are expected in the near future.

One of the anti-tumor affects of thalidomide is inhibition of angiogenesis, but the mechanism of this action remains unclear. A phase III trial by ECOG (E3598) of this agent in combination with chemoradiation for locally advanced NSCLC has also completed accrual [76]. All patients in this trial received induction paclitaxel and carboplatin every 21 days, and those with stable disease or response began chemoradiation between days 43 and 50 for a period of 6 weeks. Patients were randomized either to receive or not to receive thalidomide commenced on day 1 of induction chemotherapy and continued for 2 years. Efficacy and toxicity data have not yet been reported.

Combinations of VEGF inhibitors and chemoradiotherapy are also being investigated. The Southwestern Oncology Group (SWOG) initiated a phase I/II pilot study of induction chemoradiation (cisplatin, etoposide, and radiotherapy) with or without bevacizumab followed by consolidation docetaxel and bevacizumab for patients with newly diagnosed, locally advanced, inoperable NSCLC [76]. The primary aim of the study is to assess toxicity, and PFS, overall survival, and response are secondary endpoints. There are also several ongoing early phase trials with bevacizumab in combination with chemoradiotherapy in progress or being planned.

Clinical trials of antiangiogenic agents in small cell lung cancer

The use of antiangiogenic agents in small cell lung cancer (SCLC) has been less thoroughly evaluated than in NSCLC. The only completed phase III trial of an antiangiogenic agent in SCLC is a randomized, double-blind, placebo-controlled comparison of combination chemotherapy (cisplatin, etoposide, epidoxorubicin, and cyclophosphamide) with or without thalidomide in patients with previously untreated extensive stage disease which was conducted in France [110]. Following enrollment, all patients received two cycles of chemotherapy, and then only responding patients were randomized to either receive thalidomide or placebo concurrently with the next four cycles of chemotherapy and thalidomide was continued for up to 2 years. Of 119 patients, 97 responders went on to be randomized. There was more toxicity associated with the use of thalidomide, particularly neuropathy, constipation and requirements for red cell transfusions, and about one third of patients discontinued thalidomide due to side effects. Response rates were 81.6

and 62.8% in favor of the thalidomide arm. Overall survival also favored the thalidomide arm, with a median survival of 11.7 months versus 8.7 months ($p = 0.02$). However, it is difficult to draw any definite conclusions about the efficacy of antiangiogenic agents in SCLC from this trial because the patient number was relatively small and thalidomide has actions other than antiangiogenesis, such as immune modulatory effects.

There are a number of recently completed or ongoing trials of anti-VEGF signaling agents in previously untreated extensive stage SCLC [76]. ECOG has completed a phase II study (E3501) of first-line cisplatin, etoposide, and bevacizumab in patients with extensive stage SCLC. Results are not yet available for this trial. Another single-arm phase II study is evaluating the addition of bevacizumab to irinotecan and carboplatin as first-line treatment in patients with extensive stage disease. Those with response or stable disease after the six cycles will continue on bevacizumab for a further 6 months.

The question of incorporating bevacizumab into therapy for patients with limited stage SCLC has also been addressed in two trials. The first study in patients with limited stage SCLC evaluated chemoradiation (where the chemotherapy was four cycles of irinotecan and carboplatin) followed by single-agent bevacizumab (10 mg/kg every 2 weeks for 10 doses) as maintenance therapy for those with response or stable disease [111]. There were 60 patients enrolled. The complete and partial response rates were 27% and 53%, respectively. With a median follow-up of 24 months, the median PFS had not been reached and median OS was 17.5 months. One-year and 2-year survival rates were 70 and 29%. In a second ongoing study, patients with limited stage SCLC receive chemoradiation (with irinotecan and carboplatin for four cycles) [76] with bevacizumab given concurrently. Patients with stable disease or response after the four cycles of systemic therapy also receive single-agent bevacizumab as maintenance therapy for a further 6 months.

The NCIC-CTG has recently completed a phase II randomized trial of maintenance ZD6474 or placebo in patients with either limited or extensive stage SCLC who had a confirmed response (complete or partial) to chemotherapy with or without radiotherapy. Results from this trial have not yet been reported.

The use of anti-VEGF agents with second-line therapy for SCLC is also under study [76]. There is an ongoing phase II study in the United States of paclitaxel (90 mg/m^2 days 1, 8, and 15 of a 28-day cycle) and bevacizumab (10 mg/kg days 1 and 15) in chemosensitive relapsed SCLC, where chemosensitivity is defined as relapse more than 60 days after completion of first-line chemotherapy. Another study by the Southwest Oncology Group is investigating the use of single-agent sorafenib as second-line therapy for SCLC.

Other antiangiogenic agents

Squalamine is an aminosterol derived from the liver of the dogfish shark and has been shown to have antiangiogenic properties in vitro and in vivo. It is thought that it prevents new vessel formation by selectively inhibiting the sodium–hydrogen antiporter sodium–proton exchangers and modulating the intracellular pH of endothelial cells, resulting in inhibition of cellular proliferation [112]. Schiller and Bittner investigated the antitumor effects of squalamine with or without cytotoxic agents in human lung cancer xenografts and correlated their observations with the extent of tumor neovascularization [112]. They found that the combination of squalamine and a platinum analog had significant preclinical antitumor activity against human lung cancer. A phase I/IIa trial of squalamine with paclitaxel and carboplatin every 3 weeks as first-line treatment in 45 patients with advanced stage NSCLC was subsequently conducted [113]. The treatment was well tolerated, and there was a 28% partial response rate. To evaluate this combination further, a follow-up phase II trial of weekly squalamine, carboplatin, and paclitaxel as first-line therapy for advanced or metastatic NSCLC was performed [114]. Forty-five patients were enrolled. The treatment regimen consisted of a weekly 3-hour infusion of squalamine, with patients randomly assigned to a dose of 100 or 200 mg/m^2, combined with weekly carboplatin (AUC = 2) and paclitaxel

(75 mg/m^2), for 12 weeks. Objective responses occurred in 24% of the patients, including one patient with a complete response, and stable disease was observed in an additional 48%.

Concluding remarks

In the past three decades, antiangiogenic therapy has moved from concept to routine clinical use. The recent success of bevacizumab in combination with chemotherapy for NSCLC and other solid tumors has validated VEGF, and tumor angiogenesis, as therapeutic targets. This has resulted in a rapid escalation in the number of antiangiogenic agents under investigation for NSCLC (Table 23.2), but also has raised concerns because of unanticipated toxicities such as pulmonary hemorrhage. Several of the agents have demonstrated promising results in phase I or II testing, including the dual VEGFR/EGFR inhibitor ZD6474 and other RTK inhibitors such as sunitinib, sorafenib, and AZD2171. These agents are typically being investigated for advanced NSCLC, either in combination with chemotherapy or EGFR inhibitors. Important areas for future investigation include the application of these agents to earlier stage NSCLC (i.e., adjuvant or neoadjuvant therapy) or other thoracic malignancies (i.e., small cell lung cancer); an improved understanding of how angiogenesis inhibitors should be integrated with other treatment modalities and targeted agents; the identification of critical mediators of angiogenesis in addition to VEGF; and the development of biomarkers for identifying patients most likely to respond to treatment or experience serious toxicities. Addressing these issues will be critical for uncovering the full potential benefits that antiangiogenic therapy may offer patients with lung cancer and other malignancies.

References

1 Folkman J, Shing Y. Angiogenesis. *J Biol Chem* 1992; **267**:10931–4.

2 Folkman J, Long DM, Becker FF. Tumor behavior in isolated perfused organs: in vitro growth and metastases of biopsy material in rabbit thyroid and canine interstinal segment. *Ann Surg* 1963; **164**:491–502.

3 Gimbrone MA, Leapman SB, Cotran RS *et al*. Tumor dormancy in vivo by prevention of neovascularization. *J Exp Med* 1972; **136**:261–76.

4 Gimbrone MA, Jr, Cotran RS, Leapman SB *et al*. Tumor growth and neovascularization: an experimental model using the rabbit cornea. *J Natl Cancer Inst* 1974; **52**:413–27.

5 Thomlinson RH, Gray LH. The histological structure of some human lung cancers and the possible implications for radiotherapy. *Br J Cancer* 1955; **9**:539–49.

6 Folkman J. Tumor angiogenesis: therapeutic implications. *N Engl J Med* 1971; **285**:1182–6.

7 Fidler IJ. The organ microenvironment and cancer metastasis. *Differentiation* 2002; **70**:498–505.

8 Fidler IJ, Ellis LM. Neoplastic angiogenesis—not all blood vessels are created equal. *N Engl J Med* 2004; **351**:215–16.

9 Fontanini G, Lucchi M, Vignati S *et al*. Angiogenesis as a prognostic indicator of survival in non-small-cell lung carcinoma: a prospective study. *J Natl Cancer Inst* 1997; **89**:881–6.

10 Fontanini G, Vignati S, Boldrini L *et al*. Vascular endothelial growth factor is associated with neovascularization and influences progression of non-small cell lung carcinoma. *Clin Cancer Res* 1997; **3**:861–5.

11 Macchiarini P, Fontanini G, Dulmet E *et al*. Angiogenesis: an indicator of metastasis in non-small cell lung cancer invading the thoracic inlet. *Ann Thorac Surg* 1994; **57**:1534–9.

12 Volm M, Mattern J, Koomagi R. Expression of platelet-derived endothelial cell growth factor in non-small cell lung carcinomas: relationship to various biological factors. *Int J Oncol* 1998; **13**:975–9.

13 Giatromanolaki A, Koukourakis M, O'Byrne K *et al*. Prognostic value of angiogenesis in operable non-small cell lung cancer. *J Pathol* 1996; **179**:80–8.

14 Folkman J. Fundamental concepts of the angiogenic process. *Curr Mol Med* 2003; **3**:643–51.

15 Bouck N. Tumor angiogenesis: the role of oncogenes and tumor suppressor genes. *Cancer Cells* 1990; **2**:179–85.

16 Hanahan D, Folkman J. Patterns and emerging mechanisms of the angiogenic switch during tumorigenesis. *Cell* 1996; **86**:353–64.

17 Ausprunk DH, Folkman J. Migration and proliferation of endothelial cells in preformed and newly formed blood vessels during tumor angiogenesis. *Microvasc Res* 1977; **14**:53–65.

18 Koukourakis MI, Giatromanolaki A, Kakolyris S *et al*. Different patterns of stromal and cancer cell thymidine phosphorylase reactivity in non-small-cell lung cancer: impact on tumour neoangiogenesis and survival. *Br J Cancer* 1998; **77**:1696–703.

19 Koukourakis MI, Giatromanolaki A, O'Byrne KJ *et al*. Platelet-derived endothelial cell growth factor expression correlates with tumour angiogenesis and prognosis in non-small-cell lung cancer. *Br J Cancer* 1997; **75**:477–81.

20 Decaussin M, Sartelet H, Robert C *et al*. Expression of vascular endothelial growth factor (VEGF) and its two receptors (VEGF-R1-Flt1 and VEGF-R2-Flk1/KDR) in non-small cell lung carcinomas (NSCLCs): correlation with angiogenesis and survival. *J Pathol* 1999; **188**:369–77.

21 Han H, Silverman JF, Santucci TS *et al*. Vascular endothelial growth factor expression in stage I non-small cell lung cancer correlates with neoangiogenesis and a poor prognosis. *Ann Surg Oncol* 2001; **8**:72–9.

22 Shibusa T, Shijubo N, Abe S. Tumor angiogenesis and vascular endothelial growth factor expression in stage I lung adenocarcinoma. *Clin Cancer Res* 1998; **4**:1483–7.

23 Ito H, Oshita F, Kameda Y *et al*. Expression of vascular endothelial growth factor and basic fibroblast growth factor in small adenocarcinomas. *Oncol Rep* 2002; **9**:119–23.

24 Volm M, Koomagi R, Mattern J. PD-ECGF, bFGF, and VEGF expression in non-small cell lung carcinomas and their association with lymph node metastasis. *Anticancer Res* 1999; **19**:651–5.

25 Angeletti CA, Lucchi M, Fontanini G *et al*. Prognostic significance of tumoral angiogenesis in completely resected late stage lung carcinoma (stage IIIA-N2). Impact of adjuvant therapies in a subset of patients at high risk of recurrence. *Cancer* 1996; **78**:409–15.

26 Fontanini G, Vignati S, Lucchi M *et al*. Neoangiogenesis and p53 protein in lung cancer: their prognostic role and their relation with vascular endothelial growth factor (VEGF) expression. *Br J Cancer* 1997; **75**:1295–301.

27 Yuan A, Yu CJ, Chen WJ *et al*. Correlation of total VEGF mRNA and protein expression with histologic type, tumor angiogenesis, patient survival and timing of relapse in non- small-cell lung cancer. *Int J Cancer* 2000; **89**:475–83.

28 Yuan A, Yu CJ, Kuo SH *et al*. Vascular endothelial growth factor 189 mRNA isoform expression specifi-

cally correlates with tumor angiogenesis, patient survival, and postoperative relapse in non-small-cell lung cancer. *J Clin Oncol* 2001; **19**:432–41.

29 Yuan A, Yu CJ, Luh KT *et al*. Aberrant p53 expression correlates with expression of vascular endothelial growth factor mRNA and interleukin-8 mRNA and neoangiogenesis in non-small-cell lung cancer. *J Clin Oncol* 2002; **20**:900–10.

30 Imoto H, Osaki T, Taga S *et al*. Vascular endothelial growth factor expression in non-small-cell lung cancer: prognostic significance in squamous cell carcinoma. *J Thorac Cardiovasc Surg* 1998; **115**:1007–14.

31 Takanami I, Tanaka F, Hashizume T *et al*. Vascular endothelial growth factor and its receptor correlate with angiogenesis and survival in pulmonary adenocarcinoma. *Anticancer Res* 1997; **17**:2811–14.

32 Takanami I, Tanaka F, Hashizume T *et al*. Tumor angiogenesis in pulmonary adenocarcinomas: relationship with basic fibroblast growth factor, its receptor, and survival. *Neoplasma* 1997; **44**:295–8.

33 Semenza GL. Targeting HIF-1 for cancer therapy. *Nat Rev Cancer* 2003; **3**:721–32.

34 Giatromanolaki A, Koukourakis MI, Sivridis E *et al*. Relation of hypoxia inducible factor 1 alpha and 2 alpha in operable non-small cell lung cancer to angiogenic/molecular profile of tumours and survival. *Br J Cancer* 2001; **85**:881–90.

35 Kim SJ, Rabbani ZN, Dewhirst MW *et al*. Expression of HIF-1alpha, CA IX, VEGF, and MMP-9 in surgically resected non-small cell lung cancer. *Lung Cancer* 2005; **49**:325–35.

36 Arbiser JL, Moses MA, Fernandez CA *et al*. Oncogenic H-ras stimulates tumor angiogenesis by two distinct pathways. *Proc Natl Acad Sci U S A* 1997; **94**:861–6.

37 Konishi T, Huang CL, Adachi M *et al*. The K-ras gene regulates vascular endothelial growth factor gene expression in non-small cell lung cancers. *Int J Oncol* 2000; **16**:501–11.

38 Kieser A, Weich HA, Brandner G *et al*. Mutant p53 potentiates protein kinase C induction of vascular endothelial growth factor expression. *Oncogene* 1994; **9**:963–9.

39 Luwor RB, Lu Y, Li X *et al*. The antiepidermal growth factor receptor monoclonal antibody cetuximab/C225 reduces hypoxia-inducible factor-1 alpha, leading to transcriptional inhibition of vascular endothelial growth factor expression. *Oncogene* 2005; **24**:4433–41.

40 Hicklin DJ, Ellis LM. Role of the vascular endothelial growth factor pathway in tumor growth and angiogenesis. *J Clin Oncol* 2005; **23**:1011–27.

41 Folkman J, Heymach JV, Kalluri R. Tumor angiogenesis. In: Kufe DW, Bast RJ, Hait W *et al*. (eds). *Cancer Medicine*, 7th edn. Ontario, Hamilton, Canada: B.C. Decker, 2005.

42 Nilsson M, Heymach JV. Vascular Endothelial Growth Factor (VEGF) Pathway. *J Thorac Oncol* 2006; **1**:768–70.

43 Kaipainen A, Korhonen J, Mustonen T *et al*. Expression of the fms-like tyrosine kinase 4 gene becomes restricted to lymphatic endothelium during development. *Proc Natl Acad Sci U S A* 1995; **92**:3566–70.

44 Jemal A, Siegel R, Ward E *et al*. Cancer statistics, 2006. *CA Cancer J Clin* 2006; **56**:106–30.

45 Schiller JH, Harrington D, Belani CP *et al*. Comparison of four chemotherapy regimens for advanced non-small-cell lung cancer. *N Engl J Med* 2002; **346**:92–8.

46 Fossella F, Pereira JR, von Pawel J *et al*. Randomized, multinational, phase III study of docetaxel plus platinum combinations versus vinorelbine plus cisplatin for advanced non-small-cell lung cancer: the TAX 326 study group. *J Clin Oncol* 2003; **21**:3016–24.

47 Shepherd FA, Rodrigues Pereira J, Ciuleanu T *et al*. Erlotinib in previously treated non-small-cell lung cancer. *N Engl J Med* 2005; **353**:123–32.

48 Thatcher N, Chang A, Parikh P *et al*. Gefitinib plus best supportive care in previously treated patients with refractory advanced non-small-cell lung cancer: results from a randomised, placebo-controlled, multicentre study (Iressa Survival Evaluation in Lung Cancer). *Lancet* 2005; **366**:1527–37.

49 Herbst RS, Giaccone G, Schiller JH *et al*. Gefitinib in combination with paclitaxel and carboplatin in advanced non-small-cell lung cancer: a phase III trial–INTACT 2. *J Clin Oncol* 2004; **22**:785–94.

50 Herbst RS, Johnson DH, Mininberg E *et al*. Phase I/II trial evaluating the anti-vascular endothelial growth factor monoclonal antibody bevacizumab in combination with the HER-1/epidermal growth factor receptor tyrosine kinase inhibitor erlotinib for patients with recurrent non-small-cell lung cancer. *J Clin Oncol* 2005; **23**:2544–55.

51 Giaccone G, Herbst RS, Manegold C *et al*. Gefitinib in combination with gemcitabine and cisplatin in advanced non-small-cell lung cancer: a phase III trial–INTACT 1. *J Clin Oncol* 2004; **22**:777–84.

52 Gatzemeier U, Pluzanska A, Szczesna A *et al*. Results of a phase III trial of erlotinib (OSI-774) combined with cisplatin and gemcitabine (GC) chemotherapy in advanced non-small cell lung cancer (NSCLC). *J Clin Oncol, 2004 ASCO Annu Meet Proc (Post-Meeting Edition)* 2004; **22**:7010.

53 Sandler AB, Gray R, Perry MC *et al*. Paclitaxel-carboplatin alone or with bevacizumab for non-small cell lung cancer. *N Engl J Med* 2006; **355**:2542–50.

54 Hurwitz H, Fehrenbacher L, Novotny W *et al*. Bevacizumab plus irinotecan, fluorouracil, and leucovorin for metastatic colorectal cancer. *N Engl J Med* 2004; **350**:2335–42.

55 Giantonio BJ, Catalano PJ, Meropol NJ *et al*. High-dose bevacizumab in combination with FOLFOX4 improves survival in patients with previously treated advanced colorectal cancer: results from the Eastern Cooperative Oncology Group (ECOG) study E3200 [Abstract]. *J Clin Oncol, 2005 ASCO Annu Meet Proc* 2005; **23**:169a.

56 Johnson DH, Fehrenbacher L, Novotny WF *et al*. Randomized phase II trial comparing bevacizumab plus carboplatin and paclitaxel with carboplatin and paclitaxel alone in previously untreated locally advanced or metastatic non-small-cell lung cancer. *J Clin Oncol* 2004; **22**:2184–91.

57 Brahmer JR, Gray R, Schiller JH *et al*. ECOG 4599 phase III trial of carboplatin and paclitaxel ±bevacizumab: subset analysis of survival by gender. *J Clin Oncol, 2006 ASCO Annu Meet Proc* 2006; **24**:7063.

58 Holden SN, Eckhardt SG, Basser R *et al*. Clinical evaluation of ZD6474, an orally active inhibitor of VEGF and EGF receptor signaling, in patients with solid, malignant tumors. *Ann Oncol* 2005; **16**:1391–7.

59 Minami H, Ebi H, Tahara M *et al*. A phase I study of an oral VEGF receptor tyrosine kinase inhibitor ZD6474, in Japanese patients with solid tumors. *Proc Am Soc Clin Oncol* 2003; **22**:194.

60 Heymach J, West H, Kerr R *et al*. ZD6474 in combination with carboplatin and paclitaxel as first-line treatment in patients with NSCLC: results of the run-in phase of a two-part randomized Phase II study. *Proc 11th World Conf on Lung Cancer*, 2005.

61 Strumberg D, Richly H, Hilger RA *et al*. Phase I clinical and pharmacokinetic study of the Novel Raf kinase and vascular endothelial growth factor receptor inhibitor BAY 43-9006 in patients with advanced refractory solid tumors. *J Clin Oncol* 2005; **23**:965–72.

62 Moore M, Hirte HW, Siu L *et al*. Phase I study to determine the safety and pharmacokinetics of the novel Raf kinase and VEGFR inhibitor BAY 43-9006, administered for 28 days on/7 days off in patients with advanced, refractory solid tumors. *Ann Oncol* 2005; **16**:1688–94.

63 Eisen T, Bukowski RM, Staehler M *et al*. Randomized phase III trial of sorafenib in advanced renal cell carcinoma (RCC): Impact of crossover on survival. *J Clin Oncol, 2006 ASCO Annu Meet Proc* 2006; **24**:4524.

64 Ratain MJ, Eisen T, Stadler WM *et al*. Phase II placebo-controlled randomized discontinuation trial of sorafenib in patients with metastatic renal cell carcinoma. *J Clin Oncol* 2006; **24**:2505–12.

65 Escudier B, Szczylik C, Eisen T *et al*. Randomized Phase III trial of the Raf kinase and VEGFR inhibitor sorafenib (BAY 43-9006) in patients with advanced renal cell carcinoma (RCC) [Abstract]. *J Clin Oncol, 2005 ASCO Annu Meet Proc* 2005; **23**:LBA4510.

66 Schiller JH, Flaherty KT, Redlinger M *et al*. Sorafenib combined with carboplatin/paclitaxel for advanced non-small cell lung cancer: a phase I subset analysis. *J Clin Oncol, 2006 ASCO Annu Meet Proc* 2006; **24(Part I)**:7194.

67 Drevs J, Medinger M, Mross K *et al*. Phase I clinical evaluation of AZD2171, a highly potent VEGF receptor tyrosine kinase inhibitor, in patients with advanced tumors. *J Clin Oncol, 2005 ASCO Annu Meet Proc* 2005; **23**:3002.

68 Lorusso PM, Heath E, Valdivieso M *et al*. Phase I evaluation of AZD2171, a highly potent and selective inhibitor of VEGFR signaling, in combination with selected chemotherapy regimens in patients with advanced solid tumors. *J Clin Oncol, 2006 ASCO Annu Meet Proc* 2006; **24**:3034.

69 Laurie SA, Arnold A, Gauthier I *et al*. Final results of a phase I study of daily oral AZD2171, an inhibitor of vascular endothelial growth factor receptors (VEGFR), in combination with carboplatin (C) + paclitaxel (T) in patients with advanced non-small cell lung cancer (NSCLC): A study of the National Cancer Institute of Canada Clinical Trials Group (NCIC CTG). *J Clin Oncol, 2006 ASCO Annu Meet Proc* 2006; **24**:3054.

70 Heymach J, Johnson B, Prager D *et al*. A Phase II trial of ZD6474 plus docetaxel in patients with previously treated NSCLC: follow-up results. *J Clin Oncol, 2006 ASCO Annu Meet Proc* 2006; **24**:7016.

71 Jain RK. Normalizing tumor vasculature with anti-angiogenic therapy: a new paradigm for combination therapy. *Nat Med* 2001; **7**:987–9.

72 Yang JC, Haworth L, Sherry RM *et al*. A randomized trial of bevacizumab, an anti-vascular endothelial growth factor antibody, for metastatic renal cancer. *N Engl J Med* 2003; **349**:427–34.

73 Holash J, Davis S, Papadopoulos N *et al*. VEGF-Trap: a VEGF blocker with potent antitumor effects. *Proc Natl Acad Sci U S A* 2002; **99**:11393–8.

74 Dupont J, Schwartz L, Koutcher J *et al*. Phase I and pharmacokinetic study of VEGF Trap administered

subcutaneously (sc) to patients (pts) with advanced solid malignancies. *J Clin Oncol, 2004 ASCO Annu Meet Proc (Post-Meeting Edition)* July 15, 2004; **22(14s)**:3009.

75 Dupont J, Rothenberg ML, Spriggs DR *et al.* Safety and pharmacokinetics of intravenous VEGF Trap in a phase I clinical trial of patients with advanced solid tumors. *J Clin Oncol, 2005 ASCO Annu Meet Proc* June 1, 2005; **23(Part I of II, 16s)**:3029.

76 Available at: www.clinicaltrials.gov, October 2006.

77 Natale RB, Bodkin D, Govindan R *et al.* ZD6474 versus gefitinib in patients with advanced NSCLC: final results from a two-part, double-blind, randomized phase II trial. *J Clin Oncol, 2006 ASCO Annu Meet Proc* 2006; **24**:7000.

78 Gatzemeier U, Blumenschein G, Fosella F *et al.* Phase II trial of single-agent sorafenib in patients with advanced non-small cell lung carcinoma. *J Clin Oncol, 2006 ASCO Annu Meet Proc* 2006; **24**:7002.

79 Rosen L, Mulay M, Long J *et al.* Phase I trial of SU011248, a novel tyrosine kinase inhibitor in advanced solid tumors [Abstract 765]. *Proc Am Soc Clin Oncol* 2003; **22**:191.

80 Faivre S, Delbaldo C, Vera K *et al.* Safety, pharmacokinetic, and antitumor activity of SU11248, a novel oral multitarget tyrosine kinase inhibitor, in patients with cancer. *J Clin Oncol* 2006; **24**:25–35.

81 Motzer RJ, Michaelson MD, Redman BG *et al.* Activity of SU11248, a multitargeted inhibitor of vascular endothelial growth factor receptor and platelet-derived growth factor receptor, in patients with metastatic renal cell carcinoma. *J Clin Oncol* 2006; **24**:16–24.

82 Motzer RJ, Rini BI, Bukowski RM *et al.* Sunitinib in patients with metastatic renal cell carcinoma. *JAMA* 2006; **295**:2516–24.

83 Motzer RJ, Hutson TE, Tomczak P *et al.* Phase III randomized trial of sunitinib malate (SU11248) versus interferon-alfa (IFN-α) as first-line systemic therapy for patients with metastatic renal cell carcinoma (mRCC). *J Clin Oncol, 2006 ASCO Annu Meet Proc* 2006; **24**:LBA3.

84 Demetri G, van Oosterom AT, Garrett C *et al.* Improved survival and sustained clinical benefit with SU11248 (SU) in pts with GIST after failure of imatinib mesylate (IM) therapy in a phase III trial [Abstract 8]. *Proc 2006 Gastrointestinal Cancers Symposium*, 2006.

85 Socinski MA, Novello S, Sanchez JM *et al.* Efficacy and safety of sunitinib in previously treated, advanced non-small cell lung cancer (NSCLC): Preliminary results of a multicenter phase II trial. *J Clin Oncol, 2006 ASCO Annu Meet Proc* June 20, 2006; **24(Part I, Suppl 18)**:7001.

86 Gauler TC, Fischer B, Soria J *et al.* Phase II open-label study to investigate efficacy and safety of PTK787/ZK 222584 orally administered once daily at 1,250 mg as second-line monotherapy in patients (pts) with stage IIIB or stage IV non-small cell lung cancer (NSCLC). *J Clin Oncol, 2006 ASCO Annu Meet Proc* June 20, 2006; **24(Part I, Suppl 18)**:7195.

87 Rugo HS, Herbst RS, Liu G *et al.* Phase I trial of the oral antiangiogenesis agent AG-013736 in patients with advanced solid tumors: pharmacokinetic and clinical results. *J Clin Oncol* 2005; **23**:5474–83.

88 Ciardiello F, Caputo R, Bianco R *et al.* Inhibition of growth factor production and angiogenesis in human cancer cells by ZD1839 (Iressa), a selective epidermal growth factor receptor tyrosine kinase inhibitor. *Clin Cancer Res* 2001; **7**:1459–65.

89 Hirata A, Ogawa S, Kometani T *et al.* ZD1839 (Iressa) induces antiangiogenic effects through inhibition of epidermal growth factor receptor tyrosine kinase. PG-2554-60. *Cancer Res* 2002; **62**:2554–60.

90 Ciardiello F, Bianco R, Damiano V *et al.* Antiangiogenic and antitumor activity of anti-epidermal growth factor receptor C225 monoclonal antibody in combination with vascular endothelial growth factor antisense oligonucleotide in human GEO colon cancer cells. *Clin Cancer Res* 2000; **6**:3739–47.

91 Shaheen RM, Ahmad SA, Liu W *et al.* Inhibited growth of colon cancer carcinomatosis by antibodies to vascular endothelial and epidermal growth factor receptors. *Br J Cancer* 2001; **85**:584–9.

92 Jung YD, Mansfield PF, Akagi M *et al.* Effects of combination anti-vascular endothelial growth factor receptor and anti-epidermal growth factor receptor therapies on the growth of gastric cancer in a nude mouse model. *Eur J Cancer* 2002; **38**:1133–40.

93 Morelli MP, Cascone T, Troiani T *et al.* Anti-tumor activity of the combination of cetuximab, an anti-EGFR blocking monoclonal antibody and ZD6474, an inhibitor of VEGFR and EGFR tyrosine kinases. *J Cell Physiol* 2006; **208**:344–53.

94 Fehrenbacher L, O'Neill VJ, Belani CP *et al.* A phase II, multicenter, randomized clinical trial to evaluate the efficacy and safety of bevacizumab in combination with either chemotherapy (docetaxel or pemetrexed) or erlotinib hydrochloride compared with chemotherapy alone for treatment of recurrent or refractory non-small cell lung cancer. *J Clin Oncol, 2006 ASCO Annu Meet Proc* June 20, 2006; **24(Part I, Suppl 18)**:7062.

95 Adjei AA, Mandrekar S, Marks RS *et al.* A Phase I study of BAY 43-9006 and gefitinib in patients with refractory or recurrent non-small-cell lung cancer (NSCLC). *J Clin Oncol, 2005 ASCO Annu Meet Proc* June 1, 2005; **23(Part I of II, 16s)**:3067.

96 Mauceri HJ, Hanna NN, Beckett MA *et al.* Combined effects of angiostatin and ionizing radiation in antitumour therapy. *Nature* 1998; **394**:287–91.

97 Kozin SV, Boucher Y, Hicklin DJ *et al.* Vascular endothelial growth factor receptor-2-blocking antibody potentiates radiation-induced long-term control of human tumor xenografts. *Cancer Res* 2001; **61**:39–44.

98 Ning S, Laird D, Cherrington JM *et al.* The antiangiogenic agents SU5416 and SU6668 increase the antitumor effects of fractionated irradiation. PG-45-51. *Radiat Res* 2002; **157**:45–51.

99 Gorski DH, Mauceri HJ, Salloum RM *et al.* Potentiation of the antitumor effect of ionizing radiation by brief concomitant exposures to angiostatin. *Cancer Res* 1998; **58**:5686–9.

100 Gorski DH, Mauceri HJ, Salloum RM *et al.* Prolonged treatment with angiostatin reduces metastatic burden during radiation therapy. *Cancer Res* 2003; **63**:308–11.

101 Jain RK. Normalization of tumor vasculature: an emerging concept in antiangiogenic therapy. *Science* 2005; **307**:58–62.

102 Winkler F, Kozin SV, Tong RT *et al.* Kinetics of vascular normalization by VEGFR2 blockade governs brain tumor response to radiation: role of oxygenation, angiopoietin-1, and matrix metalloproteinases. *Cancer Cell* 2004; **6**:553–63.

103 Garcia-Barros M, Paris F, Cordon-Cardo C *et al.* Tumor response to radiotherapy regulated by endothelial cell apoptosis. *Science* 2003; **300**:1155–9.

104 Ferrara N, Gerber HP, LeCouter J. The biology of VEGF and its receptors. *Nat Med* 2003; **9**:669–76.

105 Geng L, Donnelly E, McMahon G *et al.* Inhibition of vascular endothelial growth factor receptor signaling leads to reversal of tumor resistance to radiotherapy. *Cancer Res* 2001; **61**:2413–19.

106 Gorski DH, Beckett MA, Jaskowiak NT *et al.* Blockage of the vascular endothelial growth factor stress response increases the antitumor effects of ionizing radiation. *Cancer Res* 1999; **59**:3374–8.

107 Falardeau P, Champagne P, Poyet P *et al.* Neovastat, a naturally occurring multifunctional antiangiogenic drug, in phase III clinical trials. *Semin Oncol* 2001; **28**:620–5.

108 Latreille J, Batist G, Laberge F *et al.* Phase I/II trial of the safety and efficacy of AE-941 (Neovastat) in the treatment of non-small-cell lung cancer. *Clin Lung Cancer* 2003; **4**:231–6.

109 Lu C, Komaki R, Herbst RS *et al.* A phase III study Of Æ-941 with induction chemotherapy (IC) and concomitant chemoradiotherapy (CRT) for stage III non-small cell lung cancer (NSCLC) (NCI T99-0046, RTOG 02-70, MDA 99-303): An interim report of toxicity and response. *J Clin Oncol, 2005 ASCO Annu Meet Proc* 2005; **23**:7144.

110 Pujol JL, Breton JL, Gervais R *et al.* A prospective randomized phase III, double-blind, placebo-controlled study of thalidomide in extended-disease (ED) SCLC patients after response to chemotherapy (CT): An intergroup study FNCLCC Cleo04-IFCT 00-01. *J Clin Oncol, 2006 ASCO Annu Meet Proc* June 20, 2006; **24(Part I, 18s)**:7057.

111 Patton JF, Spigel DR, Greco FA *et al.* Irinotecan (I), carboplatin (C), and radiotherapy (RT) followed by maintenance bevacizumab (B) in the treatment (tx) of limited-stage small cell lung cancer (LS-SCLC): Update of a phase II trial of the Minnie Pearl Cancer Research Network. *J Clin Oncol, 2006 ASCO Annu Meet Proc* June 20, 2006; **24(Part I, 18s)**:7085.

112 Schiller JH, Bittner G. Potentiation of platinum antitumor effects in human lung tumor xenografts by the angiogenesis inhibitor squalamine: effects on tumor neovascularization. *Clin Cancer Res* 1999; **5**:4287–94.

113 Herbst RS, Hammond LA, Carbone DP *et al.* A phase I/IIA trial of continuous five-day infusion of squalamine lactate (MSI-1256F) plus carboplatin and paclitaxel in patients with advanced non-small cell lung cancer. *Clin Cancer Res* 2003; **9**:4108–15.

114 Rose V, Schiller J, Wood A *et al.* Randomized phase II trial of weekly squalamine, carboplatin, and paclitaxel as first line therapy for advanced non-small cell lung cancer. *J Clin Oncol, 2004 ASCO Annu Meet Proc (Post-Meeting Edition)* 2004; **22**:7109.

115 Natale RB, Bodkin D, Govindan R *et al.* A comparison of the antitumour efficacy of ZD6474 and gefitinib (Iressa™) in patients with NSCLC: results of a randomized, double-blind Phase II study [Abstract O-104]. *Proc 11th World Conf on Lung Cancer*, 2005.

CHAPTER 24

Retinoids and Rexinoids in Lung Cancer Prevention and Treatment

Nishin A. Bhadkamkar and Fadlo R. Khuri

Introduction

In spite of numerous therapeutic advances over the last 20 years, particularly the advent of multimodality approaches, the 5-year survival rate of lung cancer remains less than 20% [1,2]. Although smoking cessation is clearly the most powerful intervention from a public health standpoint, new strategies are sorely needed to improve outcomes in lung cancer patients. In this context, the concept of chemoprevention has gained more attention as a new and potentially significant tool in controlling this disease. By focusing on the process of carcinogenic progression to invasive cancer rather than the treatment of frank malignancy [3], it has prompted extensive investigation of known compounds, as well as the development of novel agents. Retinoids, which have previously found widespread use in the treatment of dermatologic diseases and acute promyelocytic leukemia, have now been carefully studied in the chemopreventive and therapeutic settings for lung cancer.

Molecular biology

Retinoids are vitamin A derivatives that regulate cellular growth, differentiation, and apoptosis by in-

fluencing gene expression through a complex signaling pathway [4,5]. Cytoplasmic proteins transport them to the nucleus, where they interact with cognate receptors to form a transcription complex [6,7]. Retinoid receptors belong to the steroid-receptor superfamily, which includes vitamin D, thyroid, and peroxisome proliferator activator receptors, and function as ligand-activated transcription factors. They are classified as either retinoic acid receptors (RARs) or retinoid X receptors (RXRs). Each class of retinoid receptor is further subdivided into alpha, beta, and gamma subtypes. RAR genes have been identified on chromosomes 17q21, 3p24, and 12q13 for these respective subtypes. The RXR alpha, beta, and gamma genes have also been localized to chromosomes 9q34.3, 6p21.3, and 1q22-23, respectively. Each subtype can exist in several isoforms, which differ only in their amino-terminal domains [7]. The RARs exhibit a strong binding affinity for all-*trans*-retinoic acid (ATRA) and 9-*cis*-retinoic acid (9-*cis* RA), which are endogenous molecules, while the RXRs only bind the latter effectively [8,9]. 13-*cis*-retinoic acid (13-*cis*-RA or isotretinoin), a synthetic retinoid, is quickly converted to ATRA in vivo and thus acts primarily through RARs [10].

In the unbound state, retinoid receptors are associated with corepressors that prevent gene transcription. The binding of ligand to a retinoid receptor results in a conformational change that leads to a cascade of events, including the dissociation of corepressors and the addition of coactivating molecules [11]. Furthermore, it triggers dimerization of the retinoid receptors, forming

Lung Cancer, 3rd edition. Edited by Jack A. Roth, James D. Cox, and Waun Ki Hong. © 2007 Blackwell Publishing, ISBN: 978-1-4051-5112-2.

homodimers or heterodimers to complete the transcription complex. This complex then binds directly to specific retinoic acid response elements in gene promoter regions [7,12]. RARs must form heterodimers with an RXR in order to bind to a response element. RXRs can homodimerize or bind to other members of the steroid-receptor superfamily. In fact, these other steroid receptors (e.g., vitamin D, thyroid, etc.) must dimerize with an RXR in order to exert their effects on gene transcription. This biological arrangement leads to significant cross-talk among many cell signaling pathways [12]. The various combinations of ligand, retinoid receptor dimers, coactivators, and corepressors allow for differential gene expression and subsequent multilevel modulation of the entire retinoid signaling pathway [13,14]. In addition, RAR genes have retinoic acid response elements in their promoter regions, which allow for regulation by ATRA [15]. Genetic studies have demonstrated that deletion of a specific subtype and isoform of retinoid receptor leads to loss of endogenous activation of a specific set of genes by ATRA. This finding suggests that each receptor subtype and isoform is associated with a particular group of retinoid-responsive genes [7]. Additional studies in knockout mice have confirmed distinct and overlapping functions of individual RARs [7,16].

The target genes of retinoids play a critical role in the suppression of cell growth, the activation of apoptotic pathways [17,18], and the induction of terminal differentiation, all of which tend to counteract carcinogenic progression. More specifically, they also regulate the expression of tumor stromal factors, such as cyclin-dependent kinases [19] and matrix metalloproteinases [20], that promote tumor growth. The exact mechanisms by which this occurs are not completely understood.

Rationale for retinoids

The study of retinoids in lung cancer began with the notable observations of Wohlbach and Howe, who found an association between vitamin A deprivation of cattle and increased incidence of lung and upper aerodigestive cancers [21]. Genta *et al.* and Dogra *et al.* then revealed that vitamin A-deficient animals exposed to benzo[a]pyrene developed lung cancer more frequently compared to control animals. Enhanced binding of this tobacco carcinogen to tracheal epithelial DNA was theorized to be the mechanism of accelerated lung carcinogenesis [22,23]. These results gained further credence when vitamin A intervention studies in the laboratory setting first showed suppression or reversal of squamous metaplasia in the lung [24,25]. Observational epidemiologic studies also demonstrated an inverse correlation between dietary beta-carotene intake and overall cancer incidence [26,27].

A pivotal study by Hong and colleagues in 1986 ushered in an era of extensive clinical investigation of retinoids. Forty-four patients with oral leukoplakia were randomized to receive either high-dose 13-*cis*-retinoic acid (1–2 mg/kg) or placebo for 3 months, followed by a 6-month follow-up period. A highly statistically significant difference was observed between the two groups in terms of histologic reversal of dysplasia (13/24 patients in drug group versus 2/20 patients in placebo group) and clinical decrease in size of lesions (16 patients versus 2 patients). However, nine patients in the drug group had relapse of leukoplakia within 3 months of ending treatment [28]. A subsequent trial randomizing patients to low doses of either 13-*cis*-RA (0.5 mg/kg/day) or beta-carotene (30 mg/day) after 3 months of high dose 13-*cis*-RA (1.5 mg/kg/day) showed relative superiority of maintenance therapy with 13-*cis*-RA. Unfortunately, neither intervention demonstrated benefit with long-term follow-up [29,30]. In addition, Stich and coworkers also reported encouraging results with high-dose vitamin A intervention in Indian betel nut chewers and tobacco users with oral leukoplakia [31]. Chiesa *et al.* obtained even more dramatic results with etretinate (4-*N*-4-hydroxyphenylretinamide or fenretinide), documenting major responses in 27 of 31 patients randomized to the treatment arm of the trial [32]. In light of these encouraging results and the theory of field carcinogenesis (which proposes diffuse epithelial injury from a carcinogenic exposure and applies best to aerodigestive tumors), other researchers became intrigued by the idea of utilizing retinoids in the setting of lung cancer.

Table 24.1 Primary chemoprevention trials of retinoids in NSCLC.

	Patients (*n*)	Intervention	Endpoint	Result
ATBC [41]	29,133	β−carotene α-tocopherol	Lung cancer	Negative/harmful
Omenn *et al.* [42] (CARET)	18,314	β−carotene Retinyl palmitate	Lung cancer	Negative/harmful
Hennekens *et al.* [43] (PHS)	22,071	β−carotene	Lung cancer	Negative

At the same time, significant advances in molecular biology in the late 1980s led to the cloning of the RARs by Evans and Chambon [4]. As the role of these receptors in modulating retinoid effects became more evident, Xu *et al.* determined the expression of RARs and RXRs in 79 nonsmall cell lung cancer (NSCLC) tissue specimens by in situ hybridization with labeled probes and compared this to expression in normal bronchial epithelium. RARβ, RARγ, and RXRβ were all suppressed relative to the controls, but RARβ was most prominently affected (detectable in only 42% of NSCLC versus 90% of controls). This observation suggested that RARβ may function as a tumor suppressor [33]. Other in vivo and in vitro studies supported this idea by documenting decreased RARβ expression in human lung cancer cells [34–36]. Picard *et al.* also demonstrated suppression of RARβ in 63% of NSCLC specimens relative to normal cells. RARβ expression, however, was absent in only 6% of tumor samples (57% partial suppression). This discrepancy with respect to Xu's results may be explained by greater sensitivity of the probes and immunohistochemical compounds utilized for analysis. This study also noted decreased RXRβ expression (18% of NSCLC samples) and overexpression of RARα and RXRα (26% and 85%, respectively) [37]. More recent laboratory studies have revealed a likely mechanism for diminished RARβ expression in early stages of lung carcinogenesis. Methylation of cytosine-phospho-guanosine islands in the promoter region of the RARβ gene was shown to result in epigenetic silencing of gene expression [38,39]. In aggregate, these studies provided support for the notion that retinoids may work well as chemopreventive agents in lung cancer.

Primary chemoprevention

Primary chemoprevention in lung cancer refers to the use of chemically active agents in high-risk individuals (e.g., chronic smokers) with the goal of preventing a primary lung cancer [40]. The first large randomized trial to address the efficacy of retinoids in this setting was conducted by the Alpha-Tocopherol and Beta-Carotene Cancer Prevention Study Group (ATBC). The researchers randomized 29,133 Finnish male smokers between 50 and 69 years old to one of four arms: alpha-tocopherol (50 mg/day) alone, beta-carotene (20 mg/day) alone, both alpha-tocopherol and beta-carotene, or placebo. They followed these individuals for a median of 6.1 years with incidence of lung cancer as the primary endpoint and incidence of other malignancies as a secondary endpoint. Cancer-related mortality and overall mortality were also assessed. In the final analysis, alpha-tocopherol did not reduce the incidence of lung cancer or total mortality. Unexpectedly and alarmingly, however, subjects receiving beta-carotene had an 18% increase in lung cancer incidence and an 8% increase in total mortality. There was no statistically significant interaction between the two interventions with respect to new cases of lung cancer. The authors theorized that the follow-up period was perhaps too short, that beta-carotene may not be the major cancer-fighting component of fruits and vegetables, and that beta-carotene intake might reflect an overall lifestyle compatible with lower cancer risk [41]. In any case, the ATBC trial cast doubt on the numerous observational studies suggesting a protective benefit of beta-carotene with respect to lung cancer incidence.

These surprising results were subsequently confirmed by the Beta-Carotene and Retinol

Table 24.2 Secondary chemoprevention trials of retinoids in NSCLC.

	Patients (*n*)	Intervention	Endpoint	Result
Arnold *et al.* [44]	150	Etretinate	Squamous metaplasia	Negative
Lee *et al.* [45]	86	Isotretinoin	Squamous metaplasia	Negative
McLarty *et al.* [46]	755	β-carotene Retinol	Sputum atypia	Negative
Kurie *et al.* [47]	82	Fenretinide	Squamous metaplasia	Negative
Kurie *et al.* [48]	226	9-*cis*-RA	Squamous metaplasia	Positive

Efficacy Trial (CARET), which randomized over 18,000 heavy smokers to a daily regimen of 30 mg beta-carotene and 25,000 IU of retinyl palmitate or placebo. The trial was prematurely terminated after an interim analysis revealed a 28% increase in lung cancer incidence and 17% increase in all-cause mortality in the treatment group [42]. In addition, the Physicians' Health Study (PHS) showed no statistically significant benefit or harm with beta-carotene supplementation (50 mg on alternate days) over a 12-year period. This randomized, placebo-controlled trial included over 22,000 male physicians, half of whom were current or former smokers. No differences were observed between the treatment and placebo arms with respect to the incidence of lung cancer, death from any malignant neoplasm, or overall mortality [43].

Secondary chemoprevention

Secondary chemoprevention of lung cancer has generally focused on the reversal of premalignancy, as indicated by sputum atypia or bronchial squamous dysplasia. In the early 1990s, Arnold *et al.* randomized 150 smokers (≥15 pack-year history) with sputum atypia to receive 25 mg of the synthetic retinoid etretinate or placebo daily for 6 months. They observed no difference between the two arms with respect to the degree of sputum atypia [44]. In a subsequent study, Lee and colleagues examined the effect of isotretinoin on squamous dysplasia and metaplasia in 86 heavy smokers. These partici-

pants had bronchoscopy-proven histologic changes in more than 15% of the specimens obtained. After 6 months, both placebo and treatment groups showed a dramatic decline (approximately 50%) in squamous metaplasia on repeat bronchoscopy, as measured by the metaplasia index (MI). This quantitative index simply reflected the number of tissue samples with metaplasia divided by the total number of samples. Smoking cessation, however, proved to be the only factor associated with a reduction in metaplasia. Sixteen trial participants (10 in the 13-*cis*-RA group and 6 in the placebo group) stopped smoking during the study period [45].

These disappointing results were later echoed in a randomized, placebo-controlled trial of beta-carotene and retinol in 755 former asbestos workers. Fifty milligrams of beta-carotene daily and 25,000 IU of retinol on alternate days did not reduce the incidence or prevalence of sputum atypia, the primary endpoint of the study [46]. In addition, Kurie *et al.* randomized 82 smokers to 200 mg/day of fenretinide or placebo for 6 months. Bronchial tree biopsies were obtained from all participants before and after the intervention. The researchers assessed not only histopathology (squamous dysplasia and metaplasia) but also RARβ activity and loss of heterozygosity at chromosomes 3p, 9p, and 17p, the sites of known tumor suppressor loci. In spite of good bioavailability of fenretinide, the treatment arm did not display any change in these genotypic and phenotypic parameters [47].

Table 24.3 Tertiary chemoprevention trials of retinoids in NSCLC.

	Patients (n)	Intervention	Endpoint	Result
Pastorino et al. [50]	307	Retinyl palmitate	SPT	Positive
Van Zandwijk et al. [51] (EUROSCAN)	2592	Retinyl palmitate N-acetylcysteine	SPT	Negative
Lippman et al. [52]	1166	Isotretinoin	SPT	Negative

More recently, however, Kurie and coworkers have demonstrated a positive effect of 9-*cis*-RA on squamous metaplasia in former smokers. They randomized 226 subjects with a minimum 20 pack-year history and no tobacco use over the last 12 months to one of three arms: 9-*cis*-RA (100 mg daily), 13-*cis*-RA (1 mg/kg) plus alpha-tocopherol (1200 IU daily), or placebo. Bronchoscopic biopsies were performed at six prespecified sites in the bronchial tree before treatment and at 3 and 6 months. One hundred seventy-seven participants completed at least 3 months of therapy with the requisite bronchoscopies. Seventy percent of baseline tissue samples demonstrated RARβ activity, while 7% exhibited squamous metaplasia. The 9-*cis*-RA group, unlike the 13-*cis*-RA plus alpha-tocopherol group, showed a statistically significant upregulation of RARβ expression compared to placebo. In light of the data supporting RARβ as a marker of premalignant lesions, the researchers theorized that 9-*cis*-RA could have potential as a chemopreventive agent [48].

Tertiary chemoprevention

Tertiary chemoprevention studies of retinoids in lung cancer have focused primarily on preventing second primary tumors and local recurrences. Hong and colleagues provided the impetus for this approach with their seminal study in squamous cell carcinoma of the head and neck. One hundred and three patients free of disease after primary treatment (surgery and/or radiotherapy) were randomized to receive isotretinoin (50–100 mg/m^2) or placebo for a period of 12 months. After a median follow-up of 32 months, there was no statistically significant difference in local, regional, or distant recurrences between the two arms. However, only 2 patients in the isotretinoin group developed second primary

tumors (SPTs) versus 12 patients in the placebo group ($p = 0.005$). In fact, four placebo-treated patients had multiple SPTs during the study period [49]. This positive result spurred others to investigate the potential of retinoids in this setting in lung cancer.

Pastorino et al. conducted the first large tertiary chemoprevention trial in lung cancer. They randomly assigned 307 patients with curatively resected stage I NSCLC to receive either retinyl palmitate (300,000 IU/day) or placebo for 12 months. The intervention arm tolerated retinyl palmitate fairly well (>80% compliance) and, after a follow-up period of nearly 4 years, demonstrated a significant reduction in the incidence of SPTs relative to the placebo group. Eighteen patients in the active treatment group developed SPTs compared to 29 patients in the placebo group. In addition, a similar effect was observed when tobacco-related SPTs were assessed separately. Subjects treated with retinyl palmitate not only developed fewer tobacco-related SPTs but also enjoyed a longer disease-free interval before these tumors appeared ($p = 0.045$) [50]. Unfortunately, these encouraging results would not be duplicated in subsequent large trials.

The EUROSCAN Study was carried out to evaluate the efficacy of retinyl palmitate and N-acetylcysteine in preventing SPTs following curative treatment of squamous cell carcinoma of the head and neck and NSCLC. A total of 2592 patients (60% head and neck, 40% lung) were randomized to one of four arms in a 2 × 2 factorial design: retinyl palmitate alone (300,000 IU daily for 1 yr followed by 150,000 IU daily for 1 yr), N-acetylcysteine alone (600 mg daily), both drugs, or placebo. The subjects were followed for 4 years after a 2-year period of intervention. Ninety-four percent of them were current or former smokers, and 25% continued to smoke after being diagnosed with malignancy. Neither retinyl palmitate nor N-acetylcysteine impacted overall survival, event-free survival, or incidence of SPTs (73% tobacco-related). The placebo group actually exhibited a statistically insignificant trend toward decreased incidence of SPTs. The authors concluded that intervention with retinyl palmitate for 2 years provided no benefit in terms of SPT prevention but suggested longer follow-up periods for future trials (given the extended time course of carcinogenesis) [51].

Lippman and colleagues then conducted a National Cancer Institute (NCI) Intergroup phase III trial examining the impact of low-dose isotretinoin on prevention of SPTs in patients with curatively resected stage I NSCLC. A total of 1166 subjects were randomly assigned to receive isotretinoin (30 mg daily) or placebo for 3 years, with the primary endpoint being time to SPT and secondary endpoints being time to recurrence and death. Patients were stratified by tumor stage (T1 or T2), smoking status, and tumor histology (squamous or nonsquamous). In the overall analysis, the authors found no statistically significant differences between the isotretinoin and placebo arms with respect to SPTs, recurrence, or mortality. The multivariate analyses, however, revealed a significant interaction between isotretinoin and smoking status. Compared to placebo, current smokers treated with isotretinoin exhibited a statistically significant increase in mortality ($p = 0.04$) and a nonsignificant trend toward increased recurrence as well. Conversely, subjects with no smoking history who received isotretinoin showed a trend (not statistically significant) toward reduced mortality and recurrence [52]. These data again cast doubt on the role of retinoids in tertiary prevention and brought attention to the possible synergism between tobacco carcinogens and certain vitamin A derivatives.

Interaction between smoking and carotenoids

The preponderance of clinical evidence from lung cancer chemoprevention trials strongly suggested that vitamin A compounds may actually increase the incidence of lung cancer and overall mortality in smokers. The ATBC and CARET studies both demonstrated statistically significant harm from high-dose beta-carotene supplementation in this population [41,42]. While the PHS showed neither benefit nor harm, many researchers theorize that the administration of fairly low doses of beta carotene, as well as the atypical patient population (only 11% current smokers), likely contributed to the neutral results [43,53]. Furthermore, Lee's secondary chemoprevention trial clearly indicated a cooperative effect between isotretinoin and smoking cessation in terms of reducing squamous metaplasia. Conversely, retinoid supplementation was wholly ineffective in reversing the premalignant lesions of active smokers [45]. Finally, several large randomized trials have failed to demonstrate a role for retinoids in the setting of tertiary prevention [51,52]. Lippman's study, in fact, highlighted a negative synergistic effect between isotretinoin and smoking [52]. In summary, these findings suggested that important innate differences between smokers and former or nonsmokers result in differential effects of retinoid therapy.

Additional alarming data arrived in the form of a study in stage I NSCLC patients. Khuri *et al.* examined tissue specimens from 156 patients (nearly 90% smokers) who had undergone definitive surgical resection and received at least 2 years of clinical follow-up [54]. They determined RARβ and RXRα mRNA expression through the use of antisense probes, utilizing a technique described previously by Xu and colleagues [55]. RXRα served as a control to confirm lack of RNA degradation, since all NSCLC and normal tissue samples in Xu's earlier laboratory study expressed RXRα [33]. Given the convincing data supporting the idea that RARβ functions as a tumor suppressor [33–37], the researchers hypothesized that loss of RARβ gene expression correlates with poor clinical outcome in stage I NSCLC. Unexpectedly, their analysis revealed statistically significant worse overall survival in patients with strongly positive RARβ staining versus those with aberrant (weakly positive or absent) staining ($p = 0.045$). A trend toward worse disease-free survival was also observed in the group with strongly positive RARβ expression [54]. This surprising data prompted further investigation of the precise role of retinoid receptors in lung carcinogenesis.

Khuri and coworkers offered two possible explanations for their unexpected results. First, the RARβ gene is expressed in several isoforms based on differential splicing and utilization of alternative promoters [7,56,57]. The antisense probe used in the study, however, could not distinguish among these isoforms, which differ only in their amino-terminal domain. Li *et al.* had previously identified RARβ2 as a mediator of retinoic acid-induced apoptosis and growth arrest in lung cancer cells [12]. A subsequent in vitro study demonstrated loss of these retinoic acid properties in F9 embryonal carcinoma cells when both RARβ2 alleles were compromised [58]. In vivo studies with transgenic mice bearing antisense RARβ2 or sense RARβ4 further highlighted the importance of these isoforms in lung carcinogenesis. Transgenic mice with antisense RARβ2 developed lung tumors within 18 months after birth, suggesting that this isoform may function as a tumor suppressor [59]. On the other hand, those bearing sense RARβ4 developed alveolar epithelial hyperplasia and displayed an increased frequency of benign and malignant tumors, indicating that this isoform predisposes tissues to hyperplasia and neoplasia [60]. In aggregate, these findings support the idea that the relative expression of these two isoforms may help to predict clinical outcomes; cases with a high ratio of RARβ4 to RARβ2 may have a poorer prognosis than those with a lower ratio [54].

The second possible explanation for Khuri's findings revolves around changes in the downstream retinoid signaling pathway. Kim *et al.* demonstrated lack of response to retinoids in transformed bronchial epithelium, even with constitutive RARβ expression [61]. Other studies suggested that alterations in coactivator or corepressor level or function could contribute to loss of RARβ2 function [31,32,62,63]. Such downstream changes could prevent RARβ2 from carrying out its tumor suppressor function [63]. In light of Khuri's surprising data, RARβ expression may indeed prove useful in identifying early-stage NSCLC patients who are likely to require more aggressive treatment in the future [54].

More recently, Kim and colleagues shed additional light on the molecular basis of negative synergism between retinoids and tobacco carcinogens. They examined tissue specimens from 342 operable NSCLC patients (131 current smokers, 172 former smokers, 39 never smokers) to determine RARβ promoter methylation. Interestingly, they discovered that hypermethylation of the RARβ2 gene has a differential impact on the development of second primary lung cancers (SPLCs) in NSCLC, depending on the smoking status of the patient. In current smokers, hypermethylation correlated with a reduced incidence of SPLCs. On the other hand, SPLCs were more prevalent in former smokers with hypermethylated RARβ. Therefore, silencing of the RARβ promoter by hypermethylation seemed to have a protective effect in active smokers but the opposite effect in former smokers. The authors theorized that the persistent high oxygen tension and subsequent free radical generation in active smokers induce apoptosis, thus decreasing SPLC development. In the face of RARβ expression (unmethylated RARβ), however, endogenous retinoic acids may inhibit apoptosis. Silencing of the RARβ gene, in this case, prevents disruption of natural apoptotic pathways. In contrast, former smokers seem to benefit from the absence of this epigenetic silencing phenomenon. This intriguing data indicates that regulation of RARβ at the epigenetic level determines its effect on lung carcinogenesis. While RARβ may promote epithelial differentiation and apoptosis in former smokers, it may also inhibit apoptosis and enhance carcinogenesis in current smokers [64]. Kim's results helped to explain, at least in part, the association of RARβ expression with worse clinical outcome in Khuri's study, which involved predominantly active smokers [53].

Rexinoids

Rexinoids, or RXR-specific agonists, have come to the forefront over the last decade as a possible adjunct to existing treatment options for NSCLC. Because RARs must form heterodimers with RXRs in order to bind to retinoic acid response elements, while RXRs can homodimerize or bind a variety of

Table 24.4 Clinical trials of bexarotene in NSCLC.

	Phase	Patients (n)	Description
Miller et al. [70]	I	52*	Dose escalation only
Rizvi et al. [71]	I	60[†]	Dose escalation only
Rizvi et al. [72]	II/III	54	Maintenance therapy (stable or responsive disease after initial chemotherapy)
Govindan et al. [73]	II	146	Salvage therapy after failure of two prior chemotherapy regimens (including a platinum and a taxane)
Khuri et al. [76]	I/II	43/28[‡]	In combination with cisplatin and vinorelbine (previously untreated patients)
Edelman et al. [77]	II	48	In combination with gemcitabine and carboplatin (previously untreated patients)
Dragnev et al. [78]	I	24	In combination with erlotinib (dose escalation only)
Blumenschein et al. [86]	III	Ongoing	In combination with paclitaxel and carboplatin (treatment arm)
Jassem et al. [87]	III	Ongoing	In combination with cisplatin and vinorelbine (treatment arm)

* Twenty NSCLC patients, 32 with other solid tumors.
[†] Sixteen NSCLC patients, 43 with other solid tumors, 1 with non-Hodgkin's lymphoma.
[‡] Number of patients in each phase of the trial, respectively.

other nuclear receptors, rexinoids may prove more effective than RAR agonists in altering the expression of target genes [65]. Furthermore, multiple in vitro studies have shown that RAR-β is often silenced by promoter methylation in lung cancer [38,39], thus limiting the utility of agents acting primarily through RARs.

Brabender et al. conducted a seminal study investigating RXR expression in NSCLC. In light of previous data showing decreased RXR-β expression in NSCLC [33,37], they hypothesized that suppression of RXR expression might be a prognostic indicator of worse clinical outcome. Eighty-eight NSCLC tissue specimens from patients with completely resected disease were analyzed for RXRα, RXRβ, and RXRγ mRNA expression by reverse-transcription PCR and compared to matched controls of normal lung tissue. The authors noted that all three isoforms were decreased in malignant tissue as compared to normal tissue. Patients with RXRα suppression showed a trend toward inferior survival, but those with low RXRβ expression exhibited worse overall survival

that was highly statistically significant ($p = 0.0005$). In addition, the multivariate analysis indicated that low RXRβ expression was an independent predictor of poor clinical outcome in NSCLC ($p = 0.017$) [66]. The authors theorized that RXR suppression may occur by the same epigenetic mechanisms described for RARβ [38,39] and ultimately contribute to functional retinoid deficiency, which could allow cells to escape from normal homeostatic pathways regulated by retinoids [66].

Bexarotene, an oral synthetic rexinoid that has been FDA-approved for treatment of refractory cutaneous T-cell lymphoma, has also been studied quite extensively in the context of lung cancer. This compound has high affinity for RXRs but very limited affinity for RARs [67]. Wang et al. studied the chemopreventive efficacy of bexarotene in a murine lung cancer model. Mice with mutations in p53 or K-ras, two commonly implicated oncogenes in human lung carcinogenesis, received a single intraperitoneal injection of vinyl carbamate (a known carcinogen) at 6 weeks of age. Sixteen weeks later, bexarotene was started by gavage at a dose of 100 mg/kg/day and continued five times weekly for a total of 12 weeks. The researchers found that bexarotene reduced both tumor multiplicity and tumor volume in mice of all three genotypes (wild type, p53 mutant, and K-ras heterozygous knockout) when compared to controls. It also reduced the progression of adenoma to adenocarcinoma in the first two groups by roughly 50% [68]. In a study examining the effect of bexarotene on acquired paclitaxel resistance in NSCLC, Yen and colleagues treated cultured human NSCLC cells (Calu3) with intermittent paclitaxel alone or in combination with continuous bexarotene. The former group developed paclitaxel resistance as well as cross-resistance to P-glycoprotein substrates (vincristine, doxorubicin). The latter group, however, maintained sensitivity to all chemotherapeutic agents. These results were confirmed in a xenograft model, as Calu3 cells were implanted in athymic nude mice. The combination of bexarotene and paclitaxel reduced tumor volume by 38% relative to paclitaxel alone. It also suppressed growth of paclitaxel-resistant xenograft tumors by 40% versus paclitaxel alone, proving that resistant cells could be resensitized to paclitaxel [69].

Miller *et al.* conducted the first phase I trial of bexarotene, with 52 advanced cancer patients receiving 5–500 mg/m^2/day over 1–41 weeks. The characteristic side effects of classical retinoids, such as cheilitis, headache, and arthralgias, were not prominent. Asymptomatic elevations in liver enzymes proved to be the most common dose-limiting adverse effect, with leukopenia and hypertriglyceridemia occurring less frequently. Eight of 20 NSCLC patients exhibited sustained disease stabilization. The authors reported 300 mg/m^2 as the maximum-tolerated dose as a single agent [70]. Rizvi and colleagues undertook a similar study of bexarotene but adopted a dose range of 5–1000 mg/m^2/day. No dose-limiting side effects were noted up to 500 mg/m^2/day, but leukopenia, diarrhea, hyperbilirubinemia, and transaminase elevations became apparent at doses exceeding 650 mg/m^2/day. Again, the authors did not observe any dose-limiting toxicity from classical retinoid adverse effects. They recommended a phase II dose of 500 mg/m^2/day [71]. Rizvi later conducted a multicenter trial in which 54 advanced NSCLC patients (stage IIIB with pleural effusion, stage IV, or recurrent disease) with stable or responsive disease after first-line systemic chemotherapy were randomized to one of three arms: bexarotene 300 mg/m^2/day, bexarotene 600 mg/m^2/day, or placebo. Due to slow accrual of patients, the trial was terminated prematurely and therefore did not have the statistical power to confirm differences among the groups. Tumor progression may have been halted or delayed, however, in 5 of 16 NSCLC cases. The overall data showed increased time to progression in the bexarotene groups (82 and 128 days, respectively) versus the placebo group (56 days). The effect was even more striking in the subset of patients with a clinical response to chemotherapy [72]. More recently, Govindan *et al.* carried out a phase II trial of single-agent bexarotene in 146 patients with advanced NSCLC (stage IIIB with pleural effusion or stage IV) who had failed at least two prior chemotherapy regimens (including a platinum and a taxane). Trial participants received 400 mg/m^2/day of bexarotene, as well as a lipid-lowering agent and levothyroxine to prevent anticipated side effects of bexarotene treatment (hyperlipidemia and hypothyroidism) [73]. The goal of the study was to show a median survival of 6 months, which would represent a 50% improvement over the 4-month median survival previously documented with third-line chemotherapy regimens in advanced NSCLC [74,75]. Unfortunately, the authors reported an overall median survival of 5 months with a 1-year survival rate of 23%. Interestingly, the 26 patients who experienced bexarotene-induced hypertriglyceridemia and skin rash exhibited a median survival of 12 months with a 48% 1-year survival rate. The subset of patients with neither side effect had the worst clinical outcome, with a median survival of only 2 months [73]. These findings, in aggregate, spurred other researchers to study bexarotene in combination with cytotoxic and biologic agents.

In one of the first combination therapy trials involving bexarotene, Khuri and coworkers conducted a phase I/II study of bexarotene in combination with cisplatin and vinorelbine in advanced

NSCLC. Forty-three previously untreated patients who had stage IIIB with pleural effusion or stage IV NSCLC participated in the phase I portion of the study, which determined a daily maximum tolerated dose of 400 mg/m^2. Response rate was the primary endpoint in the phase II portion, while median survival time and 1-year survival rate were secondary endpoints. Cisplatin was administered at 100 mg/m^2 every 6 weeks, and vinorelbine was given at alternating doses of 30 mg/m^2 and 15 mg/m^2 every 2 weeks. Seven of 28 phase II patients responded to the treatment combination, and nine were still alive at a 2-year minimum follow-up; median survival was 14 months. One-year and projected 3-year survival rates were 61% and 30%, respectively. The authors reported hyperlipidemia, leukopenia, nausea, vomiting, and respiratory distress as the most common grade 3 and 4 adverse events [76].

Edelman and colleagues recently reported the results of a phase II trial of bexarotene, in combination with gemcitabine and carboplatin, for patients with untreated stage IIIB or stage IV NSCLC. Forty-eight patients were treated with up to six cycles of carboplatin (AUC = 5.0 on day 1) and gemcitabine (1000 mg/m^2 on days 1 and 8), administered every 21 days. They received 400 mg/m^2/day of bexarotene until disease progression, as well as atorvastatin 10 mg daily. The authors aimed to demonstrate a 1-year survival rate of 50%. The only significant toxicity of treatment was hypertriglyceridemia due to bexarotene, which required frequent dose adjustments of bexarotene and an increased starting dose of atorvastatin (40 mg daily). Edelman documented an overall response rate of 25% (11 partial responders and 1 complete responder). Twenty-eight patients had stable disease, while seven patients progressed on the regimen. The overall median survival was 12.7 months, and the 1-year survival rate was 53%. The median time to progression was reported as 6.7 months, compared to 3.9 months for a historical control group of 33 patients treated with two-drug, platinum-based chemotherapy ($p = 0.003$) [77].

Dragnev and colleagues conducted a phase I trial of bexarotene and erlotinib, an epidermal growth factor receptor (EGFR) inhibitor, in 24 patients with advanced aerodigestive tract cancers (19 with NSCLC) [78]. Erlotinib had previously been shown to prolong survival in chemotherapy-refractory advanced NSCLC [79,80], but only a small subset of patients achieve objective responses with this agent alone. In vitro studies had demonstrated that cyclin D1 was an important downstream effector of EGFR and served as a biomarker of response to erlotinib. EGFR inhibition by erlotinib induces G1 arrest and disrupts the normal EGFR-driven promotion of cyclin D1 transcription and expression. Therefore, it was theorized that the clinical efficacy of erlotinib could be augmented by adding a second agent that also targets cyclin D1 [81]. Utilizing an immortalized human bronchial epithelium cell line, researchers had found that both retinoids and rexinoids could suppress EGFR expression, initiate cell cycle arrest, and induce degradation of cyclin D1 through a proteasome-dependent mechanism [82–85]. In this context, Dragnev documented five objective responses (4 partial, 1 minor) among the NSCLC patients. The overall median survival was 14.1 months, and the median time to progression was 2 months. The overall 1-year survival rate proved to be 73.8%, and the corresponding value in the NSCLC subset was 72%. The phase II doses of bexarotene and erlotinib were determined to be 400 mg/m^2/day and 150 mg/day, respectively [78].

The encouraging results from phase I and II trials of bexarotene in the context of combination therapy prompted initiation of two randomized phase III trials in chemotherapy-naïve patients with advanced (stage IIIB with pleural effusion or stage IV) NSCLC. The first trial administered paclitaxel (200 mg/m^2 on day 1) followed by carboplatin (AUC = 6.0) every 3 weeks, with or without bexarotene 400 mg/m^2/day starting on day 1 [86]. In the second trial, patients receive cisplatin (100 mg/m^2 on day 1 of a 4-week cycle) and vinorelbine (25 mg/m^2 weekly), with or without bexarotene 400 mg/m^2 daily [87]. Although the results of these studies have yet to be published, the preliminary analyses suggest no overall survival benefit with the combination of bexarotene and conventional chemotherapeutic agents [78,86,87]. Preplanned subset analyses in both trials, however, suggest a significant improvement in survival in patients who develop grade 3 or 4 hypertriglyceridemia as a result of bexarotene treatment. This intriguing data could have significant impact on future clinical trials of bexarotene.

Future directions

After an initial period of optimism, retinoids have produced disappointing results thus far in the chemopreventive setting. We have much to learn in terms of the precise molecular mechanisms underlying their diverse effects. Better understanding of the retinoid signaling pathways, as well as the contextual differences determining their ultimate impact on gene expression, will help to better define a role for these compounds in treating lung premalignancy and malignancy. The effect of smoking status on retinoid action, for example, provides a glimpse of the complexities involved in the process of lung carcinogenesis. Is epigenetic silencing of RARβ an integral event on the road to malignancy or simply a marker of a much larger process involving silencing of multiple tumor suppressor genes? If demethylating agents can restore RARβ expression and retinoid responsiveness, perhaps combination chemopreventive therapy will be effective [53]. More recently, certain synthetic retinoids, such as high-dose fenretinide, have been shown to induce apoptosis through pathways independent of nuclear receptors [88,89]. These compounds may work well as chemopreventive agents, irrespective of the patient's smoking status [53].

Rexinoids have shown significant promise in phase I and II trials and seem to be much better tolerated than classical retinoids. The common side effects of hyperlipidemia, central hypothyroidism, and liver biochemical dysfunction can be anticipated and managed fairly easily. Bexarotene has yet to be fully evaluated as a single agent in refractory advanced NSCLC, and additional large randomized phase III trials are needed to better evaluate its potential as part of combination therapy. This particularly applies to patients who develop hypertriglyceridemia, a potential biomarker for benefit from rexinoid therapy. The possible synergism between bexarotene and biologic agents such as erlotinib certainly deserves further study. As tyrosine kinase inhibitors and antiangiogenesis agents, as well as other novel therapeutic classes become a part of our armamentarium, we can continue to investigate retinoids and rexinoids in both the chemopreventive and therapeutic settings.

References

1 Ginsberg RI, Vokes EE, Rosenzweig K. Cancer of the lung. Non-small cell lung cancer. In: DeVita VT, Hellman S, Rosenberg SA (eds). *Cancer: Principles and Practice of Oncology*, 6th edn. Philadelphia: Lippincott-Raven, 2001:925–83.

2 Stewart BW, Kleihues P (eds). Lung cancer. In: *World Cancer Report*. Lyon, France: IARC Press, 2003:182–7.

3 Sporn MB, Dunlop NM, Newton DL *et al*. Prevention of chemical carcinogenesis by vitamin A and its synthetic analogues. *Fed Proc* 1976; **35**:1332–8.

4 Sun SY, Lotan R. Retinoids and their receptors in cancer development and chemoprevention. *Crit Rev Oncol Hematol* 2002; **41**:41–55.

5 Gudas L, Hu L. The regulation and gene expression by retinoids in normal and tumorigenic epithelial cells. *Proc Annu Meet Am Assoc Cancer Res* 1993; **34**:588–9.

6 Morris-Kay G. Retinoic acid receptors in normal growth and development. *Cancer Surv* 1992; **14**:181–93.

7 Chambon P. A decade of molecular biology of retinoic acid receptors. *FASEB J* 1996; **10**:940–54.

8 Kastner P, Mark M, Chambon P. Nonsteroid nuclear receptors: what are genetic studies telling us about their role in real life? *Cell* 1995; **83**:859–69.

9 Mangelsdorf DJ, Umesono K, Evans RM. The retinoid receptors. In: Sporn MB, Roberts AB, Goodman DS (eds). *The Retinoids: Biology, Chemistry, and Medicine*, 2nd edn. New York: Raven Press, 1994:319–50.

10 Allenby G, Janocha R, Kazmer S *et al*. Binding of 9-cis-retinoic acid and all-trans-retinoic acid to retinoic acid receptors alpha, beta, and gamma. Retinoic acid receptor gamma binds all-trans-retinoic acid preferentially over 9-cis-retinoic acid. *J Biol Chem* 1994; **269**:16689–95.

11 Nagy L, Kao HY, Chakravarti D *et al*. Nuclear receptor repression mediated by a complex containing SMRT, mSin3A, and histone deacetylase. *Cell* 1997; **89**:373–80.

12 Li Y, Dawson MI, Agadir A *et al*. Regulation of RAR beta expression by RAR- and RXR-selective retinoids in human lung cancer cell lines: effect on growth inhibition and apoptosis induction. *Int J Cancer* 1998; **75**: 88–95.

13 Leid M, Kastner P, Chambon P. Multiplicity generates diversity in the retinoic acid signalling pathways. *Trends Biochem Sci* 1992; **17**:427–33.

14 Glass CK. Some new twists in the regulation of gene expression by thyroid hormone and retinoic acid receptors. *J Endocrinol* 1996; **150**:349–57.

15 de The H, Vivanco-Ruiz MM, Tiollais P *et al*. Identification of a retinoic acid responsive element in the retinoic acid receptor beta gene. *Nature* 1990; **343**:177–80.

16 Lotan R. Aberrant expression of retinoid receptors and lung carcinogenesis. *J Natl Cancer Inst* 1999; **91**:989–91.

17 Oridate N, Lotan D, Xu XC *et al*. Differential induction of apoptosis by all-trans-retinoic acid and N-(4-hydroxyphenyl)retinamide in human head and neck squamous cell carcinoma cell lines. *Clin Cancer Res* 1996; **2**:855–63.

18 Lu XP, Fanjul A, Picard N *et al*. Novel retinoid-related molecules as apoptosis inducers and effective inhibitors of human lung cancer cells in vivo. *Nat Med* 1997; **3**:686–90.

19 Crowe DL. Retinoic acid receptor β induces terminal differentiation of squamous cell carcinoma lines in the absence of cyclin-dependent kinase inhibitor expression. *Cancer Res* 1998; **58**:142–8.

20 Guerin E, Ludwig MG, Basset P *et al*. Stromelysin-3 induction and interstitial collagenase repression by retinoic acid. Therapeutical implication of receptor-selective retinoids dissociating transactivation and AP-1-mediated transrepression. *J Biol Chem* 1997; **272**:11088–95.

21 Wolbach SB, Howe PR. Tissue changes following deprivation of fat soluble A vitamin. *J Exp Med* 1925; **42**:753–77.

22 Genta VM, Kaufman DG, Harris CC *et al*. Vitamin A deficiency enhances binding of benzo(a)pyrene to tracheal epithelial DNA. *Nature* 1974; **247**:48–9.

23 Dogra SC, Khanduja KL, Gupta MP. The effect of vitamin A deficiency on the initiation and postinitiation phases of benzo(a)pyrene-induced lung tumourigenesis in rats. *Br J Cancer* 1985; **52**:931–5.

24 Clamon GH, Sporn MB, Smith JM *et al*. Alpha- and beta-retinyl acetate reverse metaplasias of vitamin A deficiency in hamster trachea in organ culture. *Nature* 1974; **250**:64–6.

25 Saffiotti U, Montesano R, Sellakumar AR *et al*. Experimental cancer of the lung. Inhibition by vitamin A of the induction of tracheobronchial squamous metaplasia and squamous cell tumors. *Cancer* 1967; **20**:857–64.

26 Peto R, Doll R, Buckley JD *et al*. Can dietary β-carotene materially reduce human cancer rates? *Nature* 1981; **290**:201–9.

27 Buring JE, Hennekens CH. Retinoids and carotenoids. In: Devita VT, Jr, Hellman S, Rosenberg SA (eds). *Cancer: Principles and Practice of Oncology*, 4th edn. Philadelphia: J.B. Lippincott, 1993:464–74.

28 Hong WK, Endicott J, Itri LM *et al*. 13-cis-retinoic acid in the treatment of oral leukoplakia. *N Engl J Med* 1986; **315**:1501–5.

29 Lippman SM, Batsakis JG, Toth BB *et al*. Comparison of low dose isotretinoin with beta carotene to prevent oral carcinogenesis. *N Engl J Med* 1993; **328**:15–20.

30 Jain S, Khuri FR, Shin DM. Prevention of head and neck cancer: current status and future prospects. *Curr Probl Cancer* 2004; **28**:265–86.

31 Stich HF, Hornby AP, Mathew B *et al*. Response of oral leukoplakias to the administration of vitamin A. *Cancer Lett* 1988; **40**:93–101.

32 Chiesa F, Tradati N, Marazza M *et al*. Prevention of local relapses and new localizations of oral leukoplakias with the synthetic retinoid fenretinide (4-HPR). Preliminary results. *Eur J Cancer B Oral Oncol* 1992; **28B**:97–102.

33 Xu XC, Sozzi G, Lee JS *et al*. Suppression of retinoic acid receptor beta in non-small cell lung cancer in vivo: implications for lung cancer development. *J Natl Cancer Inst* 1997; **89**:624–9.

34 Gebert JF, Moghal N, Frangioni JV *et al*. High frequency of retinoic acid receptor beta abnormalities in human lung cancer. *Oncogene* 1991; **6**:1859–68.

35 Zhang XC, Liu Y, Lee MO *et al*. A specific defect in the retinoic acid response associated with human lung cancer cell lines. *Cancer Res* 1994; **54**:5663–9.

36 Houle B, Rochette-Egly C, Bradley WE. Tumor-suppressive effect of the retinoic acid receptor β in human epidermoid lung cancer cells. *Proc Natl Acad Sci U S A* 1993; **90**:985–9.

37 Picard E, Seguin C, Monhoven N *et al*. Expression of retinoid receptor genes and proteins in non-small-cell lung cancer. *J Natl Cancer Inst* 1999; **91**:1059–66.

38 Zochbauer-Muller S, Lam S, Toyooka S *et al*. Aberrant methylation of multiple genes in the upper aerodigestive tract epithelium of heavy smokers. *Int J Cancer* 2003; **107**:612–6.

39 Virmani AK, Rathi A, Zochbauer-Muller S *et al*. Promoter methylation and silencing of the retinoic acid

receptor-beta gene in lung carcinomas. *J Natl Cancer Inst* 2000; **92**:1303–7.

40 Cohen V, Khuri FR. Chemoprevention of lung cancer. *Curr Opin Pulm Med* 2004; **10**:279–83.

41 The Alpha-Tocopherol, Beta Carotene Cancer Prevention Study Group. The effect of vitamin E and beta carotene on the incidence of lung cancer and other cancers in male smokers. *N Engl J Med* 1994; **330**:1029–35.

42 Omenn GS, Goodman GE, Thornquist MD *et al*. Effects of a combination of beta carotene and vitamin A on lung cancer and cardiovascular disease. *N Engl J Med* 1996; **334**:1150–5.

43 Hennekens CH, Buring JE, Manson JE *et al*. Lack of effect of long-term supplementation with beta carotene on the incidence of malignant neoplasms and cardiovascular disease. *N Engl J Med* 1996; **334**:1145–9.

44 Arnold AM, Browman GP, Levine MN *et al*. The effect of the synthetic retinoid etretinate on sputum cytology: results from a randomized trial. *Br J Cancer* 1992; **65**:737–43.

45 Lee JS, Lippman SM, Benner SE *et al*. Randomized placebo-controlled trial of isotretinoin in chemoprevention of bronchial squamous metaplasia. *J Clin Oncol* 1994; **12**:937–45.

46 McLarty JW, Holiday DB, Girard WM *et al*. Beta carotene, vitamin A, and lung cancer chemoprevention: results of an intermediate endpoint study. *Am J Clin Nutr* 1995; **62**:1431S–8S.

47 Kurie JM, Lee JS, Khuri FR *et al*. N-(4-hydroxyphenyl)retinamide in the chemoprevention of squamous metaplasia and dysplasia of the bronchial epithelium. *Clin Cancer Res* 2000; **6**:2973–9.

48 Kurie JM, Lotan R, Lee J *et al*. Treatment of former smokers with 9-cis retinoic acid reverses loss of retinoic acid receptor-beta expression in the bronchial epithelium. *J Natl Cancer Inst* 2003; **95**:206–14.

49 Hong WK, Lippman SM, Itri LM *et al*. Prevention of second primary tumors with isotretinoin in squamous-cell carcinoma of the head and neck. *N Engl J Med* 1990; **323**:795–801.

50 Pastorino U, Infante M, Maioli M. Adjuvant treatment of stage I lung cancer with high-dose vitamin A. *J Clin Oncol* 1993; **11**:1216–22.

51 Van Zandwijk N, Dalesio O, Pastorino U *et al*. EUROSCAN, a randomized trial of vitamin A and N-acetylcysteine in patients with head and neck cancer or lung cancer. *J Natl Cancer Inst* 2000; **92**:977–86.

52 Lippman SM, Lee JJ, Karp DD *et al*. Randomized phase III intergroup trial of isotretinoin to prevent second

primary tumors in stage I non-small-cell lung cancer. *J Natl Cancer Inst* 2001; **93**:605–18.

53 Khuri FR, Lotan R. Retinoids in lung cancer: friend, foe, or fellow traveler? *J Clin Oncol* 2004; **22**:3435–7.

54 Khuri FR, Lotan R, Kemp BL *et al*. Retinoic acid receptor-beta as a prognostic indicator in stage I non-small cell lung cancer. *J Clin Oncol* 2000; **18**:2798–804.

55 Xu XC, Ro JY, Lee JS *et al*. Differential expression of nuclear retinoid receptors in normal, premalignant, and malignant head and neck tissues. *Cancer Res* 1994; **54**:3580–7.

56 Zelent A, Mendelson C, Kastner P *et al*. Differentially expressed isoforms of the mouse retinoic acid receptor beta are generated by usage of two promoters and alternative splicing. *EMBO J* 1991; **10**:71–81.

57 Napgal S, Zelent A, Chambon P. RAR-beta-4, a retinoic acid receptor isoform, is generated from RAR-beta-2 by alternative splicing and usage of a CUG initiator codon. *Proc Natl Acad Sci U S A* 1992; **89**:2718–22.

58 Faria TN, Mendelsohn C, Chambon P *et al*. The targeted disruption of both alleles of RAR-beta-2 in F9 embryonal carcinoma cells resulted in the loss of retinoic acid-associated growth arrest. *J Biol Chem* 1999; **274**:26783–8.

59 Berard J, Gaboury L, Landers M *et al*. Lung tumors in mice expressing an antisense RAR-beta-2 transgene. *FASEB J* 1996; **10**:1091–7.

60 Berard J, Gaboury L, Landers M *et al*. Hyperplasia and tumours in lung, breast, and other tissues in mice carrying a RAR-beta-4-like transgene. *EMBO J* 1994; **13**:5570–80.

61 Kim YH, Dohi DF, Han GR *et al*. Retinoid refractoriness occurs during lung carcinogenesis despite functional retinoid receptors. *Cancer Res* 1995; **55**:5603–10.

62 Geradts J, Chen JY, Russell EK *et al*. Human lung cancer cell lines exhibit resistance to retinoic acid treatment. *Cell Growth Differ* 1993; **4**:799–809.

63 Moghal N, Neel BG. Evidence for impaired retinoic acid receptor-thyroid hormone receptor AF-2 cofactor activity in human lung cancer. *Mol Cell Biol* 1995; **15**:3945–59.

64 Kim JS, Lee H, Kim H *et al*. Promoter methylation of retinoic acid receptor b2 and the development of second primary lung cancers in non-small cell lung cancer. *J Clin Oncol* 2004; **22**:3443–50.

65 Rigas JR, Dragnev KH. Emerging role of rexinoids in non-small cell lung cancer: focus on bexarotene. *Oncologist* 2005; **10**:22–33.

66 Brabender J, Danenberg KD, Metzger R *et al*. The role of retinoid X receptor messenger RNA expression in

curatively resected non-small cell lung cancer. *Clin Cancer Res* 2002; **8**:438–43.

67 Boehm MF, Zhang L, Badea BA *et al.* Synthesis and structure-activity relationships of novel retinoid X receptor-selective retinoids. *J Med Chem* 1994; **37**:2930–41.

68 Wang Y, Zhang Z, Yao R *et al.* Prevention of lung cancer progression by bexarotene in mouse models. *Oncogene* 2006; **25**:1320–9.

69 Yen WC, Corpuz MR, Prudente RY *et al.* A selective retinoid X receptor agonist bexarotene (Targretin) prevents and overcomes acquired paclitaxel (Taxol) resistance in human non-small cell lung cancer. *Clin Cancer Res* 2004; **10**:8656–64.

70 Miller VA, Benedetti FM, Rigas JR *et al.* Initial clinical trial of a selective retinoid X receptor ligand, LGD1069. *J Clin Oncol* 1997; **15**:790–5.

71 Rizvi NA, Marshall JL, Dahut W *et al.* Phase I study of LGD1069 in adults with advanced cancer. *Clin Cancer Res* 1999; **5**:1658–64.

72 Rizvi N, Hawkins M, Eisenberg PD *et al.* Placebo-controlled trial of bexarotene, a retinoid X receptor agonist, as maintenance therapy for patients treated with chemotherapy for advanced non-small-cell lung cancer. *Clin Lung Cancer* 2001; **2**:210–15.

73 Govindan R, Crowley J, Schwartzberg L *et al.* Phase II trial of bexarotene capsules in patients with advanced non-small-cell lung cancer after failure of two or more previous therapies. *J Clin Oncol* 2006; **24**: 4848–54.

74 Massarelli E, Andre A, Liu JJ *et al.* A retrospective analysis of the outcome of patients who have received two prior chemotherapy regimens including platinum and docetaxel for recurrent non-small-cell lung cancer. *Lung Cancer* 2003; **39**:55–61.

75 Edelman MJ. Second-line chemotherapy and beyond for non-small cell lung cancer. *Clin Adv Hematol Oncol* 2004; **2**:373–8.

76 Khuri FR, Rigas JR, Figlin RA *et al.* Multi-institutional phase I/II trial of oral bexarotene in combination with cisplatin and vinorelbine in previously untreated patients with advanced non-small-cell lung cancer. *J Clin Oncol* 2001; **19**:2626–37.

77 Edelman MJ, Smith R, Hausner P *et al.* Phase II trial of the novel retinoid, bexarotene, and gemcitabine plus carboplatin in advanced non-small-cell lung cancer. *J Clin Oncol* 2005; **23**:5774–8.

78 Dragnev KH, Petty WJ, Shah S *et al.* Bexarotene and erlotinib for aerodigestive tract cancer. *J Clin Oncol* 2005; **23**:8757–64.

79 Perez-Soler R, Chachoua A, Hammond LA *et al.* Determinants of tumor response and survival with erlotinib in patients with non-small-cell lung cancer. *J Clin Oncol* 2004; **22**:3238–47.

80 Shepherd FA, Rodrigues Pereira J, Ciuleanu T *et al.* Erlotinib in previously treated non-small-cell lung cancer. *N Engl J Med* 2005; **353**:123–32.

81 Petty WJ, Dragnev KH, Memoli VA *et al.* Epidermal growth factor receptor tyrosine kinase inhibition represses cyclin D1 in aerodigestive tract cancers. *Clin Cancer Res* 2004; **10**:7547–54.

82 Lonardo F, Dragnev KH, Freemantle SJ *et al.* Evidence for the epidermal growth factor receptor as a target for lung cancer prevention. *Clin Cancer Res* 2002; **8**:54–60.

83 Boyle JO, Langenfeld J, Lonardo F *et al.* Cyclin D1 proteolysis: a retinoid chemoprevention signal in normal, immortalized, and transformed human bronchial epithelial cells. *J Natl Cancer Inst* 1999; **91**:373–9.

84 Dragnev KH, Pitha-Rowe I, Ma Y *et al.* Specific chemopreventive agents trigger proteasomal degradation of G1 cyclins: implications for combination therapy. *Clin Cancer Res* 2004; **10**:2570–7.

85 Langenfeld J, Kiyokawa H, Sekula D *et al.* Posttranslational regulation of cyclin D1 by retinoic acid: a chemoprevention mechanism. *Proc Natl Acad Sci U S A* 1997; **94**:12070–4.

86 Blumenschein GR, Khuri R, Gatzemeier U *et al.* A randomized phase III trial comparing bexarotene/carboplatin/paclitaxel versus carboplatin/ paclitaxel in chemotherapy-naïve patients with advanced or metastatic non-small cell lung cancer (NSCLC) [Abstract 7001]. *J Clin Oncol* 2007 (In press).

87 Jassem J, Zatloukal P, Ramlou P *et al.* A randomized phase III trial comparing bexarotene/cisplatin/vinorelbine versus cisplatin/ vinorelbine in chemotherapy-naïve patients with advanced or metastatic non-small cell lung cancer (NSCLC) [Abstract 7024]. *J Clin Oncol* 2007 (In press).

88 Fontana JA, Rishi AK. Classical and novel retinoids: their targets in cancer therapy. *Leukemia* 2002; **16**:463–72.

89 Lotan R. Receptor-independent induction of apoptosis by synthetic retinoids. *J Biol Regul Homeost Agents* 2003; **17**:13–28.

CHAPTER 25

Proteasome Inhibition in Nonsmall Cell Lung Cancer Therapy

Minh Huynh and Primo N. Lara Jr

Introduction

In 2006, there were be nearly 175,000 people diagnosed with lung cancer in the United States, predominantly of the nonsmall cell lung cancer (NSCLC) type [1]. The mortality from lung cancer surpassed deaths resulting from colorectal, breast, and prostate cancers combined. The vast majority of patients are diagnosed with locally advanced or metastatic disease. For many of these patients, the disease is no longer curable; therefore, treatment goals are principally palliative. Although advances in systemic treatment have been made in recent years—particularly with platinum-based combination therapy—outcomes remain suboptimal. Typically, the median survival time following platinum-based doublet therapy in metastatic NSCLC has been approximately 8–9 months [2]. Dismal outcomes have similarly been reported following salvage (or second line) systemic therapy [3–6]. Clearly, new agents with unique mechanisms of activity are needed to improve outcomes in this disease.

In recent years, the inhibition of the 26S proteasome has emerged as a rational antineoplastic strategy. The 26S proteasome is a very large proteolytic complex involved in a significant catabolic pathway—the ubiquitin–proteasome pathway—for many intracellular regulatory proteins, including IκB kinase/nuclear factor-κB (IκB/NF-κB), p53, and the cyclin-dependent kinase inhibitors p21 and p27, which contribute to the regulation of the cell cycle, apoptosis and angiogenesis [7–9] (Figure 25.1). It consists of a 19S cap on both ends, which recognizes ubiquitin-tagged proteins that are marked for degradation, and a 20S core, which contain three kinds of proteolytically active site—chymotrypsin-like, caspase-like, and trypsin-like sites [8,10]. Disrupting the ubiquitin–proteasome pathway can affect tumor growth, proliferation, and apoptosis, and is therefore an attractive target for anticancer therapy [7,11]. The inhibition of proteasome function may lead, through multiple mechanisms, to arrested growth of malignant cells, impaired tumor angiogenesis, decreased metastasis, and sensitization of cells to chemotherapeutic agents.

This chapter will review recent preclinical and clinical studies incorporating proteasome inhibition (PI) in NSCLC therapy. Specifically, work with bortezomib (PS-341)—an FDA-approved proteasome inhibitor—will be highlighted. Additionally, selected studies of this agent's activity in small cell lung cancer (SCLC) will also be discussed.

Bortezomib: potential mechanisms of anticancer activity

Bortezomib is a cell-permeable dipeptidyl boronic acid that potently inhibits the 26S proteasome.

Lung Cancer, 3rd edition. Edited by Jack A. Roth, James D. Cox, and Waun Ki Hong. © 2008 Blackwell Publishing, ISBN: 978-1-4051-5112-2.

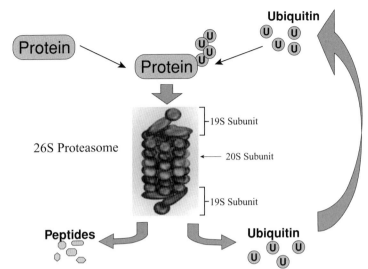

Figure 25.1 *Protein degradation by the 26S Proteasome.* The proteasome is present in both the cytoplasm and nucleus, and is comprised of two subunits, the 20S catalytic core responsible for protease activity and the 19S regulatory subunit involved in protein/ubiquitin recognition. Conjugation of ubiquitin forms a chain on selected proteins and targets them for degradation by the 26S proteasome. The ubiquitin monomers are recycled for future use.

PS-341 is highly selective and highly reversible. Because of its universal presence in mammalian cells and its predilection for disrupting malignant cells, bortezomib has been investigated for its potential antineoplastic activity in a broad range of cancers. In vitro and in vivo studies have shown activity against hematologic malignancies (specifically multiple myeloma), as well as breast, colorectal, pancreatic, prostate, and lung cancers [12,13]. In the National Cancer Institute (NCI) cell line screen, bortezomib demonstrated a unique pattern of cytotoxic activity and growth inhibition against a broad range of tumor types, with an average GI_{50} of 7 nM [13]. Analysis using the COMPARE algorithm [14] showed that cytotoxicity stemming from bortezomib was unique among all cancer drugs in its molecular mechanism of action.

Bortezomib disrupts a wide range of regulatory pathways in lung cancer including stabilization of cell growth regulators including cyclins D, E, A, the tumor suppressor gene p53, various transcription factors (e.g., c-myc, c-fos, and c-jun), several members of the apoptosis regulatory family (BAX) [15], as well as negative growth regulators including cyclin-dependent kinase inhibitors P21 and p27 [16–19].

Preliminary in vitro studies have shown that bortezomib alone can induce growth inhibition in A549, H520, H460, H358, and H322 NSCLC tumor cell lines [20–24]. A common abnormality defined in human tumors is the loss of p27 protein as a result of increased ubiquitin activity. Loss of p27 is associated with a poor prognosis in many tumor types, including NSCLC [27,28]. Conversely, overexpression of p27 triggers apoptosis in several different human cancer cell lines [29]. Meanwhile, abnormal overexpression of Bcl-2 is found in approximately 20–25% of NSCLC and is associated with resistance to chemotherapy-induced apoptosis [30].

Our group has previously reported that bortezomib therapy stabilizes p21 and p27 in NSCLC A549 cells [25]. In studies by Bold *et al.* employing MIA-PaCa-2 cells, bortezomib caused the accumulation of p21 and p27 and a decrease in Bcl-2. Resistance to chemotherapy-induced apoptosis mediated by Bcl-2 overexpression was also bypassed [26].

The p53 tumor suppressor gene has a function in cell growth arrest, apoptosis, and senescence [31]. p53 is often is mutated in advanced NSCLC [32–35]. Wild-type p53 is stabilized by proteasome inhibitors, suggesting a mechanism of bortezomib-induced apoptosis that may be relevant in suppressing lung cancer progression [31–35]. The role of p53 in promoting apoptosis after treatment with bortezomib has not been consistent across cell lines;

however, even if p53 does not play a direct role in bortezomib-induced apoptosis, p53 stabilization through PI could potentiate the activity of other cytotoxic agents [36,37].

Another pathway by which bortezomib inhibits cancer activity is through stabilization of IκB [38]. IκB is a regulatory inhibitor of NF-κB which in turn is a nuclear factor that transcriptionally regulates over 200 genes. These genes are involved in the regulation of cell adhesion, cytokines, and apoptosis. Downstream antiapoptotic factors that NF-κB regulates are BCL-2 and BcL-xL. Not surprisingly, these factors are overexpressed in both NSCLC and SCLC [39–41]. Proteasome inhibitors reduce transcription of Bcl-2 and stabilize Bax, thereby promoting apoptosis [42]. This is one proposed mechanism in which bortezomib seems to enhance sensitivity to cytotoxic chemotherapy or radiation [43]. NF-κB also appears to play a role in regulation of antiangiogenic factors including vascular endothelial growth factor (VEGF) [44,45]. In vitro studies have shown that bortezomib reduces expression of VEGF and thus angiogenesis in nude mice [44–48].

Other advantages of bortezomib therapy include the ability to circumvent multicellular drug resistance and is not a substrate for the multidrug resistance p-glycoprotein MDR1 unlike traditional antineoplastics [49]. Complete inhibition of the 26S proteasome is lethal for many cell types. In addition, malignant cells are more sensitive than normal cells to 26S proteasome inhibition, thus opening an exploitable therapeutic window for the use of proteasome inhibitors as cancer therapies [11].

Sequence specificity of combination proteasome inhibition therapy with chemotherapy

When bortezomib is combined with standard chemotherapeutic agents, an enhanced antitumor effect in NSCLC and other solid tumor cells is often observed [22,26,50–53]. Bortezomib sensitizes tumor cells to chemotherapy-induced apoptosis through mechanisms of cell-cycle dysregulation [24]. For example, bortezomib plus docetaxel has

been shown to have significant additive cytotoxicity in SKOV3 human ovarian carcinoma cells [54]. This was confirmed in an in vivo study of athymic nude mice inoculated with SKOV3 cells, in which a significantly greater reduction in tumor growth was seen in the group treated with combined bortezomib and docetaxel compared with either monotherapy group [52].

Furthermore, in vitro studies have identified the importance of administration sequence when combining bortezomib with cytotoxic chemotherapy [55–57]. Bortezomib is expected to synergize with chemotherapy drugs by lowering the apoptotic threshold of cancer cells [12]. In preclinical models, treatment with bortezomib resulted in the halting of cell cycling at the G1 and G2/M phases. In contrast, many classic chemotherapeutic agents including the taxanes exert their cytotoxic effects in the M phase of rapidly dividing cells. One hypothesis is that bortezomib exposes a cancer cell at a vulnerable phase of its cell cycle, thereby increasing cell kill. In a study employing the Calu-1 NSCLC line, bortezomib combined with docetaxel resulted in high levels of proapoptotic p27Kip1 and reduced expression of antiapoptotic BcL-2. These effects that were highly sequence specific [56]. When given in a specific sequence (i.e., docetaxel prior to bortezomib), the tumor inhibition increased from 12 to 40%. The simultaneous administration of the drug produced markedly less activity. This was echoed in a study using the A549 cell line which showed that the optimal sequence of drug administration was gemcitabine/carboplatin followed by bortezomib as opposed to the reverse sequence [56,57]. In that study, simultaneous administration of chemotherapy and bortezomib resulted in similar rates of apoptosis and cell kill as the sequence of chemotherapy followed by bortezomib.

Pharmacology of bortezomib

Circulating bortezomib is highly protein-bound in humans (approximately 83%). After intravenous administration, bortezomib is cleared rapidly from the vascular compartment and accumulates in tissues with the highest levels in the kidneys and

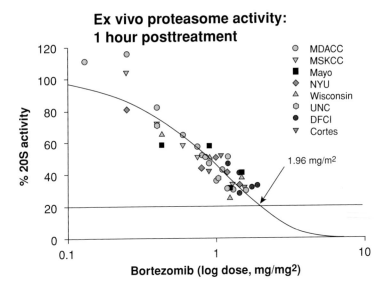

Figure 25.2 Combined proteasome activity from phase I studies according to center (provided by Millennium Pharmaceuticals).

gastrointestinal tract [58]. Because of the short plasma half-life (over 90% of the drug is cleared from the plasma within 15 min of intravenous administration), serum drug levels do not accurately reflect intracellular concentrations of the drug [59]. To aid in accurate dosing in phase I studies, an ex-vivo 20S proteasome bioassay was developed to measure the biological target of the drug, the proteasome, in whole blood, white blood cells, or tumor tissue [60]. There is dose-dependent inhibition of the 20S proteasome in blood samples taken from patients participating in phase I studies 1 hour following administration of bortezomib [12]. As seen in Figure 25.2, proteasome inhibition (PI) will exceed 80% at doses of approximately 1.96 mg/m^2. This inhibition is reversible and recovery occurs in 72 hours with little variation seen between patients or subsequent dosing. In animal studies, toxicity is directly correlated with percentage of proteasome inhibition, with treatment being well tolerated until greater than 80% PI occurs [13]. Phase I studies have also demonstrated greater toxicity with increasing proteasome inhibition [60].

Finally, bortezomib does not seem to be subjected to the same pathways of drug resistance as traditional chemotherapeutics. Bortezomib appears not to be a substrate for multidrug resistance p-glycoprotein MDR1 [49]. Bold *et al.* showed that

in a pancreatic cell line with forced overexpression of BcL-2 that rendered the cells insensitive to gemcitabine and paclitaxel, sensitivity remained high with bortezomib [26].

Early phase clinical development

Several phase I dose escalation trials of bortezomib in solid tumors have been reported [59,61–66]. In addition, large registration trials in multiple myeloma have also been completed [67,68]. Taken together, these studies have shown that the most typical dose limiting toxicities for PI are fatigue, diarrhea, neuropathy, thrombocytopenia, and electrolyte disturbances.

Single-agent bortezomib studies in advanced NSCLC

In a phase I trial of bortezomib in advanced solid tumors (8 of which included NSCLC), Aghajanian *et al.* administered bortezomib as a twice weekly IV bolus for 2 weeks, followed by a 1 week recovery period in patients with advanced solid tumor malignancies [62]. Forty-three patients were treated with bortezomib in doses ranging from 0.13 to 1.56 mg/m^2. There was one major response in a patient with refractory nonsmall cell lung carcinoma. The authors concluded the schedule used in this trial at 1.56 mg/m² biweekly was the most appropriate.

Subsequently, a phase II trial of single-agent bortezomib in advanced NSCLC has been reported [69]. Twelve patients with minimally pretreated (≤1 prior regimen) advanced NSCLC had been accrued. Patients received 1.5 mg/m² bortezomib IV infusion on days 1, 4, 8, and 11, repeated every 21 days. Preliminary results include one partial response and two stable diseases out of eight evaluable patients. Two of the patients have received >6 cycles of therapy. Toxicities were limited to grade I/II and were similar to previous studies with bortezomib.

Stevenson *et al.* conducted a lung cancer-directed phase I study [70]. In 25 patients with advanced NSCLC (≤1 prior regimen), bortezomib was given at doses ranging from 1.3 to 1.5 mg/m² on days 1, 4, 8, 11, every 21 days. There was one PR and nine SD (lasting >4 cycles in 5 patients) in 22 evaluable patients. Grade 3 toxicities included nausea/vomiting, sensory neuropathy, constipation, rash, and thrombocytopenia. The study also looked at the effects of bortezomib on NF-κB in peripheral blood mononuclear cells. A decrease in antiapoptotic signaling in the first 24 hours was seen after the first dose. This was maximal at 4 hours and was only seen in patients who experienced grade III toxicity. This suggests that the time-course of signaling effects may have significance for the scheduling of bortezomib in combination with cytotoxic chemotherapy.

An ongoing California and Pittsburg Cancer Consortium phase II trial is also investigating the role of single-agent bortezomib 1.6 mg/m² delivered on days 1 and 8, every 21 day cycles in the treatment of advanced stage bronchioloalveolar carcinoma. This NCI-sponsored study is open and accruing as of this writing.

Proteasome inhibition with chemotherapy and other agents

A number of practical issues should be considered when integrating bortezomib chemosensitization into lung cancer chemotherapy regimens. The optimal dosing schedule needs to address the

potential for DLTs (e.g., neuropathy), the optimal sequencing with various chemotherapeutic regimens, and the duration of bortezomib treatment, including the potential for cumulative toxicity with long-term administration [12].

Bortezomib plus gemcitabine

A phase I solid tumor trial of the combination of gemcitabine and bortezomib has been reported [71]. Bortezomib was administered on days 1, 4, 8, and 11 with gemcitabine infused on days 1 and 8, every 21 days. In all, 31 patients were treated at four dose levels: 1.0/500, 1.0/800, 1.0/1000, and 1.3/800. The MTD was determined to be 1.0/1000 mg/m². One heavily pretreated NSCLC patient (who had previously received gemcitabine) achieved a partial response (PR). The pharmacokinetics of bortezomib and its effect on proteasome activity in peripheral blood cells were similar to findings in single-agent studies. The pharmacokinetics of gemcitabine did not appear to be affected by bortezomib. This is especially encouraging since both bortezomib and gemcitabine commonly cause thrombocytopenia. The authors concluded that the findings of manageable toxicities and antitumor activity with bortezomib and gemcitabine warrant further investigation.

Bortezomib plus docetaxel

Docetaxel, one of three FDA-approved agents in the second-line NSCLC setting, has also been extensively studied in combination with bortezomib in clinical trials. Our group conducted a phase I trial bortezomib and docetaxel with emphasis on metastatic NSCLC [72]. Thirty-six patients were enrolled in cohorts of three over six dose levels. The MTD of the combined regimen was determined to be bortezomib 1.0 mg/m² on days 1, 4, 8, and 11 plus docetaxel 75 mg/m² on day 1, cycled every 21 days. Of these patients, 26 had NSCLC. Two patients with NSCLC achieved a PR and seven (19%) patients achieved stable disease (including six patients with NSCLC). The most common toxicities were fatigue (67%), nausea (50%), diarrhea (39%), and neutropenia (39%) with no additive toxicities observed. No patient discontinued a study drug owing to treatment-related adverse events. The overall adverse events were not unexpected in this population of patients with locally advanced or metastatic NSCLC or among patients receiving treatment with bortezomib and docetaxel. The characteristics of the study population were consistent with those seen in other phase I studies in NSCLC, with one-half of patients having relapsed or refractory cancer that had been pretreated with multiple lines of prior chemotherapy. This dose escalation study of bortezomib and docetaxel thus represented the initial clinical experiment employing this combination in patients with locally advanced or metastatic NSCLC and other solid tumors.

Messersmith *et al.* also recently published in a phase I study combining bortezomib and docetaxel in refractory solid tumor patients [73]. Patients received escalating doses of weekly docetaxel (days 1 and 8) and twice weekly bortezomib (days 2, 5, 9, and 12) in 3-week cycles. The maximum tolerated dose was docetaxel 25 mg/m^2 (days 1 and 8) with bortezomib 0.8 mg/m^2 (days 2, 5, 9, and 12) given every 21 days. Of 14 patients, four had NSCLC. Although there were no objective responses, two patients with NSCLC had SD as compared to only two others in the rest of the cohort.

The largest trial to date looking at the combination of bortezomib and docetaxel was conducted by Fanucci *et al.* [74]. In this phase II trial, patients with either stage IIIB or IV NSCLC, Karnofsky performance score (KPS) $\geq 70\%$, and one prior chemotherapy regimen were randomized to either arm A receiving bortezomib at 1.5 mg/m^2 IV bolus on days 1, 4, 8, and 11 q 21 days or arm B receiving docetaxel 75 mg/m^2 IV on day 1 and bortezomib 1.3 mg/m^2 on days 1, 4, 8, and 11 q 21 days. The primary objective was to assess response to bortezomib $\pm$ docetaxel. A total of 75 patients were enrolled in arm A and 80 were enrolled in arm B. Arm A demonstrated a PR rate of 8% and stable disease in 21%. In arm B, the PR rate was 9% and stable disease in 45%—all with manageable toxicities. Median time to progression was 1.5 months in arm A and 4.0 months in arm B with a median duration of response of 7.4 months in arm A and 7.8 months in arm B. The 1-year survival rate favored the bortezomib alone arm with 38.7% and the bortezomib + docetaxel 33.1%. Treatment was well tolerated on both arms. The most common grade 3 or worse

adverse events were fatigue, dyspnea, peripheral neuropathy and dehydration in arm A, and neutropenia, anemia, and fatigue in arm B. The authors concluded bortezomib alone demonstrates activity in patients with NSCLC and by combining both agents time to progression appears better than single-agent bortezomib.

The combination of bortezomib with docetaxel has been evaluated in several other studies, and the MTD appears to be highly dependent on the treatment schedule. In a phase I study in patients with breast cancer, the bortezomib/docetaxel combination was well tolerated, and all toxicities were manageable. DLTs were not observed in patients with breast cancer treated with 1.3/75 mg/m^2 bortezomib/docetaxel administered on the same schedule used in this study [75]. When docetaxel was given weekly for 2 weeks and bortezomib twice weekly for 2 weeks of a 21-day cycle in patients with refractory solid tumors the MTD was only 25 mg/m^2 and 0.8 mg/m^2, respectively. However, in a phase I/II study in patients with hormone-refractory prostate cancer, the MTD was not reached, and docetaxel 40 mg/m^2 on days 1 and 8 combined with bortezomib 1.6 mg/m^2 on days 2 and 9 of a 21-day cycle was well tolerated [76].

Presently, there is an ongoing National Cancer Institute-sponsored randomized phase II trial of docetaxel plus bortezomib that directly addresses the sequencing issue. This trial is being conducted by the California/Pittsburgh Cancer Consortium. In this trial, patients with advanced NSCLC who have failed one prior platinum-based chemotherapy are randomized to receive either concurrent docetaxel (day 1) plus bortezomib (on days 1 and 8) or sequential docetaxel (day 1) plus bortezomib (days 2 and 8). Cycle length is 21 days.

Bortezomib plus erlotinib

Erlotinib an epidermal growth factor tyrosine kinase inhibitor approved by the FDA for use in advanced NSCLC as a second-line agent. Although there is currently no early phase trials looking specifically at this combination in NSCLC, preclinical data were recently presented [77]. The investigators tested NSCLC cell lines for sensitivity to the combination of erlotinib and bortezomib. H-322 and H-358

Table 25.1 Summary of efficacy outcomes for S0339 (phase II trial of gemcitabine/carboplatin + bortezomib.

	n = 114 (%)
Response assessment	
Complete response (CR)	2 (2)
Partial response (PR)	22 (19)
Overall response rate (CR + PR)	24 (21)
Stable disease (SD)	51 (45)
Disease control rate (CR + PR + SD)	75 (66)
Progressive disease	21 (18)
Unknown	18 (16)
Survival	
Progression free survival	5 mo
Median survival time	11 mo

cell lines were sensitive to erlotinib (IC50 1.04 and 1.46 μM, respectively), whereas the other five had at least 10-fold higher IC50 (IC50 11.2–33.4 μM). The combination of erlotinib and bortezomib did not show additive activity. In the H-358 human bronchioloalveolar cells, the combination was more active than either agent alone but the effect was not additive. The investigators also reported that there was an optimal sequence for administration of drugs: preexposure to erlotinib for 24 hours prior to treatment with bortezomib resulted in G1 arrest thereby abrogating bortezomib-induced G2/M arrest.

Bortezomib plus platinum-based doublets

Bortezomib has also been incorporated into existing platinum-based combination regimens in advanced NSCLC. In preclinical models, gemcitabine/carboplatin activity was enhanced by the sequence-specific addition of bortezomib, where the sequence of chemotherapy following bortezomib resulted in the least optimal outcomes [22]. Data from a phase I solid tumor trial of gemcitabine/carboplatin plus bortezomib from the University of California Davis Cancer Center reported an encouraging response rate of 48%. Subsequently, a large phase II efficacy trial of this triplet was conducted by the Southwest Oncology Group

(SWOG). The initial results of this trial have been recently reported in abstract form (Table 25.1) [78].

The trial enrolled 114 eligible chemonaive stage IV and IIIB (with malignant pleural effusion) NSCLC patients. The dosing regimen included gemcitabine at 1000 mg/m^2 on days 1, 8 and carboplatin AUC = 5 on day 1, followed 1 hour later by bortezomib 1.0 mg/m^2 on days 1, 4, 8, 11, with cycles repeated every 3 weeks. Nonprogressing patients could continue bortezomib alone after 4 cycles. The overall response and stable diseases rates were 21% and 45%, respectively. Thus, the overall disease control rate (responding + stable disease) was 66%. At a median follow-up of 13 months, progression free and median survival times were 5 months and 11 months, respectively. One-year survival rate was 46%. The most common grade 3/4 toxicities included neutropenia (52%), thrombocytopenia (63%), and fatigue (13%). The 11-month median survival achieved with the addition of bortezomib to gemcitabine and carboplatin in this phase II study is unprecedented in prior SWOG trials in advanced NSCLC, and does not appear to be explained by altered patient characteristics. The toxicity profile of this regimen is favorable and a phase III trial of gemcitabine and carboplatin ± bortezomib in advanced stage NSCLC is under development.

Bortezomib in SCLC

SCLC has been classically described as responsive to frontline platinum-based chemotherapy. Unfortunately, chemotherapy resistance universally develops shortly after such therapy, mediated in part by overexpression of the antiapoptotic protein BCL-2—a frequent aberration in SCLC [79]. In preclinical models, bortezomib inhibits the growth of SCLC by inhibiting the antiapoptotic BCL-2 signaling pathway. Specifically, studies by Mortenson *et al.* in the SCLC lines H526 and H69 demonstrated that bortezomib therapy resulted in decreased transcription of the BCL-2 promoter, decreased BCL-2 levels, and induction of apoptosis. These data provided the rationale to conduct a phase II trial of bortezomib in SCLC [79]. This trial was conducted by the Southwest Oncology Group in previously treated patients with platinum-sensitive and platinum-refractory extensive stage SCLC to determine response rate, toxicity, and survival. Patients with histologically confirmed SCLC, measurable disease, Zubrod performance status 0–1, and prior treatment with platinum-based therapy were enrolled. They were stratified by platinum-sensitivity status: sensitive (relapse >90 days after platinum) or refractory (progression during or ≤90 days after platinum). Bortezomib was administered at 1.3 mg/m^2 intravenously on days 1, 4, 8 and 11, every 21 days. Of 56 eligible patients, 28 were platinum-sensitive and 28 refractory. Twenty-nine patients (52%) had received two or more prior chemotherapy regimens. One platinum-refractory patient had a confirmed partial response. A majority of evaluable patients (91%) progressed. Median progression-free survival and overall survival were 1 month and 3 months, respectively. Only 10 patients (18%) discontinued treatment due to adverse events or side effects. It was concluded that although bortezomib induced a response in a patient with platinum-refractory disease, it had limited single-agent activity in this heavily pretreated cohort. As shown in preclinical models, testing of bortezomib in combination with an apoptotic-trigger such as chemotherapy, is a rational clinical approach. A phase I/II trial of topotecan plus bortezomib has recently been initiated at UC Davis to test this concept.

Conclusion

The optimal therapy for advanced stage lung cancer remains in a state of flux. However, in the last decade, new "targeted" agents have begun to carve out specific niches in the management of this disease. Bortezomib is a proteasome inhibitor that targets many of the regulatory pathways in lung cancer including stabilization of cell growth regulators like cyclins D, E, A, the tumor suppressor gene p53, various transcription factors (e.g., c-myc, c-fos, and c-jun), several members of the apoptosis regulatory family (BAX), as well as negative growth regulators including cyclin-dependent kinase inhibitors P21 and p27. Although there has been evidence for single-agent bortezomib activity against both NSCLC and SCLC, its optimal antineoplastic application appears to be in combination with traditional cytotoxics. Clinical trials defining and confirming this paradigm are ongoing or are in development.

References

1 Jemal A, Siegel R, Ward E *et al.* Cancer statistics, 2006. *CA Cancer J Clin* 2006; **56(2)**:106–30.

2 Lara PN, Redman MW, Kelly K *et al.* Alternative measures predicting clinical benefit in advanced non-small cell lung cancer (NSCLC) from Southwest Oncology Group (SWOG) randomized trials: implications for clinical trial design. *J Clin Oncol, 2006 ASCO Annu Meet Proc Part I* 2006; **24(Suppl 18)**:7006.

3 Shepherd FA, Dancey J, Ramlau R *et al.* Prospective randomized trial of docetaxel versus best supportive care in patients with non-small-cell lung cancer previously treated with platinum-based chemotherapy. *J Clin Oncol* 2000; **8(10)**:2095–103.

4 Fossella FV, DeVore R, Kerr RN *et al.* Randomized phase III trial of docetaxel versus vinorelbine or ifosfamide in patients with advanced non–small-cell lung cancer previously treated with platinum-containing chemotherapy regimen. *J Clin Oncol* 2000; **18(12)**:2354–62.

5 Hanna N, Shepherd FA, Fossella FV *et al.* Randomized phase III trial of pemetrexed versus docetaxel in patients with non-small-cell lung cancer previously treated with chemotherapy. *J Clin Oncol* 2004; **22(9)**:1589–97.

6 Shepherd FA, Rodrigues-Pereira J, Ciuleanu T *et al.* Erlotinib in previously treated non-small-cell lung cancer. *N Engl J Med* 2005; **353(2)**:123–32.

7 Adams J. The proteasome: a suitable antineoplastic target. *Nat Rev Cancer* 2004; **4**:349–60.

8 Kisselev AF, Goldberg AL. Proteasome inhibitors: from research tools to drug candidates. *Chem Biol* 2001; **8**:739–58.

9 Myung J, Kim KB, Crews CM. The ubiquitin-proteasome pathway and proteasome inhibitors. *Med Res Rev* 2001; **21**:245–73.

10 DeMartino GN, Slaughter CA. The proteasome, a novel protease regulated by multiple mechanisms. *J Biol Chem* 1999; **274**:22123–6.

11 Adams J, Palombella VJ, Elliott PJ. Proteasome inhibition: a new strategy in cancer treatment. *Invest New Drugs* 2000; **18**:109–21.

12 Mack PC, Davies AM, Lara PN *et al.* Integration of the proteasome inhibitor PS-341 (Velcade) into the therapeutic approach to lung cancer. *Lung Cancer* 2003; **41(Suppl 1)**:89–96.

13 Adams J, Palombella VJ, Sausville EA *et al.* Proteasome inhibitors: a novel class of potent and effective antitumor agents. *Cancer Res* 1999; **59**:2615–22.

14 Weinstein JN, Myers TG, O'Connor PM *et al.* An information-intensive approach to the molecular pharmacology of cancer. *Science* 1997; **275**:343–9.

15 Adams J. The proteasome: structure, function, and role in the cell. *Cancer Treat Rev* 2003; **29(Suppl)**:3–9.

16 Tsukamoto S, Sugio K, Sakada T *et al.* Reduced expression of cell-cycle regulator p27(Kip1) correlates with a shortened survival in non-small cell lung cancer. *Lung Cancer* 2001; **34**:83–90.

17 Shoji Y, Tanaka F, Takata T *et al.* Clinical significance of p21 expression in non-small cell lung cancer. *J Clin Oncol* 2002; **20**:3865–71.

18 Hirabayashi H, Ohta M, Tanaka H *et al.* Prognostic Significance of p27KIP1 expression in resected non-small cell lung cancers: analysis in combination with expressions p16INK4A, pRB, and p53. *J Surg Oncol* 2002; **81**:177–84.

19 Komiya T, Hosono Y, Hirashima T *et al.* p21 expression as a predictor for favorable prognosis in squamous cell carcinoma of the lung. *Clin Cancer Res* 1997; **3**:1831–5.

20 Ling YH, Liebes L, Ng B *et al.* PS-341, a novel proteasome inhibitor, induces Bcl-2 phosphorylation and cleavage in association with G2-M phase arrest and apoptosis. *Mol Cancer Ther* 2002; **1**:841–9.

21 Ling YH, Liebes L, Zou Y, Perez-Soler R. Reactive oxygen species generation and mitochondrial dysfunction in the apoptotic response to Bortezomib, a novel proteasome inhibitor, in human H460 non-small cell lung cancer cells. *J Biol Chem* 2003; **278**:33714–23.

22 Mortenson MM, Schlieman MG, Virudachalam S, Bold RJ. Effects of the proteasome inhibitor bortezomib alone and in combination with chemotherapy in the A549 non-small-cell lung cancer cell line. *Cancer Chemother Pharmacol* 2004; **54**:343–53.

23 Yang Y, Ikezoe T, Saito T, Kobayashi M, Koeffler HP, Taguchi H. Proteasome inhibitor PS-341 induces growth arrest and apoptosis of non-small cell lung cancer cells via the JNK/c-Jun/AP-1 signaling. *Cancer Sci* 2004; **95**:176–80.

24 Ling YH, Liebes L, Jiang JD *et al.* Mechanisms of proteasome inhibitor PS-341-induced G(2)-M-phase arrest and apoptosis in human non-small cell lung cancer cell lines. *Clin Cancer Res* 2003; **9**:1145–54.

25 Lara PN, Jr, Davies AM, Mack PC *et al.* Proteasome inhibition with PS-341 (bortezomib) in lung cancer therapy. *Semin Oncol* 2004; **31**:40–6.

26 Bold RJ, Virudachalam S, McConkey DJ. Chemosensitization of pancreatic cancer by inhibition of the 26S proteasome. *J Surg Res* 2001; **100**:11–17.

27 Esposito V, Baldi A, De Luca A *et al.* Prognostic role of the cyclin-dependent kinase inhibitor p27 in non-small cell lung cancer. *Cancer Res* 1997; **57**:3381–5.

28 Gandara DR, Lara PN, Lau DH, Mack P, Gumerlock PH. Molecular-clinical correlative studies in non-small cell lung cancer: application of a three-tiered approach. *Lung Cancer* 2001; **34(Suppl 3)**:S75–80.

29 Katayose Y, Kim M, Rakkar AN, Li Z, Cowan KH, Seth P. Promoting apoptosis: a novel activity associated with the cyclin-dependent kinase inhibitor p27. *Cancer Res* 1997; **57**:5441–5.

30 Kim YC, Park KO, Kern JA *et al.* The interactive effect of Ras, HER2, P53 and Bcl-2 expression in predicting the survival of non-small cell lung cancer patients. *Lung Cancer* 1998; **22**:181–90.

31 Blagosklonny MV. P53: an ubiquitous target of anticancer drugs. *Int J Cancer* 2002; **98**:161–6.

32 Kubbutat MH, Vousden KH. Proteolytic cleavage of human p53 by calpain: a potential regulator of protein stability. *Mol Cell Biol* 1997; **17**:460–8.

33 Cusack JC, Liu R, Houston M *et al.* Enhanced chemosensitivity to CPT-11 with proteasome inhibitor PS-341: implications for systemic nuclear factor-kappaB inhibition. *Cancer Res* 2001; **61**:3535–40.

34 Chen F, Chang D, Goh M, Klibanov SA, Ljungman M. Role of p53 in cell cycle regulation and apoptosis following exposure to proteasome inhibitors. *Cell Growth Differ* 2000; **11**:239–46.

35 Lopes UG, Erhardt P, Yao R, Cooper GM. p53-dependent induction of apoptosis by proteasome inhibitors. *J Biol Chem* 1997; **272**:12893–6.

36 Herrmann JL, Briones F, Brisbay S *et al.* Prostate carcinoma cell death resulting from inhibition of proteasome activity is independent of functional Bcl-2 and p53. *Oncogene* 1998; **17**:2889–99.

37 An WG, Hwang SG, Trepel JB *et al.* Protease inhibitor-induced apoptosis: accumulation of wt p53, p21WAF1/CIP1, and induction of apoptosis are independent markers of proteasome inhibition. *Leukemia* 2000; **14**:1276–83.

38 Sunwoo JB, Chen Z, Dong G *et al.* Novel proteasome inhibitor PS-341 inhibits activation of nuclear factor-kappa B, cell survival, tumor growth, and angiogenesis in squamous cell carcinoma. *Clin Cancer Res* 2001; **7**:1419–28.

39 Kaiser U, Schilli M, Haag U *et al.* Expression of bcl-2—protein in small cell lung cancer. *Lung Cancer* 1996; **15**:31–40.

40 Borner MM, Brousset P, Pfanner-Meyer B *et al.* Expression of apoptosis regulatory proteins of the Bcl-2 family and p53 in primary resected non-small-cell lung cancer. *Br J Cancer* 1999; **79**:952–8.

41 Reeve JG, Xiong J, Morgan J *et al.* Expression of apoptosis-regulatory genes in lung tumour cell lines: relationship to p53 expression and relevance to acquired drug resistance. *Br J Cancer* 1996; **73**:1193–200.

42 Li B, Dou QP. Bax degradation by the ubiquitin/proteasome-dependent pathway: involvement in tumor survival and progression. *Proc Natl Acad Sci U S A* 2000; **97**:3850–5.

43 Russo SM, Tepper JE, Baldwin AS *et al.* Enhancement of radiosensitivity by proteasome inhibition: implications for a role of NF-kappaB. *Int J Radiat Oncol Biol Phys* 2001; **50**:183–93.

44 Shibata A, Nagaya T, Imai T *et al.* Inhibition of NF-kappaB activity decreases the VEGF mRNA expression in MDA-MB-231 breast cancer cells. *Breast Cancer Res Treat* 2002; **73**:237–43.

45 Huang S, Pettaway CA, Uehara H *et al.* Blockade of NF-kappaB activity in human prostate cancer cells is associated with suppression of angiogenesis, invasion, and metastasis. *Oncogene* 2001; **20**:4188–97.

46 Nawrocki ST, Bruns CJ, Harbison MT *et al.* Effects of the proteasome inhibitor PS-341 on apoptosis and angiogenesis in orthotopic human pancreatic tumor xenografts. *Mol Cancer Ther* 2002; **1**:1243–53.

47 Fujioka S, Sclabas GM, Schmidt C *et al.* Function of nuclear factor kappaB in pancreatic cancer metastasis. *Clin Cancer Res* 2003; **9**:346–54.

48 Fujioka S, Sclabas GM, Schmidt C *et al.* Inhibition of constitutive NF-kappa B activity by I kappa B alpha M suppresses tumorigenesis. *Oncogene* 2003; **22**:1365–70.

49 Frankel A, Man S, Elliott P *et al.* Lack of multicellular drug resistance observed in human ovarian and prostate carcinoma treated with the proteasome inhibitor PS-341. *Clin Cancer Res* 2000; **6**:3719–28.

50 Nawrocki ST, Sweeney-Gotsch B, Takamori R *et al.* The proteasome inhibitor bortezomib enhances the activity of docetaxel in orthotopic human pancreatic tumor xenografts. *Mol Cancer Ther* 2004; **3**:59–70.

51 Denlinger CE, Rundall BK, Keller MD *et al.* Proteasome inhibition sensitizes non-small-cell lung cancer to gemcitabine-induced apoptosis. *Ann Thorac Surg* 2004; **78**:1207–14; discussion 07–14.

52 Pink M, Pien C, Ona V *et al.* PS-341 enhances chemotherapeutic effect in human xenograft models [Abstract 787]. *Proc AACR* 2002; **43**:158.

53 Holland WS, Lara PN, Kimura T *et al.* Sequence specificity of docetaxel (Doc) and the proteasome inhibitor PS-341 combinations in androgen-independent (AI) prostate cancer (CaP). *J Clin Oncol, 2006 ASCO Annu Meet Proc (Post-Meeting Edition)* June 20, 2006; **24(Suppl 18)**:13150.

54 Millennium Pharmaceuticals. VELCADE and Taxotere in SKOV-3 human ovarian carcinoma cells. Data on file, 2001.

55 Takigawa N, Vaziri SA, Grabowski DR *et al.* Proteasome inhibition with bortezomib enhances activity of topoisomerase I-targeting drugs by NF-kappaB-independent mechanisms. *Anticancer Res* 2006; **26(3A)**:1869–76.

56 Gumerlock PH, Kawaguchi T, Moisan LP *et al.* Mechanisms of enhanced cytotoxicity from docetaxel PS-341 combination in non-small cell lung carcinoma (NSCLC) [Abstract 1214]. *Proc Am Soc Clin Oncol* 2002; **21**.

57 Davies AM, Lara PN, Mack PC *et al.* Bortezomib-based combinations in the treatment of non-small-cell lung cancer. *Clin Lung Cancer* Oct 2005; **7(Suppl 2)**: S59–63.

58 Investigators Brochure MP, Inc., November 2000.

59 Papandreou CN, Daliani DD, Nix D *et al.* Phase I trial of the proteasome inhibitor bortezomib in patients with advanced solid tumors with observations in androgen-independent prostate cancer. *J Clin Oncol* 2004; **22(11)**:2108–21.

60 Lightcap ES, McCormack TA, Pien CS *et al.* Proteasome inhibition measurements: clinical application. *Clin Chem* 2000; **46**:673–83.

61 Logothetis CJ, Yang H, Daliani D *et al.* Dose dependent inhibition of 20S proteasome results in serum Il-6 and PSA decline in patients (PTS) with androgen-independent prostate cancer (AI PCa) treated with the proteasome inhibitor PS-341 [Abstract 740]. *Proc Am Soc Clin Oncol* 2001; **20**.

62 Aghajanian C, Soignet S, Dizon D *et al.* A phase I trial of the novel proteasome inhibitor PS341 in advanced solid tumor malignancies [Abstract 338]. *Proc Am Soc Clin Oncol* 2001; **20**.

63 Orlowski RZ, Stinchcombe TE, Mitchell BS *et al.* Phase I trial of the proteasome inhibitor PS-341 in patients

with refractory hematologic malignancies. *J Clin Oncol* 2002; **20**:4420–7.

64 Hamilton AL, Eder JP, Pavlick AC *et al.* PS-341: phase I study of a novel proteasome inhibitor with pharmacodynamic endpoints [Abstract 336]. *Proc Am Soc Clin Oncol* 2001; **20**.

65 Erlichman C, Adjei AA, Thomas JP *et al.* A phase I trial of the proteasome inhibitor PS-341 in patients with advanced cancer [Abstract 337]. *Proc Am Soc Clin Oncol* 2001; **20**.

66 Ryan DP, Eder JP, Winkelmann J *et al.* Pharmacokinetic and pharmacodynamic phase I study of PS-341 and gemcitabine in patients with advanced solid tumors [Abstract 379]. *Proc Am Soc Clin Oncol* 2002; **21**.

67 Richardson PG, Sonneveld P, Schuster MW *et al.* Bortezomib or high-dose dexamethasone for relapsed multiple myeloma. *N Engl J Med* 2005; **352(24)**:2487–98.

68 Berenson JR, Yang HH, Sadler K *et al.* Phase I/II trial assessing bortezomib and melphalan combination therapy for the treatment of patients with relapsed or refractory multiple myeloma. *J Clin Oncol* 2006; **24(6)**:937–44.

69 Johnson S, Algazy K, Miller D *et al.* Phase II clinical and pharmodynamic trial of the protease inhibitor PS-341 in advanced non-small cell lung cancer [Abstract 810]. *Proc Am Soc Clin Oncol* 2003; **22**:202.

70 Stevenson J, Nho CW, Schick SW *et al.* Phase I study of a novel proteasome inhibitor with pharmodynamic endpoint [Abstract 336]. *Proc Am Soc Clin Oncol* 2001; **20**:85a.

71 Appleman LJ, Ryan DP, Clark JW *et al.* Phase I dose escalation study of bortezomib and gemcitabine safety and tolerability in patients with advanced solid tumors [Abstract 839]. *Proc Am Soc Clin Oncol* 2003; **22**.

72 Lara PN, Koczywas M, Quinn D *et al.* Bortezomib plus docetaxel in advanced non-small cell lung cancer and other solid tumors: a phase I California Cancer Consortium Trial. *J Thorac Oncol* 2006; **1(2)**:126–34.

73 Messersmith W, Baker S, Dinh K *et al.* Phase I trial of bortezomib (PS-341) in combination with docetaxel in patients with advanced solid tumors. *Clin Cancer Res* 2006; **2(4)**:1270–5.

74 Fanucci F, Fossella P, Fidias R *et al.* Bortezomib ± docetaxel in previously treated patients with advanced non-small cell lung cancer (NSCLC): a phase 2 study. *J Clin Oncol, 2005 ASCO Annu Meet Proc.* June 1, 2005; **23(Part I of II, Suppl 16)**:7034.

75 Albanell J, Baselga J, Guix M *et al.* Phase I study of bortezomib in combination with docetaxel in anthracycline-pretreated advanced breast cancer [Abstract 63]. *J Clin Oncol* 2003; **22(Suppl)**:16.

76 Dreicer R, Roth B, Petrylak D *et al.* Phase I/II trial of bortezomib plus docetaxel in patients with advanced androgen-independent prostate cancer [Abstract 4654]. *J Clin Oncol* 2004; **22**.

77 Piperdi B, Ling Y, Perez-Soler R. Schedule dependent interaction between the proteasome inhibitor bortezomib and the EGFR-PTK inhibitor, erlotinib, in human non-small cell lung cancer lines [Abstract 4010]. Presented at the 96th Annual Meeting American Association for Cancer Research 2005, April 16–20, Anaheim, CA..

78 Davies AM, McCoy J, Lara PN *et al.* Bortezomib + gemcitabine (Gem)/carboplatin (Carbo) results in encouraging survival in advanced non-small cell lung cancer (NSCLC): results of a phase II Southwest Oncology Group (SWOG) trial (S0339). *J Clin Oncol, 2006 ASCO Annu Meet Proc Part I* June 20, 2006; **24(Suppl 18)**.

79 Mortenson MM, Schlieman MG, Virudachalam S *et al.* Reduction in BCL-2 levels iby 26S proteasome inhibitor with bortezomib is associated with induction of apoptosis in small cell lung cancer. *Lung Cancer* 2005; **49**:163–70.

CHAPTER 26

Targeted Genetic Therapy for Lung Cancer

Jack A. Roth

Many studies over the past 20 years have established a genetic basis for lung cancer. Genes that suppress tumors and repair DNA can be damaged by more than 100 carcinogens contained in tobacco smoke [1]. Lung cancers show multiple genetic lesions even in histologically normal bronchial mucosa from people with a smoking history. These genetic abnormalities provide an array of targets for therapy. The *p53* tumor suppressor gene appears to play a central role in lung cancer development and was the initial focus of gene therapy approaches to lung cancer.

Mechanism of *p53* tumor suppression and rationale for *p53* gene therapy

Tumor suppressor gene expression, which inhibits cyclin-dependent kinases, induces cell cycle arrest. Two tumor suppressor genes, *Rb* (retinoblastoma gene) and *p53*, which are both regulated at the protein level by oncogenes and other tumor suppressor genes, regulate cell proliferation. The Rb protein regulates the maintenance of, and release from, the G1 phase. The p53 protein monitors cellular stress and DNA damage, either causing growth arrest to facilitate DNA repair or inducing apoptosis if DNA damage is extensive [2]. When a cell is

stressed by oncogene activation, hypoxia, or DNA damage, an intact p53 pathway may determine whether the cell will receive a signal to arrest at the G1 stage of the cell cycle, whether DNA repair will be attempted, or whether the cell will self-destruct via apoptosis (programmed cell death). Apoptosis plays a key role in numerous normal cellular mechanisms, from embryogenesis to destruction of irreparable DNA damage due to random mutations, ionizing radiation, and DNA damaging chemicals including chemotherapeutic agents. The observation that expression of a wild-type *p53* gene in a cancer cell triggers apoptosis provided the rationale for gene therapy approaches [3]. Previously, it was believed that gene therapy could not replace all the damaged genes in a cancer cell and thus would not have a significant effect. The fact that restoration of only one of the defective genes is enough to trigger apoptosis suggests that the DNA damage present in a cancer cell may prime it for an apoptotic event that can be provided through a single pathway.

The *p53* gene product is a transcription factor [4]. A major group of genes whose expression is in part regulated by *p53* are the apoptosis genes. A precisely maintained balance between two proapoptotic versus prosurvival (antiapoptotic) signals, often compared to a rheostat, determines whether apoptosis will be induced. Although these signals determine p53's actions, the expression of many of the genes that generate these critical signals is actually regulated by the activation status of *p53*, forming a complex feedback loop. p53 downregulates the prosurvival (or antiapoptotic) genes, including the

Lung Cancer, 3rd edition. Edited by Jack A. Roth, James D. Cox, and Waun Ki Hong. © 2008 Blackwell Publishing, ISBN: 978-1-4051-5112-2.

antiapoptotic genes *bcl-2* and *bcl-XL* and upregulates the proapoptotic genes *bax, bad, bid, puma*, and *noxa* [5]. Available transcripts of each of the pro and antiapoptotic genes with *bcl2* homology-3 domains interact with one another to form heterodimers, and the relative ratio of proapoptotic to prosurvival proteins in these heterodimers determines the activity of the resulting molecule, thereby determining whether the cell lives or undergoes apoptosis. p53 also targets the death-receptor signaling pathway, including DR5 and Fas/CD95, and the apoptosis machinery, including caspase-6, Apaf-1, and PIDD. It also may directly mediate cytochrome *c* release.

The p53 pathway is regulated at the protein level by other tumor suppressor genes and by several oncogenes [2]. For example, mdm2 normally binds to the N-terminal transactivating domain of *p53*, prohibiting p53 activation and leading to its rapid degradation. Under normal conditions, the half-life of p53 is only 20 minutes. In the event of genotoxic stress, resulting DNA damage causes phosphorylation of serines on p53, weakening its binding to mdm2 and destabilizing the p53/mdm2 interaction, thus prolonging the half-life of p53. The resulting increase in p53 DNA-binding activity leads to an array of downstream signals that switch other genes on or off. In normal cells, mdm2 is inhibited by expression of *p14ARF*, a tumor suppressor gene encoded by the same gene locus as *p16INK4a* but expressed as an alternate reading frame [6]. Deletion or mutation of the tumor suppressor gene *p14ARF*, which has been noted in some cancers, results in increased levels of mdm2 and subsequent inactivation of p53, resulting in inappropriate progression through the cell cycle. The expression of *p14ARF* is induced by hyperproliferative signals from oncogenes such as *ras* and *myc*, thus indicating an important role for p53 in protecting cells from oncogene activation. Importantly, *p53* also plays a central role in mediating cell cycle arrest. This function is significant as prolonged tumor stability has often been observed in clinical trials of *p53* gene replacement, suggesting that this effect is predominant over apoptosis in some tumors. p53 is involved in regulating cell cycle checkpoints, and p53 expression can promote cell senescence through its control of cell cycle effectors such as p21CIP1/WAF1.

Loss of function in the p53 pathway is the most common alteration identified in human cancer to date. About 50% of common epithelial cancers have *p53* mutations [7–9]. In some cancers, loss of *p53* also appears to be linked to resistance to conventional DNA damaging therapies that require functional cellular apoptosis to accomplish cell death.

Preclinical studies of *p53* gene replacement

The studies described above suggest that expressing a wild-type *p53* gene in cancer cells defective in p53 function could mediate either apoptosis or cell growth arrest, both of which would be of therapeutic benefit to a cancer patient. Our initial studies showed that restoration of functional *p53* using a retroviral vector suppressed the growth of some, but not all, human lung cancer cell lines [10]. Because of limitations inherent in the use of retroviruses, subsequent studies of *p53* gene replacement in lung cancer made use of an adenoviral vector (*Ad-p53*) [11]. The original adenoviral vector was a serotype 5 replication-defective vector with a deleted E1 region, which has been used in all *p53* clinical trials. The first published study of *p53* gene therapy showed suppression of tumor growth in an orthotopic human lung cancer model using a retroviral expression vector [12]. This was the first study to show that restoring the function of a single tumor suppressor gene could result in the regression of human cancer cells in vivo.

Ad-p53 also induced apoptosis in cancer cells with nonfunctional *p53* without significantly affecting the proliferation of normal cells [13]. Subsequent studies with *Ad-p53* demonstrated inhibition of tumor growth in a mouse model of human orthotopic lung cancer [14] and induction of apoptosis and suppression of proliferation in various other cancer cell lines and in vivo mouse xenograft tumor models [15–18].

Although it was first thought that the inability to transduce every cell in a tumor might limit the effectiveness of gene therapy for cancer, studies [3,19] of three-dimensional cancer cell matrices and subcutaneous xenografts proved that therapeutic genes could potentially spread beyond the injection site to untransduced tumor cells via a "bystander effect."

Bystander killing, now known to be an important phenomenon in the success of gene therapy, appears to involve regulation of angiogenesis [20,21], immune upregulation [22–24], and secretion of soluble proapoptotic proteins [25].

Clinical trials of *p53* gene replacement

The first clinical trial protocol for *p53* gene-replacement utilized a replication-defective retroviral vector expressing wild-type *p53* driven by a beta-actin promoter [26]. The gene/vector construct was injected into tumors of nine patients with unresectable nonsmall cell lung cancer (NSCLC) that had progressed after conventional therapy. Three of the nine patients showed evidence of tumor regression with no vector-related toxicity, demonstrating the feasibility and safety of *p53* gene therapy [27,28].

Subsequent *p53* clinical trials were conducted with the adenovirus *p53* vector described above. A phase I trial enrolled 28 NSCLC patients whose cancers had not responded to conventional treatments. Successful gene transfer was demonstrated in 80% of evaluable patients [29]. Expression of *p53* was detected in 46% of patients, apoptosis was seen in all but one of the patients expressing the gene, and, importantly, no significant toxicity was observed. More than a 50% reduction in tumor size was observed in two patients, with one patient remaining free of tumor more than a year after concluding therapy and another experiencing nearly complete regression of a chemotherapy- and radiation-resistant upper lobe endobronchial tumor (Figure 26.1). Additional studies in patients with head and neck cancer helped to establish *Ad-p53* gene transfer as a clinically feasible strategy resulting in successful gene transfer and gene expression, low toxicity, and strong evidence of tumor regression.

Gene replacement in combination with conventional DNA damaging agents in NSCLC

Many tumors are resistant to chemotherapy and radiation therapy and, therefore, fail initial therapeutic interventions. *p53*, often missing or nonfunctional in radiation- and chemotherapy-resistant tumors, is known to play a key role in detecting damage to DNA and either directing repair or inducing apoptosis. Once apoptosis was implicated as a mechanism of cell killing in response to these DNA damaging agents, it followed that a defect in the normal apoptotic pathway might confer resistance to some tumor cells. Due to *Ad-p53*'s low toxicity (less than a 5% incidence of serious adverse events) in initial trials, therapeutic strategies combining *Ad-p53* gene replacement and conventional DNA damaging therapies were logical extensions of earlier studies [30].

Overexpression of *p53* in wild-type *p53*-transfected cell lines induces apoptosis [31–33]. Subsequent studies that examined apoptosis in tumor cells treated with radiation or chemotherapeutic agents supported a link between apoptosis induction and functional *p53* expression [34–39]. Preclinical studies of *p53* gene therapy combined with cisplatin in cultured NSCLC cells and in human xenografts in nude mice showed that sequential administration of cisplatin and *p53* gene therapy resulted in enhanced expression of the *p53* gene product [35,40], and similar studies of *Ad-p53* gene transfer combined with radiation therapy indicated that delivery of *Ad-p53* increases the sensitivity of *p53*-deficient tumor cells to external beam radiation [17].

Numerous additional studies have generated additional supporting evidence for a critical link between radiation sensitivity and the ability of a cell to induce apoptosis [41–45]; however, the radiosensitivity of some tumor types (e.g., epithelioid tumors) does not appear to be correlated with *p53* status [46–48].

Clinical trials of tumor suppressor gene replacement combined with chemotherapy

Twenty-four NSCLC patients with tumors previously unresponsive to conventional treatment were enrolled in a phase I trial of *p53* in sequence with cisplatin [49]. Seventy-five percent of the patients had previously experienced tumor progression on

(a)

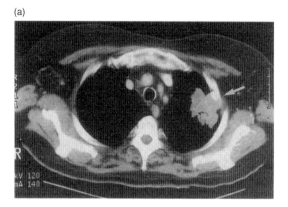

(b)

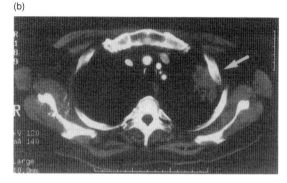

(c)

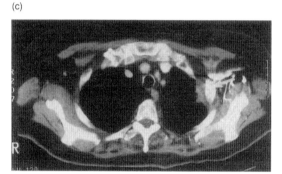

(d)

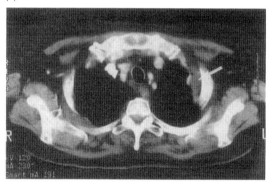

Figure 26.1 Computed tomography (CT) scans of patient following six courses of 109 plaque-forming units of *Ad-p53*, an adenoviral vector carrying the wild-type *p53* complementary DNA. (a) Before treatment, *arrow* shows recurrent left upper lobe adenocarcinoma, which progressed after 66 Gy of external beam radiation therapy and six courses of paclitaxel and carboplatin (CT scan volume: $3 \times 4 \times 5$ cm, 60 cm^3). (b) One month after treatment, *arrow* shows tumor regression after one course of *Ad-p53* treatment (CT scan volume: $2 \times 3 \times 5$ cm, 30 cm^3). (c) Eight months after treatment, image shows tumor regression following six courses of *Ad-p53* gene therapy (CT scan volume: $2 \times 2 \times 3$ cm, 12 cm^3). (d) Stable tumor 18 months after beginning treatment with *Ad-p53* (CT scan volume: $2 \times 2 \times 3$ cm, 12 cm^3). No viable tumor was found during the last 4 months of therapy (14 sequential percutaneous biopsies), and the patient was observed off all treatment for 12 months without evidence of tumor progression. Metastases developed, and the patient died 27 months after entering the study.

cisplatin- or carboplatin-containing regimens. Up to six monthly courses of intravenous cisplatin, each followed 3 days later by intratumoral injection of *Ad-p53*, resulted in 17 patients remaining stable for at least 2 months, two patients achieving partial responses, four patients continuing to exhibit progressive disease, and one patient unevaluable due to progressive disease. Seventy-nine percent of tumor biopsies showed an increase in the number of apoptotic cells, 7% showed a decrease in apoptosis, and 14% showed no change.

A phase II clinical trial evaluated two comparable metastatic lesions in each NSCLC patient enrolled in the study [50]. All patients received chemotherapy, either three cycles of carboplatin plus paclitaxel or three cycles of cisplatin plus vinorelbine, and then *Ad-p53* was injected directly into one lesion. *Ad-p53* treatment resulted in minimal vector-related toxicity and no overall increase in chemotherapy-related adverse events. Detailed statistical analysis of the data indicated that patients receiving carboplatin plus paclitaxel, the combination of drugs that provided the greatest benefit on its own, did not realize additional benefit from *Ad-p53* gene transfer. However, patients treated with the less-successful cisplatin and vinorelbine regimen experienced significantly greater mean local tumor regression, as measured by size, in the *Ad-p53*-injected lesion than in the control lesion.

Clinical trials of *p53* gene replacement combined with radiation therapy

Preclinical studies suggesting that *p53* gene replacement might confer radiation sensitivity to some tumors [17,42–45] led to a phase II clinical trial of *p53* gene transfer in conjunction with radiation therapy [51]. Patients with a poor performance status who could not undergo surgery and would be at high risk for combined chemotherapy and radiation received 60 Gy over 6 weeks with *Ad-p53* injected on days 1, 18, and 32. Nineteen patients with localized NSCLC were treated, resulting in a complete response in one patient (5%), partial response in 11 patients (58%), stable disease in three patients (16%), and progressive disease in two patients (11%). Two patients (11%) were not evaluable due to tumor progression or early death (Plate 26.1). Three months after the completion of therapy, biopsies revealed no viable tumor in 12 patients (63%) and viable tumor in three (16%). Tumors of four patients (21%) were not biopsied because of tumor progression, early death, or weakness. The 1-year progression-free survival rate was 45.5%. Among 13 evaluable patients after 1 year, five (39%) had a complete response and three (23%) had a partial response or disease stabilization. Most treatment failures were caused by metastatic disease without local progression.

In that study, biopsies of the tumor were performed before and after treatment so that detailed studies of gene expression were possible. *Ad-p53* vector-specific DNA was detected in biopsy specimens from nine of 12 patients with paired biopsies (day 18 and day 19). The ratio of copies of *Ad-p53* vector DNA to copies of actin DNA was 0.15 or higher in eight of nine patients (range, 0.05–

3.85) with four patients having a ratio >0.5. For 11 patients with adequate samples for both vector DNA and mRNA analysis, eight showed a postinjection increase in mRNA expression associated with detectable vector DNA. Postinjection increases in *p53* mRNA were detected in 11 of 12 paired biopsies obtained 24 hours after *Ad-p53* injection, with 10 of 11 increasing threefold or more. Preinjection biopsy specimens that were shown by immunohistochemistry to be negative for p53 protein expression were stained for p53 protein expression after *Ad-p53* injection. Staining results confirmed that the p53 protein was expressed in the posttreatment samples in the nuclei of cancer cells. Previous in vitro experiments in human NSCLC cell lines identified four genes (*p21*[*CDKN1A*], *MDM2*, *FAS*, and *BAK*) that showed the greatest increase in mRNA expression after induction of *p53* overexpression by *Ad-p53*. Changes in mRNA levels for these four markers were determined at various time points before and during treatment using reverse transcriptase real-time polymerase chain reaction. The study was controlled by performing a pretreatment biopsy under the same conditions as the posttreatment biopsy. The inclusion of a time point during the radiation treatment allowed for a biopsy to be performed immediately before and 24 hours after *Ad-p53* injection, thus allowing determination of the effects of the *Ad-p53* on mRNA expression during treatment. For *p21* (*CDKN1A*) mRNA, increases of statistical significance were noted 24 hours after *Ad-p53* injection and during treatment, as compared with the pretreatment biopsy. *MDM2* mRNA levels were higher during treatment than before treatment. Levels of *FAS* mRNA did not change significantly during treatment. BAK mRNA expression increased significantly 24 hours after injection of *Ad-p53* and thus appeared to be the marker most acutely upregulated by *Ad-p53* injection.

In the first randomized clinical trial of *p53* gene therapy, 90 patients with squamous cell carcinoma of the head and neck were randomly allocated to receive intratumoral injection of *Ad-p53* (10^{12} viral particles/dose/week for a total of 8 weeks) in combination with radiation therapy (70 Gy over 8 weeks) or radiation therapy alone. Complete remission was seen in 65% of patients receiving *Ad-p53* combined with radiation therapy compared with 20% of patients receiving radiation therapy alone, which was statistically significant [52].

The safety profile for intratumoral injection of *Ad-p53* has been excellent. The most frequently reported adverse events related to treatment with *Ad-p53* injection were fever and chills, asthenia, injection site pain, nausea, and vomiting. The vast majority of these events were mild to moderate. To date, no maximum tolerated dose for *Ad-p53* injection has been established.

Systemic gene therapy for metastases

Local control of cancers is important, but most patients with lung cancer die from systemic metastases. The development of a cancer vaccine to p53 is one approach. Although the p53 protein is expressed by normal cells, it has a short half-life and is thus present at low levels. Mutant p53 is conformationally altered and resists degradation in cancer cells. Thus, it has a prolonged half-life and is expressed at high levels in cancer cells. These differences in expression between normal and cancer cells suggest that p53 could function as a tumor antigen and vaccine target [53]. Several studies have shown in cultured cells and mouse models induction of anti-p53 cytotoxic lymphocytes that killed cancer cells but not normal cells [54–56]. A strategy was developed using dendritic cells, which are the most effective antigen-presenting cells, transduced with *Ad-p53* [57].

Patients with extensive-stage small cell lung cancer (SCLC) were entered into a trial. SCLC patients with extensive stage disease have a median survival of 2–4 months untreated or 6–8 months with chemotherapy. In that trial, the patients' autologous dendritic cells were treated ex vivo with *Ad-p53*, which activates the cells and results in the expression of high levels of p53 protein. Patients were first treated with conventional chemotherapy. Those who achieved at least stable disease received the vaccine biweekly for a total of three to six injections. If patients progressed, they were treated with

chemotherapy. Of the 29 patients treated, one had a partial response, seven had stable disease, and 21 had progression. Patients having progression then received second-line chemotherapy. Clinical follow-up was completed for 21 patients. Complete or partial responses to the second-line chemotherapy were observed in 61.9% of the 21 patients treated. Eleven of the patients were alive 1 year after the first vaccine treatment. These clinical responses were correlated with induction of immune responses to the vaccine. Published objective response rates for second-line chemotherapy in extensive-stage SCLC patients range from 5 to 30%.

Gene delivery to distant sites of cancer is essential for successful cancer gene therapy. Recently, the development of nanoscale synthetic particles that can encapsulate plasmid DNA and deliver it to cells after intravenous injection has been reported. This has been studied in mouse xenograft models of disseminated human lung cancer. In addition to p53, other tumor suppressor genes have been delivered using this technique. Multiple 3p21.3 genes show different degrees of tumor suppression activities in various human cancers in vitro and in preclinical animal models. One of the tumor suppressor genes at this locus is FUS1, which is not expressed in most lung cancers. When wild-type FUS1 is expressed in a lung cancer cell, apoptosis occurs. To translate these findings to clinical applications for molecular cancer therapy, we recently developed a systemic treatment strategy by using a novel FUS1-expressing plasmid vector complexed with DOTAP:cholesterol (DOTAP:Chol) liposome, termed FUS1 nanoparticle, for treating lung cancer and lung metastases [58,59]. In a preclinical trial, we showed that intratumoral administration of FUS1 nanoparticles to subcutaneous NSCLC H1299 and A549 tumor xenografts resulted in significant inhibition of tumor growth. Intravenous injections of FUS1 nanoparticles into mice bearing experimental A549 lung metastasis significantly decreased the number of metastatic tumor nodules. Lung tumor-bearing animals treated with FUS1 nanoparticles survived longer (median survival time: 80 days) than control animals. These results demonstrate the potent tumor suppressive activity of the FUS1 gene, making it a promising therapeutic agent for treatment of primary and disseminated human lung cancer [58,59]. Based on these studies, a phase I clinical trial with FUS1-mediated molecular therapy by systemic administration of FUS1 nanoparticles is now under way in stage IV lung cancer patients at The University of Texas M. D. Anderson Cancer Center in Houston, Texas.

Summary and conclusions

Current therapy such as radiation and chemotherapy controls less than 50% of lung cancers, and overall 5-year survival is only 15%. Combining existing treatments has reached a plateau of efficacy, and the addition of conventional cytoxic agents is limited because of toxicity. The clinical trials summarized in this article clearly demonstrate that, contrary to initial predictions that gene therapy would not be suitable for cancer, gene replacement therapy targeted to a tumor suppressor gene can cause cancer regression by activation of known pathways with minimal toxicity.

Gene expression has been documented and occurs even in the presence of an antiadenovirus immune response, clinical trials have demonstrated that direct intratumoral injection can cause tumor regression or prolonged stabilization of local disease, and the low toxicity associated with gene transfer indicates that tumor suppressor gene replacement can be readily combined with existing and future treatments. Initial concerns that the wide diversity of genetic lesions in cancer cells would prevent the application of gene therapy to cancer appear unfounded; on the contrary, correction of a single genetic lesion has resulted in significant tumor regression.

Studies using the transfer of tumor suppressor genes in combination with conventional DNA damaging treatments indicate that correction of a defect in apoptosis induction can restore sensitivity to radiation and chemotherapy in some resistant tumors, and indications that sensitivity to killing might be enhanced in already sensitive tumors may eventually lead to reduced toxicity from chemotherapy and radiation therapy. The most recent laboratory data demonstrating damage to tumor suppressor genes

in normal tissue and premalignant lesions suggests that these genes could someday be useful in early intervention, diagnosis, and even prevention of cancer. Preclinical studies have shown that systemic delivery for treatment of metastases can be achieved. The ready availability of gene libraries, the ability to administer genes without the extensive reformulation required of small molecules, and their specificity make this an attractive therapeutic approach. Despite the obvious promise evident in the results of these studies, though, it is critical to recognize that there are still gaps in knowledge and technology to address. The major issues for the future development of gene therapy include:

1 Development of more efficient and less toxic gene delivery vectors for systemic gene delivery.

2 Identification of the optimal genes for various tumor types.

3 Optimizing combination therapy.

4 Monitoring gene uptake and expression by cancer cells.

5 Overcoming resistance pathways.

However, given the rapid progress in the field, it is likely that many of these technological problems will be solved in the near future.

References

1 Denissenko MF, Pao A, Tang M, Pfeifer GP. Preferential formation of benzo[a]pyrene adducts at lung cancer mutational hotspots in p53. *Science* 1996; **274(5286)**:430–2.

2 Burns T, El-Deiry W. The p53 pathway and apoptosis. *J Cell Physiol* 1999; **181**:231–9.

3 Fujiwara T, Grimm EA, Mukhopadhyay T, Cai DW, Owen-Schaub LB, Roth JA. A retroviral wild-type p53 expression vector penetrates human lung cancer spheroids and inhibits growth by inducing apoptosis. *Cancer Res* 1993; **53(18)**:4129–33.

4 Raycroft L, Wu H, Lozano G. Transcriptional activation by wild-type but not transforming mutants of the p53 anti-oncogene. *Science* 1990; **249**:1049–51.

5 Adams JM, Cory S. The Bcl-2 protein family: arbiters of cell survival. *Science* Aug 28, 1998; **281(5381)**: 1322–6.

6 Kamijo T, Zindy F, Roussel MF *et al.* Tumor suppression at the mouse INK4a locus mediated by the

alternative reading frame product p19ARF. *Cell* Nov 28, 1997; **91(5)**:649–59.

7 Isobe T, Hiyama K, Yoshida Y, Fujiwara Y, Yamakido M. Prognostic significance of p53 and ras gene abnormalities in lung adenocarcinoma patients with stage I disease after curative resection. *Jpn J Cancer Res* 1994; **85**:1240–6.

8 Martin HM, Filipe MI, Morris RW, Lane DP, Silvestre F. p53 expression and prognosis in gastric carcinoma. *Int J Cancer* Apr 1, 1992; **50(6)**:859–62.

9 Quinlan DC, Davidson AG, Summers CL, Warden HE, Doshi HM. Accumulation of p53 protein correlates with a poor prognosis in human lung cancer. *Cancer Res* 1992; **52**:4828–31.

10 Cai DW, Mukhopadhyay T, Roth JA. A novel ribozyme for modification of mutated p53 pre-mrna in non-small cell lung cancer cell lines. Third Antisense Workshop sponsored by the Department of Neuro-oncology at the University of Texas M. D. Anderson Cancer Center, Houston, Texas, 1993.

11 Zhang WW, Fang X, Mazur W, French BA, Georges RN, Roth JA. High-efficiency gene transfer and high-level expression of wild-type p53 in human lung cancer cells mediated by recombinant adenovirus. *Cancer Gene Ther* 1994; **1(1)**:5–13.

12 Fujiwara T, Cai DW, Georges RN, Mukhopadhyay T, Grimm EA, Roth JA. Therapeutic effect of a retroviral wild-type p53 expression vector in an orthotopic lung cancer model (Commentary). *J Natl Cancer Inst* 1994; **86(19)**:1437–8.

13 Wang JX, Bucana CD, Roth JA, Zhang WW. Apoptosis induced in human osteosarcoma cells is one of the mechanisms for the cytocidal effect of Ad5CMV-*p53*. *Cancer Gene Ther* Oct 1995; **2(1)**:9–17.

14 Georges RN, Mukhopadhyay T, Zhang Y, Yen N, Roth JA. Prevention of orthotopic human lung cancer growth by intratracheal instillation of a retroviral antisense K-ras construct. *Cancer Res* 1993; **53(8)**:1743–6.

15 Bouvet M, Fang B, Ekmekcioglu S *et al.* Suppression of the immune response to an adenovirus vector and enhancement of intratumoral transgene expression by low-dose etoposide. *Gene Ther* Feb 1998; **5**:189–95.

16 Nielsen LL, Dell J, Maxwell E, Armstrong L, Maneval D, Catino JJ. Efficacy of p53 adenovirus-mediated gene therapy against human breast cancer xenografts. *Cancer Gene Ther* 1997; **4(2)**:129–38.

17 Spitz FR, Nguyen D, Skibber J, Meyn R, Cristiano RJ, Roth JA. Adenoviral mediated p53 gene therapy enhances radiation sensitivity of colorectal cancer cell lines. *Proc Am Assoc Cancer Res* 1996; **37**:347.

18 Xu M, Kumar D, Srinivas S *et al.* Parenteral gene therapy with p53 inhibits human breast tumors *in vivo* through a bystander mechanism without evidence of toxicity. *Hum Gene Ther* 1997; **8**:177–85.

19 Cusack JC, Spitz FR, Nguyen D, Zhang WW, Cristiano RJ, Roth JA. High levels of gene transduction in human lung tumors following intralesional injection of recombinant adenovirus. *Cancer Gene Ther* Aug 1996; **3(4)**:245–9.

20 Dameron KM, Volpert OV, Tainsky MA, Bouck N. Control of angiogenesis in fibroblasts by p53 regulation of thrombospondin-1. *Science* 1994; **265**:1582–4.

21 Miyashita T, Reed JC. Tumor suppressor p53 is a direct transcriptional activator of human bax gene. *Cell* 1995; **80(2)**:293–9.

22 Carroll JL, Nielsen LL, Pruett SB, Mathis JM. The role of natural killer cells in adenovirus-mediated p53 gene therapy. *Mol Cancer Therap* Nov 2001; 1:49–60.

23 Molinier-Frenkel V, Le Boulaire C, Le Gal FA *et al.* Longitudinal follow-up of cellular and humoral immunity induced by recombinant adenovirus-mediated gene therapy in cancer patients. *Hum Gene Ther* Sep 1, 2000; **11(13)**:1911–20.

24 Yen N, Ioannides CG, Xu K *et al.* Cellular and humoral immune responses to adenovirus and p53 protein antigens in patients following intratumor injection of an adenovirus vector expressing wild-type p53 (Ad-p53). *Cancer Gene Ther* Apr 11, 2000; **7(4)**:530–6.

25 Owen-Schaub LB, Zhang W, Cusack JC *et al.* Wild-type human p53 and a temperature-sensitive mutant induce Fas/APO-1 expression. *Mol Cell Biol* Jun 1995; **15(6)**:3032–40.

26 Roth JA, Nguyen D, Lawrence DD *et al.* Retrovirus-mediated wild-type p53 gene transfer to tumors of patients with lung cancer. *Nat Med* Sep 1996; **2(9)**:985–91.

27 Roth JA. Clinical protocol: modification of mutant K-ras gene expression in non-small cell lung cancer (NSCLC). *Hum Gene Ther* May 1, 1996; **7(7)**:875–89.

28 Roth JA. Clinical protocol: modification of tumor suppressor gene expression and induction of apoptosis in non-small cell lung cancer (NSCLC) with an adenovirus vector expressing wildtype p53 and cisplatin. *Hum Gene Ther* May 1996; **7(8)**:1013–30.

29 Swisher SG, Roth JA, Nemunaitis J *et al.* Adenovirus-mediated p53 gene transfer in advanced non-small cell lung cancer. *J Natl Cancer Inst* May 5, 1999; **91(9)**:763–71.

30 Yver A, Dreiling LK, Mohanty S *et al.* Tolerance and safety of RPR/INGN 201, an adeno-viral vector

containing a p53 gene, administered intratumorally in 309 patients with advanced cancer enrolled in phase I and II studies world-wide. *Proc Am Soc Clin Oncol* 1999; **19**:460a.

31 Ramqvist T, Magnusson KP, Wang Y, Szekeley L, Klein G. Wild-type p53 induces apoptosis in a Burkitt lymphoma (BL) line that carries mutant p53. *Oncogene* 1993; **8**:1495–500.

32 Shaw P, Bovey R, Tardy S, Sahli R, Sordat B, Costa J. Induction of apoptosis by wild-type p53 in a human colon tumor-derived cell line. *Proc Natl Acad Sci U S A* May 15, 1992; **89(10)**:4495–9.

33 Yonish-Rouach E, Resnitzky D, Lotem J, Sachs L, Kimchi A, Oren M. Wild-type p53 induces apoptosis of myeloid leukemic cells that is inhibited by interleukin-6. *Nature* 1991; **352(6333)**:345–7.

34 Dewey WC, Ling CC, Meyn RE. Radiation induced apoptosis: relevance to radiotherapy. *Int J Radiat Oncol Biol Phys* 1995; **33**:781–96.

35 Fujiwara T, Grimm EA, Mukhopadhyay T, Zhang WW, Owen-Schaub LB, Roth JA. Induction of chemosensitivity in human cancer cells *in vivo* by adenovirus-mediated transfer of the wild-type p53 gene. *Surg Forum* 1994; **45**:524–6.

36 Hamada M, Fujiwara T, Hizuta A *et al.* The p53 gene is a potent determinant of chemosensitivity and radiosensitivity in gastric and colorectal cancers. *J Cancer Res Clin Oncol* Jan 1996; **122(6)**:360–5.

37 Meyn RE, Stephens LC, Hunter NR, Milas L. Apoptosis in murine tumors treated with chemotherapy agents. *Anticancer Drugs* 1997; **6**:443–50.

38 Nguyen DM, Spitz FR, Yen N, Cristiano RJ, Roth JA. Gene therapy for lung cancer: enhancement of tumor suppression by a combination of sequential systemic cisplatin and adenovirus-mediated p53 gene transfer. *J Thorac Cardiovasc Surg* Nov 1996; **112(5)**:1372–7.

39 Roth JA. Review: clinical protocol for modification of tumor suppressor gene expression and induction of apoptosis in non-small cell lung cancer (NSCLC) with an adenovirus vector expressing wildtype p53 and cisplatin. *Hum Gene Ther* Jan 1995; **6(2)**:252–5.

40 Nguyen D, Spitz F, Kataoka M, Wiehle S, Roth JA, Cristiano R. Enhancement of gene transduction in human carcinoma cells by DNA-damaging agents. *Proc Am Assoc Cancer Res* 1996; **37**:347.

41 Akimoto T, Hunter NR, Buchmiller L, Mason K, Ang KK, Milas L. Inverse relationship between epidermal growth factor receptor expression and radiocurability of murine carcinomas. *Clin Cancer Res* 1999; **5(10)**:2884–90.

42 Broaddus WC, Liu Y, Steele LL *et al.* Enhanced radiosensitivity of malignant glioma cells after adenoviral p53 transduction. *J Neurosurg* 1999; **91(6)**:997–1004.

43 Feinmesser M, Halpern M, Fenig E *et al.* Expression of the apoptosis-related oncogenes bcl-2, bax, and p53 in Merkel cell carcinoma: can they predict treatment response and clinical outcome? *Hum Pathol* 1994; **30(11)**:1367–72.

44 Jasty R, Lu J, Irwin T, Suchard S, Clarke MF, Castle VP. Role of p53 in the regulation of irradiation-induced apoptosis in neuroblastoma cells. *Mol Genet Metab* Oct 1998; **65(2)**:155–64.

45 Sakakura C, Sweeney EA, Shirahama T *et al.* Overexpression of bax sensitizes human breast cancer MCF-7 cells to radiation-induced apoptosis. *Int J Cancer* 1996; **67(1)**:101–5.

46 Brachman DG, Becket M, Graves D, Haraf D, Vokes E, Weichselbaum RR. p53 mutation does not correlate with radiosensitivity in 24 head and neck cancer cells lines. *Cancer Res* 1993; **53**:3667–9.

47 Danielsen T, Smith-Sorensen B, Gronlund HA, Hvidsten M, Borresen-Dale AL, Rofstad EK. No association between radiosensitivity and TP53 status, G(1) arrest or protein levels of p53, myc, ras or raf in human melanoma lines. *Int J Radiat Biol* 1994; **75(9)**:1149–60.

48 Slichenmyer WJ, Nelson WG, Slebos RJ, Kastan MB. Loss of a p53-associated G1 checkpoint does not decrease cell survival following DNA damage. *Cancer Res* 1993; **53**:4164–8.

49 Nemunaitis J, Swisher SG, Timmons T *et al.* Adenovirus-mediated p53 gene transfer in sequence with cisplatin to tumors of patients with non-small cell lung cancer. *J Clin Oncol* Feb 1, 2000; **18(3)**:609–22.

50 Schuler M, Herrmann R, De Greve JL *et al.* Adenovirus-mediated wild-type p53 gene transfer in patients receiving chemotherapy for advanced non-small-cell lung cancer: results of a multicenter phase II study. *J Clin Oncol* Mar 15, 2001; **19(6)**:1750–8.

51 Swisher S, Roth JA, Komaki R *et al.* A phase II trial of adenoviral mediated p53 gene transfer (RPR/INGN 201) in conjunction with radiation therapy in patients with localized non-small cell lung cancer (NSCLC). *Am Soc Clin Oncol* 2000; **19**:461a.

52 Peng Z, Han D, Zhang S *et al.* Clinical evaluation of safety and efficacy of intratumoral administration of a recombinant adenoviral-p53 anticancer agent (Genkaxin®). *Mol Ther* 2003; **7**:422–3.

53 Chada S, Mhashilkar A, Roth JA. Development of vaccines against self-antigens: the p53 paradigm. *Curr Opin Drug Discov Dev* 2003; **6(2)**:169–73.

54 Ishida T, Chada S, Stipanov M *et al.* Dendritic cells transduced with wild type p53 gene elicit potent antitumor immune responses. *Clin Exp Immunol* 1999; **117**:244–51.

55 Mayordomo JI, Loftus DJ, Sakamoto H *et al.* Therapy of murine tumors with p53 wild-type and mutant sequence peptide-based vaccines. *J Exp Med* 1996; **183**:1357–65.

56 Nikitina EY, Clark JI, Van Beynen J *et al.* Dendritic cells transduced with full-length wild-type p53 generate antitumor cytotoxic T lymphocytes from peripheral blood of cancer patients. *Clin Cancer Res* 2001; **7**:127–35.

57 Antonia SJ, Mirza N, Fricke I *et al.* Combination of p53 cancer vaccine with chemotherapy in patients with extensive stage small cell lung cancer. *Clin Cancer Res* 2006; **12(3)**:878–87.

58 Ito I, Ji L, Tanaka F *et al.* Liposomal vector mediated delivery of the 3p FUS1 gene demonstrates potent antitumor activity against human lung cancer in vivo. *Cancer Gene Ther* Nov 2004; **11**:733–9.

59 Uno F, Sasaki J, Nishizaki M *et al.* Myristoylation of the FUS1 protein is required for tumor suppression in human lung cancer cells. *Cancer Res* 2004; **64(9)**:2969–76.

CHAPTER 27

Screening for Early Detection

James L. Mulshine

Introduction

The dismal survival of patients with lung cancer is attributable to the fact that the majority have metastatic disease at the time of initial diagnosis. With small cell lung cancer, distant metastases are almost invariably present at the time of diagnosis, making long-term survival rare even for patients with limited stage disease. Surgical resection for cure is possible for nonsmall cell lung cancer; with the chance of long-term survival greater when disease is diagnosed at an earlier stage. Historically, patients have either been diagnosed following an evaluation of symptoms suggestive of lung cancer or incidentally, by finding a pulmonary lesion on a radiographic study obtained for other reasons. Due to the high incidence of lung cancer, considerable resources have been directed at screening for early disease to improve the potential for cure. Chest radiography and sputum cytopathology, the first screening tools available, have been supplanted by newer technologies that can detect disease earlier. Promising results have recently been reported from studies employing chest computed tomography (CT) to screen various populations in centers of excellence, but long-term follow-up data are not yet available. Efforts continue to develop nonradiographic techniques, which may complement chest CT, or prove even more effective and acceptable to the population. Rather than being an exhaustive review of lung cancer screening trials, the purpose of this chapter is to (1) define the prerequisites for a successful cancer screening program, (2) discuss potential pitfalls in lung cancer screening, (3) review the modalities that have been employed in screening, using them as practical examples of the principles underlying cancer screening, (4) summarize ongoing lung cancer screening trials, and (5) provide contemporary recommendations for lung cancer screening.

Prerequisites for a lung cancer screening program

The essential ingredients of a successful screening program include a high burden of disease, a defined preclinical phase during which detection is possible, the potential for cure at some point in the disease process, acceptability, safety, and low cost [1]. A major burden of disease is apparent with lung cancer. While not the most prevalent malignancy, one in 13 Americans will be diagnosed with lung cancer during their lifetime, and it is currently the leading cause of cancer-related mortality in both men and women [2]. The American Cancer Society estimates that there will be 174,470 new cases of lung cancer diagnosed in 2006, and 162,460 cases will be fatal. Eighty-seven percent of cases are nonsmall cell lung cancers [3]. Five-year mortality is approximately 85%. While this malignancy most commonly affects older individuals, it nevertheless results in significant loss of life-years, quality-adjusted life years, and productivity. From a Centers for Disease Control and Prevention analysis of national outcomes from 1997 to 2001 among men and women, respectively,

Lung Cancer, 3rd edition. Edited by Jack A. Roth, James D. Cox, and Waun Ki Hong. © 2008 Blackwell Publishing, ISBN: 978-1-4051-5112-2.

lung cancer resulted in an average loss of about 1.1 million and 740,000 years of productive life and an estimated loss of 62 and 31 billion dollars of economic productivity [2].

Defined preclinical phase

The evolution of a single cancer cell into an invasive carcinoma is a multistage process that occurs over the course of many years. During that time, numerous genetic aberrations accumulate with corresponding histopathologic changes. This sequence, up to the point at which the patient develops symptoms, is the preclinical phase, and likely occurs over a period of at least one to two decades. This process has best been described for squamous cell carcinoma, in which dysplasia and carcinoma in situ (CIS) precede invasive cancer. Atypical alveolar hyperplasia and diffuse idiopathic neuroendocrine cell hyperplasia may be precursors of adenocarcinoma and carcinoid tumors, respectively [4]. Of more relevance is the detectable preclinical phase, which represents the time from which a preinvasive lesion or early lung cancer is detectable to the onset of symptoms. In the case of radiographic screening, the ability to detect smaller pulmonary lesions likely correlates with detecting disease at an earlier preclinical stage, thereby permitting a longer interval between screening studies, and decreasing the risk to the patient of a missed diagnosis. One study employing chest radiography demonstrated that a median delay in diagnosis of 472 days was associated with a shift of 43% of lesions from the T1 to T2 class. The median diameter of missed lesions was 16 mm [5]. Conversely, the median size of lesions missed by chest CT was less than 4 mm, and only 2% of missed lesions were larger than 7 mm [6]. An intentional delay of 1 year between chest CT studies in patients with nodules smaller than 5 mm would not have resulted in a diagnosis of cancer in any, while a similar screening interval for nodules 5–9 mm in size would have resulted in a delay [7]. The presence of a preclinical phase is necessary, but not sufficient to justify screening. The natural history of the disease must be characterized by a critical point, after which the disease becomes incurable, but before which the disease can both be detected by screening and treated effectively [8].

Potential for cure

Lung cancer is a progressive disease moving from curable localized disease to incurable metastatic disease in the absence of clinical symptoms. Five-year survival for stage I disease exceeds 65% [9–11]. There is increasing evidence that survival is improved, even within the currently defined stage IA, as tumor size decreases, in particular for tumors less than 2 cm in diameter compared to tumors ranging from 2 to 3 cm. Lesions less than 2 cm in diameter are less likely to be associated with lymph node (16% versus 27%) or distant metastases than larger lesions within the current T1 category [12,13]. Regional lymph node involvement is usually the first site involved in metastatic dissemination. In a series of resected lung cancer with lesion size less than 1 cm, the 5-year disease-free survival rate was 100% for nonsolid or part-solid lesions, and 94% for solid lesions [14]. Dividing T1 into T1a (2 cm or less) and T1b (over 2–3 cm) resulted in a division of the 5-year survival rates for the currently defined T1 class, with about 84% survival for pathologic T1a decreasing to 76% for pathologic T1b. Survival differences between cancers 2 cm or less in size compared to larger tumors within the T1 class have been noted by other investigators as well [11]. Based on data from the SEER registry, the cure rates (as assessed by 12-year survival) for tumors stratified by size in increments of 10 mm progressively decreased with increasing size, ranging from 69% for 5–15 mm tumors to 43% for tumors >45 mm [15].

Acceptability

The method of screening must be acceptable to the individual, as screening for lung cancer will mandate repeated studies over the course of many years. Over 90% of patients enrolled in a chest CT screening program returned for at least one follow-up study, with only 77 of 1000 patients declining further participation of their own accord [16]. Compliance with a program incorporating bronchoscopy, which mandates the use of sedation and time off work, and imposes the potential for discomfort and complications, will be predictably lower. Compliance with screening of blood or sputum samples would likely more closely parallel that of radiographic screening.

Safety

Some screening modalities impose direct risks to subjects. The consequences of an abnormal result on a screening test can be even more substantial however. Such a result may compromise quality of life by provoking anxiety as well as accrue the risk and cost of an invasive diagnostic procedure to confirm the suspicion of cancer. For a worthwhile screening test, the mortality benefit of finding early lung cancer must outweigh the risk inherent in the clinical management of the screening process. A major concern with chest CT screening is the high incidence of pulmonary nodules among high-risk populations, with only a small fraction of these nodules representing malignancy. An even smaller proportion of nodules would represent malignancy if screening were performed in low-risk populations or in areas with endemic fungi, exposure to which can result in pulmonary nodules. Performing biopsies of all nodules would therefore place a large number of patients at risk of complications from unnecessary diagnostic procedures. Fortunately, there are several radiographic characteristics, including a benign calcification pattern, fat attenuation, smooth borders, and size, that are associated with a low risk of malignancy. These findings may obviate the need for further follow-up, or at least the need for immediate work-up [17]. From large series, after excluding these nodules from further evaluation about 10–15% of cases remain, from which fewer than one in 10 will be found to have lung cancer [18]. One approach that balances the risk of unnecessary procedures against that of a delay in diagnosis has been the requirement for growth of the nodule prior to referral for biopsy. Measuring tumor growth, particularly for small lesions, is hard and there is no standardized approach as of yet. The standard approach of reporting a nodule's size as the average of its length and width at the point of maximal two-dimensional registration is being supplanted by the use of three-dimensional volumetric measurement in some studies [19]. The natural history of solitary pulmonary nodules in the screening setting is the subject of controversy, suggesting that further

research on the most effective approach to following small nodules is prudent.

Once the diagnosis is confirmed, the cancer must be treated. The preferred approach has been resection when possible, most often lobectomy, as this anatomic resection has been associated with improved survival compared to limited resection, which includes segmentectomy and wedge resection. Five-year survival is 75% for anatomic resection and 59% for limited resection [10]. This difference holds even for smaller lesions, with 5-year survival following resection of tumors smaller than 1 cm being 92%, 75%, and 42% for lobectomy, segmentectomy, and wedge resection, respectively [20]. A more recent study, however, demonstrated comparable local and distant recurrence rates, as well as survival, between patients undergoing limited resection, the majority of which were segmentectomies, compared to lobectomy for peripheral cancers less than 2 cm in maximal diameter [21]. Additionally, there has been no mortality or recurrence in patients undergoing resection of ground-glass opacities (nonsolid nodules), 68% of which were bronchioloalveolar carcinomas (BACs), after a median follow-up of 35 months, with 38% of these patients undergoing limited resection [22], or among a group of patients with BACs without pathologic findings of invasion who underwent limited resection, with 30 months of follow-up [23]. These more recent results are encouraging, as lung cancer survivors are at risk for second primaries as a consequence of field cancerization, and BACs are commonly multicentric, with patients more likely to tolerate a second resection if a lung-sparing operation is initially performed. A number of nonsurgical techniques, including radiofrequency ablation (RFA), external beam radiation therapy, photodynamic therapy (PDT), and brachytherapy, may also prove effective as lung-sparing alternatives, but none has demonstrated survival comparable to surgical resection. These techniques, even if less effective than surgery, may expand the reach of screening if they reduce the rate of mortality related to managing the primary tumor.

Another issue of some concern is the risk of malignancy attributable to the radiation exposure implicit in radiographic screening and cancer follow-up. An extremely conservative modeling based on follow-up of atomic bomb survivors suggests that the number of lung cancers would increase by 1.8% if half of all current and former smokers were screened from age 50 to age 75 with annual low-dose chest CT. A single CT would be associated with a risk of lung cancer of less than 0.06% over a 25-year period [24]. The clinical relevance of a radiation-induced cancer should be considered within the context of likely improvements in effective early management of lung cancer over the next 25 years. During that time, further refinement of imaging technology may not only enhance the ability to reduce radiation exposure with a screening CT but also the ability to find early curable lung cancers. While careful attention to these radiation exposure issues is prudent, research to reduce mortality from lung cancer in heavily tobacco exposed populations should not be slowed. Clinicians should share existing information about all of the safety issues discussed above with high-risk individuals considering lung cancer screening as part of the informed consent process.

Low cost

Cost-effectiveness of the screening program is the more relevant variable than cost per se. A commonly accepted cut-point for this parameter in the United States is a cost of less than $50,000 per life-year saved. Some analyses of chest CT screening have concluded that this modality can be cost-effective, with costs as low as $2500 for the baseline scan to $10,000 per life-year saved when follow-up scans are included [16,25]. Other analyses have suggested CT screening would be cost-prohibitive, with costs from ranging from $42,500 to over $100,000 per quality-adjusted life-year gained [26,27]. The disparate results of these cost-effectiveness analyses doubtless reflect differences in estimates of disease incidence, screening effectiveness, and costs associated with the diagnostic algorithm, which vary among reported modeling approaches. In general, efforts to improve the efficiency of screening will reduce its cost. Improved efficiency entails finding the relevant cancers using clinical management algorithms that subject fewer at-risk individuals to unnecessary diagnostic procedures and result in fewer thoracotomies being performed in individuals without lung cancer [18]. These are two areas for further research to improve lung cancer screening.

Pitfalls in lung cancer screening

Lung cancer screening trials are complex processes that can be confounded by a number of biases [28]. First is lead time bias, which refers to an increase in the observed survival due solely to the detection of the cancer earlier by screening than would have occurred by conventional means. An improvement in lead time is implicit in successful lung cancer screening, and an improvement in 5-year survival is necessary, but not sufficient, to prove that such screening is effective. Length-biased sampling refers to the fact that disease with a long preclinical phase is more likely to be detected in the course of screening than rapidly fatal disease. This bias will also result in an improvement in observed survival, as patients with more indolent disease will be over-represented in the screened population. These two biases can be nullified by relying on lung cancer mortality, rather than survival, as the endpoint of screening trials. Referral or selection bias reflects the enrollment into screening trials of patients with a survival advantage, whether due to being healthier at baseline, more likely to follow-up, or more likely to agree to recommended interventions [8]. This bias is more likely to be a concern in cohort studies than in randomized, controlled trials. Sticky diagnosis bias refers to the greater attribution of death to lung cancer, where another cause may have been the culprit, in patients previously diagnosed with lung cancer. This bias, unlike those above, will inflate the lung cancer mortality in a screened population [29].

The premise of screening is that it will result in a stage shift, that is, an increase in the number of early stage cancers with a concomitant decrease in advanced cancers. At baseline, the number of early and late cancers should be equivalent between individuals assigned to the screened and control groups. Over the course of the study, however, the number of early cancers should increase and advanced cancers decrease in the screened group relative to the control group. Some radiographic screening studies have demonstrated an increased number of early stage cancers, without a decrease in advanced cancers. This pattern would be expected to result in a lesser, if any, reduction in lung cancer mortality. This is an important but complex issue which would be best studied in the setting of a population-based, rather than referral-based trial, since all outcomes may be better determined.

Another potential confounder of screening studies is overdiagnosis bias, reflected by patients in whom the risk of death from lung cancer is preempted by a competing mortality risk, such as coronary artery disease. The basis for this concern arises from an autopsy study that documented the presence of unsuspected lung cancers, the majority of which had lymph node or distant metastases, in 0.8% of decedents [30]. Furthermore, as the lung cancer mortality data come from populations diagnosed conventionally, it follows that some patients who are diagnosed with early lung cancer during screening, most of whom will be at risk of respiratory or cardiovascular disease as a result of smoking, may die with lung cancer rather than from it. In particular, the natural history of BAC would be consonant with this particular type of bias, as the survival of patients with multifocal BAC (stage IIIB or IV) is on par with stage I or II non-small cell lung cancer when all nodules are completely resected and no lymph node metastases are found. Long-term survival following recurrence is also well recognized, further differentiating this subtype from other nonsmall cell lung cancers [31]. Furthermore, one study compared the survival of patients with BACs to those with adenocarcinomas with BAC components, and found no significant difference between these pathologic subtypes, with overall 5-year survival around 60% [32].

Several arguments against the relevance of overdiagnosis to lung cancer screening can be found in the literature. First, all tumors detected in the course of screening were shown to be indistinguishable from conventionally diagnosed lung cancers on pathologic examination. Only 12% of adenocarcinomas were BACs, and 78% of cancers originally described as BAC were found to have an invasive component, and thus reclassified, upon review [33]. Second, these tumors harbor the same types of genetic abnormalities as conventionally diagnosed lung cancers, and thus presumably the same potential for growth and metastasis [18]. Third, the majority of lung cancers diagnosed by screening met criteria for aggressiveness, including metastatic spread, invasion beyond the basement membrane, or doubling time less than 400 days. The percent of cancers meeting these criteria decreased from 96% for solid nodules to 67% for nonsolid nodules [34]. Fourth, mortality is high for unresected lung cancer, regardless of whether diagnosed by screening or conventionally. While the 5-year survival for patients with screening-detected lung cancer is statistically superior to those diagnosed conventionally, this survival rate is less than 30%, with further attrition resulting in 10-year survival of 10% or less [35,36]. The results from CT screening trials in the United States are even less favorable, with 5-year survival of 10% for patients with unresected stage I lung cancer [30]. These results are comparable to the 5-year survival of less than 10% for patients with unresected stage I tumors diagnosed conventionally [37,38]. While more attention to defining the exact contribution of overdiagnosis to lung cancer screening results is prudent, the last USPSTF analysis of lung cancer screening failed to find compelling evidence that overdiagnosis bias was a major problem in considering current screening results [39].

Defining the target population for lung cancer screening

An important question in lung cancer screening is, of course, who should be screened. The lifetime risk of lung cancer is about 8% for men and 6% for women [2]. Defining the target population to maximize early detection and minimize unnecessary testing is paramount. Older age and smoking history are the two strongest predictors of future risk of lung cancer. Some studies have limited enrollment to individuals 50 or 60 years or older. The incidence of lung cancer begins to increase rapidly at this point; however, 0.21% and 0.92% of individuals will be diagnosed with lung cancer between age 40 and 50 and between 50 and 60, respectively, such that individuals younger than age 55 constitute about 10% of patients diagnosed with lung cancer. A recent personal history of smoking has also been an entry requirement in some studies, but another 10% of patients diagnosed with lung cancer have never smoked [2], and the risk of lung cancer for former smokers remains greater than that of never smokers indefinitely after smoking cessation [40], such that about half of lung cancer cases occur in former smokers [41]. It becomes clear that a significant fraction of lung cancer cases will be missed by having strict age and smoking enrollment criteria. Three other examples serve to illustrate the difficulty of defining the optimal target population. First, the risk of smoking is greater with longer duration compared to increasing dose, such that individuals with the same pack-year exposure can have different risks of lung cancer [42]. Second, racial differences in susceptibility to smoking are apparent, with the risk higher for African-American and native Hawaiian, and lower for Japanese-American and Latino, than white individuals who smoke less than 30 cigarettes per day [43]. Third, although chronic obstructive pulmonary disease (COPD) and lung cancer are both predominantly smoking-related diseases, there appears to be an increased risk of lung cancer in patients with COPD compared to individuals who smoke but do not have evidence of COPD [42]. As a result of these data, one of the larger ongoing screening trials allows each participating center to devise its own entry criteria [44], and a contemporary study has replaced a lower age limit with a minimum smoking exposure history and includes individuals who have stopped smoking up to 5 years prior to entry [45].

Studying the effectiveness of lung cancer screening programs

The design of studies addressing the effectiveness of lung cancer screening programs is also problematic. The conventional wisdom is that the optimal study design would be a randomized controlled trial (RCT) in which subjects are recruited from the population that the screening program will target and randomized to screening or usual care. The major drawback of this approach is the long time required for completion of such a study. The evolution of spiral CT technology has been very rapid and even now allows the detection of smaller tumors that at its inception. Management has been changing rapidly as well to reduce the morbidity of procedures required to successfully manage these smaller tumors. The lack of flexibility intrinsic to a carefully designed RCT imposes limits on the application of technologic advances or improvements in the screening protocol over the course of the trial, with potential consequences to the applicability of any results obtained.

The RCT design serves as the basis for the National Lung Screening Trial (NLST), in which high-risk individuals have been randomized to screening with chest X-ray or chest CT. This trial has completed enrollment and is following patients for 5 years, with results anticipated in 2010. An alternate approach, exemplified by the International Early Lung Cancer Action Program (I-ELCAP), has been to screen the entire study population, which provides a measure of the chest CT to detect early stage lung cancer, and compare outcomes in patients who are selected and elect for resection to those who are either excluded from or elect not to pursue resection. Inherent in this approach is a commitment to incorporating new technology in all aspects of management, as well as incorporating refinements to the standardized management protocol based on continuous assessment of screening results.

Screening with chest radiography and cytopathology

The question of the efficacy of chest radiography in screening for lung cancer remains unanswered despite the fact that the results of the earliest studies were reported in the 1960s, with subsequent studies bringing the total number of individuals screened to well over 100,000. While this modality has proven effective at detecting early lung cancer, its impact on lung cancer mortality has not been proven, and thus its use for lung cancer screening is not recommended. A large randomized controlled study is being conducted in the United States to attempt to answer this question once and for all, with results anticipated after 2013.

One of the earliest studies of chest radiography for lung cancer screening was conducted in the United Kingdom and published in 1968, with follow-up survival data reported the following year [46]. The study population consisted of over 50,000 men, age 40 or greater. The screened group underwent chest radiography every 6 months for 3 years, while the control group only had chest radiographs performed at study entry and after 3 years. Patients with cancer diagnosed as a result of the enrollment radiograph were excluded from further participation. During the study, 101 and 76 cancers were diagnosed in the screened and control group, respectively. Overall, 44% and 29% of patients in these respective groups underwent resection. Sixty-five of the 101 cancers in the screened group were detected by screening chest radiography, with the remainder diagnosed between scheduled exams. Of these 65 cancers, 65% were resected. Five-year survival was better for patients in the screened group as a whole (23% versus 6%), as well as for the subset of patients undergoing resection (32% versus 23%), compared to the control group. Lung cancer mortality was not significantly different between groups however. While chest radiography was effective at detecting early cancer, with a greater percent of patients able to undergo resection as a result, this method clearly lacked sensitivity, missing one-third of patients later diagnosed with lung cancer. In the setting of identical lung cancer mortality rates, the survival benefit in the screened group likely resulted from lead-time bias and length-biased sampling.

The National Cancer Institute subsequently sponsored three large trials of chest radiography combined with sputum cytology for the early detection of lung cancer. Investigators at the Mayo Clinic [47], Memorial Sloan-Kettering Cancer Center [48], and Johns Hopkins Medical Institutions [49] enrolled just over 30,000 men with a history of smoking into the Cooperative Early Lung Cancer Detection Program. Patients enrolled at the Mayo Clinic underwent chest radiography and sputum cytology every 4 months, while controls were advised to have these tests performed annually. Patients at the other two sites were randomized to annual chest radiography with or without sputum cytology every 4 months. The Memorial Sloan-Kettering Study demonstrated that about one-third of lung cancers diagnosed from enrollment exams, and 14% of those diagnosed subsequently, were detected by sputum cytology. One hundred forty-four patients were diagnosed with lung cancer in each group. While cytopathology resulted in additional cases of early lung cancer being diagnosed initially, seven of 18 cancers diagnosed subsequently were advanced stage, and the lung cancer mortality rates for each group were comparable, suggesting no incremental benefit of the addition of sputum cytopathology to screening with chest radiography. This study again demonstrated the poor sensitivity of these methods for early lung cancer detection, with 39% of cancers being diagnosed between proscribed screening tests, and only just over half of cancers detected by screening being stage I. Similar results were observed in the Johns Hopkins Study, with no difference in lung cancer mortality demonstrated between groups. A majority of cancers were diagnosed between screening tests, and only 17% of these were stage I compared to 57% of cancers diagnosed by a screening test.

The design of the Mayo Lung Project was intended to permit a comparison between screening with the combination of chest radiography and sputum cytology and usual practice. A majority of control patients undertook the recommended "usual practice" which was to receive an annual chest radiograph, and therefore contaminated the subsequent comparison between this group and the screened population. Nonetheless, more cancers, particularly early stage, were detected among the screened group, with 46% of patients undergoing resection compared to 32% in the control group. Five-year survival was better for the screened group, but lung cancer mortality was not different. Of particular concern were the seven postoperative deaths among the 122 lung cancer deaths in the screened group. A specific concern for overdiagnosis resulted from the observation that the screened group had an increased number of cancers at the completion of the 6 years of screening (143 compared to 87), and this difference persisted at 11 and 28 years of follow-up (206 compared to 160 at 11 yr, and 585 and 500 at 28 yr) [29]. Controversy remains over whether these results reflect overdiagnosis or failed randomization, with the greater number of lung cancers in the screened population resulting from chance. These results again demonstrated the poor sensitivity of these methods, with 25% and 12% of cancers detected after evaluation of symptoms or by non-proscribed chest radiographs, respectively. Furthermore, only a minority of lung cancers detected by screening were resectable. This weakness resulted in an equal distribution of patients with unresectable disease among both groups, and thus a stage-shift did not occur with this method of screening.

Similar results were observed in a study of chest radiography screening conducted in Czechoslovakia [50]. This study randomized individuals to chest radiography every 6 months for 3 years or usual practice. Following this phase, all patients underwent chest radiography annually for three additional years. This study design was intended to offset the potential for overdiagnosis bias by detecting indolent cancers in the control group during this latter phase. Unexpectedly, the number of cancers detected in the screened group remained greater than that in the control group for the duration of the study and follow-up. The number of cancers detected by chest radiography during the second phase was nearly identical between groups, while an excess of interval-detected cancers was noted in the screened group, thus lung cancer mortality was not improved by screening in this study.

One study describing the lung cancer screening effort in Japan and employing a case–control study design suggested benefit from lung cancer screening with chest radiography [51]. Unique to this study was the screened population, which was population-based and included a larger number of women and never smokers. This study correlated lung cancer mortality with the interval between the diagnosis of lung cancer and the patient's most recent chest radiograph. While this relationship did not attain statistical significance across the entire study population, the odds ratio of death from lung cancer was lower among women with a short interval between chest radiograph and diagnosis (OR, 0.42; 95% CI, 0.2–0.87). Differences between the men and women with lung cancer were that 85% of the women were never smokers and about 50% were diagnosed with adenocarcinoma, both these features being less common among men.

The most recent update for the United States Preventive Health Services (USPHS), published in 2004, recommends that individuals considering screening for lung cancer should discuss the potential advantages and disadvantages of screening with their physician without making a recommendation for or against such a plan. The report summarized the above studies, in addition to several other randomized and case–control studies. The randomized controlled studies uniformly demonstrated no statistically significant benefit of chest radiography screening on lung cancer mortality but the quality of these studies is not high [39].

There is one ongoing trial evaluating the efficacy of chest radiography for lung cancer screening. The Prostate, Lung, Ovarian, and Colorectal Cancer Trial has enrolled over 100,000 individuals, selected from the general population and randomized to annual chest radiography or usual practice. Over 67,000 normal risk individuals underwent the initial chest radiograph, about 6000 of whom had an abnormal study. Just under 5000 underwent further evaluation, but only 206 eventually underwent biopsy. From these, 126 cancers were diagnosed, 108 of which were nonsmall cell lung cancers, and about half of these were stage I. Additionally observed was a higher incidence of lung cancer in former smokers, even those who had stopped smoking more than 15 years prior to study entry, than in never smokers. Lung cancer mortality results are expected in 2013 [52].

Screening with chest computed tomography

The rapidly improving resolution of chest CT, coupled with its wide availability, have made it an attractive and immediately accessible technique for lung cancer screening. This technique has largely supplanted chest radiography as a lung cancer diagnostic tool by virtue of its superior sensitivity for small pulmonary nodules. Detection of smaller tumors is more likely to result in a stage shift, but will not completely eliminate detection of advanced lung cancer, as a fraction of patients with clinical stage I disease will be found to have lymph node or distant metastases following resection [9].

Preliminary reports have already proven that chest CT is capable of detecting early lung cancer [44]. Long-term follow-up is required to determine the impact of chest CT screening on lung cancer mortality, with results of a large United States trial (the National Lung Screening Trial) anticipated in 2010.

While a number of studies have been conducted that employed chest CT for lung cancer screening, the largest number of patients come from the Early Lung Cancer Action Project (ELCAP) studies, which will be used as a backdrop for the discussion of CT screening. The first ELCAP study enrolled 1000 high-risk individuals, all of whom underwent a baseline chest radiograph and chest CT [53]. At least one pulmonary nodule was identified in 233 patients by chest CT, compared to only 68 by chest radiography. Chest CT detected 136 nodules 2–5 mm in size, compared to 11 detected by chest radiography. The specificity of chest radiography was also poor, as only 33 of the 68 nodules were confirmed by chest CT. Thirty-five percent of nodules detected by chest CT had patterns of benign calcification, representing a low risk of malignancy, and patients with such lesions were referred for annual follow-up. Patients with seven or more nodules were also referred for annual follow-up, as this pattern was defined as diffuse disease with a presumed low risk of malignancy. For patients with six or fewer noncalcified nodules, management was based on the size of the largest nodule, with those 5 mm or smaller being followed by repeat chest CT at 3, 6, 12, and 24 months, and larger ones being referred for biopsy. Only 30 of these 233 patients met the criteria for performance of a biopsy. Twenty-seven patients were diagnosed with lung cancer from these baseline studies, 85% of which were stage I, and two additional patients were diagnosed with cancer prior to the first follow-up scan. Twenty-three stage I tumors were detected by chest CT, compared to only four by chest radiography. These findings led the investigators to abandon the use of chest radiography for the remainder of the study.

The superiority of chest CT over chest radiography has been demonstrated by several other studies. Just under 1500 individuals recruited from a high-risk population in Japan underwent chest radiography and chest CT every 6 months for 2 years

[54]. About 3500 tests were performed, with lung cancer diagnosed in 15 patients by chest CT, but only four by chest radiography. Fourteen of these cancers were stage I. A second study from Japan compared the sensitivity of chest CT, chest radiography, and sputum cytology [55]. A total of 36 cases of lung cancer were detected with these methods over a 5-year period among a population of about 1600 high-risk individuals. Eleven of the 14 cases detected by baseline screening were stage I, compared to 18 of 22 detected during follow-up. Only four of these cases were detected by cytopathology alone, and none were detected only by chest radiography. A third study recruited over 5000 individuals from the general population of Japan, of whom just under 4000 completed the baseline and two annual follow-up scans. A subset of individuals with abnormal scans underwent chest radiography. Twenty-two and 34 patients were diagnosed with lung cancer from baseline and follow-up scans, respectively. A total of five cancers were detected outside the purview of screening tests. Thirty-two of the 34 cancers diagnosed during follow-up were stage I. Only about two-thirds of cancers were visible on chest radiographs reviewed retrospectively [56]. A cohort study from Japan compared the survival of patients with lung cancer detectable on chest radiography with that detectable only by chest CT. Five-year survival was 80% for CT-detected and 39% for chest radiography-detected cancer. Small cancers were more common in the CT-detected group. While this study has limitations due to its design, and lung cancer mortality was not reported, its results are consistent with the studies above [57].

Of the 1000 patients enrolled in ELCAP, 841 underwent at least one annual follow-up CT [16]. New pulmonary nodules were noted in 63 patients, 23 of which, in retrospect, were present on the baseline CT, five of which were not confirmed by high-resolution CT, and five of which occurred in the setting of multiple nodules. The 23 nodules missed on the baseline scan were all less than 5 mm in size. Of the remaining 30 patients, two died of cardiovascular disease prior to further evaluation, and nodule resolution was documented in 12 on 1-month follow-up CT. Half of the remaining 16 patients underwent biopsy, with seven diagnosed with lung cancer, and no evidence of growth on serial CT studies had been noted in the others. Five of the seven cancers were stage I. Two patients presented with symptoms that led to a diagnosis of lung cancer, one of which was nonsmall cell, in the interval between scans. Both of these were endobronchial tumors, one of which was visible on the baseline CT in retrospect, raising concern about the potential suboptimal sensitivity of chest CT for these types of cancers.

The second ELCAP study recruited an additional 1968 individuals, and the results of follow-up scans from this cohort were combined with extended follow-up of the first ELCAP study population [58]. The number of cancers diagnosed from baseline and follow-up scans were 77 and 28, respectively. Three cancers were detected in the interval between scheduled scans. Baseline scans revealed pulmonary nodules necessitating follow-up prior to 1 year in 12% of individuals, while follow-up scans had actionable findings in 6%.

Results from the International Early Lung Cancer Action Project (I-ELCAP) study have recently been reported [13,44]. This study is ongoing, but a total of 31,567 individuals have been enrolled at a number of centers, each with its own inclusion criteria. Baseline and follow-up scans required diagnostic follow-up before 1 year in 13% and 5%, respectively. Biopsies were recommended in 535 patients, with malignancy diagnosed in 492. A total of 484 patients have been diagnosed with nonsmall cell lung cancer, five outside the context of a scheduled scan. Eighty-five percent of these cancers have had no evidence of lymph node or distant metastases, with 87% of tumors being staged surgically. The proportion of cancers with nodal or distant metastases increased with increasing tumor size, from 9% of tumors less than 15 mm in size, to 45% of those 36 mm or larger. This relationship between tumor size and stage was less apparent for part-solid nodules, and no such relationship could be demonstrated for nonsolid nodules. Specifically, none of the nonsolid nodules had evidence of nodal or distant metastases regardless of size. The proportion of early stage cancers within each size grouping is higher in this study than comparable groupings from the SEER database, even when the part- and nonsolid nodules detected in this study are excluded

from the comparison [59]. Five- and ten-year year survival are estimated at about 84% and 80%, respectively, for the entire cohort of patients with lung cancer, with 92% estimated 10-year survival for patients with resected clinical stage I cancer. Operative mortality was 0.5%. None of the eight patients with stage I cancer who did not receive any therapy survived for 5 years.

A study conducted at the Mayo Clinic enrolled just over 1500 individuals who underwent baseline and four annual follow-up chest CT scans and submitted a sample for sputum cytology concurrently [60]. This study employed a four-detector row scanner, and at least one noncalcified pulmonary nodule was found in 74% of the individuals over the course of the study. Of these nodules, 61% were smaller than 4 mm. Nearly 35% of nodules on baseline scans were initially missed and identified only after review at the time of a follow-up scan. Nonsmall cell lung cancer was definitively diagnosed in 57 patients, 29 from the baseline scan, and 28 during follow-up, with up to three of these being diagnosed outside the context of screening tests. Two cancers, one baseline and one follow-up, were detected by sputum cytology alone. Twenty-two of the 29 baseline cancers, and 17 of the 28 follow-up cancers, were stage I. This study protocol obtained a 68% incidence of early stage disease, but 13 individuals underwent negative surgical biopsies, suggesting that the diagnostic algorithm could be further optimized.

The Lung Screening Study (LSS), a pilot study of the National Lung Screening Trial, randomized about 3200 individuals to baseline and 1-year follow-up chest CT or chest radiography screening. Eighteen percent of patients in the CT screening group, compared to 9% in the chest radiography group, had a positive baseline study, defined as at least one noncalcified nodule 4 mm or greater in size, and new findings on the 1-year follow-up study were noted in 18% and 7% of patients in these respective groups. The diagnostic work-up was at the discretion of each patient's primary care physician and resulted in the detection of 40 lung cancers in the chest CT group and 20 in the chest radiography group. In the CT group, 20 cancers were detected at baseline, 8 at 1-year follow-up, and 2 between screening studies, compared to 7 baseline, 9 follow-up, and 4 interval cancers in the chest radiography group. While more early stage cancers were detected with chest CT, the number of advanced cancers was also higher in this group, suggesting that the stage-shift, if any, was no greater with this more sensitive technique than with chest radiography. The investigators recognized the possibility that additional cases of lung cancer would be diagnosed in the chest radiography group over time, but this study was not designed with the goal of long-term follow-up [61]. One other study that recruited 449 high-risk individuals who underwent baseline and two annual follow-up chest CT scans reported a low yield of screening. Two lung cancers were detected on baseline scan, three on follow-up, and one was diagnosed between scans. Only two of these tumors were definitively diagnosed as nonsmall cell lung cancers, both stage I, but the pathologic subtype of the advanced, interval-detected tumor was unknown [62]. The disparate results of the LSS pilot compared to the I-ELCAP study illustrate the impact of the diagnostic management protocol on the efficacy of the screening program. As discussed previously, the major hurdle in lung cancer screening is the high incidence of pulmonary nodules, the vast majority of which, even among high-risk populations, will not be malignant. CT screening programs must therefore be designed to balance safety and efficiency in the subsequent evaluation of these nodules. Again, the ELCAP studies serve as an example of how observations in earlier studies can result in the evolution of more effective diagnostic pathways, the current iteration of which is employed by all centers participating in the I-ELCAP study.

An observation from the first and second ELCAP studies was that, among individuals completing 1 year of follow-up, none of the nodules less than 5 mm on baseline CT scan demonstrated growth on any scans performed through the first annual follow-up, and no diagnoses of cancer were made among nodules of this size within that time frame [7]. A small number of patients with nodules between 5 and 9 mm did experience tumor growth, and were subsequently diagnosed with lung cancer, prior to the 1-year follow-up scan however. In these studies, pulmonary nodules were found on 24% and 38% of scans performed on single- and multidetector scanners, respectively. As about 13% of baseline CT scans demonstrated nodules less than 5 mm in size, the number of scans could have been reduced about 50% by recommending no further follow-up of such nodules until the first annual follow-up, with minimal risk of a delay in diagnosis of lung cancer. This recommendation was incorporated into the I-ELCAP study protocol [63] and served as the basis for the recently published Fleischner Society guidelines for the management of small pulmonary nodules detected by chest CT outside the context of a screening trial. Specifically within these guidelines, repeat chest CT is recommended only after 1 year for nodules less than 5 mm in size in high-risk individuals, and no further evaluation is required for low-risk individuals with such nodules, as the risk of malignancy in this case is less than 1% [64]. A second observation from the first two ELCAP studies was that a significant number of nodules detected on either baseline or follow-up scans resolved or decreased in size, suggesting either an infectious or inflammatory etiology [65]. Some patients, particularly those with multiple or nonsolid nodules, were therefore prescribed antibiotics and underwent a repeat CT within 2 months of the abnormal study. This group of patients was selected for by reviewing all cases in which a patient had undergone a chest CT within 2 months of either a baseline or follow-up CT. Lesions were classified based on appearance as either a nodule or patchy infiltrate and by whether it had been detected on the baseline or a follow-up scan, and the lesions within each subgroup were assessed for change in size within the 2-month follow-up window. Eighty percent of patchy infiltrates decreased in size within 2 months of a baseline scan, and 95% improved within 2 months of a follow-up scan. Only 13% of nodules found on a baseline scan improved within 2 months, but 55% improved if first noted on a follow-up scan. These results led to the recommendation to prescribe antibiotics and obtain a follow-up CT within 2 months in the event that a patchy infiltrate was detected on any scan, or a nodule was newly detected on a follow-up scan, which has been incorporated into the I-ELCAP protocol as an alternative to previously recommended radiographic follow-up based on nodule size.

Several new technologies offer the potential to improve the detection and management of pulmonary nodules in a lung cancer screening program. As noted above, despite the high sensitivity of chest CT for pulmonary nodules, studies report missing 9–34% of small pulmonary nodules [16,60]. Computer-aided diagnosis (CAD) systems have the potential to improve the sensitivity of CT for nodule detection, in particular detection of small, isolated nodules. Currently, such programs are limited by suboptimal sensitivity and specificity, the former hampered by difficulty detecting nodules adjacent to other anatomic structures. While most studies report the sensitivity of these systems below that of radiologists, they can augment the sensitivity of the radiologist interpretation. CAD systems that can help differentiate malignant from benign lesions based on a combination of image characteristics are also in development. Computer-assisted measurement, both in two and three dimensions, is becoming integrated into contemporary screening trials. Volumetric measurement is generally regarded as more accurate than two-dimensional measurement in assessing nodule growth, with inter- and intraobserver variability around 2% for nodules 5 mm or larger [6].

Noninvasive techniques to select patients with suspicious pulmonary nodules for biopsy are in common practice, and include contrast-enhanced CT and positron emission tomography (PET). Malignant lesions are more likely to demonstrate contrast enhancement following intravenous injection of such media. An increase of more than 15 Hounsfield units (HU) is 98% sensitive for malignancy, but the specificity of this cut-point is only 58%. Malignant lesions are also more likely to demonstrate uptake of a radioactively labeled glucose molecule, commonly F-18-fluorodeoxyglucose (FDG). The sensitivity and specificity of this technique have been reported as 90–95% and 80–90%, respectively. Of concern in the context of lung cancer screening, however, is the decreased sensitivity of this technique for nodules less than 1 cm in size, as well as for bronchioloalveolar cell cancers [6]. This limitation notwithstanding, PET has been employed in several lung cancer screening programs. In one study, this technique was employed on nodules 7 mm and

larger, but the mean size of lung cancers was 21 mm on baseline CT scan and 15 mm on follow-up scan. PET scans were performed on 29 of 56 individuals with baseline abnormal CT scans, and 13 of 34 individuals with abnormal follow-up scans. A total of 22 lung cancers were diagnosed, two of which occurred in patients in which PET scanning was not performed. The sensitivity and specificity of PET, in this trial, which defined a positive test as an SUVmax of 2 or above, were 90% and 82%, respectively, with four false-positive and two false-negative PET results, the former of which subjected four patients to unnecessary biopsies [66]. A second study performed PET scans on nodules larger than 10 mm, or 7 mm if demonstrating growth. Of the 911 individuals enrolled, 131 had suspicious nodules at baseline. Nonsmall cell lung cancer was diagnosed in 10 of these patients. Two additional cancers were detected among the 424 patients completing at least one follow-up CT scan. Twenty-five nodules in 23 patients were evaluated with PET. Eleven nodules were positive, defined as any detectable 18-FDG uptake in this study, and 14 were negative. One definite false-positive and four false-negative results were obtained, yielding a sensitivity and specificity of 69% and 91%, respectively, and subjecting only one individual to an unnecessary biopsy. Nine cancers were diagnosed 3 months earlier than they likely would have been had PET scanning not been employed. All nonsmall cell lung cancers were stage I [67].

Another potential refinement is the application of electromagnetic guidance bronchoscopy, in place of percutaneous CT-guided biopsy, in the diagnostic algorithm. Although significant complications have not been reported in CT screening studies, percutaneous biopsy can be associated with a 30% incidence of pneumothorax [68]. While only a minority of patients require any intervention (tube thoracostomy) as a consequence, wider application of CT screening will lead to more biopsies being performed in centers with less experience with this procedure, particularly for the subcentimeter lesions that will be detected. Standard transbronchial biopsy is performed with the use of fluoroscopy, with poor sensitivity for visualization of small lesions detected by CT (even with advanced knowledge of their exact location) and limited ability to guide the biopsy forceps to the lesion of interest, resulting in a yield of 14% for lesions smaller than 2 cm in the periphery (outer third) of the lung. The combination of software to generate three-dimensional images from CT data ("virtual bronchoscopy"), a steerable probe, and a real-time positioning system permits the bronchoscopist to place the probe in a lesion of interest (peripheral lung nodule or lymph node). A biopsy forceps, cytology brush, or needle can then be advanced directly to the site in order to obtain diagnostic specimens. In a study of 60 patients, the yield of this technique for peripheral lung lesions was found to be 74%. The average lesion size was 22.8 mm, although lesion size ranged from 8 to 78 mm. Fifty-seven percent of lesions were smaller than 2 cm, but the number smaller than 1 cm was not reported. The yield was not statistically different between larger and smaller lesions, using cutoffs of 2 cm and 3 cm. Importantly, the distance between the virtual lesion and the actual lesion ranged from 2.9 to 13.8 mm, which has some implications for sampling error with smaller lesions. Pneumothorax occurred in two patients (3.5%) [69].

As is evident from the above, controversy exists over the use of chest CT for lung cancer screening, with some studies showing minimal improvement in the detection of early stage disease, and none of the studies having sufficient long-term follow-up to report lung cancer mortality results. Table 27.1 illustrates the enhanced performance of chest CT over chest radiography in several areas relevant to lung cancer screening, providing support for the continuing study of chest CT screening. Results from two large randomized trials will be available within the next 5 years and are hoped to provide definitive answers regarding the efficacy of chest CT in lung cancer screening. The National Lung Screening Trial enrolled around 50,000 patients who were randomized to annual four-detector row chest CT or chest radiography at study entry and then annually for 2 years. Enrollment was complete in 2004, and the first analysis of lung cancer mortality is expected in 2009 [70]. The Dutch-Belgian NELSON trial is an ongoing multicenter trial in Europe that will enroll about 20,000 individuals who will be randomized to 16-detector row CT at baseline, 1, 2, and 4 years or

Table 27.1 Comparison between chest radiography (CXR) and chest CT screening.

Variable	CXR	CT	References
Pulmonary nodule detected at baseline (%)	7	23	[53]
Nodules missed on baseline exam (%)	19	4	[5,16]
Median size of missed nodules (mm)	16	≤5	[5,16]
Interval cancers (%)	39	6	[44,48]
Clinical stage I cancers (%)			[16,48,53]
Baseline exam	35	85	
Follow-up exam*	58	83	
Estimated survival (%)			[44,48]
5 yr	35	85	
10 yr	30	80	

*Excludes interval cancers.

usual practice. As discussed above, the entry criteria were carefully devised to maximize the number of high-risk patients enrolled [45], and the diagnostic pathway will largely parallel that of the I-ELCAP study, but with the use of volumetric measurement to assess nodule growth. This study opened in 2003 and will be completed in 2010 [71,72].

Direct visualization of abnormal tissue

Unless CT is performed at high resolution, the sensitivity of chest CT for endobronchial tumors may be suboptimal. Bronchoscopy, particularly AFB, can potentially offset this specific weakness. While squamous cell carcinoma has been declining in frequency in the United States and Canada as compared to Europe, this subtype continues to account for a significant fraction of nonsmall cell lung cancers. Incorporating AFB, which is capable of detecting premalignant as well as malignant airway lesions, into a chest CT screening program would likely increase efficacy. Unfortunately, several factors conspire against the cost-effectiveness of this technique, specifically its high cost and high rate of false-positive results.

The principle behind AFB is that normal respiratory mucosa fluoresces green when exposed to light in the blue-violet spectrum (400–450 nm), whereas there is progressive loss of green fluorescence with increasing degrees of cellular atypia, resulting in a red-brown appearance of abnormal mucosa [73]. As about 10% of moderately dysplastic lesions and 40–83% of severely dysplastic ones will progress to invasive cancer, AFB provides an opportunity to detect premalignant lesions that have been shown to be amenable to endobronchial (lung-sparing) therapies. Five-year survival for patients with CIS exceeds 90% when treated with PDT, electrocautery, YAG laser, or surgery [74]. An early study compared the sensitivity of white-light bronchoscopy (WLB) with that of AFB. WLB was performed, followed by AFB, and biopsies were taken from areas that appeared suspicious by each method. Additional biopsies of normal-appearing areas were also taken. The sensitivity of WLB and AFB for detecting areas of moderate dysplasia or worse was 25% and 67%, and the specificity for normal mucosa was 90% and 66%, respectively [75]. In another study, the sensitivity of WLB and AFB for high-grade dysplasia or worse was 40% and 88%, respectively [73]. Two additional studies compared a specific AFB system, LIFE, with WLB in high-risk individuals. One study showed that LIFE was more sensitive than WLB for detecting areas of high-grade dysplasia or worse, with comparable specificity, but all three cancers diagnosed from the group of 55 subjects were also detected by WLB [76]. The second study also demonstrated improved sensitivity of LIFE over WLB for detection of preinvasive lesions [74].

Two studies employed AFB in combination with chest CT for lung cancer screening. The first study enrolled high-risk patients, all of whom had automated quantitative cytometry (AQC) performed on an induced sputum sample. This test quantifies the number of hyperdiploid nuclei per sample, with five or more considered atypical in this study. Patients were subsequently randomized to chest CT with or without AFB. Fourteen lung cancers were detected among the 561 patients. Only one patient with lung cancer had a normal AQC, but 75% of all subjects had an abnormal AQC. Chest CT detected 10 cancers, and AFB detected four [77]. The second study recruited high-risk individuals who underwent sputum cytology, chest CT, and AFB. Thirteen lung cancers, 11 of which were nonsmall cell, were diagnosed among the 169 subjects who completed follow-up. Chest CT was negative in 3 of the 11 nonsmall cell cancers, and AFB was negative in 8 [78]. Together, these studies provide confirmation that the sensitivity of chest CT for endobronchial tumors is poor.

The poor specificity of AFB is, at least in part, due to abnormal fluorescence in areas of inflammation. High-magnification bronchoscopy is a technique that permits characterization of mucosal vascular patterns. This procedure was used to correlate the vascular patterns observed in areas that had previously been examined by AFB with the underlying histopathologic findings at each site. Vascular networks of increased density and complexity characterized dysplastic lesions, and the presence of complex, tortuous vessels was 71% sensitive and 91% specific for dysplasia, as opposed to bronchitis, in areas of abnormal fluorescence [79]. The specificity of AFB may therefore be improved with the concurrent use of high-magnification bronchoscopy.

Due to its poor sensitivity for peripheral lung cancer, AFB cannot be recommended for use as an independent lung cancer screening modality. The studies above demonstrate an improvement in lung cancer detection when this technique is added to chest CT screening however. Cost-effectiveness, patient acceptability, and limited availability are several obstacles that stand in the way of AFB becoming integrated into contemporary lung cancer screening programs. Advances in chest CT technology have result in improved sensitivity for endobronchial tumors, which is likely to restrict the development of AFB to more specialized research or clinical management situations.

Detection of abnormal amounts of or defective DNA

A final approach to lung cancer screening focuses on detection of specific genetic abnormalities or host responses associated with early lung cancer. These methods have been developed for detection of abnormalities present in blood, sputum, bronchoscopic samples, or exhaled breath. While some of these methods would likely be as, if not more, acceptable to patients as chest CT screening, few have demonstrated the ability to selectively identify patients with early stage disease, and none has yet been tested in the context of a screening trial.

Blood

Lung cancer cells have been shown to release DNA into the circulation. A case–control study demonstrated higher levels of circulating DNA in patients with lung cancer compared to controls, including current and former smokers as well as never smokers [80]. Serum DNA levels were measured by quantitative PCR of a sequence of the human telomerase reverse transcriptase gene (*hTERT*). The median value for patients with cancer was 24.3 ng/mL compared to 6.3 for controls. A cutoff value of 4 provided a sensitivity and specificity of 97% and 60%, while a cutoff of 25 resulted in respective values of 46% and 99%. Unfortunately, the amount of circulating DNA did not correlate with pathologic stage, but the median level decreased in patients who underwent tumor resection, and the reduction was greater among those who were relapse-free at follow-up. A study incorporating serum DNA measurements with chest CT is underway.

Promoter hypermethylation is one mechanism whereby gene expression can be silenced and has been observed in tumor suppressor genes of lung cancer cells. In a study including 22 patients with nonsmall cell lung cancer, promoter hypermethylation of at least one of four tumor suppressor genes was noted in 68% of the primary tumors, with 73% of the matched serum samples demonstrating similar abnormalities [81]. Promoter hypermethylation was detected in 70% of stage I, all stage II, and 62% of stage III cancers. The only stage IV cancer and bronchioloalveolar cell cancer both had normal methylation status. Due to the small number of cancers of each stage, it is not possible to draw conclusions about the sensitivity of this technique for the detection of early stage disease, nor was it possible from the data reported to determine the impact of promoter hypermethylation on mortality.

Two other types of genetic abnormalities have been observed in lung cancer cells. Microsatellite instability refers to replication errors in short tandem repeat sequences, and loss of heterozygosity (LOH) refers to deletion of a section of a chromosome. Several studies have attempted to detect these abnormalities in blood samples from patients with lung cancer. In a study including 21 patients with nonsmall cell lung cancer, at least one genetic abnormality was detected in 12 of the primary tumors, and nine of the matched serum samples [82]. Again, due to the small group sizes, no correlation between tumor stage or outcome and the presence of a detectable genetic abnormality could be discerned. A second study evaluated primary tumors and serum samples from 64 patients with stage I–III nonsmall cell lung cancer using a panel of three molecular markers—p53 mutations, fragile histidine triad (FHIT) LOH, and 3p microsatellite instability or LOH [83]. Just over half of the serum samples demonstrated at least one abnormality, but about one-third were negative in the setting of a positive result from the primary tumor. The investigators noted that they had found no false-positive results with this panel among 43 controls, including eight smokers, in a previous study. One other study tested for the presence of microsatellite instability or LOH at several loci in samples from 87 patients with stage nonsmall cell lung cancer and 14 controls [84]. At least one abnormality was detected in 40% of serum samples and 56% of the primary tumors. Abnormal serum samples were found in 43% of stage I compared to 67% of stage IIIB–IV cancers. Forty-five percent of patients with tumors 2 cm or smaller had an abnormal serum sample. Cancer recurrence was detected in 15 patients, but this outcome did not correlate with the presence of an abnormal serum sample.

Tumor-associated antibodies have also been used to detect and screen for lung cancer. Serum from patients with early lung cancer and high-risk controls was used to identify highly discriminatory tumor antigens from a previously generated pool. A test devised from these antigens was applied to blood samples collected from individuals enrolled in the Mayo Clinic CT screening trial. The combination of five of these antigens attained optimal performance, with 83% sensitivity and 87% specificity for the diagnosis of cancer within 5 years [85].

Sputum

Promoter hypermethylation of a number of genes was assessed in sputum samples obtained from patients prior to a diagnosis of lung cancer and matched controls [86]. Abnormalities were detected in the majority of both cases and controls, with the best discrimination between cases and controls observed at six loci. The presence of promoter hypermethylation of three or more of these genes had 65% sensitivity and specificity for the subsequent diagnosis of cancer. This study lends strong but indirect support to the hypothesis that sputum samples will be more sensitive that blood for detecting early lung cancer.

Similar to the above-mentioned tumor-associated antibody approach, tumor antigens can be directly assayed from clinical specimens. One of the better studied tumor antigens is the heterogeneous nuclear ribonucleoprotein A2/B1 (hnRNP A2/B1). Individuals from two high-risk populations, patients who had undergone lung cancer resection and tin miners from China, were enrolled in a study to determine the utility of this antigen for lung cancer surveillance and screening [87]. Sputum samples were examined for cytopathologic changes and stained with a monoclonal antibody against hnRNP A1/B2. Among the patients who had previously undergone lung cancer resection, the presence of this antigen was 77% sensitive and 82% specific for the subsequent diagnosis of lung cancer, compared to respective values of 8% and 100% for cytopathology. Among the group of tin miners, the sensitivity and specificity were 82% and 65% for the presence of the antigen, and 22% and 100% for cytopathology, respectively. A challenge with these cellular techniques is scaling the demanding analysis from a small volume setting to the vast number of evaluations required in a true population-based application. For a variety of biomarker assays this barrier is a significant challenge.

Bronchoscopic samples

The presence of hnRNP A2/B1 was also assessed in bronchoalveolar lavage (BAL) samples from a subset of 195 patients referred to a lung cancer clinic [88]. Cytopathologic examination was performed, and samples demonstrating malignant or metaplas-

tic cells were subjected to antibody staining. Only 1 of 23 samples with malignant cells did not stain positive for hnRNP A2/B1. Eighty of the remaining 172 samples demonstrated metaplastic cells, and 41 stained positive for the antigen. Thirty-three of these individuals were diagnosed with lung cancer at the time of initial evaluation or within 8 months. Of the 39 patients with negative hnRNP A2/B1 staining, only one was subsequently diagnosed with lung cancer.

Fluorescence in situ hybridization (FISH) is a technology that permits visualization of specific gene sequences in cell samples or tissue sections. BAL and bronchoscopic brushing samples from 137 individuals with suspected lung cancer were examined for cytopathologic changes and underwent FISH. Eighty-nine of these individuals were subsequently diagnosed with lung cancer, 71 with non-small cell. The sensitivity and specificity of FISH on BAL samples were 49% and 95%, respectively, with respective values of 71% and 83% for bronchoscopic brushing samples. The sensitivity of cytopathology was intermediate between that of FISH on BAL and bronchoscopic brushing samples. FISH was more sensitive for detecting peripheral tumors, but not for detecting early disease, although the combination of FISH on bronchoscopic brushing samples and cytopathology was more sensitive than cytopathology alone for detecting early disease [89].

BAL samples from patients with lung cancer and controls were assessed for the presence of LOH at eight loci, an abnormality at one or more of which had previously been demonstrated in over 95% of lung cancer cells [90]. LOH at one of four of these loci proved to have the best test performance, attaining 74% sensitivity and 76% specificity. Unfortunately, no association was found between LOH at these loci and tumor stage.

Exhaled breath

The detection of lung cancer based on exhaled breath analysis of volatile organic compounds (VOCs) by a sensor array ("electronic nose") is possible, with one study demonstrating a sensitivity of 71% and specificity of 92% [91]. This study had only small numbers of patients of each stage, and its utility for detection of early stage disease was not

Table 27.2 Points about screening for lung cancer to share with patients.

No data are available from randomized trials, which are ongoing; results are expected in 3–4 yr

Results from observational studies of CT screening among high-risk patients (i.e., those with a history of heavy smoking) indicate a high rate of diagnosis of lung cancer in stage 1 (a relatively curable stage)

CT screening reveals many noncalcified nodules, only a fraction of which will be found to be lung cancer

Costly invasive procedures that are associated with serious risks may be required to evaluate some nodules

A diagnostic workup should be done by physicians experienced in such evaluation

The selection of a facility with physicians who are experienced and credentialed in multidisciplinary fields (including thoracic surgeon, pathology, and pulmonology) is critical to an optimal outcome

The most effective way for smokers to improve their health is to stop smoking

There is an increased risk of subsequent lung cancers after curative resection of lung cancer, so ongoing surveillance is essential

Screening-management trials are available for the evaluation of CT screening

---

Adapted from [18].

specifically addressed. The mass spectrometry backbone of this technique is expensive and not applicable to mass screening at this time.

Conclusion

Screening clearly has the potential to impact mortality in lung cancer, as effective methods, particularly chest CT exist to detect early disease, and surgical resection is associated with long-term survival in this setting. Long-term follow-up from large spiral CT studies is just beginning to emerge. Spiral CT does detect smaller and frequently earlier stage cancers with relatively few missed diagnoses. Concern about overdiagnosis exists, as with other forms of cancer screening, but this is not a contraindication

to early detection research. While the biologic behavior of screening-detected cancers appears to be comparable to that of those detected conventionally, more research about screening benefit in the setting of competing mortality risks among high-risk populations would be useful. Safety and cost-effectiveness concerns are legitimate, but may be ameliorated by the improved diagnostic algorithm arising from the ELCAP studies. Should ongoing trials show that chest CT screening programs are able to decrease lung cancer mortality, additional questions will remain. These include whether incorporation of other techniques, specifically AFB, PET, or serum or lung markers, can improve effectiveness, economy, or safety. Until definitive results are available, however, the recommendations of the American Cancer Society [92] and United States Preventive Health Service [39] are appropriate. Individuals considering screening should discuss the risks and potential benefits with an experienced healthcare provider and have screening performed in the context of a multidisciplinary program for the evaluation and management of high-risk individuals (Table 27.2).

References

1 Bastarrika G, Pueyo J, Mulshine J. Radiologic screening for lung cancer. *Expert Rev Anticancer Ther* 2002; **2**:385–92.

2 Ries L, Harkins D, Krapcho M *et al. SEER Cancer Statistics Review, 1975–2003*, Vol. 2006. Bethesda, MD: National Cancer Institute, 2006.

3 Society AC. *Cancer Facts and Figures 2006*. Atlanta: American Cancer Society, 2006.

4 Hirsch F, Franklin W, Gazdar A, Bunn P. Early detection of lung cancer: clinical perspectives of recent advances in biology and radiology. *Clin Cancer Res* 2001; **7**:5–22.

5 Quekel L, Kessels A, Goei R, van Engelshoven J. Miss rate of lung cancer on the chest radiograph in clinical practice. *Chest* 1999; **115**:720–4.

6 Ko J. Lung nodule detection and characterization with multi-slice CT. *J Thorac Imaging* 2005; **20**:196–209.

7 Henschke C, Yankelevitz D, Naidich D *et al.* CT screening for lung cancer: suspiciousness of nodules according to size on baseline scans. *Radiology* 2004; **231**:164–8.

8 Gordis L. *Epidemiology*. Philadelphia: W.B. Saunders Company, 2000:258–76.

9 Mountain C. Revisions in the international system for staging lung cancer. *Chest* 1997; **111**:1710–7.

10 Martini N, Bains M, Burt M *et al.* Incidence of local recurrence and second primary tumors in resected stage I lung cancer. *J Thorac Cardiovasc Surg* 1995; **109**:120–9.

11 Port J, Kent M, Korst R, Libby D, Pasmantier M, Altorki N. Tumor size predicts survival within stage IA non-small cell lung cancer. *Chest* 2003; **124**:1828–33.

12 Flieder D, Port J, Korst R *et al.* Tumor size is a determinant of stage distribution in T1 non-small cell lung cancer. *Chest* 2005; **128**:2304–8.

13 Yankelevitz D. *International Early Lung Cancer Action Program I-ELCAP*. Chicago, IL, 2006.

14 Asamura H, Suzuki K, Watanabe S, Matsuno Y, Maeshima A, Tsuchiya R. A clinicopathological study of resected subcentimeter lung cancers: a favorable prognosis for ground glass opacity lesions. *Ann Thorac Surg* 2003; **76**:1016–22.

15 Wisnivesky J, Yankelevitz D, Henschke C. The effect of tumor size on curability of stage I non-small cell lung cancers. *Chest* 2004; **126**:761–5.

16 Henschke C, Naidich D, Yankelevitz D *et al.* Early lung cancer action project: initial findings on repeat screening. *Cancer* 2001; **92**:153–9.

17 Ost D, Fein A, Feinsilver S. The solitary pulmonary nodule. *N Engl J Med* 2003; **348**:2535–42.

18 Mulshine J, Sullivan D. Lung cancer screening. *N Engl J Med* 2005; **352**:2714–20.

19 Yankelevitz D, Reeves A, Kostis W, Zhao B, Henschke C. Small pulmonary nodules: volumetrically determined growth rates based on CT evaluation. *Radiology* 2000; **217**:251–6.

20 Miller D, Rowland C, Deschamps C, Allen M, Trastek V, Pairolero P. Surgical treatment of non-small cell lung cancer 1 cm of less in diameter. *Ann Thorac Surg* 2002; **73**:1545–51.

21 Okada M, Koike T, Higashiyama M, Yamato Y, Kodama K, Tsubota N. Radical sublobar resection for small-sized non-small cell lung cancer: a multicenter study. *J Thorac Cardiovasc Surg* 2006; **132**:769–75.

22 Suzuki K, Asamura H, Kusumoto M, Kondo H, Tsuchiya R. "Early" peripheral lung cancer: prognostic significance of ground glass opacity on thin-section computed tomographic scan. *Ann Thorac Surg* 2002; **74**:1635–9.

23 Yamato Y, Tsuchida M, Watanabe T *et al.* Early results of a prospective study of limited resection for bronchioloalveolar adenocarcinoma of the lung. *Ann Thorac Surg* 2001; **71**:971–4.

24 Brenner D. Radiation risks potentially associated with low-dose CT screening of adult smokers for lung cancer. *Radiology* 2004; **231**:440–5.

25 Wisnivesky J, Mushlin A, Sicherman N, Henschke C. The cost-effectiveness of low-dose CT screening for lung cancer: preliminary results of baseline screening. *Chest* 2003; **124**:614–21.

26 Mahadevia P, Fleisher L, Frick K, Eng J, Goodman S, Powe N. Lung cancer screening with helical computed tomography in older adult smokers: a decision and cost-effectiveness analysis. *JAMA* 2003; **289**:313–22.

27 Manser R, Dalton A, Carter R, Byrnes G, Elwood M, Campbell D. Cost-effectiveness analysis of screening for lung cancer with low dose spiral CT (computed tomography) in the Australian setting. *Lung Cancer* 2005; **48**:171–85.

28 Mulshine J, Tockman M, Smart C. Considerations in the development of lung cancer screening tools. *J Natl Cancer Inst* 1989; **81**:900–6.

29 Marcus P, Bergstralh E, Zweig M, Harris A, Offord K, Fontana R. Extended lung cancer incidence follow-up in the Mayo Lung Project and overdiagnosis. *J Natl Cancer Inst* 2006; **98**:748–56.

30 Strauss G, Gleason R, Sugarbaker D. Chest x-ray screening improves outcome in lung cancer. A reappraisal of randomized trials on lung cancer screening. *Chest* 1995; **107**:270–9.

31 Roberts P, Straznicka M, Lara P *et al.* Resection of multifocal non-small cell lung cancer when the bronchioloalveolar subtype is involved. *J Thorac Cardiovasc Surg* 2003; **126**:1597–602.

32 Ebright M, Zakowski M, Martin J *et al.* Clinical pattern and pathologic stage but not histologic features predict outcome for bronchioloalveolar carcinoma. *Ann Thorac Surg* 2002; **74**:1640–7.

33 Flieder D, Vazquez M, Carter D *et al.* Pathologic findings of lung tumors diagnosed on baseline CT screening. *Am J Surg Pathol* 2006; **30**:606–13.

34 Henschke C, Shaham D, Yankelevitz D *et al.* CT screening for lung cancer: significance of diagnoses in its baseline cycle. *J Clin Imaging* 2006; **30**:11–15.

35 Motohiro A, Ueda H, Komatsu H, Yanai N, Mori T. Prognosis of non-surgically treated, clinical stage I lung cancer patients in Japan. *Lung Cancer* 2002; **36**:65–9.

36 Sobue T, Suzuki T, Matsuda M, Kuroishi T, Ikeda S, Naruke T. Survival for clinical stage I lung cancer not surgically treated: comparison between screen-detected and symptom-detected cases. *Cancer* 1992; **69**:685–92.

37 Vrdoljak E, Mise K, Sapunar D, Rozga A, Marusic M. Survival analysis of untreated patients with non-small-cell lung cancer. *Chest* 1994; **106**:1797–800.

38 Capewell S, Sudlow M. Performance and prognosis in patients with lung cancer: the Edinburgh Lung Cancer Group. *Thorax* 1990; **45**:951–6.

39 Humphrey L, Teutsch S, Johnson M. Lung cancer screening with sputum cytologic examination, chest radiography, and computed tomography: an update for the US Preventive Services Task Force. *Ann Intern Med* 2004; **140**:740–53.

40 Enstrom J. Smoking cessation and mortality trends among two United States populations. *J Clin Epidemiol* 1999; **52**:813–25.

41 Ganti A, Mulshine J. Lung cancer screening. *Oncologist* 2006; **11**:481–7.

42 van Klaveren R, de Koning H, Mulshine J, Hirsch F. Lung cancer screening by spiral CT: what is the optimal target population for screening trials? *Lung Cancer* 2002; **38**:243–52.

43 Haiman C, Stram D, Wilkins L *et al.* Ethnic and racial differences in the smoking-related risk of lung cancer. *N Engl J Med* 2006; **354**:333–42.

44 Henschke C, Yankelevitz D, Libby D, Pasmantier M, Smith J, Miettinen O. Survival of patients with stage I lung cancer detected on CT screening. *N Engl J Med* 2006; **355**:1763–71.

45 van Iersel C, de Koning H, Draisma G *et al.* Risk-based selection for the general population in a screening trial: selection criteria, recruitment and power for the Dutch-Belgian randomised lung cancer multi-slice CT screening trial (NELSON). *Int J Cancer* 2007; **120**:868–74.

46 Brett G. Earlier diagnosis and survival in lung cancer. *Br Med J* 1969; **4**:260–2.

47 Fontana R, Sanderson D, Woolner L *et al.* Screening for lung cancer: a critique of the Mayo Lung Project. *Cancer* 1991; **67**:1155–64.

48 Melamed M, Flehinger B, Zaman M, Heelan R, Perchick W, Martini N. Screening for early lung cancer: results of the Memorial Sloan-Kettering Study in New York. *Chest* 1984; **86**:44–53.

49 Tockman M. Survival and mortality from lung cancer in a screened population. *Chest* 1986; **89**:324S.

50 Kubik A, Parkin D, Khlat M, Erban J, Polak J, Adamec M. Lack of benefit from semi-annual screening for cancer of the lung: follow-up report of a randomized controlled trial on a population of high-risk males in Czechoslovakia. *Int J Cancer* 1990; **45**:26–33.

51 Sobue T, Suzuki T, Naruke T. A case–control study for evaluating lung-cancer screening in Japan. *Int J Cancer* 1992; **50**:230–7.

52 Oken M, Marcus P, Hu P *et al.* Baseline chest radiograph for lung cancer detection in the randomized prostate, lung, colorectal and ovarian cancer screening trial. *J Natl Cancer Inst* 2005; **97**:1832–9.

53 Henschke C, McCauley D, Yankelevitz D *et al.* Early lung cancer action project: overall design and findings from baseline screening. *Lancet* 1999; **354**:99–105.

54 Kaneko M, Eguchi K, Ohmatsu H *et al.* Peripheral lung cancer: screening and detection with low-dose spiral CT versus radiography. *Radiology* 1996; **201**:798–802.

55 Sobue T, Moriyama N, Kaneko M *et al.* Screening for lung cancer with low-dose helical computed tomography: Anti-Lung Cancer Association Project. *J Clin Oncol* 2002; **20**:911–20.

56 Sone S, Li F, Yang Z-G *et al.* Results of three-year mass screening programme for lung cancer using mobile low-dose spiral computed tomography scanner. *Br J Cancer* 2001; **84**:25–32.

57 Kashiwabara K, Kohshi S. Outcome in patients with lung cancer invisible on chest roentgenograms but detected only by helical computed tomography. *Respirology* 2006; **11**:592–7.

58 Henschke C, Yankelevitz D, Smith J *et al.* CT screening for lung cancer: assessing a regimen's diagnostic performance. *J Clin Imaging* 2004; **28**:317–21.

59 Henschke C, Yankelevitz D, Miettinen O. Computed tomographic screening for lung cancer: the relationship of disease stage to tumor size. *Arch Intern Med* 2006; **166**:321–5.

60 Swensen S, Jett J, Hartman T *et al.* CT screening for lung cancer: five-year prospective experience. *Radiology* 2005; **235**:259–65.

61 Gohagan J, Marcus P, Fagerstrom R *et al.* Final results of the lung screening study, a randomized feasibility study of spiral CT versus chest X-ray screening for lung cancer. *Lung Cancer* 2005; **47**:9–15.

62 MacRedmond R, McVey G, Lee M *et al.* Screening for lung cancer using low dose CT scanning: results of 2 year follow up. *Thorax* 2006; **61**:54–6.

63 IELCAP (International Early Lung Cancer Action Program). *Enrollment and Screening Protocol*, New York, 2006.

64 MacMahon H, Austin J, Gamsu G *et al.* Guidelines for management of small pulmonary nodules detected on CT scans: a statement from the Fleischner Society. *Radiology* 2005; **237**:395–400.

65 Libby D, Wu N, Lee I *et al.* CT screening for lung cancer: the value of short-term CT follow-up. *Chest* 2006; **129**:1039–42.

66 Pastorino U, Bellomi M, Landoni C *et al.* Early lung-cancer detection with spiral CT and positron emission tomography in heavy smokers: 2-year results. *Lancet* 2003; **362**:593–7.

67 Bastarrika G, Garcia-Velloso M, Lozano M *et al.* Early lung cancer detection using spiral computed tomography and positron emission tomography. *Am J Respir Crit Care Med* 2005; **171**:1378–83.

68 Tan B, Flaherty K, Kazerooni E, Iannettoni M. The solitary pulmonary nodule. *Chest* 2003; **123**:89–96.

69 Gildea T, Mazzone P, Karnak D, Meziane M, Mehta A. Electromagnetic navigation diagnostic bronchoscopy: a prospective study. *Am J Respir Crit Care Med* 2006; **174**:982–9.

70 Institute NC. *National Lung Screening Trial*, Vol. 2006. Bethesda, MD: National Cancer Institute, 2006.

71 Mulshine J. Screening for lung cancer: in pursuit of pre-metastatic disease. *Nat Rev Cancer* 2003; **3**:65–73.

72 Xu D, Gietema H, de Koning H *et al.* Nodule management protocol of the NELSON randomised lung cancer screening trial. *Lung Cancer* 2006; **54**:177–84.

73 Feller-Kopman D, Lunn W, Ernst A. Autofluorescence bronchoscopy and endobronchial ultrasound: a practical review. *Ann Thorac Surg* 2005; **80**:2395–401.

74 Lam S, MacAulay C, leRiche J, Palcic B. Detection and localization of early lung cancer by fluorescence bronchoscopy. *Cancer* 2000; **89**:2468–73.

75 Lam S, Kennedy T, Unger M *et al.* Localization of bronchial intraepithelial neoplastic lesions by fluorescence bronchoscopy. *Chest* 1998; **113**:696–702.

76 Hirsch F, Prindiville S, Miller Y *et al.* Fluorescence versus white-light bronchoscopy for detection of preneoplastic lesions: a randomized study. *J Natl Cancer Inst* 2001; **93**:1385–91.

77 McWilliams A, Mayo J, MacDonald S *et al.* Lung cancer screening: a different paradigm. *Am J Respir Crit Care Med* 2003; **168**:1167–73.

78 Loewen G, Natarajan N, Tan D *et al.* Autofluorescence bronchoscopy for lung cancer surveillance based on risk assessment. *Thorax* 2007; **62**:335–40.

79 Shibuya K, Hoshino H, Chiyo M *et al.* Subepithelial vascular patterns in bronchial dysplasias using a high-magnification bronchovideoscope. *Thorax* 2002; **57**:902–7.

80 Sozzi G, Conte D, Leon M *et al.* Quantification of free circulating DNA as a diagnostic marker in lung cancer. *J Clin Oncol* 2003; **21**:3902–8.

81 Esteller M, Sanchez-Cespedes M, Rosell R, Sidransky D, Baylin S, Herman J. Detection of aberrant promoter hypermethylation of tumor suppressor genes in serum DNA from non-small cell lung cancer patients. *Cancer Res* 1999; **59**:67–70.

82 Cuda G, Gallelli A, Nistico A *et al.* Detection of microsatellite instability and loss of heterozygosity in serum DNA of small and non-small cell lung cancer patients: a tool for early diagnosis? *Lung Cancer* 2000; **30**:211–4.

83 Andriani F, Conte D, Mastrangelo T *et al.* Detecting lung cancer in plasma with the use of multiple genetic markers. *Int J Cancer* 2004; **108**:91–6.

84 Sozzi G, Musso K, Ratcliffe C, Goldstraw P, Pierotti M, Pastorino U. Detection of microsatellite alterations in plasma DNA of non-small cell lung cancer patients: a prospect for early diagnosis. *Clin Cancer Res* 1999; **5**:2689–92.

85 Zhong L, Coe S, Stromberg A, Khattar N, Jett J, Hirschowitz E. Profiling tumor-associated antibodies for early detection of non-small cell lung cancer. *J Thorac Oncol* 2006; **1**:513–9.

86 Belinsky S, Liechty K, Gentry F *et al.* Promoter hypermethylation of multiple genes in sputum precedes lung cancer incidence in a high-risk cohort. *Cancer Res* 2006; **66**:3338–44.

87 Tockman M, Mulshine J, Piantadosi S *et al.* Prospective detection of preclinical lung cancer: results from two studies of heterogeneous nuclear ribonucleoprotein A2/B1 overexpression. *Clin Cancer Res* 1997; **3**:2237–46.

88 Fielding P, Turnbull L, Prime W, Walshaw M, Field J. Heterogeneous nuclear ribonucleoprotein A2/B1 up-regulation in bronchial lavage specimens: a clinical marker of early lung cancer detection. *Clin Cancer Res* 1999; **5**:4048–52.

89 Halling K, Rickman O, Kipp B, Harwood A, Doerr C, Jett J. A comparison of cytology and fluorescence in situ hybridization for the detection of lung cancer in bronchoscopic specimens. *Chest* 2006; **130**:694–701.

90 Liloglou T, Maloney P, Xinarianos G *et al.* Cancer-specific genomic instability in bronchial lavage: a molecular tool for lung cancer detection. *Cancer Res* 2001; **61**:1624–8.

91 Machado R, Laskowski D, Deffenderfer O *et al.* Detection of lung cancer by sensor array analyses of exhaled breath. *Am J Respir Crit Care Med* 2005; **171**:1286–91.

92 Society AC. *Detailed Guide: Lung Cancer—Non-Small Cell*, Vol. 2006. Atlanta: American Cancer Society, 2006.

CHAPTER 28

Natural Agents for Chemoprevention of Lung Cancer

Amir Sharafkhaneh, Suryakanta Velamuri, Seyed Javad Moghaddam, Vladimir Badmaev, Burton Dickey, and Jonathan Kurie

Introduction

Lung cancer is the most common type of cancer and the leading cause of cancer death in adults. Tobacco smoking is the major risk factor leading to lung cancer and an important risk factor for cancer in general. Furthermore, the presence of chronic obstructive pulmonary disease (COPD) increases the risk of lung cancer. Chronic inflammation, such as occurs with COPD, plays a role in epithelial carcinogenesis. In fact, data have suggested that airway and parenchymal inflammation is the link between tobacco smoke and lung cancer. However, much is yet to be learned about the role of inflammation, the major biochemical factors involved in the translation of this effect to cancer, and what factors, in concert with smoking, put an individual at increased risk.

Intervention in the form of chemoprevention is an attractive approach to reducing the number of deaths caused by lung cancer. Notably, recent results have shown the beneficial effects of chemoprevention for breast, colon, and prostate cancers. However, the available data on the chemoprevention of lung cancer have thus far not been promising [1]. Recent data have suggested that natural agents with a significant anti-inflammatory effect may reduce the occurrence of carcinogenesis and play a chemopreventive role while also providing the necessary safety profile for long-term use. An ideal natural agent to use in lung cancer chemoprevention is one that reduces the incidence of the lung cancer at a safe dose range and duration. In this chapter, we briefly review the role of inflammation in lung cancer and then review the potential natural agents that may be useful as chemopreventive intervention in lung cancer.

The relation between consumption of vegetables and fruits and daily supplementation with plant compounds in lowering risk of respiratory pathology and malignancy has been well established [2–7]. The lower risk with consumption of vegetables and fruits is consistently seen for the both sexes and strata of age, education, alcohol and tobacco consumption, and total nonalcohol energy intake [2]. In one study, low intakes of vegetable and fruit were contributing factors in 65% and 54%, respectively, of oral and pharyngeal cancer cases [3]. While a diet rich in eggs, red meat, and processed meat increased the risk of oral and pharyngeal cancer, the addition of fruits and/or vegetables to the diet and diet diversity were inversely related to the risk of oral and pharyngeal cancer [3]. Furthermore, there is epidemiological evidence of beneficial effect of high intake of vegetables and fruits, particularly in heavy smokers and alcohol drinkers [4].

Lung Cancer, 3rd edition. Edited by Jack A. Roth, James D. Cox, and Waun Ki Hong. © 2008 Blackwell Publishing. ISBN: 978-1-4051-5112-2.

Additionally, the risk of lung cancer for persons who seldom consumed vegetables and/or fruits was about twice that of those who consumed vegetables and/or fruits frequently, both among nonsmokers, smokers, and former smokers after adjustment for the amount of tobacco exposure [5]. Increasing levels of intake of fruit and vegetables showed a favorable effect on the prognosis in lung cancer patients [6].

It has been recognized that the response to any cancer prevention or therapy may depend on the genetic predisposition of the patient [7]. Accordingly, the role of cruciferous vegetables in lung cancer was studied after stratifying by GSTM1 and GSTT1 status, two genes implicated in the elimination of isothiocyanates. Isothiocyanates are principal chemopreventive compounds derived from cruciferous vegetables. Weekly consumption of cruciferous vegetables protected against lung cancer in people who were GSTM1 null, GSTT1 null, or both. No protective effect was seen in those who were both GSTM1 and GSTT1 positive [7].

The benefit–risk ratio of the natural chemopreventive and/or chemotherapeutic compounds should be carefully considered, since the mechanisms by which they inhibit carcinogenesis are incompletely understood [8]. Experimental data indicate that some compounds may inhibit certain cancers while being ineffective against or even promoting other forms of cancer. This phenomenon is sometimes referred to as speciation of the compound, i.e., inherent mechanism of a nutrient for a specific cancer. Therefore, any prevention or intervention guidelines with natural compounds should be carefully applied based on the type of tumor, ethnic variations, and the complete data on efficacy and safety of the compounds and potential drug–nutrient interaction.

The use of selected plants and plant compounds, including botanicals and minerals, will be briefly discussed in this overview as preventive and/or therapeutic measures in respiratory cancer based on the potential mechanism and data on in vitro, preclinical and clinical use. Table 28.1 provides a summary list of natural agents and their mechanism(s) of action.

Table 28.1 Natural agents with potential in cancer chemoprevention.

Mechanism	Agent
CYP enzyme modifiers	Resveratrol
	Indole-3-carbinol
	Hypericin
	Piperine
	Quercitine
	Z-guggulsterone and E-guggulsterone
Cyclooxygenase-2 enzyme inhibitors	Curcumin
	Gingerol,
	Beta-elemene
	Zerumbone
	Catechins
	Berberine
NF-κB inhibitors	Curcumin
	Boswellic acids
	Guggulsterone Z and E and ferulates
	Genistein and daidzein
	Glabridin and glycyrrhetic acid
	Casuarinin
Enhancement of selenoproteins	Selenium
Adaptogen mechanism	Whitanolids
	Ginsenosides

Cytochrome P450 enzyme modifiers

Resveratrol

Resveratrol (trans-3,4′,5-trihydroxystilbene) is phytoalexin, a diphenolic antioxidant found in grapes, mulberry, and numerous other plants and in plant-derived products, especially red wine. Resveratrol may possess broad anticancer properties, as indicated by its striking inhibition of diverse cellular events associated with tumor initiation, promotion, and progression. An in vitro study performed with the human bronchial epithelial cell line BEP2D showed that resveratrol has chemopreventive and chemotherapeutic potential by regulation of the constitutive and the induced expression of metabolizing enzymes: CYP1A1 and CYP1B1 genes' expressions were inhibited in metabolism of polycyclic aromatic hydrocarbons, whereas expression of the mEH (microsomal epoxide hydrolase) gene was increased in response to resveratrol with no change in the expression of GSTP1 (glutathione S-transferase P1) gene [9]. Dietary flavonoids, including resveratrol, were tested for their effect on CYP1A1 expression in vitro. Human hepatocytes were treated with resveratrol, apigenin, curcumin, kaempferol, green tea extract (GTE), (−)-epigallocatechin gallate (EGCG), quercetin, and naringenin. Of these flavonoids, resveratrol produced the greatest increase in CYP activation [10]. Oxyresveratrol, a derivative of resveratrol found in mulberry wood, may have higher biological potential with lower toxicity as assessed in in vitro experiments [11].

Indole-3-carbinol

Indole-3-carbinol (I-3-C) is a natural chemopreventive and chemotherapeutic compound derived from vegetables of the Cruciferae family, such as cabbage and broccoli. The I-3-C-receptor complex activates the gene of CYP1A1 enzyme (isoenzyme of cytochrome P450-dependent monoamine oxidase), which enhances the 2-hydroxylation of selected estrogens and leads to inactivation of certain carcinogens. The lowered level of estrogens inhibits the growth of hormone-dependent tumors or prevents their appearance. The I-3-C also inhibits expression of the cyclin-dependent kinase 6 (CDK6) by indole-3-carbinol, leading to cell cycle arrest in G1 phase [12]. In a preclinical experiment, pretreatment with I-3-C of A/J mice previously challenged with a tobacco-specific nitrosamine (NNK), a potent lung carcinogen in these mice, resulted in inhibition of tumor multiplicity, decreased DNA adducts in lung, and increased DNA adducts in liver, due to induction of hepatic activation of NNK. Reducing NNK-induced lung tumorigenesis and decreased delivery of NNK to lung has been explained as a result of enhanced hepatic CYP activity with the I-3-C [13].

Hypericin

Hypericin is a compound derived from plants of the genus *Hypericum*, most commonly from St John's wort (*Hypericum perforatum* L.). Hypericin exerts inhibitory effects on enzymes such as MAO (monoaminoxidase), PKC (protein kinase C), dopamine-beta-hydroxylase, reverse transcriptase, telomerase and CYP (cytochrome P450) [14]. The effect on CYP enzymes may be inhibitory (e.g., CYP2C6) or stimulatory (e.g., CYP2D2 and CYP3A2) [15]. In an in vitro experiment, hypericin blocked cigarette smoke condensate (CSC)-induced tumor metastases by blocking activity of PKC. CSC is known to increase invasion and metastasis of tumor cells by activating PKC [16]. Hypericin is a photosensitizing compound. Its tumoricidal properties with photodynamic therapy reduced primary tumor development and significantly prolonged the survival of tumor-bearing mice with a highly metastatic adenocarcinoma (DA3Hi) and anaplastic squamous cell carcinoma tumors in vivo [17].

Most recent studies indicate that in vitro treatment of NIH-H460 human lung cancer cells with *Hypericum* plant extract modulates subcellular localization of retinoid X receptor-alpha (RXRα) (relocalization of RXRα from the nucleus to the cytoplasm) and induces cancer cell apoptosis [18].

Piperine

Piperine is a pungent principle and alkaloid found in fruits of black pepper, *Piper nigrum* Linn, and long pepper, *Piper longum* Linn, inhibits both the drug transporter P-glycoprotein and the major xenobiotic-metabolizing enzyme CYP3A4. Piperine administration to mice with benzo[a]pyrene-induced tumors significantly increased the activities of mitochondrial enzymes [19].

In another study, dietary supplementation of piperine to mice administered benzo(a)pyrene decreased the total protein and protein-bound carbohydrate (hexose, hexosamine, and sialic acid) levels of lung cancer-bearing animals in initiation and postinitiation phases. Piperine may exert its chemopreventive and chemotherapeutic mechanism in experimental lung cancer by lowering protein bound carbohydrate levels, one of the indicators of tumorigenesis [20]. In another related study of experimental lung cancer, supplementation with piperine enhanced the phase II detoxification enzymes, showed antiperoxidative effects, reduced DNA damage, and decreased DNA–protein cross links in animals with lung cancer [21].

Quercitine

Quercitine is a bioflavonoid, a polyphenolic compound widely distributed in the plant kingdom and concentrated in fruits and vegetables. The intake of quercetin is inversely related to the lung cancer incidence. In an in vitro study, quercetin inhibited CYP1A1 enzyme and bioactivation of certain pro-carcinogens [22]. In an in vivo study, after 90 days of administration of quercetin to mice challenged with benzo[a]pyrene, the degree of pulmonary precancerous pathologic changes in the quercetin-treated animals decreased significantly compared with the control group. The cytochrome CYP1A1-linked activities in lung of the mice decreased as the dose of quercetin increased [22]. In a separate in vitro study, quercetin decreased apoptosis via caspase-3 cascade in a dose and time-dependent manner in a human lung cancer cell line NCI-H209 [23].

Numerous plants, foods, and derived compounds have the potential to inhibit the metabolizing activity of the P450 (CYP) enzymes. An in vitro study evaluated the inhibitory potential of plant extracts on six major human drug-metabolizing enzymes, i.e., CYP1A2/2C8/2C9/2C19/2D6 and 3A4. The following plant extracts were identified as CYP inhibitors: devil's claw root (*Harpagophytum procumbens*), feverfew herb (*Tanacetum parthenium*), fo-ti root (*Polygonum multiflorum*), kava–kava root (*Piper methysticum*), peppermint oil (*Mentha piperita*), eucalyptus oil (*Eucalyptus globulus*), red clover blossom (*Trifolium pratense*), and grapefruit juice (*Citrus paradisi*) [24].

Z-guggulsterone and E-guggulsterone

Z-guggulsterone and E-guggulsterone, plant sterols from myrrh gum–resin of the guggul tree, *Commiphora muku* Wighti, exemplify natural compounds with chemopreventive and chemotherapeutic potential and which preferentially stimulate CYP enzymes. In vitro study showed that guggulsterone-mediated activation of the pregnane X receptor (PXR) induced the expression of CYP3A genes in both rodent and human hepatocytes [25]. Plants showing stimulatory effects on phase I and II enzyme systems included *Tinospora cordifolia* Miers and *Adathoda vasica* Ness [26].

Natural agents with anti-inflammatory effect

A large amount of epidemiologic data supports the role of chronic inflammation in epithelial carcinogenesis. The strongest association has been found in the gastrointestinal tract, where chronic ulcerative colitis leads to a greatly increased incidence of colon cancer, and chronic infection of the stomach with the bacterium *Helicobacter pylori* leads to stomach cancer [27]. In the lung, more than 10 separate studies have found that smokers with COPD, an inflammatory disease of the airways and alveoli, have an increased risk of lung cancer (1.3- to 4.9-fold) compared with smokers with comparable cigarette exposure but without COPD [28–30]. Despite the fact that smoking causes most cases of COPD, only 15–20% of smokers develop COPD, and the variable susceptibility to COPD is thought to reflect genetic variation in the inflammatory response to inhaled smoke and to microorganisms colonizing the injured airways of smokers [31,32].

Evidence for a role for inflammation in mouse models of lung cancer comes from both loss-of-function and gain-of-function experiments [33]. In models in which an activated K-ras allele is selectively expressed in airway secretory cells, an inflammatory infiltrate composed mostly of macrophages and neutrophils accompanies the development of adenenocarcinoma, suggesting that recruitment of inflammatory cells contributes to tumor progression [34,35]. This is supported by a reduction in tumor progression with neutralizing antibody against CXCR2 [36]. Further, mice deficient in neutrophil elastase showed reduced tumor progression, pointing to the contribution of a specific inflammatory cell macromolecule [37]. In a gain-of-function experiment, mice expressing activated K-ras in airway secretory cells that were exposed repetitively to an aerosolized lysate of nontypeable *Hemophilus influenza* showed increased tumor progression [38], indicating that tumor-induced inflammatory mechanisms are not fully sufficient to support maximal tumor progression in the K-ras model and supporting a causal link underlying the epidemiologic data relating COPD and lung cancer. The inflammatory response to cigarette smoke and microbial pathogens could potentially activate multiple growth-promoting and antiapoptotic pathways, and precise elucidation of the causal roles of these pathways in tumor progression could provide targets for lung cancer prevention. Because many natural agents have anti-inflammatory properties, targeting inflammation with natural agents is one preventive strategy that can be considered. The following is a partial list of natural agents that share the ability to inhibit inflammation through diverse actions on proinflammatory mediators including NFκB, cyclooxygenase-2 (COX-2), cytokines, and others. While we have grouped them together for the purposes of this review, many of these agents have other biological properties and thus are not strictly anti-inflammatory agents.

Curcumin and curcuminoids

Curcumin (diferuloylmethane), a β-diketone derived from the plant *Curcuma longa*, has substantial properties that make it an excellent potential agent in cancer chemoprevention. Tumorigenesis is a multistep pathway, and the potential of curcumin as a chemopreventive agent stems from its ability to inhibit various processes in this pathway, from tumor initiation to tumor progression. This includes effects on signaling mechanisms, angiogenesis, nuclear transcription, and apoptosis. Curcumin has potent antioxidant and anti-inflammatory properties, which may also play an important role in its anticarcinogenic effect.

Chemoprevention of lung cancer: Many authors have found that curcumin alters the metabolic activation and detoxification of mutagens. In lung cancer specifically, curcumin inhibits the mutagenicities of unfractionated mainstream cigarette smoke. In mouse tissues, topical pretreatment with curcumin decreased the levels of bulky aromatic DNA adducts generated by exposure to total particulate matter from smoke of cigarettes. Kalpana and Menon evaluated the protective effects of curcumin on lipid peroxidation and antioxidant status in BAL fluid and specimens from nicotine-treated Wistar rats. The results suggested that curcumin exerts its protective effect against nicotine-induced lung toxicity by modulating biochemical marker enzymes and lipid

peroxidation and by augmenting the antioxidant defense system [39,40].

Biochemical effects in cells: Curcumin affects signaling mechanisms critical for tumor growth, including expression and activation of some receptor tyrosine kinases. Her2/neu, a receptor tyrosine kinase member of the epidermal growth factor receptor family, is overexpressed in different types of tumors, including breast cancer. Curcumin inhibits the level of protein expression and the tyrosine kinase activity of HER2/neu in HER2/neu-overexpressing cells and other tumor cell lines [41].

Curcumin inhibits endothelial and vascular smooth muscle cell proliferation and invasion in vitro and angiogenesis in vivo. Curcumin inhibits the expression of the adhesion molecules ICAM-1, VCAM-1, and E-selectin on endothelial cells. In the human hepatocellular carcinoma cell line, curcumin inhibited invasion and migration in vitro. Curcumin blocks VEGF induction by transforming growth factor-β1 in murine osteoblasts and also inhibited VEGF production by human melanoma cells [42,43].

NF-κB activation by carcinogens causes it to translocate into the nucleus, where it induces expression of genes that can block apoptosis, promote proliferation, and mediate tumorigenesis. Curcumin is a potent inhibitor of NF-κB. Biswas *et al.* [44] showed that curcumin inhibits NF-κB activation in alveolar epithelial cells. Shishodia *et al.* investigated the effect of curcumin on cigarette smoke (CS)-induced NF-κB activation and NF-κB-regulated gene expression in human nonsmall cell lung cancer (NSCLC) cells [45]. The exposure of cells to CS-induced persistent activation of NF-κB, and pretreatment with curcumin abolished the CS-induced DNA-binding of NF-κB. AP-1 is implicated in tumorigenesis by its effects on the regulation of genes involved in apoptosis, repression of tumor-suppressor genes, and promotion of transition of tumor cells from an epithelial to a mesenchymal pattern. Curcumin suppresses the AP-1 activation process downregulated by curcumin. These mechanisms may account for the inhibitory effects of curcumin on the proliferation of various tumor cell lines [41,46–49].

Chen *et al.* [50] showed the anti-invasive gene expression profile of curcumin in lung adenocarcinoma cells. Several invasion-related genes were suppressed by curcumin, including MMP14, the neuronal cell adhesion molecule, and integrin alpha6/beta4 complex. In addition, several heat-shock proteins (Hsp27, Hsp70, and Hsp40-like protein) were induced by curcumin. On the basis of these data, it can be concluded that curcumin might be an effective antimetastatic agent with a mechanism of anti-invasion via the regulation of gene expression.

Curcumin also inhibits proliferation or induces apoptosis in a wide variety of tumor cells, including cells from human colon, breast, prostate, kidney, and liver and from human melanomas, sarcomas, lymphomas, and leukemias. In contrast, nonmalignant cells including mouse and rat embryonic fibroblasts, human foreskin fibroblasts, and mammary epithelial cells are relatively unaffected by curcumin [41].

Other antitumor effects in animals: Many animal studies support the role of curcumin in tumor prevention. Curcumin prevents tumor formation in genetically predisposed animals, such as C57BL/6J-Min/+ mice, a model for familial adenomatous polyposis (FAP). Dietary curcumin inhibited tumor growth in these animals by 63% [51]. Curcumin also inhibits polyp formation and growth, in part by affecting arachidonic acid metabolism in a manner similar to that of traditional NSAIDs and the selective inhibitors of cyclooxygenase-2 (COX-2). The ability of curcumin to inhibit tumor development in response to various carcinogens has also been shown in other animal models [52]. In C57BL/6 mice inoculated in the tail vein with B16F10 melanoma cells, dietary curcumin reduced the number of lung tumor nodules by 89% compared with controls. Curcumin was also associated with a 143.8% increase in mean survival in tumor-bearing animals [53].

Human studies of curcumin: Early human trials showed a beneficial effect of curcumin in chemoprevention and therapy. Cheng *et al.* [54] investigated the toxicity and pharmacokinetics of curcumin (purity, 99.3%) in 25 patients with precancerous lesions. There was no treatment-related toxicity, although high doses were too bulky for patient comfort. Two out of 25 patients (8%) developed frank malignancies, but seven patients (28%) showed histologic improvement in their precancerous lesions. Although this trial had a small sample size and no placebo control, these results support the role of curcumin in chemoprevention.

In a dose-escalation study of 15 patients with advanced colorectal cancer refractory to standard treatment, study subjects received doses of 440–2200 mg/day of curcuma extracts (containing 36–180 mg of curcumin) daily for 4 months [55]. Orally administered curcuma extracts were well tolerated, with no dose-limiting toxicity. Radiologically stable disease was obtained during treatment for 2–4 months in five patients [56]. This study showed that curcumin is safe and well tolerated and suggested a biologic effect in the chemotherapy of cancer [54].

These in vitro, animal, and early human studies show the immense potential of curcumin in the chemoprevention of cancers. Further human studies are still required on the effect of curcumin in chemoprevention and chemotherapy of many different cancers, including lung cancer.

Gingerol, beta-elemene, and zerumbone

Gingerol, beta-elemene, and zerumbone are active principles from the roots of *Zingiber officinale* Roscoe and *Zingiber zerumbet* Smith, respectively. [6]-Gingerol inhibited COX-2 expression by blocking the p38 MAP kinase-NF-κB signaling pathway in mice [57]. Zerumbone, found in subtropical ginger *Zingiber zerumbet* Smith, exhibited antiproliferative and anti-inflammatory activities by suppressing NF-κB activation induced by cigarette smoke condensate and other inducers and inhibited the NF-κB-regulated gene products, including COX-2 [58]. Beta-elemene, a novel compound extracted from the ginger root, triggered apoptosis in NSCLC cells, possibly through a mitochondrial release of the cytochrome c-mediated apoptotic pathway [59].

Catechins

Catechins of green tea (*Camellia sinesis* Griff) have inhibitory effects on the expression of COX-2 enzyme activity. Epigallocatechin-3-gallate (EGCG), the most potent of the four major catechins, significantly inhibited constitutive COX-2 mRNA and protein overexpression in cancer cells in vitro [35]. The signaling pathways controlling COX-2 expression showed decreased COX-2 promoter activity via inhibition of nuclear factor kappaB (NF-κB) activation. EGCG also promoted rapid mRNA decay mediated through the COX-2 3'untranslated region (3'UTR) [60]. Cotreatment with EGCG plus celecoxib strongly induced apoptosis and expression of apoptosis-related genes, especially growth arrest and DNA damage-inducible 153 (GADD153) gene in the human lung cancer cell line PC-9. Neither EGCG nor celecoxib alone produced similar changes in PC-9 cells. EGCG did not enhance GADD153 gene expression or apoptosis induction in PC-9 cells in combination with N-(4-hydroxyphenyl) retinamide or with aspirin. This experiment also showed that high upregulation of GADD153 is a key requirement for cancer prevention with EGCG [61]. A phase I study with total of 17 patients with advanced lung cancer was designed to establish maximum tolerated dose of green tea extract. Seven patients had stable disease ranging from 4 to 16 weeks; no patient remained on therapy longer than 16 weeks due to the development of progressive disease. This study suggests that green tea extract is relatively nontoxic at a dose of 3 g/m^2/day [61]. The green tea extract maybe considered as a chemopreventive and chemotherapy-enhancing compound.

Berberine

Berberine, a bitter alkaloid found in many plants (e.g., *Berberis aristata*) was evaluated for its anticancer potential in KB cancer cell culture [62]. Berberine induced apoptosis in KB cells and inhibited expression of COX-2 and Mcl-1, but not Bcl-2, in a dose-dependent manner. PGE2 added to the cell culture reversed the apoptotic effect and induced COX-2 and Mcl-1 expression. The PGE2 had no effect on total Akt but slightly reversed the phosphorylated Akt, which was decreased by berberine. Berberine-induced apoptosis may be COX-2-dependent.

In another in vitro study, berberine exerted a dose- and time-dependent inhibitory effect on the motility and invasion ability of highly metastatic

A549 cells under noncytotoxic concentrations [63]. In the A549 cell culture matrix, berberine inhibited degrading proteinases, including matrix metalloproteinase-2 and urokinase-plasminogen activator. It also exerted its action via regulating tissue inhibitor of metalloproteinase-2 and urokinase-plasminogen activator inhibitor. The mechanism of berberine likely involved c-jun, c-fos, and NF-κB. Berberine may have antimetastatic potential in NSCLC, because cancer cell migration and the invasion process require matrix-degrading proteinases.

Oral administration of berberine for 14 days in mice significantly inhibited the spontaneous mediastinal lymph node metastasis produced by orthotopic implantation of Lewis lung carcinoma (LLC) into the lung parenchyma in a dose-dependent manner but did not affect the tumor growth at the implantation site of the lung [64]. Combined treatment with berberine and an anticancer drug, CPT-11, resulted in a marked inhibition of tumor growth at the implantation site and of lymphatic metastasis, as compared with either treatment alone. Antiactivator protein-1 (anti-AP-1) transcriptional activity of noncytotoxic concentrations of berberine inhibited the invasiveness of LLC cells through the repression of expression of urokinase-type plasminogen activator.

Isoliquiritigenin

Isoliquiritigenin is a flavonoid derived from the roots of licorice, *Liqueritia glabra* L., shallot, and bean sprouts. Isoliquiritigenin (ILTG) has been reported to be a strong suppressor of the COX-2 pathway as well as an inducer of apoptosis in cancer cells [65]. Susceptibility to apoptosis by ILTG is inversely proportionate to the level of COX-2 expressed by the cancer cells. This dependency was enhanced by inhibition of the lipoxygenases (LOXs)-mediated metabolic pathway and attenuated by addition of a number of prostaglandins and thromboxanes. Isoliquiritigenin significantly inhibited the proliferation of A549 lung cancer cells in a dose- and time-dependent manner and inhibited the cell cycle progression at G2/M phase [66]. Furthermore, isoliquiritigenin enhanced the expression of p21(CIP1/WAF1), a universal inhibitor of cyclin-dependent kinases.

Myo-inositol

Myo-inositol (phytic acid) is ubiquitous in plants; its ferulic acid derivatives suppressed the COX-2 promoter activity in a concentration-dependent manner. In vitro treatment resulted in a 50% decrease of COX-2 promoter activity without a cytotoxic effect [67]. The potential of butylated hydroxyanisole (BHA), myo-inositol, curcumin, esculetin, resveratrol, and lycopene-enriched tomato oleoresin as chemopreventive agents against experimentally induced (tobacco smoke carcinogens) lung tumor in A/J mice was evaluated. Among the compounds tested, myo-inositol was the most effective anticarcinogen treatment.

A phase I, open-label, dose-escalation clinical study was conducted to assess the safety, tolerability, maximum tolerated dose, and potential chemopreventive effect of myo-inositol in smokers with bronchial dysplasia [68]. The study enrolled 26 smokers between 40 and 74 years of age with the dose of myo-inositol ranged from 12 to 30 g/day for 3 months. The maximum tolerated dose was 18 g/day with mild, mainly gastrointestinal in nature side effects. The study showed a significant rate of regression of preexisting dysplastic lesions. However, larger studies are needed to establish the efficacy of the agent as a chemopreventive medication.

Boswellic acids

Boswellic acids are pentacyclic terpenoid compounds derived from frankincense gum resin of the tree *Boswellia serrata* Roxb. These compounds are well established as effective and safe (no gastrointestinal side effects) nutritional supplements against a large number of inflammatory diseases, including cancer, arthritis, chronic colitis, ulcerative colitis, Crohn's disease, and bronchial asthma. Among four major beta boswellic acids, the acetyl-11-keto-beta-boswellic acid (AKBA) is the most potent anti-inflammatory and anticancer compound [69]. In an in vitro study with several cancer cell cultures, including human lung cancer cell line (human lung adenocarcinoma H1299 cells), AKBA potentiated the apoptosis induced by TNF and chemotherapeutic agents (doxorubicin, 5-FU). AKBA downregulated expression of NF-κB-regulated antiapop-

totic, proliferative, and angiogenic gene products and suppressed both inducible and constitutive NF-κB activation in cancer cells, most likely via inhibition of Akt [69]. The compound prevented NF-κB activation induced by several biological factors, including cigarette smoke carcinogens. The results of the study indicate that AKBA enhances apoptosis induced by cytokines and chemotherapeutic agents, inhibits tumor invasion, and should be considered an important chemotherapeutic compound for clinical studies.

Guggulsterone Z and E and ferulates

Guggulsterone Z and E and ferulates derived from myrrh gum–resin of the tree *Commiphora mukul* Wighti have been recently found in clinical studies to lower validated serum markers of inflammation, i.e., serum levels of malondialdehyde (MDA) and high sensitivity c-reactive protein hs-crp (Badmaev, V. personal communication 2004). In an in vitro study utilizing several cancer cell lines, guggulsterone suppressed DNA-binding NF-κB induced by TNF, phorbol ester, okadaic acid, cigarette smoke condensate, hydrogen peroxide, and interleukin-1 [70]. Guggulsterone also suppressed constitutive NF-κB activation expressed in most tumor cells. Through inhibition of IκB kinase activation, this plant sterol blocked IkappaBalpha phosphorylation and degradation, thus suppressing p65 phosphorylation and nuclear translocation. Guggulsterone decreased the expression of gene products involved in antiapoptosis (IAP1, xIAP, Bfl-1/A1, Bcl-2, cFLIP, and survivin), proliferation (cyclin D1 and c-Myc), and metastasis (MMP-9, COX-2, and VEGF). This finding correlated well with the enhancement of apoptosis induced by TNF and chemotherapeutic agents. Guggulsterone suppresses NF-κB and NF-κB-regulated gene products, which may explain its anti-inflammatory and potential chemotherapeutic role.

The recent analytical chemistry study of a standardized *Commiphora* gum–resin extract revealed new bioactive compounds, two ferulates, with an unusual skeleton determined by spectral and chemical methods, including NMR, GC-MS, and chemical derivatization. This new fraction containing the two ferulates displayed moderate scavenging effects against 2,2-diphenyl-1-picrylhydrazyl (DPPH) radicals and cytotoxic activity against several cancer cell lines [71].

Genistein and daidzein

Genistein and daidzein are two major soy-derived isoflavones and phytoestrogens. The utility of soya isoflavones is debated in the prevention and treatment of cancer is currently debated. Several mechanisms for the chemopreventive action of genistein have been proposed in the literature. These mechanisms include "weak" estrogen activity competing with "strong" estrogens, antioxidant effects, inhibition of tyrosine kinase enzyme activity, inhibition of topoisomerase II enzyme activity, induction of apoptosis, induction of cell differentiation, and inhibition of angiogenesis. Genistein was tested on diffuse large cell lymphoma (DLCL), a common subtype of non-Hodgkin's lymphoma, for its potential inhibitory effect on the expression of NF-κB [72]. Genistein increased the Bax:Bcl-2 ratio, decreased DNA-NF-κB binding, and induced apoptosis of cancer cells. Genistein also inhibited DNA-NF-κB binding in vivo. In addition, genistein potentiated the anticancer mechanism of chemotherapeutic drugs.

Epidemiological studies have confirmed the usefulness of a soy-based diet in the prevention of lung cancer [73]. Chinese women, who are unique in having a high incidence of lung cancer despite a low smoking prevalence and high intake of soy, were the subjects of the study. A hospital-based case–control study was performed among Singapore Chinese women, comprising 303 cases and 765 age-matched controls (176 cases and 663 controls were lifetime nonsmokers). The study showed an inverse association between intake of fruit or cruciferous and noncruciferous vegetables and the risk of lung cancer. A higher intake of soy foods significantly reduced the risk of lung cancer among lifetime nonsmokers but not among smokers.

The chemotherapeutic usefulness of soy isoflavones was evaluated in in vitro and in vivo studies [74]. Chemotherapeutic drugs are known to induce NF-κB activity in tumor cells, resulting in lower cell killing and in drug resistance. In contrast, genistein has been shown to inhibit the activity of NF-κB and the growth of various cancer cells without causing systemic toxicity. PC-3 (prostate), MDA-MB-231 (breast), H460 (lung), and BxPC-3 (pancreas) cancer cell cultures were pretreated with 15–30 mmol/L genistein for 24 hours and then exposed to low doses of chemotherapeutic agents, i.e., cisplatin, docetaxel, and doxorubicin, for an additional 48–72 hours. This combined therapy in vitro resulted in significantly greater inhibition of cell growth and induction of apoptosis compared with the agents alone. These results were also supported by results of animal experiments, which showed that NF-κB was affected in vivo. Clinical trials of soy isoflavones in combination with chemotherapeutic agents are needed to evaluate efficacy of isoflavones in treatment of human cancer.

Glabridin and glycyrrhetic acids

Glabridin and glycyrrhetic acids are two compounds derived from the roots of licorice, *Liqueritia glabra* L.Glabridin possesses anti-inflammatory, antimicrobial, and cardiovascular protective activities. Glabridin inhibited intercellular adhesion molecule-1 (ICAM-1) expression in TNF-α-stimulated human umbilical vein endothelial cells (HUVECs) [75]. Glabridin inhibited THP-1 cell adhesion to HUVECs stimulated by TNF-α and cell surface expression of ICAM-1 in TNF-α-stimulated HUVECs. The mRNA expression of adhesion molecules was also suppressed by glabridin. Further study demonstrated the inhibition of NF-κB DNA binding, inhibition of the chain reaction leading to translocation and activation of NF-κB. Glabridin treatment of a variety of cell lines showed that its inhibitory effect on NF-κB activation is not cancer cell type specific. Glabridin inhibits both inducible and constitutive NF-κB. In addition, TNF-α-induced phosphorylation of Akt and extracellular signal-regulated kinase (ERK) was blocked by the treatment.

Beta-glycyrrhetinic acid (GA), a saponin isolated from licorice roots, displayed inhibitory action on TNF-α-induced IL-8 production in human colonic epithelial cells [75]. Interleukin (IL)-8 plays a central role in inflammatory responses, and its function requires activation of NF-κB. GA inhibited

TNF-α-induced phosphorylation of p38 MAPK and ERK, IκB alpha degradation, and NF-κB activation. These results suggest that GA has inhibitory effects on TNF-α-induced IL-8 production in the intestinal epithelial cells through the inhibition of phosphorylation of MAPKs, following I kappa B alpha degradation and NF-κB activation.

Fewer than 20% of habitual smokers develop lung cancer, which suggests that genetic, environmental, and nutritional factors contribute to the risk for developing this disease. Recently, five enzymes were shown to initiate the detoxification of nicotine-derived nitrosamine ketone (NNK), the most potent carcinogen present in tobacco. Four of these enzymes are potently inhibited by glycyrrhetinic acid [76].

Casuarinin

Casuarinin is a hydrolyzable tannin isolated from the bark of *Terminalia arjuna*. This compound inhibited IκB kinase (IKK) activity in lipopolysaccharide (LPS)-activated murine macrophages. This mechanism indicates the anti-inflammatory and chemopreventive/chemotherapeutic potential of casuarinin by suppressing the activation and expression of NF-κB [77]. Casuarinin was found in vitro to inhibit human NSCLC A549 cells, by blocking cell cycle progression in the G0/G1 phase and inducing apoptosis [78]. The G0/G1 phase arrest is due to p53-dependent induction of p21/WAF1. An enhancement in Fas/APO-1 and the two forms of Fas ligand (FasL), membrane-bound FasL and soluble FasL, might be responsible for the apoptotic effect induced by casuarinin.

Enhancement of selenoproteins

Selenium is an essential trace element, and its target molecules are various selenoproteins with specialized functions in the body. In a recent study, a supplementation trial in a selenium-deficient population of China showed that full expression of selected selenoprotein, i.e., glutathione peroxidase was achieved with 37 μg of elemental selenium per day as selenomethionine. However, full expression of selenoprotein P was not achieved at this dose of supplemental selenium [79]. On the other hand, the North American study population, generally considered selenium replete, benefited in lung, colon, and prostate cancer prevention when supplemented with 200 μg of elemental selenium (derived from selenized yeast—80% as selenomethionine) daily for 10 years versus the nonsupplemented study group [80]. Total cancer mortality (RR, 0.50; 95% CI, 0.31–0.80), total cancer incidence (RR, 0.63; 95% CI, 0.47–0.85), and incidences of lung, colorectal, and prostate cancers were significantly lower in selenium arm compared to control arm [80].

In addition to chemopreventive selenium, there is also increased discussion of a pharmacological dose of selenium to treat active conditions. We predicted the need for a pharmacological dose of selenium in 1996 [81]; 10 years later, we published a clinical paper reporting administration of 2200 μg of elemental selenium (selenomethionine) combined with irinotecan (125 mg/m^2/week) in cancer patients [82]. Unexpected responses and disease stabilizations were noted in a highly refractory population treated with this high dose of selenium, including a stable disease in NSCLC for 24 weeks. The coadministration of selenomethionine significantly reduced the irinotecan biliary index, which has been associated with gastrointestinal toxicity. No side effects related to selenium administration was reported in course of the study, with the exception of transient garlicky breath, which is characteristic of high-dose selenium supplementation. Further escalation of the selenomethionine dose is recommended in future clinical trials.

In addition to the dose of supplemental selenium, the chemical form of the selenium compound emerges as an important consideration in effective chemopreventive or chemotherapeutic selenium delivery. In a murine model in which the mice received various forms of supplemental selenium in the diet against tobacco-related lung tumorigenesis, only two compounds resulted in significant tumor reduction: selenazolidine-4(2-oxo)-carboxylic acid and selenocystine. Also, only these two compounds showed ubiquity of changes, elevating both selenium levels and glutathione peroxidase activity in both liver and RBC.

Adaptogen mechanism

Cancer, including lung cancer, can be seen as a stress-related or stress-aggravated condition. One of the most comprehensive approaches in dealing with psychological and physical stress was practiced in the ancient medical systems of the Orient. A group of rejuvenating herbs and minerals named in Sanskrit as *Rasayanas* or vitalizers was purposefully used there against stress-related conditions.

The concept of *Rasayanas* inspired the contemporary idea of adaptogen, a term that was proposed in the 1950s by Lazarev and Brekhman. Brekhman and Fulder [83] described the ideal characteristics of pharmacological agents considered as adaptogens: (a) Safety of the adaptogen's action on the organism; (b) a wide range of regulatory activity, but manifesting its action only against the actual challenge to the system; (c) action through an increase in a non-specific adaptation energy (resistance) to harmful influences of an extremely wide spectrum of physical, chemical, and biological factors causing stress; and (d) a normalizing action irrespective of the direction of the foregoing pathological changes.

Whitanolids

Whitanolids are steroidal lactones, active principles of a standardized extract of *Withania sominifera* Dunnal roots (ver. Ashwagandha). Ashwagandha is considered to be a classic example of Rasyana herb. In an in vivo study, male Swiss albino mice challenged with benzo[a]pyrene received no treatment or paclitaxel and paclitaxel along with *Withania sominifera* [84]. The results of the experiment suggest that paclitaxel, administered with *Withania sominifera*, may exert its chemotherapeutic effect through modulating protein-bound carbohydrate levels and marker enzymes, i.e., aryl hydrocarbon hydroxylase, gamma-glutamyl transpeptidase, 5'-nucleotidase, lactate dehydrogenase, and protein-bound carbohydrate components (hexose, hexosamine, and sialic acid).

Withanolide D (one of withanolids) and *Withania sominifera* standardized extract were studied for its antimetastatic activity using B16F-10 melanoma cells in C57BL/6 mice [85]. Administration of *Withania* extract and withanolide significantly inhibited the metastatic colony formation of the melanoma in lungs: 72.58% of mice treated with extract and 69.84% of those treated with withanolide had increased in survival time, compared with untreated controls. Lung collagen hydroxyproline, hexosamine, and uronic acid, which were elevated in cancer-challenged controls, were lower in mice that received the combined extract-withanaloide treatment. Prophylactic administrations of both extracts as well as withanolide were ineffective in inhibiting the metastasis of B16F-10 melanoma cells.

Ginsenosides

Ginsenosides, like withanaloids, belong to the class of steroidal lactones and adaptogenic principles found in the roots of *Panax ginseng* C.A. Meyer. Redginseng administered in drinking water to A/J mice challenged with the tobacco-specific carcinogen benzo[a]pyrene had tumor multiplicity that was 36% lower and tumor load that was 70% lower compared with values for untreated controls [86].

The chemopreventive action of *Panax ginseng* extract was evaluated in Swiss albino mice [87]. Newborn mice (less than 24 h old) were challenged with a single injection of benzo[a]pyrene to induce lung adenomas. Pulmonary histopathology, chromosomal aberrations, and micronuclei induction were evaluated in bone marrow cells. The oral administration of ginseng extract significantly reduced the number of adenomas and the weight of the carcinogen-challenged lungs as compared with animals not treated with ginseng. Tumor multiplicity was significantly lower in treated mice than in untreated animals. The extract-treated group had significantly lower frequencies of chromosomal aberrations and micronuclei induced by carcinogen administration.

In a cohort study with 5 years of follow-up conducted in the red ginseng cultivation area, ginseng users had a decreased relative risk of gastric and lung cancer compared with nonusers [88]. In case–control studies, odds ratios of cancers of the lip, oral cavity and pharynx, larynx, lung, esophagus, stomach, liver, pancreas, ovary, and colorectum were significantly reduced among ginseng users compared with nonusers. These findings strongly suggest that red ginseng has nonorgan-specific cancer preventive effects against various cancers. Furthermore, several fractions of fresh and red ginseng and four semisynthetic ginsenosides (Rh1, Rh2, Rg3 and Rg5, the major saponin components in red ginseng) were prepared; administration of Rg3 and Rg5 showed statistically significant reduction of lung tumor incidence, and Rh2 showed only a tendency to decrease the tumor incidence [88].

References

1 Shaipanich T, McWilliams A, Lam S. Early detection and chemoprevention of lung cancer. *Respirology* 2006; **11(4)**:366–72.

2 Soler M, Bosetti C, Franceschi S *et al.* Fiber intake and the risk of oral, pharyngeal and esophageal cancer. *Int J Cancer* 2001; **91(3)**:283–7.

3 Levi F, Pasche C, La Vecchia C, Lucchini F, Franceschi S, Monnier P. Food groups and risk of oral and pharyngeal cancer. *Int J Cancer* 1998; **77(5)**:705–9.

4 Tavani A, Gallus S, La Vecchia C *et al.* Diet and risk of oral and pharyngeal cancer. An Italian case–control study. *Eur J Cancer Prev* 2001; **10(2)**:191–5.

5 Rylander R, Axelsson G. Lung cancer risks in relation to vegetable and fruit consumption and smoking. *Int J Cancer* 2006; **118(3)**:739–43.

6 Skuladottir H, Tjoenneland A, Overvad K, Stripp C, Olsen JH. Does high intake of fruit and vegetables improve lung cancer survival? *Lung Cancer* 2006; **51(3)**:267–73.

7 Brennan P, Hsu CC, Moullan N *et al.* Effect of cruciferous vegetables on lung cancer in patients stratified by genetic status: a Mendelian randomisation approach. *Lancet* 2005; **366(9496)**:1558–60.

8 Lee BM, Park KK. Beneficial and adverse effects of chemopreventive agents. *Mutat Res* 2003; **523–524**:265–78.

9 Berge G, Ovrebo S, Botnen IV *et al.* Resveratrol inhibits benzo[a]pyrene-DNA adduct formation in human bronchial epithelial cells. *Br J Cancer* 2004; **91(2)**:333–8.

10 Allen SW, Mueller L, Williams SN, Quattrochi LC, Raucy J. The use of a high-volume screening procedure to assess the effects of dietary flavonoids on human cyp1a1 expression. *Drug Metab Dispos* 2001; **29(8)**:1074–9.

11 Lorenz P, Roychowdhury S, Engelmann M, Wolf G, Horn TF. Oxyresveratrol and resveratrol are potent antioxidants and free radical scavengers: effect on nitrosative and oxidative stress derived from microglial cells. *Nitric Oxide* 2003; **9(2)**:64–76.

12 Preobrazhenskaia MN, Korolev AM. Indole derivatives in vegetables of the family Cruciferae. *Bioorg Khim* 2000; **26(2)**:97–111.

13 Morse JM. Expired research. *Qual Health Res* 2003; **13(5)**:595–6.

14 Kubin A, Wierrani F, Burner U, Alth G, Grunberger W. Hypericin—the facts about a controversial agent. *Curr Pharm Des* 2005; **11(2)**:233–53.

15 Dostalek M, Pistovcakova J, Jurica J *et al.* Effect of St John's wort (Hypericum perforatum) on cytochrome P-450 activity in perfused rat liver. *Life Sci* 2005; **78(3)**:239–44.

16 Gopalakrishna R, Chen ZH, Gundimeda U. Tobacco smoke tumor promoters, catechol and hydroquinone, induce oxidative regulation of protein kinase C and influence invasion and metastasis of lung carcinoma cells. *Proc Natl Acad Sci U S A* 1994; **91(25)**:12233–7.

17 Blank M, Lavie G, Mandel M, Keisari Y. Effects of photodynamic therapy with hypericin in mice bearing highly invasive solid tumors. *Oncol Res* 2000; **12(9–10)**:409–18.

18 Zeng JZ, Sun DF, Wang L *et al.* Hypericum sampsonii induces apoptosis and nuclear export of retinoid X receptor-alpha. *Carcinogenesis* 2006; **27(10)**:1991–2000.

19 Selvendiran K, Thirunavukkarasu C, Singh JP, Padmavathi R, Sakthisekaran D. Chemopreventive effect of piperine on mitochondrial TCA cycle and phase-I and glutathione-metabolizing enzymes in benzo(a)pyrene induced lung carcinogenesis in Swiss albino mice. *Mol Cell Biochem* 2005; **271(1–2)**:101–6.

20 Selvendiran K, Prince Vijeya SJ, Sakthisekaran D. In vivo effect of piperine on serum and tissue glycoprotein levels in benzo(a)pyrene induced lung carcinogenesis in Swiss albino mice. *Pulm Pharmacol Ther* 2006; **19(2)**:107–11.

21 Selvendiran K, Banu SM, Sakthisekaran D. Oral supplementation of piperine leads to altered phase II enzymes and reduced DNA damage and DNA-protein cross links in Benzo(a)pyrene induced experimental lung carcinogenesis. *Mol Cell Biochem* 2005; **268(1–2)**:141–7.

22 Jin NZ, Zhu YP, Zhou JW *et al.* Preventive effects of quercetin against benzo[a]pyrene-induced DNA damages and pulmonary precancerous pathologic changes in mice. *Basic Clin Pharmacol Toxicol* 2006; **98(6)**:593–8.

23 Yang JH, Hsia TC, Kuo HM *et al.* Inhibition of lung cancer cell growth by quercetin glucuronides via G2/M

arrest and induction of apoptosis. *Drug Metab Dispos* 2006; **34(2)**:296–304.

24 Unger M, Frank A. Simultaneous determination of the inhibitory potency of herbal extracts on the activity of six major cytochrome P450 enzymes using liquid chromatography/mass spectrometry and automated online extraction. *Rapid Commun Mass Spectrom* 2004; **18(19)**:2273–81.

25 Brobst DE, Ding X, Creech KL, Goodwin B, Kelley B, Staudinger JL. Guggulsterone activates multiple nuclear receptors and induces CYP3A gene expression through the pregnane X receptor. *J Pharmacol Exp Ther* 2004; **310(2)**:528–35.

26 Singh RP, Banerjee S, Kumar PV, Raveesha KA, Rao AR. Tinospora cordifolia induces enzymes of carcinogen/drug metabolism and antioxidant system, and inhibits lipid peroxidation in mice. *Phytomedicine* 2006; **13(1–2)**:74–84.

27 Karin M, Lawrence T, Nizet V. Innate immunity gone awry: linking microbial infections to chronic inflammation and cancer. *Cell* 2006; **124(4)**:823–35.

28 Brody JS, Spira A. State of the art. Chronic obstructive pulmonary disease, inflammation, and lung cancer. *Proc Am Thorac Soc* 2006; **3(6)**:535–7.

29 Ballaz S, Mulshine JL. The potential contributions of chronic inflammation to lung carcinogenesis. *Clin Lung Cancer* 2003; **5(1)**:46–62.

30 Schabath MB, Delclos GL, Martynowicz MM *et al.* Opposing effects of emphysema, hay fever, and select genetic variants on lung cancer risk. *Am J Epidemiol* 2005; **161(5)**:412–22.

31 Barnes PJ. Small airways in COPD. *N Engl J Med* 2004; **350(26)**:2635–7.

32 Hogg JC. Pathophysiology of airflow limitation in chronic obstructive pulmonary disease. *Lancet* 2004; **364(9435)**:709–21.

33 Malkinson AM. Role of inflammation in mouse lung tumorigenesis: a review. *Exp Lung Res* 2005; **31(1)**:57–82.

34 Ji H, Houghton AM, Mariani TJ *et al.* K-ras activation generates an inflammatory response in lung tumors. *Oncogene* 2006; **25(14)**:2105–12.

35 Wislez M, Spencer ML, Izzo JG *et al.* Inhibition of mammalian target of rapamycin reverses alveolar epithelial neoplasia induced by oncogenic K-ras. *Cancer Res* 2005; **65(8)**:3226–35.

36 Wislez M, Fujimoto N, Izzo JG *et al.* High expression of ligands for chemokine receptor CXCR2 in alveolar epithelial neoplasia induced by oncogenic kras. *Cancer Res* 2006; **66(8)**:4198–207.

37 Houghton AM, Marconcini LA, Ji H, Wong KK, Shapiro SD. Neutrophil elastase causes increased mortality, angiogenesis, and lung tumor growth in a murine model of lung cancer [Abstract]. *Proc Am Thorac Soc* 2006; **3**:A479.

38 Moghaddam SJM, Tuvim M, DeMayo FJ, Dickey BF. Promotion of lung cancer progression by stimulation of innate immunity [Abstract]. *Proc Am Thorac Soc* 2006; 3: A458.

39 Kalpana C, Menon VP. Modulatory effects of curcumin on lipid peroxidation and antioxidant status during nicotine-induced toxicity. *Pol J Pharmacol* 2004; **56(5)**:581–6.

40 Kalpana C, Menon VP. Curcumin ameliorates oxidative stress during nicotine-induced lung toxicity in Wistar rats. *Ital J Biochem* 2004; **53(2)**:82–6.

41 Aggarwal BB, Kumar A, Bharti AC. Anticancer potential of curcumin: preclinical and clinical studies. *Anticancer Res* 2003; **23(1A)**:363–98.

42 Han SS, Chung ST, Robertson DA, Ranjan D, Bondada S. Curcumin causes the growth arrest and apoptosis of B cell lymphoma by downregulation of egr-1, c-myc, bcl-XL, NF-kappa B, and p53. *Clin Immunol* 1999; **93(2)**:152–61.

43 Piwocka K, Zablocki K, Wieckowski MR *et al.* A novel apoptosis-like pathway, independent of mitochondria and caspases, induced by curcumin in human lymphoblastoid T (Jurkat) cells. *Exp Cell Res* 1999; **249(2)**:299–307.

44 Biswas SK, McClure D, Jimenez LA, Megson IL, Rahman I. Curcumin induces glutathione biosynthesis and inhibits NF-kappaB activation and interleukin-8 release in alveolar epithelial cells: mechanism of free radical scavenging activity. *Antioxid Redox Signal* 2005; **7(1–2)**:32–41.

45 Shishodia S, Potdar P, Gairola CG, Aggarwal BB. Curcumin (diferuloylmethane) down-regulates cigarette smoke-induced NF-kappaB activation through inhibition of IkappaBalpha kinase in human lung epithelial cells: correlation with suppression of COX-2, MMP-9 and cyclin D1. *Carcinogenesis* 2003; **24(7)**:1269–79.

46 Singh S, Aggarwal BB. Activation of transcription factor NF-kappa B is suppressed by curcumin (diferuloylmethane) [corrected]. *J Biol Chem* 1995; **270(42)**:24995–5000.

47 Baldwin AS. Control of oncogenesis and cancer therapy resistance by the transcription factor NF-kappaB. *J Clin Invest* 2001; **107(3)**:241–6.

48 Garg A, Aggarwal BB. Nuclear transcription factor-kappaB as a target for cancer drug development. *Leukemia* 2002; **16(6)**:1053–68.

Chapter 28

49 Giri DK, Aggarwal BB. Constitutive activation of NF-kappaB causes resistance to apoptosis in human cutaneous T cell lymphoma HuT-78 cells. Autocrine role of tumor necrosis factor and reactive oxygen intermediates. *J Biol Chem* 1998; **273(22)**:14008–14.

50 Chen HW, Yu SL, Chen JJ *et al.* Anti-invasive gene expression profile of curcumin in lung adenocarcinoma based on a high throughput microarray analysis. *Mol Pharmacol* 2004; **65(1)**:99–110.

51 Perkins S, Verschoyle RD, Hill K *et al.* Chemopreventive efficacy and pharmacokinetics of curcumin in the min/+ mouse, a model of familial adenomatous polyposis. *Cancer Epidemiol Biomarkers Prev* 2002; **11(6)**:535–40.

52 Mahmoud NN, Carothers AM, Grunberger D *et al.* Plant phenolics decrease intestinal tumors in an animal model of familial adenomatous polyposis. *Carcinogenesis* 2000; **21(5)**:921–7.

53 Menon LG, Kuttan R, Kuttan G. Inhibition of lung metastasis in mice induced by B16F10 melanoma cells by polyphenolic compounds. *Cancer Lett* 1995; **95(1–2)**:221–5.

54 Cheng AL, Hsu CH, Lin JK *et al.* Phase I clinical trial of curcumin, a chemopreventive agent, in patients with high-risk or pre-malignant lesions. *Anticancer Res* 2001; **21(4B)**:2895–900.

55 Ireson C, Orr S, Jones DJ *et al.* Characterization of metabolites of the chemopreventive agent curcumin in human and rat hepatocytes and in the rat in vivo, and evaluation of their ability to inhibit phorbol ester-induced prostaglandin E2 production. *Cancer Res* 2001; **61(3)**:1058–64.

56 Sharma RA, McLelland HR, Hill KA *et al.* Pharmacodynamic and pharmacokinetic study of oral Curcuma extract in patients with colorectal cancer. *Clin Cancer Res* 2001; **7(7)**:1894–900.

57 Kim SO, Kundu JK, Shin YK *et al.* [6]-Gingerol inhibits COX-2 expression by blocking the activation of p38 MAP kinase and NF-kappaB in phorbol ester-stimulated mouse skin. *Oncogene* 2005; **24(15)**:2558–67.

58 Takada Y, Murakami A, Aggarwal BB. Zerumbone abolishes NF-kappaB and IkappaBalpha kinase activation leading to suppression of antiapoptotic and metastatic gene expression, upregulation of apoptosis, and downregulation of invasion. *Oncogene* 2005; **24(46)**:6957–69.

59 Wang G, Li X, Huang F *et al.* Antitumor effect of beta-elemene in non-small-cell lung cancer cells is mediated via induction of cell cycle arrest and apoptotic cell death. *Cell Mol Life Sci* 2005; **62(7–8)**:881–93.

60 Suganuma M, Kurusu M, Suzuki K, Tasaki E, Fujiki H. Green tea polyphenol stimulates cancer preventive effects of celecoxib in human lung cancer cells by upregulation of GADD153 gene. *Int J Cancer* 2006; **119(1)**:33–40.

61 Laurie SA, Miller VA, Grant SC, Kris MG, Ng KK. Phase I study of green tea extract in patients with advanced lung cancer. *Cancer Chemother Pharmacol* 2005; **55(1)**:33–8.

62 Kuo CL, Chi CW, Liu TY. Modulation of apoptosis by berberine through inhibition of cyclooxygenase-2 and Mcl-1 expression in oral cancer cells. *In Vivo* 2005; **19(1)**:247–52.

63 Peng PL, Hsieh YS, Wang CJ, Hsu JL, Chou FP. Inhibitory effect of berberine on the invasion of human lung cancer cells via decreased productions of urokinase-plasminogen activator and matrix metalloproteinase-2. *Toxicol Appl Pharmacol* 2006; **214(1)**:8–15.

64 Mitani N, Murakami K, Yamaura T, Ikeda T, Saiki I. Inhibitory effect of berberine on the mediastinal lymph node metastasis produced by orthotopic implantation of Lewis lung carcinoma. *Cancer Lett* 2001; **165(1)**:35–42.

65 Takahashi T, Baba M, Nishino H, Okuyama T. Cyclooxygenase-2 plays a suppressive role for induction of apoptosis in isoliquiritigenin-treated mouse colon cancer cells. *Cancer Lett* 2006; **231(2)**:319–25.

66 Ii T, Satomi Y, Katoh D *et al.* Induction of cell cycle arrest and p21(CIP1/WAF1) expression in human lung cancer cells by isoliquiritigenin. *Cancer Lett* 2004; **207(1)**:27–35.

67 Hosoda A, Ozaki Y, Kashiwada A *et al.* Syntheses of ferulic acid derivatives and their suppressive effects on cyclooxygenase-2 promoter activity. *Bioorg Med Chem* 2002; **10(4)**:1189–96.

68 Lam S, McWilliams A, LeRiche J, Macaulay C, Wattenberg L, Szabo E. A phase I study of myo-inositol for lung cancer chemoprevention. *Cancer Epidemiol Biomarkers Prev* 2006; **15(8)**:1526–31.

69 Takada Y, Ichikawa H, Badmaev V, Aggarwal BB. Acetyl-11-keto-beta-boswellic acid potentiates apoptosis, inhibits invasion, and abolishes osteoclastogenesis by suppressing NF-kappa B and NF-kappa B-regulated gene expression. *J Immunol* 2006; **176(5)**:3127–40.

70 Shishodia S, Aggarwal BB. Guggulsterone inhibits NF-kappaB and IkappaBalpha kinase activation, suppresses expression of anti-apoptotic gene products, and enhances apoptosis. *J Biol Chem* 2004; **279(45)**:47148–58.

71 Zhu N, Rafi MM, DiPaola RS *et al*. Bioactive constituents from gum guggul (Commiphora wightii). *Phytochemistry* 2001; **56(7)**:723–7.

72 Mohammad RM, Al Katib A, Aboukameel A, Doerge DR, Sarkar F, Kucuk O. Genistein sensitizes diffuse large cell lymphoma to CHOP (cyclophosphamide, doxorubicin, vincristine, prednisone) chemotherapy. *Mol Cancer Ther* 2003; **2(12)**:1361–8.

73 Seow A, Poh WT, Teh M *et al*. Diet, reproductive factors and lung cancer risk among Chinese women in Singapore: evidence for a protective effect of soy in nonsmokers. *Int J Cancer* 2002; **97(3)**:365–71.

74 Li Y, Ahmed F, Ali S, Philip PA, Kucuk O, Sarkar FH. Inactivation of nuclear factor kappaB by soy isoflavone genistein contributes to increased apoptosis induced by chemotherapeutic agents in human cancer cells. *Cancer Res* 2005; **65(15)**:6934–42.

75 Kang OH, Kim JA, Choi YA *et al*. Inhibition of interleukin-8 production in the human colonic epithelial cell line HT-29 by 18 beta-glycyrrhetinic acid. *Int J Mol Med* 2005; **15(6)**:981–5.

76 Maser E. Significance of reductases in the detoxification of the tobacco-specific carcinogen NNK. *Trends Pharmacol Sci* 2004; **25(5)**:235–7.

77 Pan MH, Lin-Shiau SY, Ho CT, Lin JH, Lin JK. Suppression of lipopolysaccharide-induced nuclear factor-kappaB activity by theaflavin-3,3′-digallate from black tea and other polyphenols through down-regulation of IkappaB kinase activity in macrophages. *Biochem Pharmacol* 2000; **59(4)**:357–67.

78 Kuo PL, Hsu YL, Lin TC, Chang JK, Lin CC. Induction of cell cycle arrest and apoptosis in human non-small cell lung cancer A549 cells by casuarinin from the bark of Terminalia arjuna Linn. *Anticancer Drugs* 2005; **16(4)**:409–15.

79 Xia Y, Hill KE, Byrne DW, Xu J, Burk RF. Effectiveness of selenium supplements in a low-selenium area of China. *Am J Clin Nutr* 2005; **81(4)**:829–34.

80 Clark LC, Combs GF, Jr, Turnbull BW *et al*., for Nutritional Prevention of Cancer Study Group. Effects of selenium supplementation for cancer prevention in patients with carcinoma of the skin. A randomized controlled trial. *JAMA* 1996; **276(24)**:1957–63.

81 Badmaev V, Majeed M, Passwater RA. Selenium: a quest for better understanding. *Altern Ther Health Med* 1996; **2(4)**:59–7.

82 Li L, Xie Y, El Sayed WM, Szakacs JG, Franklin MR, Roberts JC. Chemopreventive activity of selenocysteine prodrugs against tobacco-derived nitrosamine (NNK) induced lung tumors in the A/J mouse. *J Biochem Mol Toxicol* 2005; **19(6)**:396–405.

83 Brekhman II, Fulder S. *Man and Biologically Active Substances: The Effect of Drugs, Diet, and Pollution on Health*. New York: Pergamon, 1980.

84 Senthilnathan P, Padmavathi R, Magesh V, Sakthisekaran D. Chemotherapeutic efficacy of paclitaxel in combination with Withania somnifera on benzo(a)pyrene-induced experimental lung cancer. *Cancer Sci* 2006; **97(7)**:658–64.

85 Leyon PV, Kuttan G. Effect of Withania somnifera on B16F-10 melanoma induced metastasis in mice. *Phytother Res* 2004; **18(2)**:118–22.

86 Yan Y, Wang Y, Tan Q *et al*. Efficacy of polyphenon E, red ginseng, and rapamycin on benzo(a)pyrene-induced lung tumorigenesis in A/J mice. *Neoplasia* 2006; **8(1)**:52–8.

87 Panwar M, Samarth R, Kumar M, Yoon WJ, Kumar A. Inhibition of benzo(a)pyrene induced lung adenoma by panax ginseng extract, EFLA400, in Swiss albino mice. *Biol Pharm Bull* 2005; **28(11)**:2063–7.

88 Yun TK. Experimental and epidemiological evidence on non-organ specific cancer preventive effect of Korean ginseng and identification of active compounds. *Mutat Res* 2003; **523–524**:63–74.

Index